THE ELEMENTS

								Helium **He** **4·00** 2
			III A	**IV A**	**V A**	**VI A**	**VII A**	
			5 Boron **B** **10·81** 2,3	6 Carbon **C** **12·01** 2,4	7 Nitrogen **N** **14·01** 2,5	8 Oxygen **O** **16·00** 2,6	9 Fluorine **F** **19·00** 2,7	10 Neon **Ne** **20·18** 2,8
			13 Aluminium **Al** **26·98** 2,8,3	14 Silicon **Si** **28·09** 2,8,4	15 Phosphorus **P** **30·97** 2,8,5	16 Sulfur **S** **32·06** 2,8,6	17 Chlorine **Cl** **35·45** 2,8,7	18 Argon **Ar** **39·95** 2,8,8
28 Nickel **Ni** **58·71** ,8,16,2	29 Copper **Cu** **63·55** 2,8,18,1	30 Zinc **Zn** **65·38** 2,8,18,2	31 Gallium **Ga** **69·72** 2,8,18,3	32 Germanium **Ge** **72·59** 2,8,18,4	33 Arsenic **As** **74·92** 2,8,18,5	34 Selenium **Se** **78·96** 2,8,18,6	35 Bromine **Br** **79·90** 2,8,18,7	36 Krypton **Kr** **83·80** 2,8,18,8
46 alladium **Pd** **106·4** ,8,18,18	47 Silver **Ag** **107·87** 2,8,18,18,1	48 Cadmium **Cd** **112·40** 2,8,18,18,2	49 Indium **In** **114·82** 2,8,18,18,3	50 Tin **Sn** **118·59** 2,8,18,18,4	51 Antimony **Sb** **127·75** 2,8,18,18,5	52 Tellurium **Te** **127·60** 2,8,18,18,6	53 Iodine **I** **128·90** 2,8,18,18,7	54 Xenon **Xe** **131·30** 2,8,18,18,8
78 latinum **Pt** **195·09** 18,32,17,1	79 Gold **Au** **196·97** 2,8,18,32,18,1	80 Mercury **Hg** **200·59** 2,8,18,32,18,2	81 Thallium **Tl** **204·37** 2,8,18,32,18,3	82 Lead **Pb** **207·2** 2,8,18,32,18,4	83 Bismuth **Bi** **208·98** 2,8,18,32,18,5	84 Polonium **Po** **[209]** 2,8,18,32,18,6	85 Astatine **At** **[210]** 2,8,18,32,18,7	86 Radon **Rn** **[222]** 2,8,18,32,18,8

63 uropium **Eu** **151·96** ,18,25,8,2	64 Gadolinium **Gd** **157·25** 2,8,18,25,9,2	65 Terbium **Tb** **158·93** 2,8,18,27,8,2	66 Dysprosium **Dy** **162·50** 2,8,18,28,8,2	67 Holmium **Ho** **164·93** 2,8,18,29,8,2	68 Erbium **Er** **167·26** 2,8,18,30,8,2	69 Thulium **Tm** **168·93** 2,8,18,31,8,2	70 Ytterbium **Yb** **173·04** 2,8,18,32,8,2	71 Lutetium **Lu** **147·97** 2,8,18,32,9,2

95 mericium **Am** **[243]** ,18,32,24, 9,2	96 Curium **Cm** **[247]** 2,8,18,32,25, 9,2	97 Berkelium **Bk** **[247]** 2,8,18,32,26, 9,2	98 Californium **Cf** **[251]** 2,8,18,32,27, 9,2	99 Einsteinium **Es** **[254]** 2,8,18,32,28, 9,2	100 Fermium **Fm** **[257]** 2,8,18,32,29, 9,2	101 Mendelevium **Md** **[258]** 2,8,18,32,30, 9,2	102 Nobelium **No** **[255]** 2,8,18,32,31, 9,2	103 Lawrencium **Lr** **[256]** 2,8,18,32,32, 9,2

A value given in brackets denotes the mass number of the isotope of longest known half-life.

Cathy Farrell

NURSING SCIENCE

MATTER AND ENERGY IN THE HUMAN BODY

NURSING SCIENCE

MATTER AND ENERGY IN THE HUMAN BODY

Ray Hickman and Martin Caon School of Nursing Studies The Flinders University of South Australia

M

First published 1991 by
THE MACMILLAN COMPANY OF AUSTRALIA PTY LTD
107 Moray Street, South Melbourne 3205
6 Clarke Street, Crows Nest 2065

Associated companies and representatives
throughout the world

National Library of Australia
cataloguing in publication data

Hickman, Raymond John St. Clair.
Nursing science.

Includes index.
ISBN 0 7329 0521 4.
ISBN 0 7329 0191 X (pbk.).

1. Biophysics. 2. Biochemistry. I. Caon, Martin,
1955– II. Title.

612.014

Set in Times by
Superskill Graphics, Singapore
Printed in Hong Kong

Contents

Preface

This book has been written to increase the range of suitable physical science textbooks available for use by students and staff in Australian tertiary nursing courses. In it we have attempted to make a number of physical science topics which are relevant to nursing more accessible to people who have not previously, or recently, studied either physics or chemistry. This has been our priority, but we have also tried to write in a way, and about things, which might catch the interest of people who have had some previous experience of these two subjects.

During the fifteen or so years in which we have been teaching nursing students we have often been asked the question 'Why do nurses need to know anything about physics and chemistry?' The answer is that without some knowledge of physics and chemistry it is simply not possible to deliver safe and effective care in some very common nursing situations. For example, without a knowledge of some basic electrical principles it is not possible for nurses to guarantee their own, or a client's, safety in situations where electric shock may occur. In such situations nurses who have no knowledge of the basic principles of electricity will be forced to proceed in their workplaces in a 'monkey see, monkey do' fashion. This means that they will have to rely on someone to show them exactly what to do and what not to do in every new situation in which they work. Nurses who possess a sound understanding of the basic principles of electricity will be in a much better position to change their own behaviour as they move between different work situations.

Another good example of the usefulness of physical science occurs in the common nursing situation of intravenous solution administration. These solutions have a property called 'tonicity' which determines their effect on the movement of water into and out of cells. Tonicity is a critical property of an intravenous solution and it must be taken into account when selecting the solution and deciding upon its route and rate of administration. Without a knowledge of atoms, molecules, ions and their behaviour in water it is not possible to judge the tonicity of a solution or the appropriateness of instructions that have been given for its administration.

An answer which we have often given to this question of the relevance of physical science for nurses is that it has a great capacity to set nurses free from the tyranny of modern technology. This technology has its basis in the sciences of physics, chemistry and biology. Nurses who must use the technology without an understanding of the science on which it is based will always be dominated by it and frightened of it. On the other hand, nurses who understand the science will be able to use the technology, with confidence and without fear, to improve the quality of the care they provide.

The task of writing for a readership as diverse as the group of people who enter Australian nursing courses has been a demanding one. We have tackled it by using a number of different tactics. Wherever possible we have introduced concepts by referring to everyday experiences. Thus, our discussion of the role played by surfactants in the body is introduced by reference to the soaps and detergents used for washing dishes and clothes. In some instances we have adopted an intuitive approach to topics which are often dealt with in a highly formal way. For example, the action of buffer solutions is explained in terms of neutralisation as a process which can be viewed as a contest of strength between an acid and a base. From this intuitive foundation we have been able to proceed quite quickly to a description of a buffer solution as one which contains appreciable quantities of a weak acid and a weak base, and then go on to give a convincing explanation of the most important properties of buffer solutions. Where understanding can be achieved via a short route we have followed that rather than use a longer one. Thus, we give an account of ionic and covalent bond formation which does not require the writing of electron structures. At every opportunity we have attempted to demystify scientific language by connecting it with everyday language, or by explaining its origins. Force, buffer, conjugation are all examples of terms used in science and which have related meanings in everyday affairs. Most important of all, we have adopted at every opportunity the tactic of illustrating physical science concepts with examples from the structure and function of the human body, or from practical nursing situations.

Each chapter includes near the beginning a list of learning objectives, and we strongly advise students to keep referring to these objectives as they work through the chapter. At the completion of each chapter students should look back at the learning objectives and check what they know and understand in relation to each one. Some chapters include study exercises and all chapters have a set of study questions at the end. Answers to many, but not all, of these questions are presented in the *Answers to Exercises and Questions*. By attempting the exercises and questions, and then checking the answers obtained, students will receive valuable feedback on the extent to which they have mastered the important ideas of each chapter.

This book is suitable for use in courses where physics and chemistry topics are combined in single units, where the topics are organised as separate physics or chemistry units, and where the physics and chemistry topics are integrated fully with biological science topics.

We wish to acknowledge the patience of our families over the long period of time during which we were distracted by the demands of writing. We are also grateful to our colleagues Peter Brinkworth, Carl Cepurneek, Jury Mohyla, Jane Neill and Trevor White who read our initial draft and offered constructive criticism of it. Their advice has improved the accuracy and quality of this final product. Of course, we are entirely responsible for the errors and inadequacies which remain. Both of us are grateful to Janet Stone who prepare most of the figures. One of us (R.H.) is grateful to Wendy Hickman who typed parts of the manuscript and assisted with compilation of the index.

Being optimists we expect to write a second edition in the not too distant future and so we would be very grateful to hear from readers with suggestions about how the book might be improved.

Martin Caon, Ray Hickman
School of Nursing Studies
Flinders University of SA
Bedford Park 5042
June 1991

CHAPTER 1

The Physical World

The physical world includes all living things although it does not include all aspects of living things. The human body is a part of the physical world, but the human spirit is not, and so physical science has a lot to say about the human body but nothing to say about the human spirit. For this reason nurses need to know a lot more about human beings than physical science or biological science can ever tell them. Nevertheless, physical and biological sciences do contribute to the technical competence of the nurse and there are situations where this type of knowledge is essential for the delivery of effective care.

In this first chapter we deal with several quite different topics at a very general level. There is a section on the nature of matter and this provides a foundation for Chapter 2, 'Atoms, Ions and Molecules: Particles that Matter'. Another section deals with measurement. It has been included because nurses routinely perform a variety of measurements in their work and because measurement is the foundation of physical science.

A striking feature of science is the capacity of scientists to acquire detailed knowledge from each other across distance and time. This is largely due to the special nature of scientific language and some insights into the nature of this language are provided in a section which deals with scientific language and literature.

Learning Objectives

At the completion of this chapter you should be able to:

1. Describe the three different states of matter and account for their main characteristics in terms of the particle theory of matter.
2. Distinguish between mixtures and pure substances; elements and compounds; physical change and chemical change.
3. Distinguish between qualitative, semi-quantitative and quantitative measurements.
4. Outline the essential features of the Australian Metric System of Units and its relationship to the SI system.
5. Explain the meaning of the terms accuracy, precision, random error, systematic error, parallax error, absolute error, percentage error, calibration, significant figure.
6. Describe some differences and similarities between scientific language and ordinary language.
7. Describe some ways in which the human body acts as a transformer of matter and energy.

1.1 The Physical World

The physical world is a world of **matter** and **energy**. Matter is the stuff out of which all the objects in the world are made. Tables, chairs, water and the body of a human being are all examples of objects composed of matter. We may define matter by saying that it is **anything which has mass and occupies space**. **Mass** is the measure of the amount of matter which is present in an object. The simplest way to measure mass is by means of a balance such as the one illustrated in Figure 1.1. It consists of a rod which is pivoted on a sharp edge. A pan hangs from each end of the rod and when both pans are empty the rod is horizontal (Figure 1.1a). If some object is placed in the left-hand pan then the rod will tilt to the left (Figure 1.1b). If we were now to add sand to the right-hand pan we would find that eventually the rod would begin to move back towards the horizontal position and if we added the sand in small enough portions we could restore it to a perfectly horizontal position (Figure 1.1c). When we have done this the object in the left-hand pan and the sand in the right-hand pan both have the same mass. If, instead of sand, we had a series of standard masses (objects of known mass) varying in size from very small to large we could restore the balance by adding these to the right-hand pan. The mass of the object in the left-hand pan would then be obtained by adding together all the standard masses which had been placed on the right-hand pan.

You may be thinking that balances are devices used to measure something called 'weight', not mass. It is certainly true that we often talk about the weight of an object and when we do it can usually be taken that we actually mean mass. However, there is an important difference between mass and weight. To see that there must be, we only need to think about the well-known experiences of the astronauts and cosmonauts. They become 'weightless' once their spaceships are in orbit around the earth, but it is obvious that their bodies are still intact and contain just as much matter as they do on earth. This shows that weight is something that depends on an object being located near the surface of the earth whereas mass does not. Weight is a force and the relationship which exists between the mass of an object and its weight is discussed in more detail in Chapter 4, 'Biomechanics'.

The mass of an object makes it resist a change in its state of motion. Objects at rest resist being set in motion and moving objects resist any change in the speed or direction of their motion. The greater the mass of an object the greater its resistance to any change in its state of motion.

Once we have accepted that matter is anything which resists being moved it is easy for us to accept that tables, chairs, water and the human body are all matter. We know this because of the effort that is needed to move them about. Air is also matter but its mass is not so obvious to us. We have to think a bit harder about our everyday experiences to convince ourselves that air has mass and is matter.

The fact that air has mass is responsible for the phenomenon of wind resistance. As any object moves through air it must push the air aside as it goes. This involves the air in a change in its state of motion and its resistance to this change (wind resistance) shows that it has mass. Wind resistance is a very important factor to be taken into account in the design of vehicles which move through air. Its magnitude depends on the shape of the vehicle and the speed with which it moves. Fast-moving vehicles, such as cars and planes, have shapes which minimise the push needed to move air out of their way as they travel through it. On the other hand, the vehicles used to travel from earth orbit to the

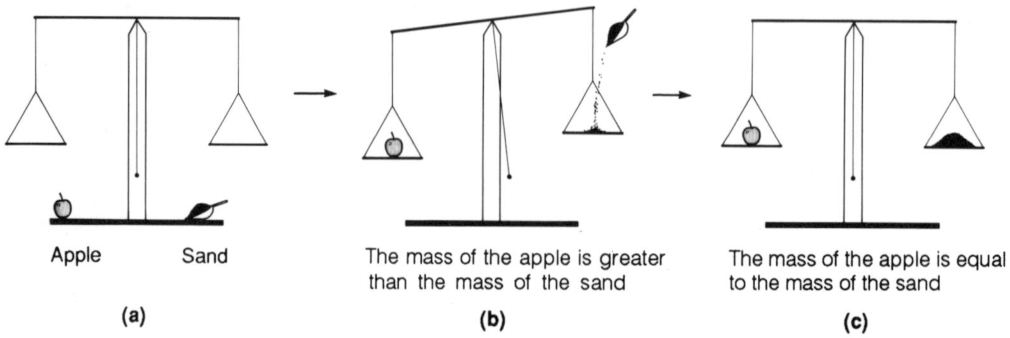
Apple
Sand
(a)
The mass of the apple is greater than the mass of the sand
(b)
The mass of the apple is equal to the mass of the sand
(c)

Figure 1.1 *A simple balance for the measurement of mass. See text for explanation of (a), (b) and (c)*

moon and back move at great speeds but are designed with no regard to wind resistance because they travel through empty space and so have no matter to push aside as they go.

What about sunlight? Our commonsense tells us that this also exists in the world, but sunlight is not matter. It offers no resistance to the movement of objects. An aircraft moving through the darkness encounters no more and no less resistance to its progress than when it moves through bright sunlight. Sunlight is an example of energy and energy may be thought of as the **mover of matter**. For example, sunlight evaporates water from the surface of the oceans. This water then moves with air currents (which are also set up by the action of sunlight) to different parts of the world where it falls to the ground as rain. Much of it then runs into creeks and rivers which eventually flow back into the oceans. All this movement is caused by sunlight, a form of energy. There are other forms of energy and some familiar examples of these are: **heat**, which we associate with cold and warm objects, the burning of fuels, with melting, boiling and so on; **electricity**, which we know activates a large number of the gadgets in our homes; **nuclear energy**, which most of us have little experience of, but hear and read a great deal about. If you now reconsider the statement that 'energy is the mover of matter' you will realise that heat, electricity and nuclear energy all meet this criterion: they are all capable of causing motion. The topic of energy is discussed in more detail in Chapter 5, 'Energy', but we need to say something more about heat and its relationship to the familiar (but poorly understood) property, **temperature**.

Heat is a form of energy but temperature is not. Heat is the energy associated with the motion of particles within matter. Temperature is a measure of the **intensity of heat** which an object possesses. As the temperature rises the motion of the particles in a sample of matter increases and the intensity of the heat increases (for further discussion of this point see Sections 5.7 and 5.8). The importance of temperature is that it tells us the direction in which heat energy will flow when objects are brought into contact with each other. This is, *from* the object of higher temperature (greater intensity of heat energy) *to* the object of lower temperature (lower intensity of heat energy).

1.1.1 *The States of Matter*

Matter may be solid, liquid or gas and these are called the three states of matter (there is a fourth state of matter called the plasma state which will not concern us). Solids have fixed shapes and volumes and usually exist in the form of **crystals**. These are pieces of matter having a regular geometrical shape. For example, common table salt exists as cubic crystals, although the crystals are too small to be distinguished easily with the naked eye. Liquids have fixed volumes, but shapes which vary according to the shapes of the containers in which they are placed. Gases do not maintain either their shape or their volume and always adopt both the shape and volume of the container in which they have been placed.

Changes of State. Many types of matter can be made to change their state by altering the temperature. For example, below 0 °C water is a solid (ice), between 0 °C and 100 °C it exists as a liquid and above 100 °C it exists as a gas (steam).

The change of a solid into a liquid is called **melting** or **fusion** and the change of a liquid into a solid is called **freezing**. The temperature at which these two changes occur is called the **melting point** and **freezing point** respectively. For a particular type of matter, melting point and freezing point are the same. Thus, ice has a melting point of 0 °C and water has a freezing point of 0 °C. The change of a liquid into a gas is called **boiling** or **vaporisation** while the change of a gas into a liquid is called **condensation**. The temperature at which these changes occur is called the **boiling point** and this term is normally used regardless of whether it is boiling or condensation which is occurring.

It is possible for matter to change from the solid state to the gas state without first forming a liquid and this is known as **sublimation**. The reverse process, in which a gas forms a solid, is called **crystallisation**. Two well-known types of matter which sublime are naphthalene and carbon dioxide. Naphthalene is used as mothballs and we all know that mothballs eventually disappear from the drawers and cupboards in which we have placed them. The reason for this is that once mothballs are removed from their container the naphthalene of which they are composed begins to

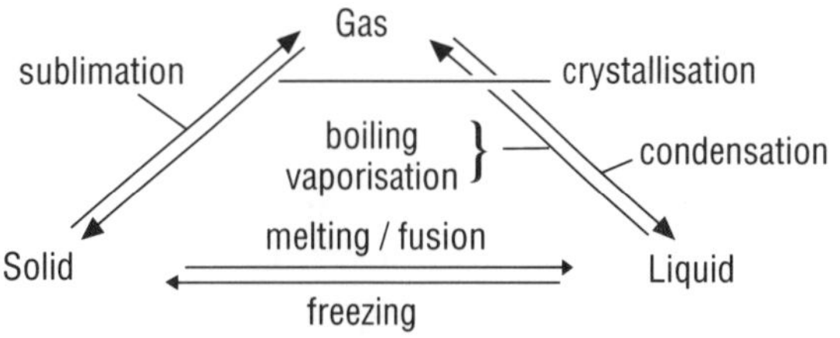

Figure 1.2 *Changes of state*

disperse into the atmosphere due to sublimation. Carbon dioxide is used as 'dry ice'. At temperatures above –78 °C it changes straight from a solid to a gas. Solid carbon dioxide is called dry ice because it is very cold (like ice, only much colder) and it leaves no liquid behind after it has changed state. All these changes of state have been summarised in Figure 1.2.

1.1.2 *The Particle Theory of Matter*

Imagine that you have the means of dividing a lump of matter into smaller and smaller pieces. There are two possibilities for what may occur as you continue to carry out the division. You may go on forever, dividing the matter into smaller and smaller pieces but never reaching a stage where you could go no further. If this happened you might conclude that there is no piece of matter so small that it cannot be made still smaller. If this were the case we would say that matter is **continuous**. The other possibility is that you might reach a stage where the piece of matter which you had could not be made any smaller and we would then say that matter is **discontinuous**, or that it consists of **particles**.

At first sight, matter appears to be continuous and so you may be somewhat surprised to be told here that matter consists of particles. The evidence for the existence of these particles is indirect but it is, nevertheless, convincing. For example, it is very difficult to see how it would be possible for us to move if the air was continuous. Where would the air go to as we displaced it? How could salt dissolve in water if both were continuous? In what way are the three states of matter different if all matter is continuous? To explain these common observations,while maintaining that matter is continuous, we would have to make some very strange assumptions. For example, to explain the ability of salt to dissolve in water we would have to say that different pieces of matter are capable of occupying and completely filling the same space at the same time.

The familiar properties of matter are much easier to understand if we accept that it consists of particles. For example, we can account for the existence of the three states of matter and their different characteristics as follows.

Solids. The particles of a solid are packed tightly together in a regular arrangement. They occupy fixed positions with respect to each other and their only movement is vibration about the positions which they occupy. The tight packing of particles and their inability to move from place to place within the solid explains why solids have fixed shapes and volumes. The fact that solids usually exist as crystals is due to the regular packing of particles within the solid.

Liquids. These have their particles packed closely together but in a random fashion. The closeness of the packing explains why liquids have fixed volumes (provided that the temperature is constant). Although the particles of a liquid are closely packed they are not held as tightly together as the particles of a solid and so are able to move from place to place within the liquid. This explains why a liquid will flow and adopt the shape of its container.

Gases. The particles are widely separated from each other and move about quite independently. The distance between particles is much greater than the size of the particles themselves. Because of the large amount of space between gas particles gases are easily compressed. The ability of gas particles to move independently

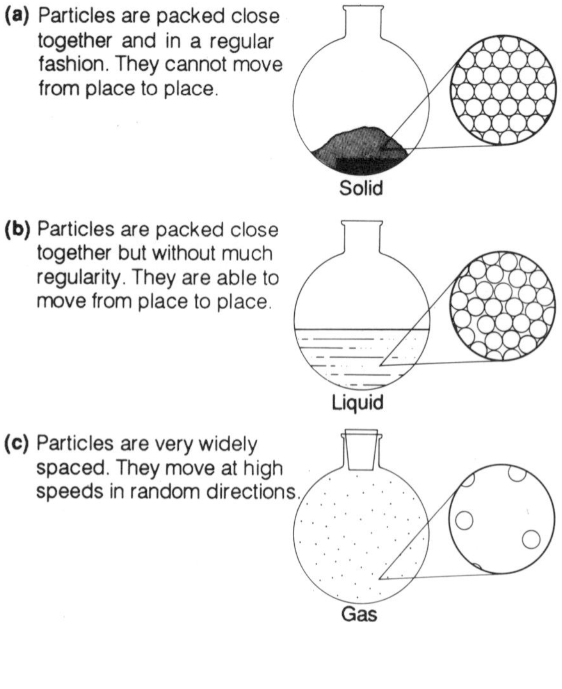

(a) Particles are packed close together and in a regular fashion. They cannot move from place to place.
Solid
(b) Particles are packed close together but without much regularity. They are able to move from place to place.
Liquid
(c) Particles are very widely spaced. They move at high speeds in random directions.
Gas

Figure 1.3 *The arrangement and motion of particles in the three states of matter: (a) solid; (b) liquid; (c) gas*

of one another allows them to spread throughout any container no matter what its size or shape.

This description of matter as consisting of particles in constant motion is called the **Kinetic Theory of Matter** and it is discussed further in Section 5.8, 'Temperature and Kinetic Theory'. Differences between the arrangement and motion of particles in solids, liquids and gases are illustrated in Figure 1.3.

Increasing the temperature of a substance may cause it to change from solid to liquid, or liquid to gas, or solid to gas. The reason for this is that the temperature increase involves an increase in the speed at which the particles of the substance move. If this increase is sufficient (that is, if the temperature is made high enough) the particles will be able to overcome the forces holding them in a solid or liquid state and become liquid or gas.

1.1.3 *Mixtures and Pure Substances*

The ideas of **mixed** and **pure** are commonsense ideas forming a part of everyday language and thought. If you apply these commonsense ideas to a cup of tea which has had sugar added to it you will have no difficulty concluding that the cup of tea is a mixed thing rather than a pure thing. Even without the sugar, tea is obviously mixed. It contains water and other matter originating from the tea leaves which were used to make it. But what about sugar? Is this mixed or pure?

Most people will say that sugar is pure, but with less confidence than when they say that a cup of tea is mixed. If they have no knowledge of chemistry they probably base their statement on advertisements which declare that sugar is a pure and healthy food, or on some notion that 'natural' things (sugar is obtained from plants) are always pure. In this particular case they happen to have guessed right, sugar is pure. However, in other similar cases this sort of commonsense reasoning leads to the wrong answer.

Nearly all foodstuffs are claimed by their growers or manufacturers to be pure but, with very few exceptions (such as sugar), foodstuffs are mixed. What the growers and manufacturers mean is that their products contain nothing that it is harmful. This is fair usage of the term pure because, in ordinary language, it implies such things as 'good', 'harmless', 'beneficial'. In chemistry, though, the term pure has nothing to do with being good, harmless or beneficial. It simply means a single type of matter, unmixed with other different types of matter. It is quite possible for something to be pure and deadly. An example of this would be strychnine which, like sugar, is obtained from a plant. However, a cup of tea which contains a teaspoon or so of strychnine would kill the person drinking it.

Most of the matter in the world is mixed and we say that such matter exists in the form of **mixtures**. Sea water, tap water, air, soil and living tissue are all examples of mixtures containing many different types of matter. Over the centuries, human beings have learned how to separate the components of mixtures from each other. Once a particular type of matter has been separated from all the other types of matter with which it was originally mixed we say that it has been obtained in the form of a **pure substance**. The task of separating pure substances from mixtures is an important part of the science of **chemistry** — so important, in fact, that chemistry is sometimes referred to as **the art of separation**.

1.1.4 *Homogeneous and Heterogeneous Matter*

If a sample of matter has the same properties throughout it is said to be **homogeneous.** If its properties vary from place to place it is said to be **heterogeneous**. Mixtures are usually heterogeneous while pure substances are usually homogeneous, but there are many exceptions to this generalisation, particularly in the case of mixtures. Thus, a cup of tea to which sugar has been added without stirring is a heterogeneous mixture. The first few sips from this cup of tea will taste different from the last few and so this property of the tea varies from place to place. Once the tea has been stirred its taste (and all its other properties) become the same throughout. It is still a mixture but now it is homogeneous. Another example of a mixture which is usually homogeneous is sea water, although it may vary in its composition if samples are taken from widely separated parts of the sea.

In the case of mixtures, homogeneity or heterogeneity often depends on the size of the sample which is considered, and its history. For example, freshly drawn blood is a homogeneous mixture provided that we consider portions bigger than about 1 mm^3. In portions of this size the proportion of each blood component present is the same from one portion to the next. However, if we consider portions of blood which are more than a million times smaller than this we would find that different portions varied in the proportion of blood components which they contained. In particular, some of these portions might contain five erythrocytes (red blood cells), others might contain three or six. On this scale, then, blood is heterogeneous. If a blood sample is left to stand it becomes heterogeneous because the cell component begins to settle out and fewer cells are found in portions taken from the top of the sample than in those taken from the bottom.

A pure substance will usually be homogeneous because no matter what portion of it is taken it will contain particles of just the one type and these will usually be distributed uniformly throughout the space which the substance occupies. However, it is quite possible to have different states of matter existing in contact with each other. Each state is homogeneous but, since particles are distributed differently in different states of matter, we will have a sample of a pure substance which is heterogeneous whenever we take a portion containing both of the states which are present. All of this can be illustrated by considering the familiar example of a kettle which contains boiling water. The only matter inside the kettle is water (all the air has been replaced by steam). If we take our sample of matter to be just the liquid water in the kettle then this is a homogeneous sample because all the particles which it contains are of the one type and they are spread uniformly throughout the space which the sample occupies. If we take our sample of matter to be just the steam inside the kettle this also is homogeneous. However, if we take our sample of matter to be all the water inside the kettle (liquid water and steam) then the sample is heterogeneous because the water particles are spread much more thinly in the steam than in the liquid water.

1.1.5 *The Separation of Mixtures*

The components of a mixture are separated from each other by using some difference in their properties. By way of illustration let us consider the formation of pure water from sea water by **distillation**. This method makes use of the difference in boiling points between water and salt, which is the other main component of sea water. Water boils at 100 °C and salt boils at 1465 °C. When sea water is heated to a temperature of slightly more than 100 °C the water in it boils and changes to a gas. However, the salt, which has a boiling point much higher than 100 °C, does not boil. The gaseous water is then allowed to pass through a condenser where it is cooled and forms liquid water again. This liquid water contains none of the salt present in sea water and so it is a sample of pure water. As this process continues, more and more water is removed from the sea water. Eventually it is observed that crystals form in the sea water and these crystals are pure salt.

The question which arises now is: 'How can we be sure that the water and salt really are pure substances?' The answer is that the water and salt obtained in this way have properties which are different from those of the sea water from which they were obtained and these properties do not change further when the water and salt are put through the same procedure again and again. For example, sea water may have a freezing point of –2 °C, a boiling point of 100.3 °C and a density of 1.03 g/ml (we say that sea water *may* have these properties because its composition does vary slightly from place to place). When water is obtained from this sea water by distillation the sea water left behind has different properties from the original sea water. Furthermore, its properties continue to change as more and more water is removed from it by distillation. The water obtained as a result of distillation has a freezing point of 0 °C, a boiling point of 100 °C and a density of 1.000 g/ml (or values very close to these). Now, if we subject this water to another distillation we find that there is no further change in these properties and we take this to indicate that we have obtained water in its pure form. Likewise, if we were to re-dissolve the salt in some pure water, repeat the distillation, recover the salt as before and find that its properties were unchanged we would take this as an indication that it was also a pure substance. To summarise all this we may say that *a pure substance is a sample of matter with properties which do not change as it is subjected to further attempts at purification.*

The complete separation of mixtures and the attainment of an absolutely pure substance are ideals rarely (if ever) achieved in practice. Mixtures are separated and substances purified to the extent which is convenient or warranted by the circumstances. Tap water is pure enough to be used in the radiator of a car but distilled water must be used to top up the battery. For some scientific applications water needs to be distilled not once, but several times before it is used.

There are other methods besides distillation which can be used to separate the components of a mixture. Sometimes it is a difference in solubility between components which is used as the basis for separation. Marie Curie used this approach to obtain a pure radium substance from a mixture which contained vastly greater amounts of other types of matter.

The components of a mixture may also be separated by bringing it into contact with a finely divided powder in the form of a column or layer. The components of the mixture adhere (stick) to the powder but some components are stuck more tightly than others. When a suitable liquid is run through the powder it washes the components of the mixture along with it at different rates determined by the solubility of that component in the liquid and the tightness with which it sticks to the powder. As a result of this different rate of movement the components of the mixture separate from each other on the column or layer of powder. This is the basis of a separation technique known as **chromatography**.

1.1.6 *Physical and Chemical Properties*

All the properties described in the previous section, and which served as the basis for separating the components of mixtures, are **physical properties**. These are properties which can be observed without changing the nature of a substance. When we determine the boiling point of water we do not alter its chemical nature. We know that the water which is converted into steam can be easily recovered by cooling. Similarly, when we observe that salt is soluble in water we are observing a physical property. The act of dissolving the salt does not alter its nature and we can easily recover it afterwards.

Chemical properties are those which can only be observed by arranging for a substance to change into another different type of matter. It is usually more difficult to recover a substance after observing one of its chemical properties. For example, the fact that petrol floats on water is a physical property which may be observed without changing the nature of petrol. After the observation the petrol is easily recovered. The fact that petrol burns is a chemical property. In order to observe this property one must set light to some petrol and change it into some completely different substances (carbon dioxide and water). The petrol which has been burned cannot be recovered, except with great difficulty.

As well as talking about physical and chemical properties it is common for us to talk about the closely related ideas of **physical change** and **chemical change**. Thus, the change which a sample of matter undergoes as we observe one of its physical properties is called a physical change and the change which it undergoes as we observe one of its chemical properties is called a chemical change.

When mixtures form, or are separated into their components, the changes involved are all physical changes. Although the physical properties of one component of a mixture may obscure some physical properties of another component it is generally true that the components of a mixture retain their properties after the mixture has formed. For example, the tastes of sugar and salt are still evident in most mixtures which contain them.

1.1.7 *Pure Substances from Mixtures*

Modern chemistry has provided us with a vastly increased number of new types of matter to be used in meeting our needs. Some idea of the impact which new types of matter have had upon our lives may be obtained by comparing the substances used 200 years ago to construct buildings, make clothing and fight disease with some which are available today for the same purposes.

Two centuries ago buildings were made almost entirely of wood and stone. Some glass and metal was also used, but in limited amounts and for mainly ornamental purposes. Today we construct our buildings using steel and aluminium as well as stone and wood. Glass is used to a much greater extent and a whole range of plastics is available for many different building purposes.

Two centuries ago all clothing was made from wool, or silk, or the hides of animals. Today, much of our clothing is made from plastics which are cheaper and, in many respects, superior to the natural materials.

The medicines available to the physician two centuries ago were few in number and limited in their effectiveness. Surgery was a tactic of last resort because effective anaesthetics were not available. Most infections were simply allowed to run their course. No effective methods were available for the treatment of cancers. People suffering from mental illness were often just locked away in the most terrible conditions and forgotten. Today, surgery is a common technique which people face quite readily, knowing that they will have the benefit of safe, effective anaesthetics. Effective medicines are available for the treatment of most bacterial infections and there are also medicines which can be used to cure, or control, some cancers. A large proportion of mental illness is now treated using medicines which often allow the person affected to lead a fairly normal life.

Nearly all these useful substances originate from mixtures and are made available by subjecting the mixtures to physical changes which separate their components from one another. In many instances these separated components must then be subjected to chemical changes in order to obtain the desired substance. Three pure substances which are obtained like this are aluminium, nylon and penicillin.

Aluminium. Prior to 1886, aluminium was a laboratory curiosity not seen in the outside world. It could only be obtained in relatively small quantities via an expensive and dangerous process. Its cost was approximately $330/kg (in 1886 dollars). In 1886, two scientists, Charles Hall of the United States and Paul Heroult of France, independently discovered a method for obtaining aluminium from the common mineral, bauxite. Bauxite is a mixture of several different substances. One of these is alumina which can be separated from the other components of bauxite by making use of the fact that it has different solubility properties. Once alumina is obtained as a pure substance it can be subjected to a series of chemical changes which transform it into aluminium. The process developed by Hall and Heroult saw the cost of making aluminium drop from $330/kg to $0.40/kg overnight and the substance became available for use on a massive scale.

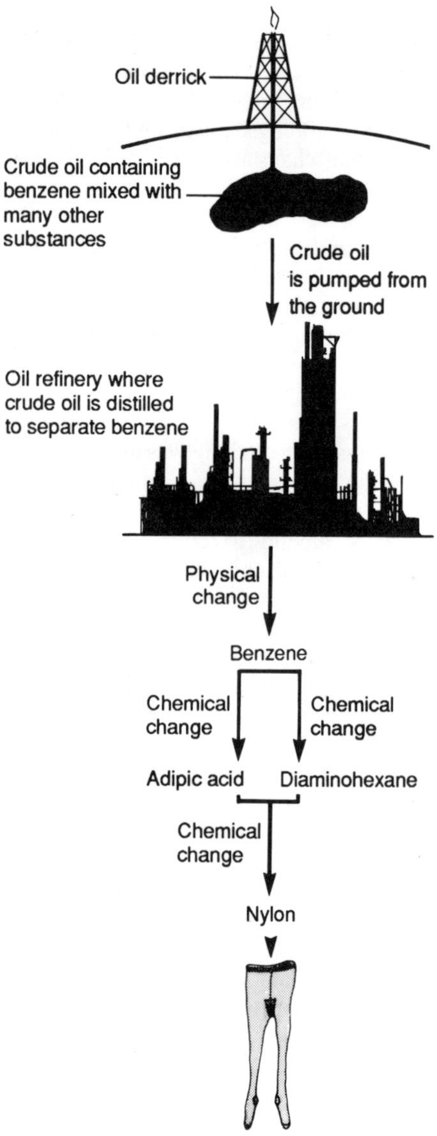

Figure 1.4 *From petroleum to pantyhose*

Nylon. This is the best known example of a synthetic fibre. It was first made in the United States in 1934. The ultimate source of nylon is crude petroleum. This is a mixture of many different pure substances, one of which is benzene, a colourless liquid with a boiling point of 80 °C. Benzene is separated from the other substances present in crude petroleum using a distillation technique. It is then subjected to two different series of chemical changes. One of these series converts it into a different pure substance called adipic acid. The other series of chemical changes converts benzene into diaminohexane. The combination of adipic acid with diaminohexane in yet another chemical change produces nylon. This remarkable transformation is outlined in Figure 1.4.

Penicillin. In 1929 the British scientist, Alexander Fleming reported that the mould *Penicillium notatum* produced a substance which was capable of destroying a wide range of disease-causing organisms. Fleming named this substance penicillin and attempted its separation from the complex mixture on which the mould grew. He was not successful and turned his attention to other things. In 1939, Howard Florey, an Australian, and Ernst Chain, a German, took up where Fleming left off and they eventually succeeded in obtaining penicillin as a pure substance. It turned out to be the most effective anti-bacterial agent ever discovered and in the time since it first became available (1943) it has saved millions of lives.

1.1.8 *Elements and Compounds*

Elements. There is an enormous number of different pure substances that have been separated from the mixtures occurring naturally in the world. There is also an enormous number of pure substances obtained from other pure substances by subjecting them to chemical change. The great diversity in the types of matter which exist and the fact that matter often changed from one type to another were both noticed by the ancients. They explained this apparent complexity in their world by saying that there were only four fundamentally different types of matter: earth, air, fire and water. They believed that all the different types of matter in the world were formed by interaction between two or more of these four fundamental types of matter.

Today we also believe that the vast number of different types of pure substance which exist are formed out of a relatively small number of fundamental types of matter which we call the **chemical elements**. The number of chemical elements is not four but more than 100. Of these only 90 occur naturally on earth. The chemical elements do not include any of the four elements in which the ancients believed.

The systematic identification of chemical elements was made possible when the seventeenth century Irish scientist, Robert Boyle, pointed out that such a substance would not be capable of separation into simpler substances. This is the essence of our modern definition which states that *an element is a pure substance not capable of being broken down into simpler forms by ordinary physical or chemical means.* The definition specifies 'ordinary' physical or chemical means of conversion into simpler forms because it is possible to change one element into two others using nuclear reactors and other high-energy devices.

Using Boyle's criterion, scientists were able to identify more and more chemical elements and to show that some substances previously thought to be elements were not elements at all.

As an example of the type of experiment and reasoning involved in the process of deciding whether or not a pure substance is an element, let us consider the behaviour of water. If electricity is passed between two oppositely charged electrodes immersed in water it is observed that a gas forms at each electrode. These gases can be collected separately using an arrangement such as the one illustrated in Figure 1.5. The gas which forms at the negative electrode is called **hydrogen** and that which forms at the positive electrode is called **oxygen**. The volume of hydrogen formed is always twice that of oxygen.

The properties of hydrogen and oxygen are different from one another and different from those of gaseous water. These properties are not affected by typical physical changes such as condensation or dissolving and so we can be confident that hydrogen and oxygen are both pure substances. We may also conclude that the passage of electricity through water brings about a chemical change. This process of causing chemical change by the passage of electricity through a liquid is called **electrolysis**. During the nineteenth century, electrolysis played a part in the discovery of many elements.

When hydrogen and oxygen are formed as illustrated in Figure 1.5 it is obvious that they have come from the water (it contains no significant quantity of anything else except a tiny quantity of acid which is added to promote the passage of the electricity). Furthermore, when a mixture of hydrogen and oxygen is ignited the two gases combine (explosively!) to form water. This shows clearly that water can be transformed into two other pure substances (hydrogen and oxygen) which come entirely from the water and so must be simpler forms of matter than water is. We can conclude from this that water is not one of the chemical elements.

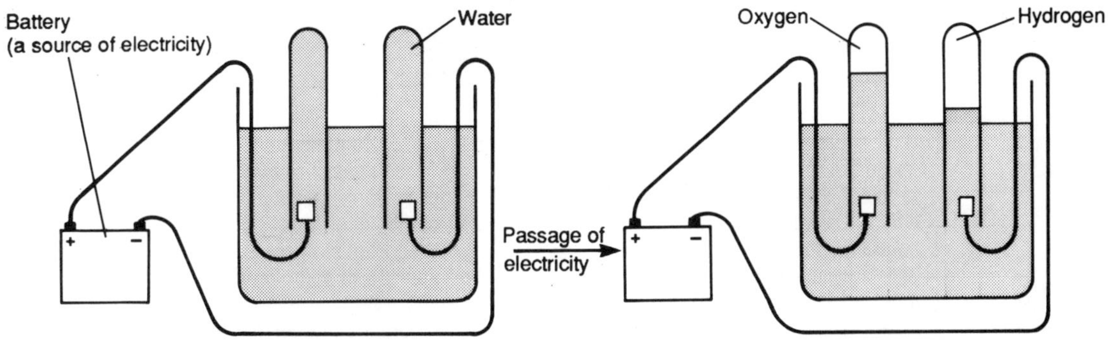

Figure 1.5 *Conversion of water into hydrogen and oxygen*

Let us now turn to oxygen and hydrogen. No one has ever performed an experiment in which either hydrogen or oxygen is converted into simpler forms of matter. At the same time there are many substances which, like water, can be made to undergo chemical changes and form either hydrogen or oxygen. These observations had, by 1781 in the case of hydrogen and 1774 in the case of oxygen, convinced virtually all scientists that the two substances must be elements. By 1939 the 90 naturally occurring elements had been discovered. Since that time a number of other elements have been found among the products formed under very drastic conditions such as those existing inside nuclear reactors. These conditions are able to bring about changes in matter which do not take place under the milder conditions which apply when physical and chemical changes occur.

Compounds. The 90 elements which occur naturally on earth are able to combine and form what appears to be an unlimited number of additional, pure substances. These pure substances are called **compounds** and water is just one example. Compounds may be defined as *matter in which two or more elements are combined in fixed proportions*. The main differences between compounds and mixtures are that:

1. the components of a mixture may be present in varying proportion (for example, a salt-water mixture may contain 5% salt, or 6% salt or 10% salt and so on), whereas the elements making up a compound are always present in a fixed proportion (for example, water always contains one gram of hydrogen for every eight grams of oxygen);
2. the components of a mixture retain their properties when present in the mixture (for example, the taste of salt is still noticeable after it has formed a salt-water mixture), whereas the properties of the elements making up a compound are lost while the elements remain in the form of a compound (for example, hydrogen ignites when in the form of the element but not while it is combined in water).

Several of the relationships existing between different forms of matter are shown in Figure 1.6.

1.1.9 *The Electrical Nature of Matter*

Electricity is something most people take for granted. This is not surprising because we are surrounded by electrical devices. We use them for lighting, heating, cooling, cooking, entertainment, communication, traffic control and for many other purposes. In a modern city the loss of the electricity supply can bring business activity and traffic movement to a virtual halt. While the numerous electrical devices we use are all products of human ingenuity, electricity itself is a part of the physical world.

We are regularly treated to displays of natural electricity in the form of lightning. The common experiences of feeling a jolt when stepping out of a car

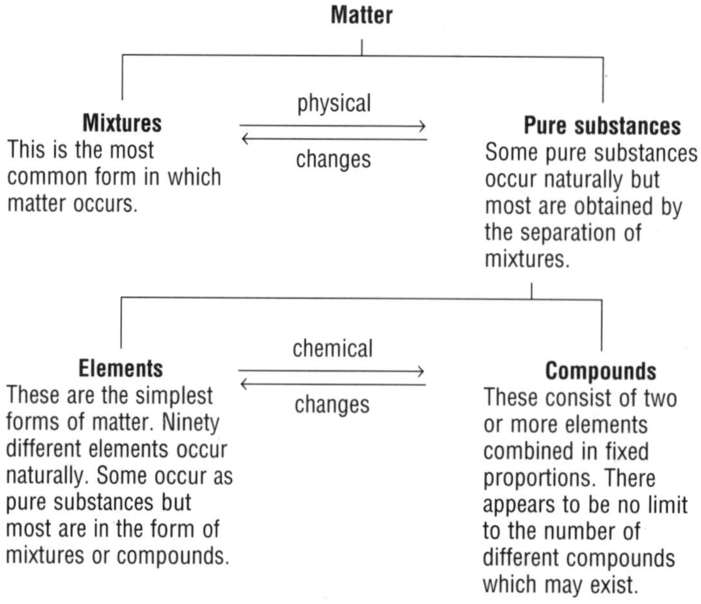
Matter
Mixtures
This is the most common form in which matter occurs.
physical
changes
Pure substances
Some pure substances occur naturally but most are obtained by the separation of mixtures.
Elements
These are the simplest forms of matter. Ninety different elements occur naturally. Some occur as pure substances but most are in the form of mixtures or compounds.
chemical
changes
Compounds
These consist of two or more elements combined in fixed proportions. There appears to be no limit to the number of different compounds which may exist.

Figure 1.6 *Relationships between different forms of matter*

or touching a door handle are also examples of natural electricity. So is the crackling which occurs when some types of clothing are removed. If the clothes are removed in a darkened room we also see light produced and this is lightning on a small scale.

Most of us have at some time or other rubbed a piece of plastic with a cloth and then seen that the plastic will attract a piece of paper. This is an electrical effect and we say that the rubbing has **electrified** the plastic. Electrification achieved in this simple fashion can be used to illustrate something very important about electricity.

Let us consider the situation depicted in Figure 1.7a. Two rods are both made of glass and both have been rubbed vigorously with silk. Both are suspended by fine strings so that they are free to rotate horizontally. When they are brought near to each other, *but without touching*, we notice that they rotate *away from* each other (they repel each other). It is important to realise that the two glass rods must be the same as each other because each has been rubbed with the same material. When we replace either the glass rods or the silk with other materials and repeat this exercise we find that there are many other combinations of materials which behave in the same way as glass and silk do. As long as the two rods are of the same material and have been rubbed with the same type of cloth all we see is repulsion between them.

When we carry out the same exercise using rods composed of different materials, but electrified by rubbing with the same cloth (see Figure 1.7b) we observe some examples of attraction between them, as well as some examples of repulsion. This is also the case when the rods are composed of the same material electrified by rubbing with different cloths. However, there are no instances of electrified rods which are neither attracted nor repelled by each other. The simplest explanation for this behaviour is that there are two, and only two, different types of electrified object and that repulsion occurs between electrified objects of the same type while attraction occurs between electrified objects of different types.

The question which now arises is: 'How does rubbing objects electrify them?' The answer is that matter is fundamentally electrical in nature. It consists ultimately of electrical particles. We usually say that these particles possess an **electrical charge**. There are

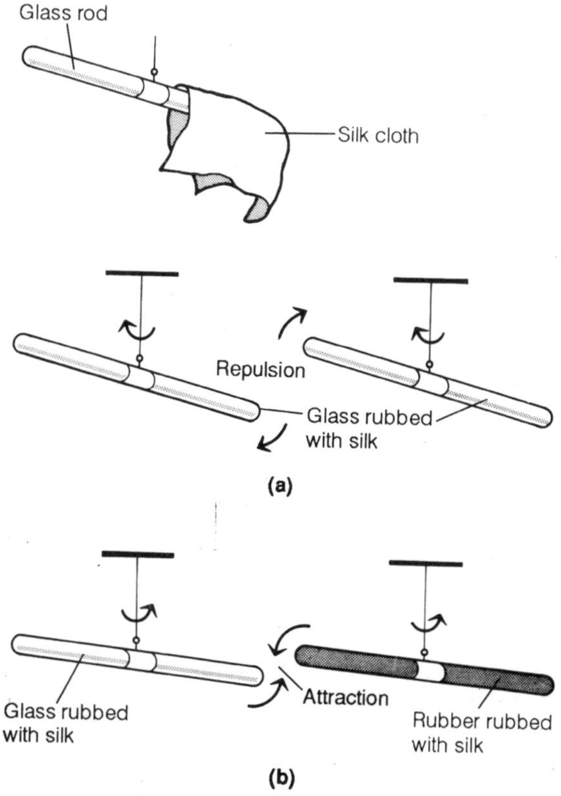

Figure 1.7 *Repulsion and attraction between electrified objects. See text for explanation of (a) and (b)*

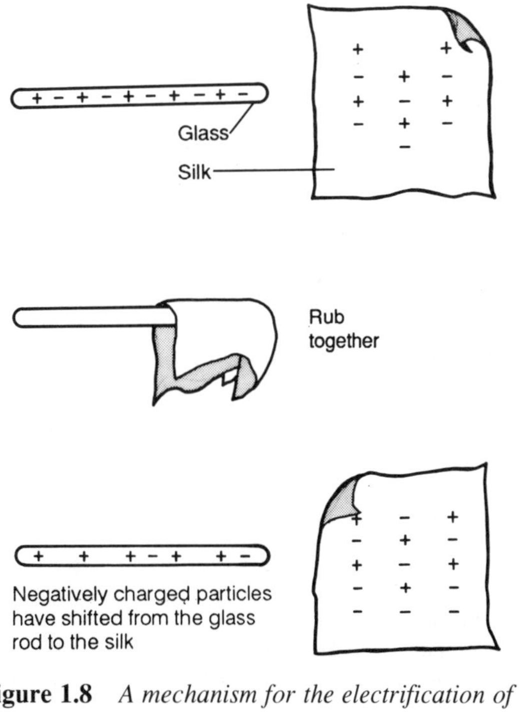

Figure 1.8 *A mechanism for the electrification of objects*

two types of charge and they are simply designated as **positive** and **negative**.

Matter is not normally electrified and this is because it contains an equal number of charges of each type. Rubbing objects together sometimes causes electrification because it transfers one type of electrically charged particle (this is always the negative particle) from one object to the other. In this way one of the objects obtains an excessive amount of electrical charge of one type while the other object obtains an excessive amount of the other type. This is illustrated in Figure 1.8.

We introduced the phenomenon of electrification by referring to the simple observation that an electrified piece of plastic will attract paper. The paper is not an electrified object and so we need to account for the ability of the plastic to attract it. The explanation involves a process called **induction**. This occurs because as the plastic approaches the paper it causes the particles in the paper of opposite charge to its own charge to accumulate on the surface which is nearer to it (see Figure 1.9). This accumulation of electrical charge on the surface of the paper closer to the approaching plastic causes the attraction which is observed.

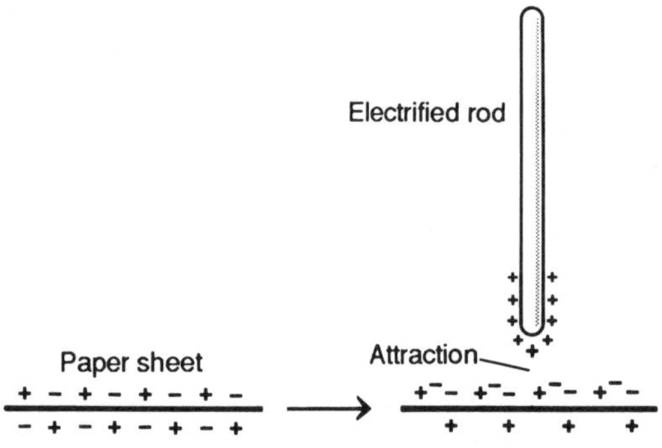

Figure 1.9 *Induction caused by an electrified object*

1.1.10 *The Human Body as a Transformer of Matter and Energy*

The air which we breathe is a mixture of oxygen, nitrogen and small quantities of other gases including carbon dioxide and water vapour. In Table 1.1 the composition of air which we breathe in (inspired air) is compared with the composition of the air which we breathe out (expired air).

The nitrogen component of air is not used by the body and we simply breathe out all that we breathe in. For this reason the percentages in Table 1.1 have been calculated ignoring nitrogen. You can see that our bodies remove oxygen from the air and add carbon dioxide and water to it.

Table 1.1 *Comparison of the compositions of inspired and expired air (nitrogen has been ignored)*

	Inspired air	Expired air
oxygen	96.3	61.1
carbon dioxude	0.2	14.2
water vapour	3.5	24.7

Oxygen is one of the chemical elements while carbon dioxide and water are both compounds of oxygen. In our bodies oxygen is transformed into these compounds by chemical changes in which it combines with other substances present to form the carbon dioxide and water. Most of the water in our bodies, and that which we expire, comes from the food and drink that we consume, but water formed by chemical changes involving oxygen also accounts for a significant proportion of it.

The other main processes involved in the flow of matter through our bodies are the elimination of faeces and urine. Faeces are a very complex mixture consisting of water, fragments of tissue (from the lining of the gastrointestinal tract), bacteria and undigested food. Urine is also a complex mixture, but three of its components dominate the others in terms of quantity. Of course, one of these is water. Another is **urea**, which is a compound of the elements carbon, hydrogen, nitrogen and oxygen. Urea forms in the body as a result of chemical changes undergone by compounds known as **proteins**, which are major components of food. Each day, an adult male on a normal diet produces about 25 g of urea in his urine. The third major component of urine is salt. Like a lot of the water which flows through our bodies the salt in urine enters the body as the salt content of the food and drink that we consume. Our bodies do not subject it to chemical changes on its way through.

Let us now consider energy flow through the human body. We know from our everyday experience that when a warm object (higher temperature) is brought into contact with a cooler one (lower temperature) the warm object becomes cooler and the cool one becomes warmer. We say that there has been a flow of heat (energy) *from* the warmer object *to* the cooler one, causing the warm object to cool because it has lost heat and the cool object to warm because it has gained heat.

No one has ever witnessed a situation in which a warm object stays warm while it is in contact with a cooler object, unless the warm object is constantly supplied with energy to replace that lost to the cooler object with which it is in contact. For example, a kettle full of boiling water sitting on a gas flame will only maintain its warmth as long as the flame remains lit and continues supplying the water with heat to replace that which it loses to its cooler surroundings.

The human body is another example of an object which remains warmer than its surroundings. Our bodies stay warm even when the surrounding air is much cooler. There must be a constant flow of heat away from the body in this circumstance and so the question which arises is: 'From what source is this loss made up?' The answer is: 'From food'. Just as the kettle receives heat from the chemical change undergone by the gas when it combines with oxygen (to form carbon dioxide and water), so our bodies constantly receive heat from the chemical changes undergone by food as it combines with oxygen in our tissues (to form carbon dioxide and water). This heat keeps the body warm. Of course, as the body's surroundings get colder and colder the rate of the heat loss gets greater and greater. Eventually this will overwhelm the body's capacity to replace the heat being lost and the body will start to grow cold. When this happens life is threatened.

So, we see that matter and energy flow through our bodies. In fact, it is this flow which keeps us alive and as soon as it stops we die.

1.2 Units and Measurement

Human beings are creatures which think and talk and **measure**. A measurement involves some comparison with a scale and it allows us to rank things on that scale. Any device used to carry out a measurement is called a **measuring instrument**. For example, the measurement of mass is carried out using a **balance** and the measurement of temperature is carried out using a **thermometer**.

The British physicist, William Thomson (Lord Kelvin) once said:

> I often say that if you can measure that of which you speak, and can express it by a number, you know something of your subject; but if you cannot measure it, your knowledge is meagre and unsatisfactory.
>
> Lord Kelvin, 1824–1907

These words are an expression of the fact that measurements give us confidence in the validity of our ideas and help us make correct decisions. They also impose a strict discipline, because in any field where ideas are expressed in terms of things which can be measured it is much more difficult to conceal or distort the truth and much easier to recognise ideas which are wrong. There are many measuring instruments which are capable of distinguishing between things which are very similar. For example, a typical set of clinical scales is capable of detecting the change in a person's mass from (say) 71.0 to 71.2 kg. A clinical thermometer is capable of detecting changes in a person's temperature that are as small as 0.1 °C. There are many instruments used in physical science which are capable of detecting differences even smaller than these.

Physical science, more than any other human activity, consists of ideas which can be tested by measurement. For this reason the knowledge which it gives us of the nature of the physical world is regarded as the most reliable knowledge which human beings possess.

Measurements are not only useful to physical scientists. They are also performed by nurses who use them as a basis for decision making. In the course of a day's work a nurse is likely to perform measurements which include mass (weight), height, blood pressure, temperature, medicine dosage, blood or urine volume, pulse rate and many others. These measurements fall into one of three categories.

1. Qualitative Measurements. This type of measurement simply involves a report of the presence or absence of some characteristic. When a person is described as being obese or feverish or depressed or thin or tall or dehydrated or in shock or confused or as having glucose in their urine a qualitative measurement has been made. All these characteristics may exist in a person to a greater or lesser degree but no indication has been given of this degree. A single qualitative measurement does not normally supply very much information about a person's condition although several different qualitative measurements may be highly informative if they are considered together.

2. Semi-quantitative Measurements. These give some indication of the magnitude of the characteristic which is being measured and allow things to be ranked in order of magnitude of that characteristic. Making a measurement semi-quantitative may simply involve using a series of words or symbols to form a scale for the characteristic. For example, the level of glucose in a person's urine may be measured by dipping a test strip into the urine and observing the colour which forms on the strip. The range of colours observed is from blue, when little or no glucose is present, through green to brown as the amount of glucose increases. The colour on the strip is compared to a series of standard colours and a set of corresponding symbols, 0, +, ++, +++, ++++. According to the colour seen the measurement is then reported using one of these symbols. Knowing that the level of glucose in a person's urine has been rated as +++ is much more useful than simply knowing that glucose is present. Even so, this semi-quantitative scale is quite ambiguous. In the case of many measurements the colour observed will be in between the colours which correspond to the different reference points on the scale and so different people performing the measurement (and even the same person repeating the measurement) will often come up with a different rating.

3. Quantitative Measurements. When numbers are used to express a measurement it is said to be a quantitative measurement. This type of measurement requires the use of instruments which have a well-defined and widely accepted scale on which there are many clearly distinguished reference points. Every reference point on the scale of instruments used in quantitative measurements can have a number assigned to it and this often makes it possible to distinguish between measurements which are very similar in their magnitudes. For example, a clinical thermometer has about 70 reference points and a set of clinical scales has more than 1000. Quite often the difference between semi-quantitative and quantitative measurement is simply that the semi-quantitative measurement has been performed using a scale which has relatively few divisions.

Quantitative measurements are the most informative and useful of all measurements. For a given characteristic it is always better to have a quantitative measure than a semi-quantitative or qualitative measure.

In quantitative measurement the units used are of great importance. Being told that a person has a mass of 114 is of no use unless we are are also told whether the units are kilograms or pounds. Scientists have taken a great deal of trouble to define units for the various measurements which they perform. This has resulted in the development of a set of units which are used by scientists all over the world and which have the same meaning wherever they are used.

1.2.1 *SI Units*

In 1960 the International Bureau of Weights and Measures, which is based in France, adopted a set of units which can be used to measure all physical quantities. It was called the *Système International d'Unites* (International System of Units) and became known as the SI system.

The SI system has seven **base units** and two **supplementary units**. They are all listed in Table 1.2.

Table 1.2 *Base and supplementary units of the SI system*

Physical quantity	SI unit	
	Name	Symbol
Base units		
length	metre	m
mass	kilogram	kg
time	second	s
electric current	ampere	A
temperature	kelvin	K
amount of substance	mole	mol
luminous intensity	candela	cd
Supplementary units		
plane angle	radian	rad
solid angle	steradian	sr

There are many more physical quantities than the nine listed in Table 1.2, for example area, volume, speed, concentration, pressure and energy. All these additional quantities are combinations of two or more of the quantities listed in Table 1.2. Area is the quantity obtained when one length is multiplied by another. The unit of area in the SI system is the **square metre** and its symbol is $\mathbf{m^2}$. Speed is a measure of how quickly something moves and it is a quantity obtained by measuring the distance moved and the time taken. The distance is then divided by the time. The SI unit for speed is **metre per second** and its symbol is **m/s** or $\mathbf{m.s^{-1}}$.

In the SI system, quantities which are obtained by the combination, through multiplication and division, of two or more of the base or supplementary quantities are known as **derived quantities** and their units are said to be **derived units**. A number of examples of derived quantities and their units are presented in Table 1.3. Some derived units have names and symbols which are combinations of the names and symbols for the corresponding base or supplementary units. These names are said to be **compound names**. Other derived units have special names and symbols but these are always capable of being expressed as compound names and symbols. Special names usually honour the achievements of some person who made an outstanding contribution in the field of science where the unit is important. Thus, the unit of force is called the newton in honour of Sir Isaac Newton who discovered the force of gravity. Where a unit has been named after a person its symbol always commences with a capital but the name of the unit does not. Thus, we would write that the SI unit of force is the newton (no capital) and report a force as 7 N. The symbols for SI units are *never* given a plural ending and it would be incorrect to report a force as 7 Ns.

Table 1.3 *Names and symbols for some common derived units*

Quantity	Unit name (symbol)	
area	square metre (m^2)	
volume	cubic metre (m^3)	
speed	metre per second (m/s or $m.s^{-1}$)	
density	kilogram per cubic metre (kg/m^3 or $kg.m^{-3}$)	
frequency	hertz (Hz)	special names and symbols
force	newton (N)	special names and symbols
pressure	pascal (Pa)	special names and symbols
energy	joule (J)	special names and symbols
electric charge	coulomb (C)	special names and symbols

Prefixes for SI Units. Where a quantity being measured is of a magnitude much greater or much smaller than the SI unit for that quantity then prefixes are used with the unit name and symbol. The full set of prefixes used in conjunction with SI units is given in Table 1.4. They are used to represent magnitudes which are different by some multiple of 10 and the meaning of a prefix is the same regardless of the SI unit with which it is being used. The prefixes most commonly encountered in nursing are marked with an asterisk.

Table 1.4 *Prefixes used with SI units*

Prefix name	Symbol	Magnitude
exa	E	10^{18}
peta	P	10^{15}
tera	T	10^{12}
giga	G	10^{9}
mega	M	10^{6}
kilo*	k	10^{3}
hecto	h	10^{2}
deka	da	10
deci	d	10^{-1}
centi*	c	10^{-2}
milli*	m	10^{-3}
micro*	μ	10^{-6}
nano	n	10^{-9}
pico	p	10^{-12}
femto	f	10^{-15}
atto	a	10^{-18}

* A prefix likely to be encountered in nursing.

Prefixes are useful because they allow any measurement to be stated as a number of familiar magnitude. The prefix normally chosen is one that allows the measurement to be quoted as a number between 0.1 and 1000. Thus, a person's height would most often be stated as 180 cm, sometimes as 1.80 m but never as 1800 mm or 0.0018 km. Likewise, a person's mass (weight) is always stated as 72 kg and never as 72 000 g.

1.2.2 *The Australian Metric System of Measurement*

In 1970, the Australian Parliament passed the *Metric Conversion Act* which defined the Australian Metric System of Measurement as measurement using:

1. units of the SI system;
2. decimal multiples of SI units;
3. such other units as the minister declares, from time to time by notice published in *The Gazette*, to be within the metric system.

Part 3 of the definition allows for custom and convenience by providing for the use of non-SI units where the circumstances warrant. People get very used to using a particular set of units, and making a complete change in a nation's system of measurement is one of the most difficult things to achieve smoothly. Just imagine how difficult it would be to convince people that they should give up measuring time in days, hours and minutes and use decimal multiples of the second as time units! The units which are included in the metric system as a result of ministerial declaration are called **declared units** and some common examples which are available for general use in Australia are given in Table 1.5.

Table 1.5 *Declared units of the Australian Metric System having general application*

Physical quantity	Declared unit	Symbol
volume	megalitre	Ml
	kilolitre	kl
	litre	l*
	millilitre	ml
	microlitre	μl
time	day	d
	hour	h
	minute	min
speed	kilometre per hour	km/h
temperature	degree celsius	°C

* In Australia it is quite common for 'L' to be used in place of 'l' as the symbol for litre.

There are some units which have been specifically excluded from the Australian Metric System and these are known as **excluded units**. Some examples are given in Table 1.6 together with the names and symbols of the metric units which should be used in their place. Excluded units include the centimetre of mercury which is a unit of pressure. The designation of this unit as an excluded unit means that it is officially forbidden for use in Australia. This has not stopped use of the closely related unit millimetre of mercury which is still the preferred unit for the measurement of blood pressure. It is one thing for a government to say that a unit should not be used and another thing altogether for the government to prevent its use where the use occurs in private settings not subject to government control. The Calorie, a unit for energy, is still encountered in many popular publications which include sections on food and diet. However, this excluded unit is becoming less and less common as it is replaced by the kilojoule.

Table 1.6 *Units excluded from the Australian Metric System*

Physical quantity	Excluded unit	Metric unit (symbol)
pressure	centimetre of mercury	kilopascal (kPa)
pressure	atmosphere	kilopascal (kPa)
energy	calorie	joule (J)
energy	Calorie	kilojoule (kJ)

Physical Quantities in Nursing. Physical quantities which nurses routinely encounter include:

mass (weight)	electric current
liquid volume	voltage
length	frequency (rate)
gas pressure	energy
solution concentration	temperature

When communicating with one another, Australian health professionals should use the appropriate Australian metric unit or SI unit for any measurement which is part of the communication. This is done in most settings where nurses work, although you can expect blood pressure to be reported in millimetres of mercury, rather than kilopascals, for many years yet.

When health professionals communicate with members of the public they should keep in mind that they have a responsibility to ensure that they are understood. Many elderly people have no idea of the meaning of metric units and still think in terms of imperial units. If you check the births column of your daily newspaper you will find that most birth announcements include the child's mass (weight) expressed in the imperial units of pounds and ounces rather than in the metric unit of kilogram. The reason for this is that, aside from the parents, the people most interested in the birth of a new child are its grandparents. Most people old enough to be grandparents still think about weight in terms of imperial units, not metric units. For several very common physical quantities a nurse should take the trouble to know the relationship between imperial and metric units. In Table 1.7 the imperial and metric units for several of these quantities are listed, together with the corresponding conversion factors.

Table 1.7 *Interconversion of metric and imperial units*

Physical quantity	Metric unit	Imperial unit	Conversion factors
length	metre	foot	1 m = 3.28 feet
		yard	1 m = 1.09 yard
	centimetre	inch	1 cm = 0.39 inch
mass	kilogram	pound	1 kg = 2.2 pound
		stone	1 kg = 0.16 stone
		hundredweight	1 kg = 0.02 h/weight
	gram	ounce	1 g = 0.035 ounce
volume	litre	pint	1 l = 1.76 pint
		gallon	1 l = 0.22 gallon
	millilitre	fluid ounce	1 ml = 0.35 fluid ounce
energy	kilojoule	calorie	1 kJ = 240 calorie
		Calorie	1 kJ = 0.24 Calorie

1.3 Errors of Measurement

1.3.1 *Accuracy and Precision*

The words accuracy and precision are commonly encountered in ordinary language, where their meanings are very similar. In science, though, an important distinction is made between the two. Accuracy refers to the closeness of a measurement to the *true value* for the particular physical quantity which is being measured. Precision refers to the *reproducibility* of a measurement. A measurement is said to be precise if the same value is obtained when it is repeated several times. It is possible to have a situation in which a physical quantity can be measured precisely but not accurately. This will be the case if there is something about the measuring instrument or the procedure used which causes the measurement to be out by the same amount each time it is performed. On the other hand, if a measurement can be performed accurately then precision is guaranteed because an accurate measurement is one which is close to the true value and there can be only one true value. Therefore, each time an accurate measurement is made the same value must be obtained (unless the quantity changes in between measurements).

1.3.2 *The Inevitability of Error*

It is impossible to measure physical quantities with complete accuracy unless the measurement simply involves counting. The quantity of students in a lecture theatre can be measured with complete accuracy provided that they all agree to stay in their places while the measurement is performed. There is no possibility of the quantity of students being a fractional number and this type of situation is described by saying that the number of students is a **discontinuous** quantity. However, most quantities can have any value and are said to be **continuous**. When they are measured the value is read from a scale and the accuracy of the measurement is determined by the size of the smallest interval on this scale. For illustration, let us consider the measurement of length using a rule which has a scale divided into intervals of 1 mm. With this rule we might obtain a value such as 108 mm for the length of some object. This would mean that when we laid the rule alongside the object and noted the position of its end we made the judgement that it was closer to the 108 mm mark than to either the 107 or 109 mm marks. This is illustrated in Figure 1.10.

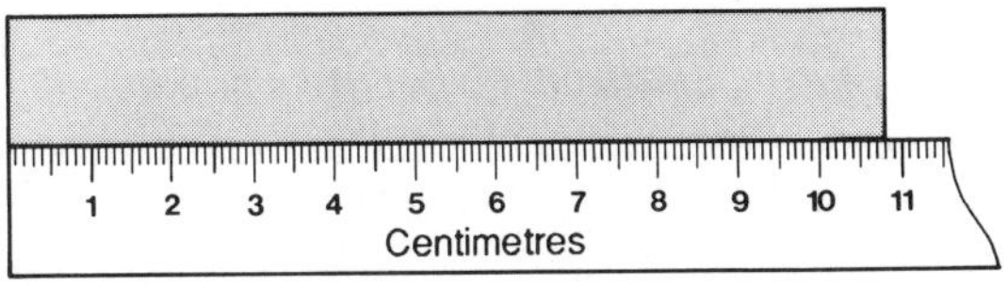

Figure 1.10 *Reading length from a scale*

If we repeated the measurement illustrated in Figure 1.10 several times, or if we got someone else to do it, then it is quite likely that the value of 108 rather than 107 or 109 would be obtained each time. However, if we were to ask different people to estimate the length to the nearest 0.1 mm using the same rule it would be quite a different story. Now they would have to assign a number to a position on the scale within an interval and there would be no lines within the interval to help them. In this situation we would find that different people reported different values for the measurement. One might report 107.8 mm, another 107.9 mm, another 108.1 mm and so on. If we needed to know the length of this object to within 0.1 mm of its true length then we would need to use an instrument having intervals on its scale no more than this distance apart. However, no matter how small we make the intervals on a scale it will still be possible for a measured quantity to lie within one of these intervals and so complete accuracy will always elude us. The inevitable discrepancy between the true value for a measurement and the value obtained is called the **error of observation**.

Although physical scientists attach great significance to measurements they do not get too depressed by the fact that it is impossible to achieve complete accuracy in the measurement of physical quantities. As a matter of fact, scientists will often accept a value for a physical quantity knowing that it would be possible to obtain a much more accurate value for the same quantity.

In performing measurements the aim is not necessarily to make the error as small as possible. A relatively large error may be acceptable provided that it is not so large as to affect any conclusions drawn from the measurement or any actions based upon it. Extreme accuracy should not be sought except when it is needed. Procedures necessary to attain high levels of accuracy may take more time and effort than is warranted. For example, a value for body temperature of 39.347 °C is of no more use to a clinician than a value of 39.3 °C. Either value would lead a clinician to draw the same conclusions and take the same actions.

1.3.3 *Classification of Errors*

Errors have many causes. Even the same person using the same piece of equipment several times to measure the same quantity will not always obtain the same value. This may be due to some lack of uniformity of the equipment, some variation in the person's behaviour as they perform the measurement or to changes in other factors which influence the quantity being measured. It is common to classify errors of measurement as either **random errors** or **systematic errors**.

Random Errors. These errors are inevitable and are not due to faults in the equipment or measuring technique. They can be detected by repeating a measurement several times. Random errors have the following characteristics:

1. Small variations in the measurement occur much more frequently than larger ones.
2. Measurements which are too large by a certain amount occur with about the same frequency as measurements which are too small by the same amount.

These two characteristics of random errors are illustrated in Figure 1.11.

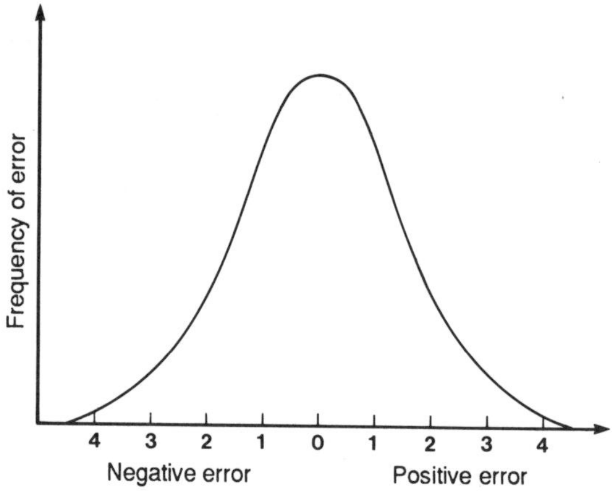

Figure 1.11 *Characteristics of random errors*

Systematic Errors. These arise from some particular fault in the measuring instrument or in the way that a person carries out the measurement. A systematic error will cause a measurement to be out by the same amount and in the same direction each time the measurement is performed. This means that a systematic error will affect the accuracy of a measurement but not its precision.

Measurements of mass are prone to systematic error because most balances have a means of adjusting the zero setting. It is easy for this setting to be accidentally shifted so that the balance either registers a mass when there is nothing on it (positive error) or must have something placed on it in order for it to show zero (negative error). Where this is the case all mass measurements made with the balance will yield values which are either too large or too small by the same amount. To avoid this systematic error a nurse should always check the zero setting on clinical scales when he or she is measuring a person's mass (weight).

Systematic errors can be detected readily if there is a standard quantity available to be measured using the instrument. For example, many balances are provided with a set of standard masses. These can be used at any time to check that the balance is operating correctly. You will find that many pieces of measuring equipment are provided with some means of checking the accuracy of the measurements which they provide and where this is so the checking procedure should be carried out at regular intervals. In some situations it may be necessary to carry out this procedure every time the instrument is used. This checking that an instrument is providing the expected readings is called **calibration**.

Error of Parallax. This is a very common error of technique. It arises because the reading obtained from a simple scale is influenced by the relationship which exists between the point on the scale from which the reading is to be taken and the position adopted by the person performing the measurement. This is illustrated in Figure 1.12.

In Figure 1.12 the correct readings are those obtained from positions marked B. The other readings are in error and this error is called the **error of parallax**. To avoid it, a person should adopt a position such that the straight line drawn from their eye to the point on the scale from which the measurement is to be taken is perpendicular to the scale. This is what we are doing when we raise a medicine glass up to the level of our eyes as we pour liquid into it. A well-made measuring instrument will be designed to minimise the likelihood of parallax errors. This is the case with clinical thermometers (see Section 1.3.5).

1.3.4 *Estimating Errors*

We have seen that errors are inevitable and so we need a way of deciding when an error might be large enough to cause us concern. This decision is made by taking account of the size of the smallest intervals on the scale of the measuring instrument and saying that all readings taken from this scale (by a careful person who has been properly instructed in reading scales) are subject to errors which will be no larger than half the smallest scale interval which can be clearly distinguished. This is called the **absolute error of measurement**. This definition is simply based on the commonsense notion that a person will always be able to tell that any measurement lies closer to one end of an interval than to the other or that it lies in the middle of the interval. In adopting this criterion we are being rather conservative and saying that the error could be larger than it is in many cases. Let us consider a (careful, well-instructed) person taking the measure-

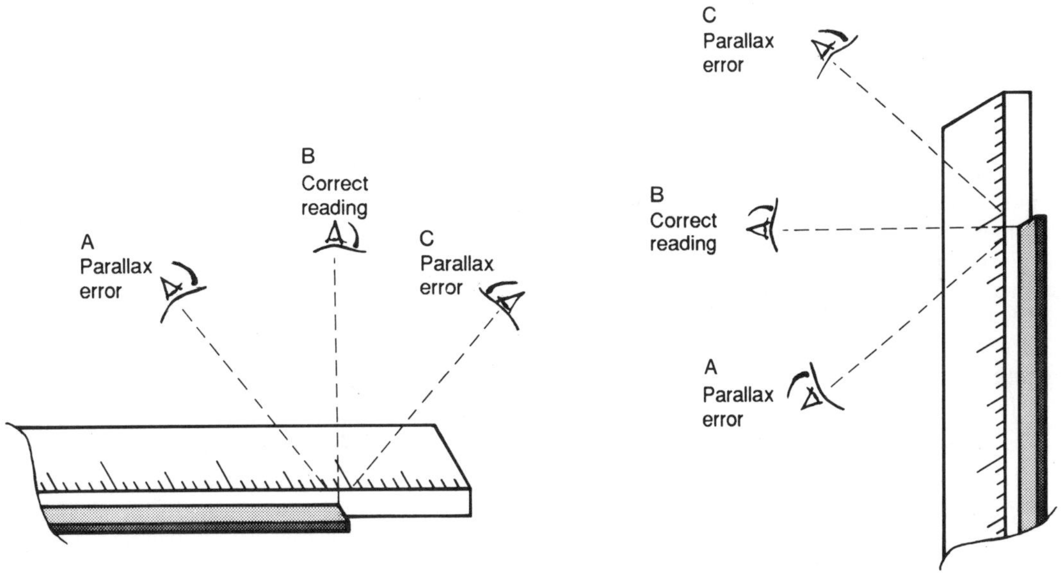

Figure 1.12 *The error of parallax*

ment of length illustrated in Figure 1.10. The absolute error of the measurement is half of 1 mm (0.5 mm) and if the person stated the measurement as being 108 ± 0.5 mm we could be very confident that the true value for the measurement would lie within this range (between 107.5 and 108.5 mm). Of course, we would be assuming that the rule is correctly calibrated. Even where a measurement falls in the middle of an interval it can be stated as (say) 107.5 ± 0.5 mm and we could still be confident that the true value lies within the stated range.

Whether or not an absolute error is large enough for us to be concerned about will be influenced by the magnitude of the measurement being performed. For this reason it is common to express the absolute error as a percentage of the magnitude of a measurement and obtain the **percentage error of measurement**. Thus,

$$\text{percentage error} = \frac{\text{absolute error}}{\text{magnitude of measurement}} \times 100$$

For the case of the measurement stated as 108 ± 0.5 mm this expression becomes:

$$\text{percentage error} = \frac{0.5}{108} \times 100$$
$$= 0.5$$

When an absolute error is expressed as a percentage of the measurement which has been performed we get a much better impression of its significance. In the case above we know that it represents about half of one per cent of the measurement. In most situations this would be quite acceptable. As the percentage error of a measurement gets larger and larger we have more and more reason for being concerned.

A point to emphasise about absolute error is that it is a property of the measuring instrument being used and on most instruments (but not all) it does not vary from one measurement to another. On the other hand, percentage error is influenced by the magnitude of the measurement as well as by the absolute error. If we obtained a measurement of 2 mm from a scale on which the absolute error is 0.5 mm then the percentage error would be 0.5/2 × 100 = 25 and we would have good reason to be concerned about its accuracy.

1.3.5 *Simple Measuring Devices*

Medicine Glass. A typical medicine glass is represented in Figure 1.13 and there is more to this simple device than first meets the eye. It has a cone shape and a non-linear scale on which the intervals are smaller at the bottom than at the top (it is an example of an instrument for which the absolute error is not constant). These features help ensure that all volumes measured with the glass are subject to about the same percentage errors.

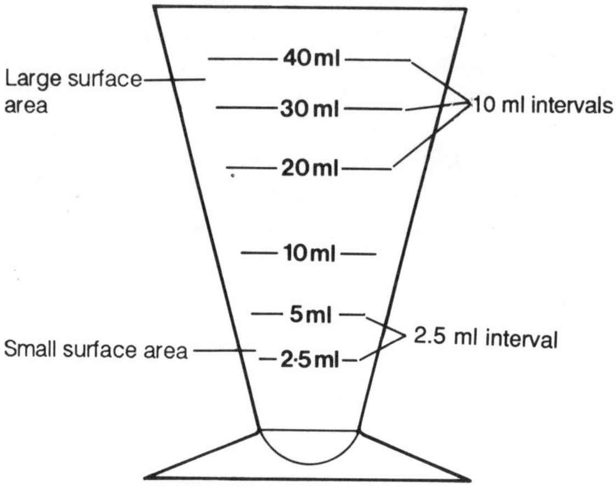

Figure 1.13 *Medicine glass with scale*

Whenever a volume of liquid is measured out with a medicine glass some judgement must be made about the closeness of the liquid level to one of the scale marks on the side of the glass. The glass may be filled slightly more or slightly less than it should and this will produce an error in the volume. This error is the absolute error of measurement. It is smaller when smaller volumes are measured because there are more scale marks at the bottom of the scale to assist in judging when the glass has been filled to the required depth. Also the narrowness of the cone there means that any error in judging the depth corresponds to a relatively small error in the volume. Conversely, a small error in volume is easier to detect because the liquid level changes more. The reduction in absolute error which occurs as smaller volumes are measured keeps the percentage error about the same as it is when larger volumes are measured out. This is important because the dose of a medication for a child is usually smaller than that for an adult but the percentage error in the dose which can be safely tolerated is the same for both.

Clinical Thermometer. A typical clinical thermometer covers the temperature range 35–42 °C in intervals of 0.1 °C and is constructed so that it must be held directly in front of the eyes in order for a reading to be taken. If it is not held in this position the mercury thread of the thermometer is simply not visible. This eliminates the error of parallax. Another feature of the instrument's construction is that the reading does not alter after it has been removed from contact with the body until it is given a sharp flick. This ensures that the reading seen when the measurement is taken is exactly the same as it was when the thermometer was in contact with the body. Of course, before every temperature measurement the thermometer must be flicked to restore the mercury to a level well below that of the reading last taken, otherwise the next reading obtained will be at least as high as the previous one no matter what the person's temperature really is.

1.3.6 *Errors in Quantities Depending on Several Measurements*

Quite often a physical quantity is obtained by a calculation which involves two or more separate measurements. *In such situations it is very important to realise that the accuracy with which the physical quantity is known cannot be any greater than that of the least accurate measurement used in the calculation.*

To illustrate this, let us consider a solution which has been prepared by measuring out 4.6 g of glucose, using a balance on which the smallest scale interval is 0.1 g, and dissolving it in 120 ml of water measured out using a graduated vessel on which the smallest scale interval is 10 ml. The absolute errors in these two measurements are 0.05 g and 5 ml respectively. The percentage errors are 1% and 4% respectively. The measurements of mass and volume are used to calculate the concentration of the solution from the expression:

$$\text{concentration} = \frac{\text{mass}}{\text{volume}} = \frac{4.6}{120}$$

If we perform the calculation using a calculator we might obtain a value for the concentration which is 0.0383333. However, if we reported this as the concentration we would be claiming that the absolute error in the concentration was 0.00000005 and the percentage error in the concentration would be given by

$$\begin{aligned}\text{percentage error} &= \frac{0.00000005}{0.0383333} \times 100 \\ &= 0.00013\end{aligned}$$

We would be claiming that we have determined the concentration with an accuracy much greater than that of the measurements on which it is based. This would be quite wrong! The concentration must be subject to an error of at least 4%. If we calculate 4% of 0.0383333 we obtain 0.0015 and we must concede that as soon as we reach the fourth digit to the right of the decimal point there is no way that we can be confident of its accuracy and so we should not include this digit, or others even further to the right, when we report the value for the concentration. It would be much more honest of us to report it as 0.038 or, better still, as 0.038 ± 0.0015.

There is an easier way to decide the number of digits which should appear in a value for a physical quantity and this is through the use of **significant figures**.

Measurements and Significant Figures. A significant figure may be defined as *a figure which is known with confidence*. To illustrate some important features of a significant figure we shall consider the case of a measurement performed with a ruler which is 1 m long and divided into 1 mm intervals. We could perform a measurement of length with this ruler and obtain a value of 68 mm. We could have confidence in the 6 and in the 8 and so this measurement has two significant figures. However, we could express this length in metres by dividing by 1000 and we would obtain 0.068 m. How many significant figures do we have now? To answer this question we need only realise that expressing the measurement in metres rather than millimetres cannot possibly make a difference to the confidence which we have in the measurement. Therefore, it would not make sense to say that there are any more or any less significant figures, even though we have used more figures in writing the value out. The extra figures which we have used are zeros and they have appeared simply because we decided to change the units for our measurement. For this reason they are not significant figures and in general it may be said that *any zero which appears in a number before the first non-zero digit is not a significant figure.*

Significant figures can be used to make the decision about how many figures should appear in a value which has been obtained using two or more measurements. The number of significant figures should be the same as the number present in the measurement which has the fewest significant figures. To illustrate this we shall return to our example of the solution prepared by dissolving 4.6 g of glucose in 120 ml of water.

When we measure out 4.6 g of glucose with a balance having a smallest scale interval of 0.1 g, we can be confident of the 4 and the 6. The measurement has two significant figures. When we measure out the 120 ml of water with a graduated vessel having smallest scale intervals of 10 ml we can be confident of the 1, the 2 but not the 0. This measurement also has two significant figures. Therefore, when we calculate the concentration using these values for mass and volume we should only include two significant figures in our answer. Our calculator might give us an answer of 0.0383333 but we know that we should only include two significant figures in the answer and so we would write the value as 0.038. Remember, zeros appearing before the first non-zero digit are not significant. What has been done here is often described by saying that the answer has been *rounded off to the second significant figure*. Rounding off involves looking at the value of the digit immediately to the right of the last significant figure. If its value is less than five the last significant figure is left as it is. If its value is five or more, the last significant figure is increased by one. Thus the number 0.03873604 becomes 0.039 when rounded off to two significant figures.

Sometimes it can be hard to tell if a zero is significant. An example of this would be when a number is written without a decimal point and has one or more zeroes at its right-hand end. For example, if we are told that the annual salary for a job is $24 000 we might suspect that one or more of the zeroes appearing in the number is not significant. Our suspicion would be based on the knowledge that when people talk about salaries they often round them off to the nearest thousand dollars (although they are not usually so ready to do this when it comes to what is actually paid out). This just serves to emphasise the value there is in taking the trouble to use the appropriate number of significant figures when reporting a quantity.

1.4 The Language and Literature of Science

1.4.1 *Words and Their Meanings in Science*

Science has developed from everyday experience and there are many connections which can be made between everyday language and the language of science. These connections form in both directions. Sometimes a word used first in science becomes a part of ordinary language and sometimes a word used in ordinary language is given a new meaning through its use in science. In Table 1.8 there is a list of words which are all commonly used in ordinary language as well as scientific language. The scientific meaning of each word is compared with one of its ordinary meanings adapted from *The Concise Oxford Dictionary* and the comparison makes it quite clear that scientific meaning is closely related to ordinary meaning.

Table 1.8 *Scientific and ordinary meanings for words*

	Scientific meaning	Ordinary meaning
buffer	a chemical system for reducing the effect which acids and bases have on solutions	an apparatus for reducing the effect of a collision
compound	a substance made up of two or more elements joined in fixed proportions by mass	something made up of several ingredients
electrify	charge a body with electricity causing it to behave or be capable of behaving in new ways	startle or excite a person into some new action or utterance
element	a pure substance which cannot be converted into simpler forms	a fundamental component of something. Wool is an element of Australia's wealth
quantum	a discrete quantity of energy	a portion or share of something

The difference between the use of words in ordinary language and in science is that in science they have meanings which are much more restricted. For example, let us consider the case of a person who has spent all day pushing and pulling a tree stump in his front garden in an attempt to remove it from the ground, but without success. In the ordinary sense of the word it would be agreed that this person had put in a hard day's work. We would not be surprised to hear him say, at the end of the day, that he had done a lot of work and was very tired. However, in the scientific sense this person has done no work because as far as science is concerned pushing and pulling things is not work unless it has the effect of moving them about. If this person had spent his day picking up bricks and carrying them from one place to another then he would have done some work in the scientific sense of the word. We would say that by pushing and pulling on the bricks he applied a force which has overcome the force of gravity and caused them to move.

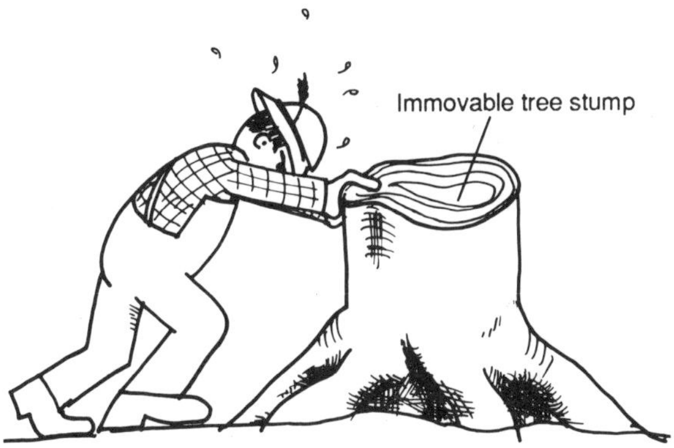

Figure 1.14 *Getting tired without working*

The reason why science restricts the work done by pushing and pulling to situations where objects are moved is that this involves something that can be reliably measured. We can measure the mass of the bricks and the distance that they are moved. From the mass of the bricks we are able to calculate the force of gravity which acts on them and so determine the magnitude of the force needed to move them. This is done simply by multiplying the mass by 9.8. The work involved can then be calculated using the simple expression

$$\text{work} = \underbrace{\text{mass} \times 9.8}_{\text{force}} \times \text{distance}$$

This expression, and the origin of the number 9.8, which it includes, is discussed in more detail in Section 5.1. The expression has been introduced here simply to emphasise that 'scientific' work is easily measured whereas the changes which occur when a person pushes or pulls something without moving it are much more difficult to measure. This is not to say that scientists would want to argue that a person who complains of feeling tired after pushing and pulling something all day without moving it is a hypochondriac. Scientists know perfectly well, from their commonsense, that this person's tiredness is just as real as the tiredness of a man who has spent his day doing something more useful, such as loading a furniture van. It is more the case that a decision has been made to put the sort of work done by the first person in the 'too hard basket'. The sort of measurements which would have to be carried out to obtain information about this work are of a completely different type from the measurement of mass and distance. They might involve the measurement of muscle tensions, chemical composition of body fluids, the rate of oxygen consumption and the rate of heat loss from the body's surface. Such measurements can be done but they are very different from measurements of mass and distance. Furthermore, there is no simple relationship which allows them to be used to calculate work.

By agreeing that work must involve a force being applied *and* causing movement, and by further agreeing that the quantity of work involved is the product of the force and the distance, scientists have removed all ambiguity from their concept of work. This ensures that when they speak and write to one another about work there is no doubt about what they mean. The removal of ambiguity is a feature of scientific language. It is achieved by clearly defining the meaning of words and through the use of mathematics for the expression of relationships. In the next section some commonly used mathematical techniques are described.

1.4.2 *Common Mathematical Techniques*

Equations and Their Manipulation. The great Italian Scientist, Galileo Galilei, said: 'Nature is written in the language of mathematics'. We see the truth of this statement in the form of a large number of mathematical equations which, in a few symbols, are able to describe the relationship between the numerical values for many different sets of physical quantities. Thus, the expression for work is an equation which can be written as:

$$\underset{\text{work}}{\underset{\uparrow}{W}} \quad \underset{\text{equals}}{=} \quad \underset{\text{force}}{\underset{\uparrow}{F}} \quad \overset{\text{multiplied by}}{\overset{\downarrow}{\times}} \quad \underset{\text{distance}}{\underset{\uparrow}{D}} \qquad (1.1)$$

Some other equations which you will encounter in

later chapters of this book, and elsewhere, are set out below:

$$\text{K} = {}^{\circ}\text{C} + 273 \tag{1.2}$$

K ↑ temperature in kelvins; °C ↑ temperature in degrees Celsius

$$C = \frac{m}{V} \times 100 \tag{1.3}$$

C ↑ per cent concentration of a solution; m ↓ mass of dissolved material; V ↑ volume of solution

$$R = \frac{V}{I} \tag{1.4}$$

R ↑ resistance; V ↓ voltage; I ↑ current

$$Q = s \times m \times \Delta T \tag{1.5}$$

Q ↑ energy; s ↑ specific heat; m ↓ mass; Δ ↓ this symbol means 'the change in'; T ↑ temperature

It is common for students to be frightened by the mathematical expressions for relationships. If you are such a person it may be a help for you to know that these relationships can always be expressed in words and doing this is a good way to begin using them. For example, Equation 1.5 is a statement about the relationship which exists between the amount of energy (Q) which is involved when an object with a certain mass (m), composed of a substance having a certain specific heat (s) undergoes a temperature change (ΔT). It tells us that the quantity of energy is always the product of the numerical values for mass, specific heat and temperature change. All these, and other physical quantities, are often referred to as **variables** when their relationships with each other are being discussed.

Exercise 1.1

(a) Express Equation 1.4 in words.

(b) The cardiac output is equal to the stroke volume times the heart rate. Express this relationship as an equation.

Now, you might want to ask: 'If mathematical equations can always be expressed in words, why do we bother to use the mathematical expressions?' The answer is that mathematics provides us with more reliable and efficient ways of manipulating relationships than those available for the manipulation of ordinary language. Any person who knows the rules for adding, subtracting, multiplying and dividing can manipulate mathematical equations such as those set out above. It is only necessary to keep in mind two additional rules which apply to equations. These are:

1. If $a = b$ then $b = a$. For example, using Equation 1.4:

$$R = \frac{V}{I} \text{ and so } \frac{V}{I} = R$$

2. The two sides of an equation can be subjected to addition, subtraction, multiplication and division without altering its validity provided that both sides are subjected to exactly the same set of operations.

This second rule may be understood in terms of the operation of a balance such as the one illustrated in Figure 1.1. If the balance is properly balanced to begin with and we add or subtract the same mass to both sides, then it will remain properly balanced. It will

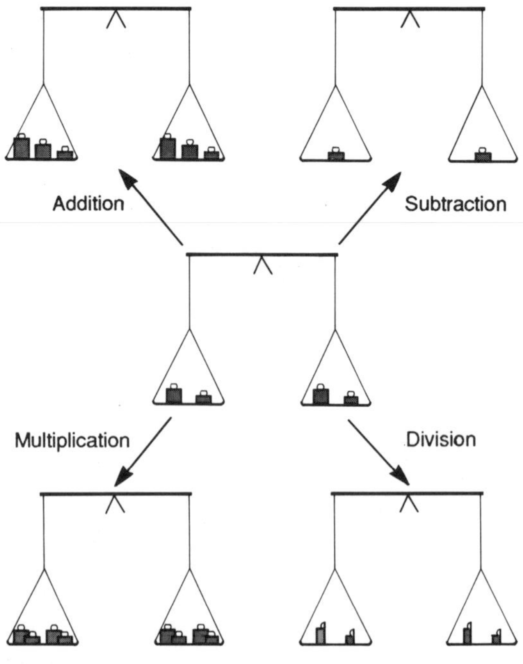

Figure 1.15 *A physical illustration of the 'balancing' of equations*

also remain properly balanced if we double the mass in each pan or halve it. If we add or subtract mass from one pan of the balance without doing the same to the other, or if we multiply or divide the mass in one pan without doing the same to the other, then the balance will swing out of balance. This is illustrated in Figure 1.15.

To illustrate how useful it is to be able to manipulate equations let us begin by considering the equation which relates temperature measured in kelvins to temperature measured in degrees Celsius.

$$\underset{\substack{\uparrow \\ \text{temperature} \\ \text{in kelvins}}}{\mathrm{K}} = \underset{\substack{\uparrow \\ \text{temperature} \\ \text{in degrees Celsius}}}{{}^{\circ}\mathrm{C}} + 273 \qquad (1.2)$$

If we are told that the temperature in degrees Celsius (°C) is 50 then we could use Equation 1.2 to decide that the same temperature measured in kelvins is 50 + 273 = 323. But if we are told that the temperature measured in kelvins is 440 how would we decide on the value for the corresponding Celsius temperature? If we are to use our equation we need it to be written as:

$$^{\circ}\mathrm{C} = ?$$

Since we want the symbol °C to be on the left-hand side of the equation we can achieve this by making use of rule 1 above and writing:

$$^{\circ}\mathrm{C} + 273 = \mathrm{K}$$

Now we need to remove the + 273 from the left-hand side of the equation. We could do this by subtracting 273 but we must do this to both sides of the equation in order to ensure that it remains valid (this is rule 2). This would give us:

$$^{\circ}\mathrm{C} + 273 - 273 = \mathrm{K} - 273$$

and then:

$$^{\circ}\mathrm{C} = \mathrm{K} - 273$$

Now the relationship allows us to say confidently that a temperature of 440 K is the same as 440 – 273 = 167 °C. You may now be saying to yourself: 'What are they on about? I didn't have to use that long-winded method, I just *knew* that I needed to subtract 273 from 440'. If this is so then perhaps you will find this next example a bit more convincing.

Let us suppose that we are in a situation where we have to make some decisions about solutions, using Equation 1.3.

$$\underset{\substack{\uparrow \\ \text{per cent} \\ \text{concentration} \\ \text{of a solution}}}{C} = \frac{\overset{\substack{\text{mass of} \\ \text{dissolved material} \\ \downarrow}}{m}}{\underset{\substack{\uparrow \\ \text{volume of} \\ \text{solution}}}{V}} \times 100 \qquad (1.3)$$

The equation written out in this form will allow us to calculate concentration if we know values for mass and volume (provided, of course, that we know the rules for multiplying and dividing numbers). But suppose we already know the concentration and the volume and wish to determine the mass. To do this we really need to have the relationship written as

$$m = ?$$

We could make a start on getting to this situation by using rule 1 above and writing:

$$\frac{m}{V} \times 100 = C$$

Now we need to get rid of the volume term and the 100 from the left-hand side of the equation. We can get rid of the V by multiplying both sides by V (remember we must always do the same thing to both sides of the equation in order for it to remain valid). This gives us:

$$V \times \frac{m}{V} \times 100 = C \times V$$

The V now cancels out on the left-hand side and we get:

$$m \times 100 = C \times V$$

If we now divide both sides by 100 we obtain:

$$\frac{m \times 100}{100} = \frac{C \times V}{100}$$

Now the 100 cancels out on the left-hand side and we have:

$$m = \frac{C \times V}{100}$$

This is what we need. It is a valid statement of the relationship between concentration, mass and volume and is in a form which permits us to calculate the mass easily when we know values for concentration and volume. We obtained this different expression for the relationship simply through the application of multiplication and division to the original expression. The same approach can be used when we need to calculate volume from known values for concentration and mass. We would end up using the expression:

$$V = \frac{m}{C} \times 100$$

It is always possible to rearrange an equation in as many different ways as there are different variables in the equation. All that is needed is some flexible thinking and the use of the two rules set out above. A final point to be made concerns units for physical quantities obtained by substituting numerical values for other physical quantities into an equation. For example, the concentration variable in Equation 1.3 must be measured in g/100 ml. This requires the mass to be measured in grams and the volume of the solution to be measured in millilitres. If mass and volume are specified in units other than these then they must be converted into grams and millilitres prior to, or during, the calculation.

Exercise 1.2
Write out the different forms of Equations 1.1, 1.4 and 1.5.

Drawing and Interpreting Graphs. Quite often a scientific investigation will involve the study of the effect changing one physical quantity has upon the value of another. For example, we might be interested in the effect moving further and further away from a source of radiation has on the intensity of the radiation which we experience. If so, we would obtain a radiation source, a means of measuring radiation intensity, a means of measuring distance and carry out a series of measurements. Table 1.9 contains a set of values obtained in this way.

Table 1.9 *Variation in the intensity of radiation as the distance from the radiation source increases*

Intensity of radiation (counts per minute)	Distance from the source (cm)
3100	1
2000	2
1450	3
1100	4
900	5
750	6
600	7
550	8
450	9
400	10

Anyone asked to look at the values in Table 1.9 and interpret them will quickly be able to say they show that the intensity of radiation gets smaller as the distance from the source gets larger. However, if there is anything more to be said about the relationship between radiation intensity and distance it is not easy to see from the information as it has been presented in Table 1.9. Let us now consider the set of measurements presented in Table 1.10. These have been obtained by taking 25 ml of solution A and measuring its pH (don't worry about what pH is, just accept that it is a property of solution A which can be measured) as known volumes of another solution (solution B) are added to it.

Table 1.10 *Variation in the pH of solution A as solution B is added*

pH of solution A	Volume of solution B added (ml)
4.1	0
4.6	1
4.8	2
4.9	4
5.0	8
5.2	12
5.5	16
6.9	20
8.1	21
9.5	22
10.5	23
10.8	24
11.0	26
11.3	28
11.4	30
11.6	32

Now, a person glancing at the measurements in Table 1.10 would be able to say that the pH increases as the volume increases. But, as was the case with the measurements in Table 1.9, this person would have to look long and hard at the measurements to see more than this, even though there is more to be seen.

The difficulty which we have in seeing the full significance of the way in which one quantity is affected by changes in another is one of the reasons why scientists often take the trouble to display the measurements which they have made in the form of a **graph**. The values in Tables 1.9 and 1.10 are displayed as graphs in Figure 1.16.

Looking at Figure 1.16 you will probably agree that graphical displays create an immediate impression

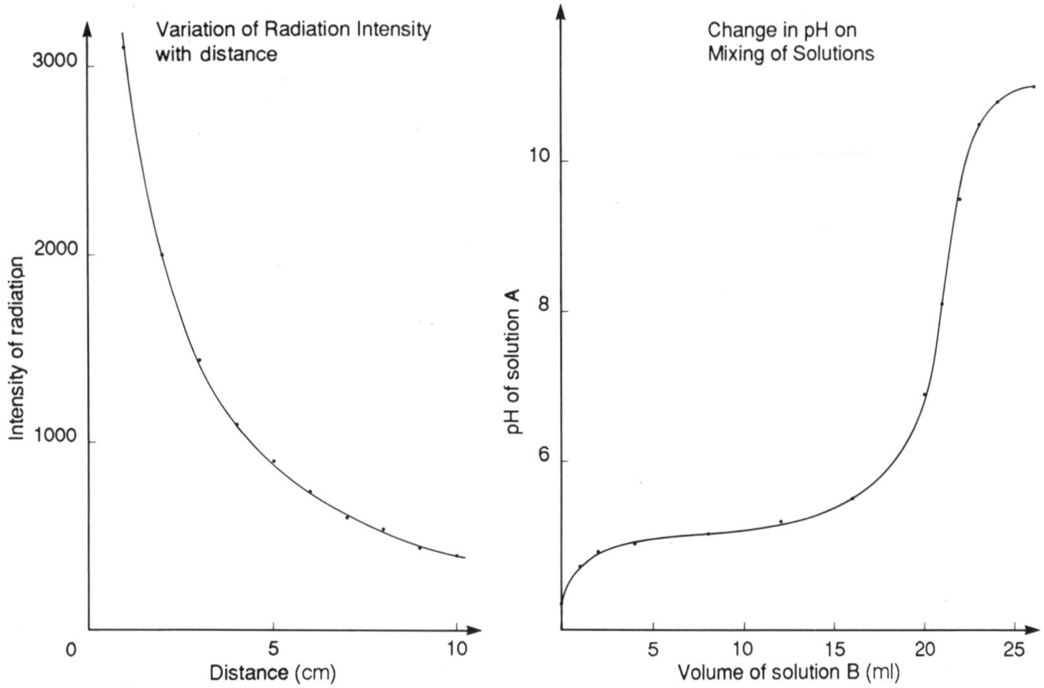

Figure 1.16 *Graphical display of the measurements in Tables 1.9 and 1.10*

when they are seen. Even a quick glance is enough to reveal that radiation intensity does not simply decrease as distance from the source increases. Likewise, it is immediately apparent from the graph that the pH of solution A does more than just increase as more and more of solution B is added. When we look at a graph, compared to a table of measurements, it is rather like looking at a person's face compared to looking at a photograph of the same person's face which has been cut into pieces (the photograph, that is) and shown to us one piece at a time. By the time we have seen the last piece of the photograph our recollection of the first piece has faded and we have great difficulty forming the total picture.

The essential feature of the graphs in Figure 1.16 (and all simple graphs) is that the magnitude of a measurement is represented by distance from a reference point on a scale. To facilitate this representation graphs are usually drawn on special paper which has many evenly spaced lines drawn horizontally and vertically upon it.

A simple procedure which may be followed to construct a graph of the relationship which exists between two different quantities is set out below:

1. Look at the two measurements which you have and decide if one of them has been set by the investigator. If so this is called the **independent variable** and it is customary to display this quantity along the horizontal edge (called the horizontal axis) of the graph paper. The other measurement is called the **dependent variable** and is displayed along the vertical edge (called the vertical axis) of the graph paper.
2. For each measurement choose a scale to represent it so that all the values which you have can be accommodated on your graph paper and differentiated clearly from one another. Choosing a scale simply involves looking at the range of values you have to deal with and at the number of divisions there are along the edge of your graph paper.
3. Label each axis with the name of the physical quantity which is to be represented on it and the units in which it has been measured.
4. Take one pair of measurements (often called a **data pair**) in turn. Make a clear mark on the graph paper at the position which is vertically above the position on the horizontal axis corresponding to the value of the measurement being represented on that axis, and horizontally across from the position on the vertical axis corresponding to the value of the measurement being represented there.
5. Once all data pairs have been represented on

the graph paper you will have to make a judgement as to the general shape of the graph. It may be a simple straight line or it may be a curve. In either case you will often find that you cannot draw a single straight line or smooth curve which passes through all your data points. You must draw what is called a **line of best fit**. This is the straight line or the smooth curve which passes as close as it can to as many data pairs as it can. Finally, the graph should be given a brief, descriptive title.

Many of these features of graphs are illustrated in Figure 1.17, using one of the graphs from Figure 1.16.

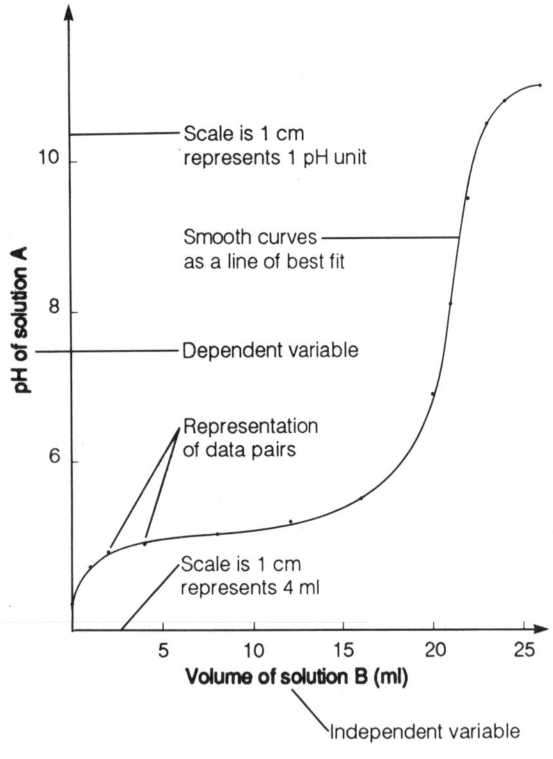

Figure 1.17 *The main features of graphs*

One of the most common errors made in drawing graphs is to ignore the advice given in (5) above and draw the graph so that it passes through all the data pairs. Often people will draw a straight line from one position to the next and so end up with many different lines joined end to end. In Figure 1.18 the graphs shown in Figure 1.16 have been redrawn in this way.

Graphs drawn in the manner shown in Figure 1.18 imply that the relationships which they represent change suddenly at certain points. This could possibly be the case but there is a much simpler way of explaining why all the members of a set of data pairs do not fall exactly on a single straight line or smooth curve. This is that when the data pairs consist of measurements the values will, like all measurements, be subject to error. This error will cause them to **scatter** to some extent around the line on which the true values would have fallen perfectly. As a general rule in science the simplest explanation is always preferred and unless there is good reason (as there sometimes is) for believing that you are dealing with more than one relationship you should draw graphs of physical quantities as *single* straight lines or smooth curves.

Exercise 1.3
Draw a graph of the set of measurements given below.

Concentration (g/100 ml)	Specific gravity (no units)
1	1.007
2	1.014
3	1.021
4	1.029
5	1.035
6	1.043
7	1.050
8	1.058
9	1.065
10	1.073

Using Decimal Numbers and Powers of 10. We usually represent numbers as **decimals**. The digits appearing in a decimal number have values which differ according to the position of the digit in relation to the decimal point. This is illustrated below.

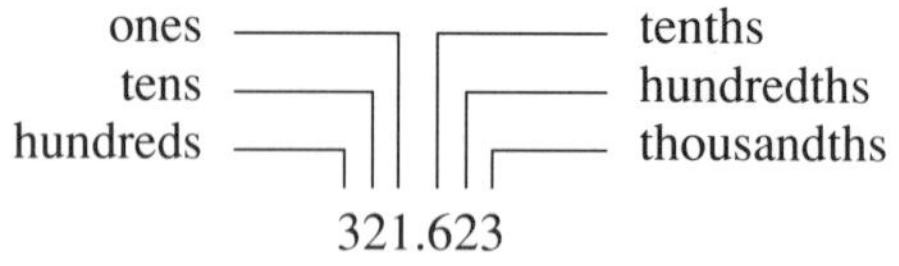

Shifting the decimal point in a decimal number alters its value in a simple way. Each position moved alters the value by a factor of 10 (makes the number 10 times bigger or 10 times smaller). Movement to the left decreases the value of the number and movement to the right increases it. For example:

$\overrightarrow{307.862}$ ⟶ 30786.2
(multiplication by 10 × 10 = 100)

$\overleftarrow{307.862}$ ⟶ 0.307862
(division by 10 × 10 × 10 = 1000)

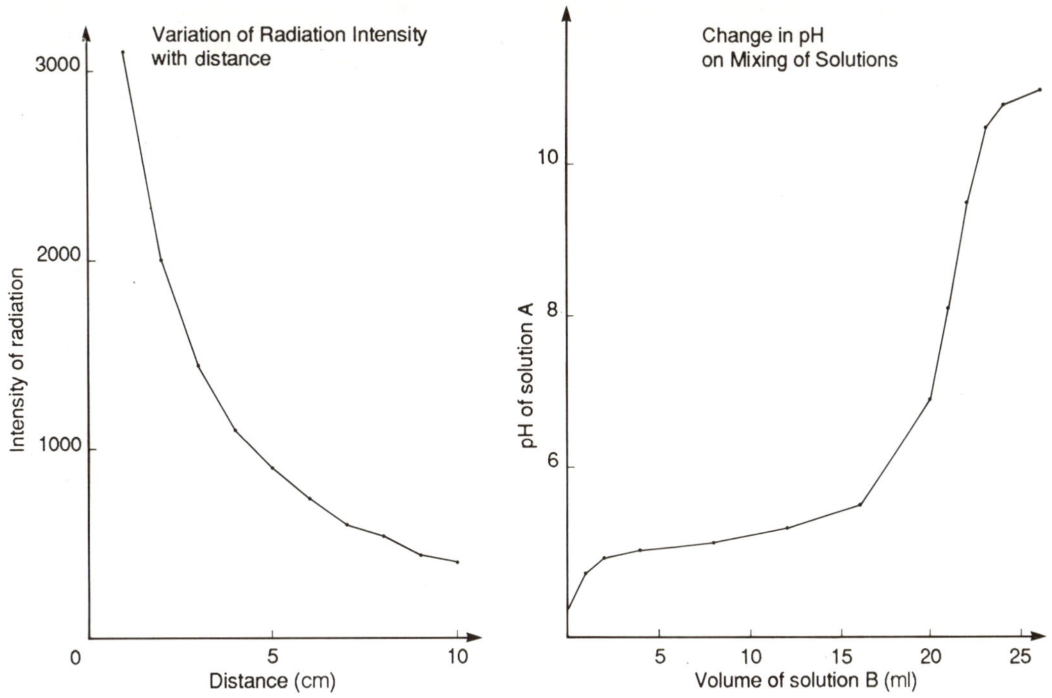

Figure 1.18 *Graphs drawn incorrectly*

There is always more than one way to write a number and this may be illustrated by reference to some familiar numbers such as 100, 1000, 0.1. These could be written as:

$$100 = 10 \times 10$$
$$1000 = 10 \times 10 \times 10$$
$$0.1 = 1 \div 10$$

We wouldn't often write the numbers this way because it is too much trouble. However, it is also a lot of trouble to write out Australia's current account deficit as \$16 000 000 000 per annum and so it is clear that the method which we use to write out familiar numbers such as 100 and 1000 becomes very cumbersome when we need to represent a very large number. It also becomes very cumbersome when it is used to represent a very small number. This is a particularly important problem for scientists who must deal with very big and very small numbers. Physicists, for example, must deal with numbers such as 10 000 000 000 000 000 (the distance, in metres, from the earth to the next star beyond our own sun) and 0.000 000 000 000 000 001 (the diameter of some small particles of matter, also measured in metres). Mathematics provides us with a method of representing very large and very small numbers much more conveniently than this. With this method the numbers 100 and 1000 are represented as 10^2 and 10^3 respectively and we say that they are being represented as **powers of 10**. The number written to the upper right of the 10 is called the **power** or the **exponent**. The 10 itself is called the **base**.

10^3 ⟵ the power or exponent
↗
the base

Table 1.11 contains numbers represented as powers of 10, and in other ways. You can see that representing the numbers in the table as powers of 10 is, in nearly all cases, simpler than the other methods. There is a clear pattern in the way that the exponent varies as the magnitude of the numbers alter: for each factor of 10 by which the number increases or decreases the value of the exponent increases or decreases by one respectively. Another advantage of this representation is that the numbers become much simpler to multiply and divide. Multiplication is accomplished by adding the exponents and division by subtracting them. Thus,

$$10^4 \times 10^5 = 10^{4+5} = 10^9$$
$$10^6 \div 10^8 = 10^{6-8} = 10^{-2}$$

These answers may be confirmed by working in a long-hand fashion. Thus,

$$10^4 \times 10^5 = 10 \times 10 \times 10 \times 10 \times 10 \times 10 \times 10 \times 10 \times 10 = 10^9$$

$$10^6 \div 10^8 = \frac{10 \times 10 \times 10 \times 10 \times 10 \times 10}{10 \times 10 \times 10 \times 10 \times 10 \times 10 \times 10 \times 10} = \frac{1}{10 \times 10} = 10^{-2}$$

Table 1.11 *Different ways of expressing numbers*

$10 \times 10 \times 10 \times 10 \times 10 \times 10$	=	$1000\,000 = 10^6$
$10 \times 10 \times 10 \times 10 \times 10$	=	$100\,000 = 10^5$
$10 \times 10 \times 10 \times 10$	=	$10\,000 = 10^4$
$10 \times 10 \times 10$	=	$1000 = 10^3$
10×10	=	$100 = 10^2$
10	=	$10 = 10^1$
1	=	$1 = 10^0$
$\frac{1}{10}$	=	$0.1 = 10^{-1}$
$\frac{1}{10 \times 10}$	=	$0.01 = 10^{-2}$
$\frac{1}{10 \times 10 \times 10}$	=	$0.001 = 10^{-3}$
$\frac{1}{10 \times 10 \times 10 \times 10}$	=	$0.0001 = 10^{-4}$
$\frac{1}{10 \times 10 \times 10 \times 10 \times 10}$	=	$0.00001 = 10^{-5}$
$\frac{1}{10 \times 10 \times 10 \times 10 \times 10 \times 10}$	=	$0.000001 = 10^{-6}$

Logarithms. The numbers in between 1, 10, 100, 1000 and so on can also be expressed as powers of 10. If 316 lies between 10^2 and 10^3 then it is reasonable to assume that 315 is 10 raised to some power between 2 and 3. The actual value of the power is 2.5. Thus, we may write $316 = 10^{2.5}$. The number 0.025 when expressed as a power of 10 will have an exponent which lies between –1 and –2. Its value is –1.6 and we may write $0.025 = 10^{-1.6}$. The value of the exponent when a number is expressed as a power of 10 is called the **logarithm of the number to the base 10**. The phrase 'to the base 10' is included because it is possible to express any number as a power of any other number. If we express numbers as powers of 2 then the exponents are logarithms to the base 2. For example, 8 may be expressed as 2^3 and the logarithm of 8 to the base 2 is therefore 3. Base 10 logarithms are used more than other logarithms and it is common for them to simply be called logarithms without the base being stated. This is what we shall do on the few occasions where logarithms come up in later chapters of this book. In Table 1.12 some numbers are expressed as powers of 10 with their logarithms listed alongside. You only need to think of logarithms as being another way of writing numbers.

Table 1.12 *Numbers and their base 10 logarithms*

Number	Logarithm	Number	Logarithm
10^5	5	10^{-1}	–1
10^4	4	$0.025 = 10^{-1.6}$	–1.6
10^3	3	10^{-2}	–2
$316 = 10^{2.5}$	2.5	10^{-3}	–3
10^2	2	10^{-4}	–4
10^1	1	10^{-5}	–5
10^0	0	10^{-6}	–6

There are a number of important physical quantities which are expressed as logarithms. One of these is pH which is a measure of the acidity of a solution (see Section 7.7.7). The well-known Richter Scale which is used to measure the severity of earthquakes is a logarithmic scale. An earthquake which is measured as 5 on the Richter Scale is more than ten times as powerful as one which is rated 4.

Standard or Scientific Notation. Take a *quick* look at the two numbers written below. Which is the bigger number, the one on the left or the one on the right?

37 629 870.04   5 876 607.40

You probably found it difficult to tell the difference with a quick look but if you look carefully you will be able to see that the number on the left is bigger. To tell which number is bigger we have to compare the number of digits in each and check the location of the decimal point. *The number which has more digits to the left of the decimal point is always the larger number.* Now look what happens if we shift the decimal point in each number until there is only one digit on its left. We get

3.762 987 004   and   5.876 607 40

In the case of the first number we have shifted the decimal point 7 positions towards the left. Each position moved reduces the value of the number by a factor of

10 and so movement of 7 positions reduces it by the factor 10 × 10 × 10 × 10 × 10 × 10 × 10. This is equivalent to dividing the number by 10^7. The second number has had its decimal point shifted 6 positions towards the left and so been divided by 10^6. We can restore each number to its original value by multiplying by these same powers of 10. This would give us

$3.762\,987\,004 \times 10^7$ and $5.876\,607\,40 \times 10^6$

With the numbers written in this form we can tell immediately which is larger. All we have to do is look at the exponents in the two numbers (that is, 7 and 6 respectively). Whichever has the larger exponent is the larger number. The two numbers have now been written out in what is called **standard notation** or **scientific notation**. This can be defined as *the expression of a number as the product of a number between 1 and 10 and the appropriate power of 10*. The numbers used in the example above are not typical numbers and they contain many more digits than would normally be encountered. Even so, it is still the case that the use of numbers expressed in the standard notation is of real value in keeping track of their size, particularly during multiplication and division. It is very easy to end up with an answer which is 10 or 100 times bigger or smaller than it should be. For example, consider the following series of multiplications.

$26.32 \times 107.8 \times 0.027$

Can you tell the approximate size of the answer? Is it about 10, 100, 1000? Most people would have some trouble deciding this and if they made a mistake in performing the calculation might not realise that their answer was wrong. What happens when we write the numbers out in their standard forms? We get

$2.632 \times 10^1 \times 1.078 \times 10^2 \times 2.7 \times 10^{-2}$

This shows us that our answer will be

$2.632 \times 1.078 \times 2.7 \times 10^{1+2-2}$

which becomes

$2.632 \times 1.078 \times 2.7 \times 10^1$

If we round our decimal numbers up or down to the nearest whole number we obtain $3 \times 1 \times 3 \times 10^1 = 9 \times 10^1 = 90$ and we can see the approximate value our answer should have. Working this way makes it more likely that we would notice a mistake made in performing the calculation. The correct answer is 7.7 (two sig. figs).

Proportion and Ratio. According to *The Concise Oxford Dictionary* the word proportion means 'correct relation between one thing and another or between parts of a thing'. There are many situations in science where proportion is important and there are a number of different ways in which proportion is expressed. The most common method used is to express the proportions of things as a **ratio**.

An example of a relationship expressed as a ratio would be:

Martin's age : Ray's age = 2 : 3

In this statement the colon (:) stands for 'compared to' and, in ordinary language, the statement reads 'Martin's age compared to Ray's age is the same as 2 compared to 3'. It is important to realise that the statement does not say that Martin's age is 2 and Ray's is 3. This is just one possibility. Martin could be 10 years old and Ray could be 15, or Martin could be 60 and Ray 90. Ratios can be manipulated in a number of ways. For example, we could write:

Ray's age : Martin's age = 3 : 2

Ratios may also be stated as fractions. For example:

$$\frac{\text{Martin's age}}{\text{Ray's age}} = \frac{2}{3} \text{ or } = \frac{\text{Ray's age}}{\text{Martin's age}} = \frac{3}{2}$$

There may be more than two quantities which exist in a ratio relationship. For example:

Martin's age : Ray's age : June's age = 2 : 3 : 1

In later chapters of this book you will encounter ratios in the discussion of: chemical formulae for compounds; specific gravity; buffer solutions.

1.4.3 *The Scientific Literature*

The scientific literature is the collection of books and journals which contain an account of the experiments, observations, theories and laws of science. Some people would say that the term 'scientific literature' is inherently contradictory. Furthermore, they would have *The Concise Oxford Dictionary* on their side. This defines scientific as meaning 'according to rules laid down in exact science for performing observations and testing soundness of conclusions' and literature as 'writings whose value lies in beauty of form or emotional effect'.

The gap which exists between scientific writing and literature is well illustrated by the two samples of writing given below.

> . . . the atoms are not in a stable state, since particles smaller than the atom are emitted. The atom, indivisible from the chemical point of view, is divisible here, and the sub-atoms are in movement. The radioactive material then undergoes a chemical transformation which is the source of the radiated energy; but it is certainly not an ordinary chemical transformation, for ordinary chemical transformations leave the atom unchanged. In the radioactive material, if there is something that is altered, it is necessarily the atom, since it is to the atom that radioactivity is attached.
>
> (Marie Curie, 1900, translated from the French by Robert Wolke)

> When they reached the mountain's summit, even Clancy took
> a pull ——
> It well might make the boldest hold their breath;
> The wild hop scrub grew thickly and the hidden ground was
> full
> Of wombat holes, and any slip was death.
> But the man from Snowy River let the pony have his head,
> And he swung his stockwhip round and gave a cheer,
> And he raced him down the mountain like a torrent down
> its bed,
> While the others stood and watched in very fear.
>
> (Andrew Barton (Banjo) Paterson, 1899, 'The Man From Snowy River ')

Marie Curie was writing about one of the most dramatic developments in the history of science, something that would change the world forever, but there is no sense of this in her choice of words or expression. Her writing is plain and dispassionate. She sticks to the rules and writes entirely in terms of accepted scientific concepts and relationships even though she knows that her work must bring them into question. Furthermore she must have been very excited about this prospect. Banjo Paterson was writing about an event in the everyday life of a simple bushman and yet his writing transformed it into something quite beautiful and unforgettable. The choice of words and their arrangement re-creates the excitement of the occasion and conveys the emotions of those who witnessed it.

The scientific literature is probably better described as the **scientific record**. This would be more in keeping with the fact that scientific writing is usually stripped of all emotion. It is confined to facts and the relationships which might exist between them. However, this should not be taken as an indication that scientists are completely unemotional about their work and never excited by it. Science is exciting and scientists feel the excitement of their work just as other people do. This excitement is deliberately kept out of the written accounts which scientists give of their work in the scientific books and journals. The purpose is to ensure that communication between scientists about the facts and relationships which they have discovered is as efficient as it can be.

Science, more than any other human activity, is cumulative. The scientists of today are in possession of all the facts and all the insights discovered by those who have gone before them. Sir Isaac Newton is widely acknowledged as the greatest scientist who has ever lived, but, speaking of his achievements, he once said: 'If I have seen further than others, it is because I have stood on the shoulders of giants'. By giants, Newton meant other scientists whose ideas he made use of. They were available to him because they had been written into the scientific record. Today this record still serves the same purpose as it did in Newton's time. It provides a means by which any scientist can learn about the work of any other scientist. The scientific record is steadily accumulating and a great deal of trouble is taken to ensure that this record is available to scientists working in different parts of the world and living at different times. Marie Curie embarked on the work which resulted in the discovery of radium after she had read Henri Becquerel's account of his discovery of a new type of radiation emitted by compounds of uranium.

About 40 years later, Howard Florey and Ernst Chain decided that they would conduct a search for naturally occurring substances which might be effective in controlling bacterial infections. What was needed was a substance which would kill or prevent the growth of the offending bacteria, but have a low toxicity for the person infected. At the time it was well known that many naturally occurring substances did affect the growth of bacteria but very few had been isolated and none was effective for controlling infections in human beings.

Florey and Chain decided to look carefully back over the scientific literature of the previous 60 years at all the reports which had been made of bacterial inhibition by naturally produced substances. They found many more examples than they expected and among these was Alexander Fleming's account of bacterial inhibition by the mould *Penicillium notatum*. Florey and Chain decided that this was a promising observation and they set out to isolate the substance which was responsible for the mould's anti-bacterial action. In this way penicillin was made available to the world.

In their search for information Florey and Chain did not have to read all the scientific literature which had been published in the previous 60 years. They did not even have to read all the literature of biology, which is the broad field of science encompassing the types of phenomena in which they were interested. If scientists had to do this every time they wanted to find out all that was known about a particular matter it would be impossibly difficult. The scientific literature could not be read in a whole lifetime.

It is only possible for scientists to make effective use of the scientific literature because, as it accumulates, it is subjected to systematic analysis which identifies the most important facts and ideas contained in each contribution. These facts and ideas are indexed in catalogues which are rather similar to library catalogues but which, in many cases, are more detailed. If a scientist knows what facts and ideas she is looking for she can use these catalogues to compile a list of all the articles in which they feature prominently. This list may also include a summary of each article and, if so, this can be used to decide if it is worthwhile obtaining a copy of the entire article. By this means any scientist with access to the services of a large, modern library can find out a great deal about any scientific matter in a short time.

There is no other body of writing which is as accessible as the scientific literature. This accessibility is only possible because of the effort which is devoted to the analysis and indexing of scientific writing as it accumulates. In turn, this effort is only effective because science imposes a strict discipline on the writing of its individual practitioners. This discipline has produced a uniformity of meaning for scientific concepts and this greatly facilitates the task of analysis and indexing. It also makes most scientific writing unattractive but this is accepted because the primary purpose of scientific writing is unambiguous communication across distance and time.

Bibliography

Bickel, L. *Rise up to Life*. Angus and Robertson, London, 1972.

Hewitt, P. G. *Conceptual Physics* (sixth edition). Scott, Forsman and Company, Boston, 1989.

Hill, J. W. *Chemistry for Changing Times* (third edition). Burgess Publishing Company, Minneapolis, 1980.

Metric Conversion Board. *A Metric Handbook. Australia's Metric System.* Metric Conversion Board, St Leonards, New South Wales.

Øgrim, O. and Vaughan, A. E. *Quantities and Units in Science*. Science Press, Marrickville, New South Wales, 1977.

Wolke, R. L. 'Marie Curie's Doctoral Thesis: Prelude to a Nobel Prize', *Journal of Chemical Education*, **65**(7), July, 1988.

Questions

1. Which of the following samples of matter is an example of a heterogeneous, pure substance?
   - J. sea water
   - K. milk chocolate
   - L. air
   - M. melting ice
2. Of the four different types of matter listed below which is *not* an example of an element?
   - J. hydrogen
   - K. oxygen
   - L. water
   - M. gold
3. A certain pure substance, A, when heated is changed into two quite different pure substances, C and D. Which of the following statements *must be true*?
   - J. A is a compound.
   - K. C and D are not elements.
   - L. A, C and D are all compounds.
   - M. C and D are elements.
4. Which of the following statements involves a *qualitative measurement*?
   - J. James has a height of 170 cm.
   - K. Barry's blood pressure is elevated.
   - L. Gino was born in Italy.
   - M. More than 5% of Australians receive a pension.
5. In the Australian Metric System of measurement the prefix milli stands for
   - J. one thousandth
   - K. one thousand
   - L. one millionth
   - M. one million
6. The millimetre of mercury is a unit commonly used for the measurement of blood pressure. Which of the following statements about this unit is *true*?
   - J. It is part of the Australian Metric System but not part of the SI system.
   - K. It is part of the SI system but not part of the Australian Metric System.
   - L. It belongs to both the SI system and the Australian Metric System.
   - M. It does not belong to either the SI system or the Australian Metric System.
7. Which of the following imperial units for mass (weight) is closest to the kilogram in magnitude?
   - J. ounce

K. pound
L. stone
M. hundredweight

8. Categorise the following changes as being physical or chemical changes:
(a) The glucose present in a drink becomes glucose in the bloodstream of a person who has consumed the drink.
(b) Glucose in the bloodstream becomes glycogen in liver and muscle tissue.
(c) Water evaporates from the surface of the lungs and is exhaled.

9. Write a paragraph which makes clear the meaning of the following terms:
mixture
pure substance
element
compound

10. What do the two processes **sublimation** and **boiling** have in common? What is different about them?

11. A quantity called the **Body Mass Index** (BMI) is obtained by measuring a person's height (in metres) and mass (in kilograms). The BMI is obtained by substituting these measurements in the expression:

$$\text{Body Mass Index} = \frac{\text{body mass}}{\text{height}^2}$$

In a particular case, a person had their height determined as 1.63 m using a scale on which the smallest interval was 1.0 cm and their mass determined as 60.5 kg on a balance with a scale on which the smallest interval was 0.1 kg.
(a) State the absolute errors in the measurement of height and mass.
(b) Calculate the percentage errors in the measurement of height and mass.
(c) Calculate the BMI and report your answer using the appropriate number of significant figures.

12. During a clinical teaching session an experienced nurse educator gets her group of six novice students to determine the specific gravity of a urine sample using a urinometer. The measurement is read from a scale which covers the range 0–60 in intervals of 2. Her students report the following values for the same urine sample: 26, 25, 24, 25, 15, 24. When the instructor performs the measurement herself she obtains the value 26.
(a) If you were asked to state what you think is the best estimate for the true value of the measurement, what would you say? How would you justify this?
(b) What do you think about the accuracy and precision of the set of measurements obtained by the students?
(c) Is there anything about the measurements performed by the students which allows you to conclude anything about the type of errors they have made?

13. What are some important differences between scientific writing and literature? What effects do these differences have?

14.

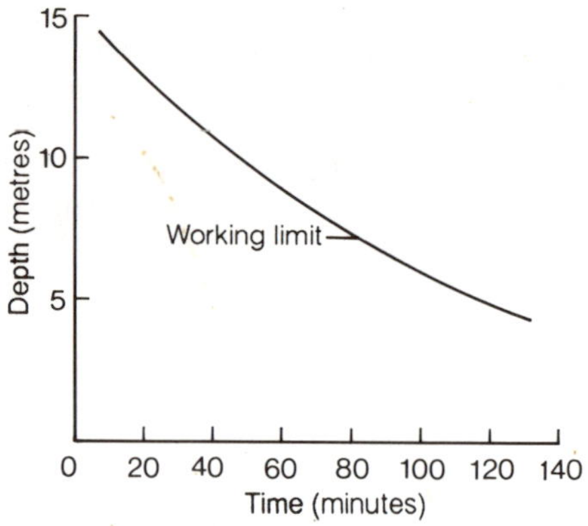

The graph shown above is a **working limit curve** used to determine the length of time that a person breathing pure oxygen may work underwater at various depths without undue risk. Combinations of time and depth which lie above the working limit curve are unsafe while those which lie below the line are safe. For each of the combinations below decide whether it is safe or unsafe.
(a) 40 minutes at 15 metres
(b) 60 minutes at 6 metres
(c) 80 minutes at 9 metres
(d) 10 minutes at 3 metres

15. Some drugs are administered in microgram quantities, others in milligram quantities. It is often recommended that prescriptions for drugs which are required to be administered in microgram quantities should have the word microgram written out in full rather than as the metric symbol μg. Why do you think this is?

16. The English poet Lord Macauley once said:

> . . . when men, in treating of things which cannot be circumscribed by precise definitions . . . talk of power, happiness, misery, pain, pleasure motives, objects of desire, as they talk of lines and numbers, there is no end to the contradictions and absurdities into which they can fall.

What do you think that Macauley meant by this?

CHAPTER 2

Atoms, Molecules and Ions: Particles That Matter

So far, material things have been described as consisting of particles, but nothing has been said about the exact nature of these particles. In this chapter we shall go beyond this level of description and talk in considerable detail about particles called atoms. We shall be concerned with their methods of arrangement and with the forces which maintain these arrangements intact. This provides a means of understanding some of the more applied topics which are to be encountered later on. Examples are osmosis, acid–base balance, organic compounds in the body and the action of some medicines.

Learning Objectives

At the completion of this chapter you should be able to:

1. Name the three main sub-atomic particles, describe their main properties and their distribution within the atom.
2. Define the terms atomic number, mass number and isotope.
3. Describe the basis of the arrangement of elements in the Periodic Table and use the table to determine the number of electrons present in any atom.
4. List the main properties of metals and non-metals.
5. Describe the difference between molecular and non-molecular arrangements of atoms.
6. List the main properties of molecular and non-molecular compounds.
7. Describe the essential features of ionic and covalent bonds.
8. Use the Periodic Table to:
   (a) predict whether the bonding in a particular compound is ionic or covalent;
   (b) predict the valency of a particular atom, i.e. the number of electrons it uses to form bonds with other atoms.
9. Predict the formula for a compound formed by combination of a particular pair of elements.
10. Give an account of the properties of molecular and non-molecular compounds in terms of the type of bond which operates within the material.
11. Explain the meaning of the terms essential element, macromineral and trace element.
12. Explain what is meant by the terms deficiency disease and toxicity disease and describe at least one example of each.
13. State the property of carbon responsible for its ability to form the vast numbers of different compounds found in living creatures.
14. Outline the natural cycles through which the elements carbon, oxygen and nitrogen constantly pass and define the terms photosynthesis, respiration and nitrogen fixation.

2.1 Atoms

We have seen in Chapter 1, 'The Physical World', that there are millions of different types of matter, called compounds, which form by the combination of two or more of a small number of chemical elements. This combination must ultimately involve the joining of whatever particles make up the elements and it is now time for us to consider this in more detail.

The particles of which an element is composed are called **atoms**, and atoms of one particular element are different to those of all the other elements. As a set of elements combine with each other to form a compound their atoms join together to form a new arrangement which is characteristic of the compound. By way of illustration, let us consider the combination of the elements hydrogen (H) and oxygen (O). This usually results in the formation of water, which is a compound consisting of particles (called **molecules**) in which two atoms of hydrogen are joined to one atom of oxygen. These particles are represented as H_2O.

hydrogen + oxygen ⟶ water
2 atoms of H + 1 atom of O ⟶ H_2O

Hydrogen and oxygen may combine in a different way to this and form a completely different compound, hydrogen peroxide, which consists of particles having two atoms of hydrogen joined to two of oxygen.

hydrogen + oxygen ⟶ hydrogen peroxide
2 atoms of H + 2 atoms of O ⟶ H_2O_2

In Table 2.1 some properties of water and hydrogen peroxide are compared. The existence of these two compounds of hydrogen and oxygen, and the striking differences in their behaviour, make it clear that the properties of a compound depend not only on the identity of the elements which are present, but also on the ratio of their atoms. Hydrogen and oxygen only combine in the two different ways described above, but other sets of elements, particularly those which include the element carbon, may combine in hundreds of different ways. This makes it possible to form millions of different particles from a small number of different types of atoms.

If you find this a bit hard to believe just pause for a minute and consider the English alphabet which consists of 26 different letters and a few punctuation marks. These are sufficient to describe all that human beings have seen and done and thought. There is no limit to the number of distinctive stories that can be told using the English alphabet and there is no limit to the number of distinctive particles that can be formed by the combination of atoms.

Table 2.1 *Comparison of the properties of water and hydrogen peroxide*

Property	Water	Hydrogen peroxide
density	1 g/ml	1.47 g/ml
melting point	0 °C	−0.4 °C
boiling point	100 °C	151 °C
stability to heat	stable below 2000 °C	concentrated solutions are explosively unstable even at quite low temperatures
bleaching action	none	powerful bleaching agent
toxicity	none	highly toxic

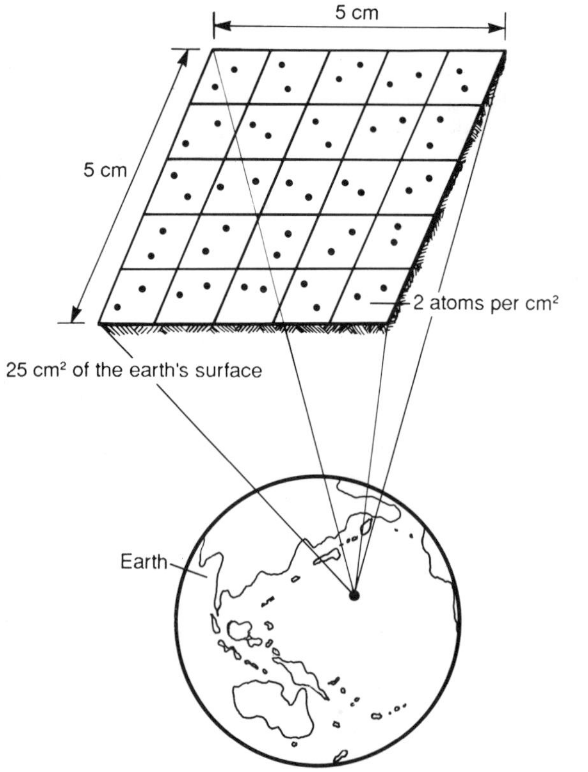

Figure 2.1 *An illustration of the smallness of atoms*

Atoms are very tiny particles. In one milligram of iron, which is considerably less than the amount found in the head of a pin, there are about 10^{19} atoms. This is a number so large that if these atoms were spread uniformly over the entire surface of the earth there would be at least two atoms on every square centimetre of land and water. The situation is illustrated in Figure 2.1.

If an object as small as the head of a pin contains more than 10^{19} atoms it is clear that a single atom must be tiny indeed! Atoms are so tiny that, until recently, it was not possible to see them, using even the most powerful microscopes. However, images of individual atoms have been obtained using modern instruments with magnifying powers much greater than any microscope previously available. Even so, this development has not meant much as far as our confidence in the existence of atoms is concerned. For decades now scientists have been convinced of the existence of atoms and finally being able to see them is not a matter of any great importance. Furthermore, the images which can be seen provide no detail of the structure of atoms. This prompts many new students of chemistry to ask: 'If scientists could not see atoms how could they have been so sure of their existence?' The answer is that confidence in the existence of atoms was based on the fact that they provided the best explanation available for the behaviour of material things. The atom was not a thing at all but an idea which worked extremely well. This is still substantially true.

You may consider all this to be a bit fanciful and perhaps you are beginning to think that the science of chemistry rests on rather shaky foundations: ideas about things that cannot be seen! Nothing could be further from the truth. It is quite common for us to invent ideas which then play a central role in our understanding of things. Think for a moment about the idea of an attitude. None of us will ever see an attitude but we will see human beings perform acts which we can only understand by using our idea of an attitude. Until recently no one had ever seen an atom but there was an enormous amount of the behaviour of material things which could only be understood in terms of atoms.

The first important question about atoms which we shall consider is: 'What makes atoms of one type, say, gold, different from atoms of another type, say, iron?' The sections which follow provide an answer to this question in the form of an historical survey of the development of our modern ideas about the nature of atoms. Even if you know the answer to the question you may still find it interesting to read these sections and they will probably add to your understanding. However, if you are confident that your understanding is already clear enough you can proceed directly to Section 2.3, 'The Composition of Atoms', and take the story up from that point.

2.2 History of the Atom

2.2.1 *Differences Between Atoms*

The idea that the world is composed of atoms can be traced back more than 2000 years to the Greek philosopher, Democritos. He believed that atoms differed from each other in their shape, some being spherical, others being flat and so on.

This was still the view held 20 centuries later and the idea of atoms did not increase much in popularity or usefulness throughout all this time. It was not until the beginning of the nineteenth century that atoms came into their own. In 1808, the English schoolmaster John Dalton published an account of the atomic theory having as its central theme the belief that matter consisted of indestructible atoms which differed from one another in their weights. He described them as solid, impenetrable spheres and on the matter of their indestructibility he was emphatic. Dalton said: 'We might as well attempt to introduce a new planet into the solar system or to annihilate one already in existence, as to create or destroy a particle of hydrogen.'

Dalton's theory represented a significant advance over earlier versions of atomic theory because it assigned to atoms a property that could be measured. Wait a minute! Only a few paragraphs back some trouble was taken to point out that atoms are so tiny as to be invisible even under quite powerful microscopes. How then could John Dalton, in 1808, have hoped to measure their weights? Well, the weights which Dalton determined were not **absolute weights**. They were **relative weights** and he obtained them in a manner which is illustrated below for the two atoms hydrogen and chlorine.

When hydrogen and chlorine combine with each other it is observed that for each gram of hydrogen consumed about 36 g of chlorine are also consumed. Given this information (and a lot of experimental data of this sort was available at the start of the nineteenth century) Dalton would have assumed that the combination of hydrogen and chlorine involved the joining of atoms of these two elements. He would have further assumed (unless he had reason to believe otherwise) that one atom of hydrogen combined with one atom of chlorine. This would have allowed him to say that a chlorine atom must weigh 36 times as much as a hydrogen atom. Dalton, and others, applied this reasoning to many pairs of atoms and this allowed the assignment of numbers to the individual atoms which expressed their weights relative to each other. These numbers became known as **atomic weights**.

Some of Dalton's assumptions about the way in which atoms combined were not correct and so some of his conclusions about the relative weights of atoms were contradictory. Nevertheless, he is rightly given full credit for reviving the idea of atoms, and for realising that they differed from each other in their weights. By the end of the nineteenth century a reliable set of atomic weights had been compiled and it was perfectly clear that each atom did have a unique weight. It became accepted, for a time, that this was the most important property distinguishing one atom from another. However, we shall see that early in the twentieth century it became necessary to abandon this idea.

2.2.2 *Atomic Weights and the Periodic Law*

As atomic weights were determined for more and more atoms, chemists became intrigued by the possibility that there might be some relationship between atomic weight and chemical behaviour. It was clear that some sets of elements were very similar in their properties, for example the elements lithium, sodium, potassium, rubidium and caesium. This set of elements, known as the **alkali metals**, was one of several groups in which the members had very similar properties and so were obviously related to each other in some way. However, the nature of the relationship did not start to become clear until the middle of the nineteenth century.

When the known elements were listed in increasing order of their atomic weights it was noticed that the members of groups such as the alkali metals appeared in the list at regular intervals of seven or some multiple of seven (see Table 2.2).

Table 2.2 *Alkali metals and their positions in the list of atomic weights*

Element	Symbol	Position in the list of atomic weights
lithium	Li	2
sodium	Na	9
potassium	K	16
rubidium	Rb	30
caesium	Cs	44

In 1868–69 two chemists, Julius Lothar Meyer of Germany, and Dmitri Mendeleeff of Russia, took this regularity to indicate the existence of what they called the **Periodic Law**. This law may be stated as follows: *the properties of the elements vary in a periodic manner with the atomic weight.* Meyer and Mendeleeff used the Periodic Law to construct a table in which many elements having similar properties fell naturally into the same vertical columns once they had been arranged in increasing order of their atomic weights. At some positions in the table Meyer and Mendeleeff were forced to leave gaps because no known elements had the properties which were expected for those positions. They predicted that elements would be discovered to fill these gaps and Mendeleeff even predicted values for some of the physical properties of these yet-to-be-discovered elements. At other positions in the table it was necessary to reverse the positions which some elements occupied when listed according to their atomic weights. This was in order to have them occupy the same vertical columns of the table as other similar elements.

The confident predictions of Mendeleeff and Myer concerning undiscovered elements were vindicated in spectacular fashion. Elements corresponding to some of the gaps which had been left in the table were found and their properties were very close to those which had been predicted by Mendeleeff. For example, he had predicted the existence of an element of atomic weight 72 which he called ekasilicon. In 1886, a new element was discovered by the German chemist Clements Winkler. This is the element now known as germanium and in Table 2.3 its properties are compared to those which Mendeleeff had predicted for ekasilicon.

Table 2.3 *Properties predicted for ekasilicon compared with those found for germanium*

	Mendeleeff's ekasilicon	Winkler's germanium
atomic weight	72	72.6
specific gravity of the element	5.5	5.5
specific gravity of the oxide of the element	4.7	4.7

As convincing as this was it still left unsettled the matter of those elements which occupied positions that were not consistent with their atomic weights. The only explanation which could be given for this was that the atomic weights of the elements must be incorrect. However, this could not be shown to be the case, and so these elements served as a constant reminder of the fact that atomic weight values did not provide the perfect means of accounting for the observed regularities in the behaviour of the chemical elements.

As the end of the nineteenth century drew near, the atomic theory of John Dalton became very firmly entrenched in scientific thought. It had led to the determination of atomic weights and these had provided a basis for predicting the behaviour of elements and even for predicting the existence of elements which were yet to be discovered. In spite of this success the last years of the nineteenth and early years of the twentieth centuries brought developments which clearly showed that atoms were very different from the description which Dalton had given.

2.2.3 *Radioactivity and the Electron*

These major developments in our understanding of the nature of atoms began with the discoveries of radioactivity, in 1896, by Henri Becquerel and the electron, in 1897, by Joseph Thomson.

Becquerel noticed the emission of a new type of radiation from a substance known to contain uranium. The radiation, which was produced spontaneously and steadily, was capable of passing through many materials and it affected photographic plate in the same way as X-rays did. This phenomenon became known as **radioactivity**. The study of radioactivity was taken up by Marie Curie in 1895 and she was assisted in her early researches by her husband, Pierre. She showed that all materials which contained uranium were radioactive. In this way she established that radioactivity was a property of particular atoms and did not depend upon the other atoms which happened to be present in the material. Marie Curie achieved enduring fame through her scientific work and particularly for her discovery of the new radioactive element, radium, which provided the first effective means of treating cancer.

Although Marie Curie is the best known of the early researchers into radioactivity it was a field which attracted many others and, in the early years of this century, it led to the most dramatic conclusions concerning the nature of atoms. Whereas John Dalton, and everyone before him, had considered atoms to be indestructible, the research into radioactivity showed that radioactive atoms were subject to a steady, spontaneous disintegration. The effect of this disintegration is the conversion of the radioactive atom into a different atom, with the simultaneous release of radiation.

Thomson's discovery of the electron was made during his investigation of **cathode rays**. These rays had been discovered much earlier in the nineteenth century during experiments in which electrical discharges were being made to occur between metal electrodes in a highly evacuated glass tube. Under these conditions it was observed that the negative electrode (the **cathode**) emitted radiation. Thomson showed that cathode rays were streams of negatively charged particles of mass about one two-thousandth the mass of the lightest known atom, hydrogen. The significance of his discovery was that it proved the existence of a particle much smaller than an atom. Furthermore, it was shown that the same particle could be produced from many different types of cathode material. This indicated very clearly that the particle must be a component of all atoms. An atom, therefore, could not be the solid, impenetrable sphere which Dalton had described. About 40 years earlier another great physicist, James Clerk Maxwell, had predicted the existence within atoms of a small, electrically charged particle which became known as the **electron**. This was the name given to the particle discovered by Thomson and it continues in use today.

2.2.4 *The Nuclear Model of the Atom*

In normal circumstances chemical materials have no net electrical charge and yet Thomson's discovery of the electron showed that negative particles existed within atoms. This meant that positive electricity must also be present within the atom. Thomson himself proposed a model of the atom known as the 'plum-pudding' model in which the electrons of the atom were embedded in a larger mass over which a positive charge was uniformly distributed (Figure 2.2).

Not long after it had been proposed by Thomson, this model of the atom was abandoned because it could not explain some important observations. For example, it could not explain some observations made by Charles Wilson in 1897, during his study of **alpha radiation**. This was a component of the radiation emitted by the newly discovered radioactive materials.

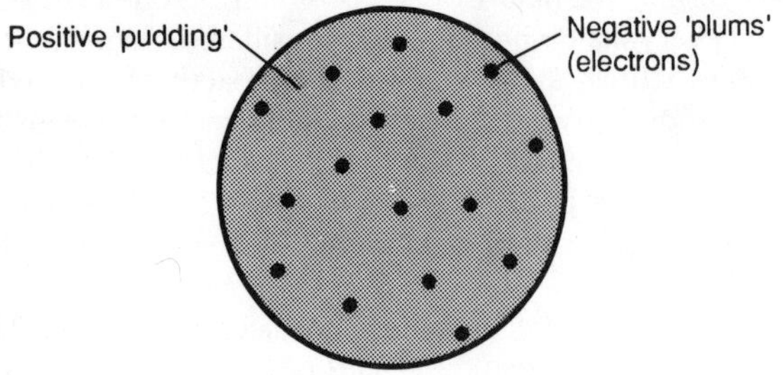

Figure 2.2 *Thomson's 'plum-pudding' model of the atom*

Alpha radiation had already been shown to consist of positive particles and Wilson studied the passage of these particles through the air in a **cloud chamber**. This air was saturated with water which condensed like a cloud along the path followed by each alpha particle to form tracks which were readily visible. In most cases the tracks were straight, but, occasionally, they showed an alpha particle undergoing a large deflection from its straight-line path. In 1906, Ernest Rutherford, using quite different apparatus, also observed the deflection of alpha particles which had been 'fired' at thin sheets of gold foil. Most of the particles passed straight through the foil as if it were not there. However, a few of them were deflected from their straight-line paths and some did not pass through the foil at all, but bounced back in the direction from which they had come. Rutherford's experiment is represented in Figure 2.3.

Rutherford, considering his own observations, and those of Wilson, formed the brilliant insight that atoms have a very open structure. He concluded that the structure must include a small, central **nucleus** having a positive charge and containing most of the atom's mass. Around this nucleus the light-weight, negative electrons circulated, sweeping out a volume many millions of times greater than the volume of the nucleus.

Rutherford's model accounted for the ability of alpha particles to travel unhindered through matter and for the occasional large deflection which a few of them always suffered. These were the few which came close enough to the tiny, positively charged nucleus to be deflected by it. The rest of the alpha particles simply travelled through the largely empty space surrounding the nucleus.

Rutherford's model of the atom has often been compared to the solar system. The nucleus corresponds to the sun, the orbiting planets to the electrons and

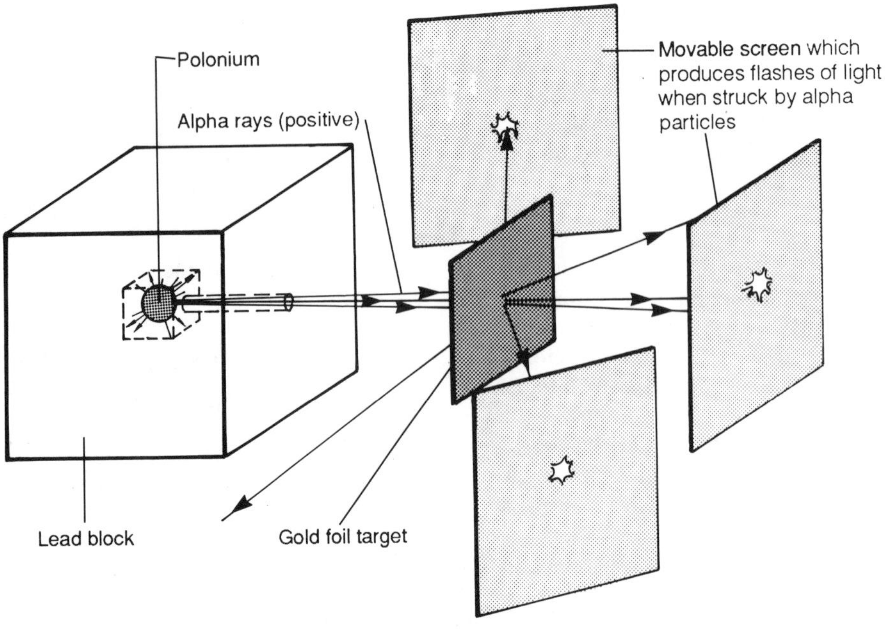

Figure 2.3 *Rutherford's scattering experiment*

most of the solar system is empty space. However, the sun and its planets form a flat disc whereas atoms are spherical.

The nuclear model of the atom has undergone a great deal of refinement in the time since Rutherford first proposed it. In 1913, Henry Moseley discovered a way of establishing the number of electrons which circulate around the nucleus of an atom. His work eventually led to the realisation that the nuclei of atoms contain positively charged particles, now called **protons**. The electric charge carried by each proton is positive and equal in magnitude to the negative charge carried by each electron. The number of protons in the nucleus is normally equal to the number of electrons which surround the nucleus and this explains why atoms are normally neutral.

Moseley introduced the term **atomic number** to describe atoms. This is the number of protons present in the atom's nucleus and is also the number of electrons circulating around the nucleus of the neutral atom. Moseley's work finally made clear the relationship between atoms of different elements: they correspond to a one-at-a-time increase in the number of protons present in the nucleus. Hydrogen, the simplest atom, has one proton in its nucleus. Uranium, the most complex of the naturally occurring atoms, has 92. Each of the other naturally occurring atoms has between one and 92 protons in its nucleus.

When the elements are listed in increasing order of atomic number the sequence obtained is similar to that obtained using atomic weights but there are a few very significant differences. These differences occur at exactly those points where Mendeleeff and Meyer had found it necessary to alter the atomic weight sequence in order to fit elements into vertical columns of the Periodic Table containing other similar elements. This provides a clear indication that it is the atomic number, and not the atomic weight, of an atom which is its most fundamental property. This is what we accept today. Once the significance of the atomic number was realised it became possible to predict, with absolute certainty, the maximum number of elements, less complex than uranium, which could be present on earth. All the missing elements were eventually discovered, the last being francium which was discovered in 1939 by Marguerite Perey.

The final detail of atomic structure which is of interest to us was determined in 1932 by James Chadwick of Cambridge University. He provided an explanation for a puzzling feature of the relationship between the atomic numbers of atoms and their atomic weights. Hydrogen, the lightest element, had an atomic number of 1 and an atomic weight of approximately 1. Oxygen had an atomic number of 8 but an atomic weight of approximately 16. While the number of protons in the nucleus of an oxygen atom was eight times as great as hydrogen, its weight was sixteen times as great. This was the general rule when the atomic number and weight of hydrogen were compared with the atomic number and weight of a more complex atom. It was as if the nuclei of the more complex atoms contained more than just the number of protons corresponding to their atomic numbers.

The initial explanation for this was that the nuclei of all atoms other than hydrogen contained extra protons which accounted for the additional weight. According to this view the nucleus also contained additional electrons to maintain the electrical neutrality of the atom. Chadwick did not accept the existence of separate protons and electrons in the nucleus and he proposed instead the existence of another type of particle having about the same mass as a proton but no electrical charge. He called these particles **neutrons** and was able to show that streams of them formed when certain elements were bombarded by high-energy alpha radiation.

So far, this chapter has been concerned with an account of the main developments in our understanding of the nature of atoms. These were developments which occurred in the period 1800–1932. Since the end of that period there have been further developments and an entirely up-to-date description of atoms would be much more sophisticated than the one which has been outlined in the preceding pages. However, it is not necessary for us to take account of all that is now known about atoms in order to establish an adequate foundation for later topics and so we can leave the remainder of the story untold.

In the next few sections a summary of the composition of atoms is presented and used to account for the existence of isotopes and the form of the Periodic Table.

2.3 The Composition of Atoms

From the way that atoms behave it has been concluded that they have the following features:

1. They are very small particles (10^{-10} m in diameter), composed of a number of even smaller particles, the most important of which are protons, neutrons and electrons. Protons and neutrons are about equal in their mass and are about 1870 times as massive as an electron. Protons, neutrons and electrons are often referred to as **sub-atomic particles**.

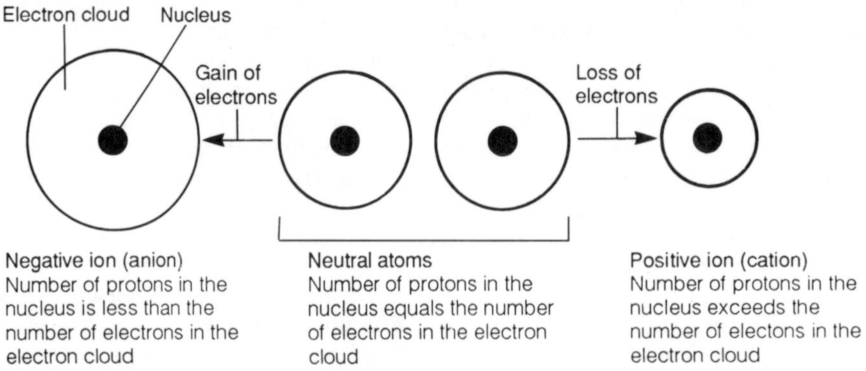
Electron cloud
Nucleus
Gain of electrons
Loss of electrons
Negative ion (anion)
Number of protons in the nucleus is less than the number of electrons in the electron cloud
Neutral atoms
Number of protons in the nucleus equals the number of electrons in the electron cloud
Positive ion (cation)
Number of protons in the nucleus exceeds the number of electons in the electron cloud

Figure 2.4 *Formation of ions from neutral atoms*

2. They have a small, central region (10^{-14} m in diameter), called the nucleus, in which the protons and neutrons are located. The electrons exist in an electron 'cloud' which surrounds the nucleus and occupies a much bigger region of space.

3. They are electrical in nature. Protons have a positive charge and electrons have a negative charge of the same magnitude. Neutrons are electrically neutral.

Atoms may contain the same number of electrons as protons and when this is the case they are electrically neutral. However, it is quite common for an atom to gain or lose a small number of electrons, and when this happens the atom becomes electrically charged and is called an **ion**. Atoms that lose electrons form positively charged ions and these are called **cations**. Atoms that gain electrons form negatively charged ions called **anions**. The formation of ions from neutral atoms is illustrated in Figure 2.4.

2.3.1 *Atomic Number, Mass Number and Isotopes*

The number of protons in the nucleus of an atom is called its atomic number and this determines its nature. Thus, all atoms of atomic number 7 are atoms of nitrogen. Nitrogen is present in the atmosphere as the uncombined element, in which form it is very unreactive. All atoms of atomic number 8 are atoms of oxygen, which is also present in the atmosphere as the uncombined element. Oxygen in this form, though, is quite reactive and it supports the burning of many materials. All atoms of a particular element have the same atomic number and behave in the same way in most respects.

The sum of the number of protons and neutrons in the nucleus of an atom is called its **mass number**. Atoms which have the same number of protons as each other and which are therefore atoms of the same element may, nevertheless, have different numbers of neutrons. When this is the case, the atoms are said to be **isotopes** of that particular element. For example, some atoms of oxygen contain 8 neutrons in the nucleus and so have a mass number of $8 + 8 = 16$. Other atoms of oxygen have nine neutrons and a mass number of $8 + 9 = 17$. These two types of oxygen atoms are said to be isotopes of oxygen. Isotope is a word derived from the two Greek words, *isos*, meaning 'same' and *topes*, meaning 'place'. It was introduced by Frederick Soddy to describe the fact that isotopes were different atoms but had properties so similar that they had to be assigned to the same place in the Periodic Table.

Isotopes are identical in their chemical properties but differ in their physical properties. For example, some isotopes are radioactive. This particular property has been extensively exploited in medicine where use is made of the fact that all isotopes of a particular element are processed in the same way by the body. Furthermore, much of the radiation emitted by radioactive atoms is capable of penetrating tissue. When radioactive atoms are introduced into the body they are distributed in the same way as non-radioactive atoms of the same element are, but the radiation they emit makes it possible to detect them with equipment located outside the body. In this way a great deal of information can be quickly obtained about body structure and function. Techniques of this type are discussed more fully in Chapter 14, 'Nuclear Medicine'.

The existence of isotopes provides an explanation for a curious feature of the atomic weight values for the elements. Most of these are very close to being simple whole numbers but there are some which have values in between. For example, chlorine has an atomic weight of 35.45. Simple whole number values for atomic weights fit in nicely with the idea that each atom contains a simple whole number of relatively heavy protons and neutrons in its nucleus. These particles are roughly equal in mass and, being many times more massive than electrons, are responsible for virtually all the mass of any atom. The lightest atom, hydrogen, has one proton in its nucleus and an atomic weight value of one. This suggests that any other atom should have an atomic weight very close to a simple whole number because each proton and neutron in its nucleus should contribute one unit to its atomic weight. On this basis the atomic weight of chlorine seems to be out of place but it can be readily accounted for by the existence of isotopes.

Chlorine consists of a mixture of two isotopes having the mass numbers 35 and 37. The proportions of these two isotopes are 77.5 and 22.5% respectively. The weight of each isotope, relative to that of hydrogen, is very close to a simple whole number but the atomic weight of chlorine reflects the existence of both isotopes and is an average of their individual weights. This average is calculated by taking account of the proportion of each isotope present. The calculation is set out below.

Table 2.4 *Symbolic representation of atoms*

	Phosphorus	Cobalt	Iodine	Chlorine	Hydrogen
Symbol	${}^{32}_{15}P$	${}^{60}_{27}Co$	${}^{131}_{53}I$	${}^{35}_{17}Cl$	${}^{1}_{1}H$
Protons	15	27	53	17	1
Neutrons	17	33	78	18	0
Electrons	15	27	53	17	1

Consider a sample of 1000 chlorine atoms. This will consist of:

775 atoms of mass 35. Total mass = 775 × 35
= 27125

225 atoms of mass 37. Total mass = 225 × 37
= 8325

Total mass of 1000 atoms = 27125 + 8325
= 35450

Average mass of a single atom $= \frac{35450}{1000}$
= 35.45 (atomic weight)

The term 'atomic weight' has now been replaced by the term 'relative atomic mass' (RAM) and this is the term which we shall use from now on.

2.3.2 *Symbolic Representation of Atoms*

A common method used to represent atoms, and give details of their structures, is illustrated in Table 2.4. The symbol for the element is written with the atom's mass number to the upper left and its atomic number to the lower left.

The element potassium may be used to illustrate most of the points made so far about atoms and their composition. Atoms of potassium have the symbol K and they all contain 19 protons, that is, the atomic number of potassium is 19. Of the potassium atoms which occur naturally about 93% have a mass number of 39 (${}^{39}_{19}K$), about 6.9% have a mass number of 41 (${}^{41}_{19}K$) and a very small percentage have a mass number of 40 (${}^{40}_{19}K$). Thus, there are three naturally occurring isotopes of the element potassium and this gives the element a relative atomic mass of 39.10. The potassium isotope of mass number 40 is radioactive, whereas the other two are not. There are several other isotopes of potassium which have been produced in nuclear reactors and all of these are radioactive.

Potassium is an important component of human tissue, and in this situation consists of the same set of potassium isotopes that is found in minerals and natural waters. Furthermore, potassium obtained from all these different sources contains the same isotopes present in the same proportions. When it exists in tissue (and in all other circumstances where it has combined with other elements) potassium is in the form of a cation which carries a single, positive charge. This cation forms as a result of the loss of one electron from a potassium atom and it is represented by the symbol, K^+.

2.3.4 *The Arrangement of Electrons in Atoms*

The electrons in the electron clouds of all atoms are arranged in the same general way: they are organised into clusters located at different distances from the nucleus. These clusters are often described as **electron shells**. The shell closest to the nucleus is designated K, the next one out as L, the next M and so on. The maximum number of electrons that each shell may hold is shown below.

K	2 electrons
L	8 electrons
M	18 electrons
N	32 electrons

The most important feature of the electron arrangement within a particular type of atom is the number of electrons in the shell located at the outside of the electron cloud. This is because atoms may only interact with each other at the fringes of their electron clouds (see Figure 2.5). More substantial interaction between atoms is prevented by forces of repulsion which come into play as they approach each other.

In many introductory chemistry textbooks the electron arrangement in atoms is described in considerable detail. It can be used to account for chemical formulae and explain chemical bonding. However, we shall not be adopting this approach but will, instead, achieve the same aims by using the Periodic Table of the Elements. One version of this table is at the front of this book.

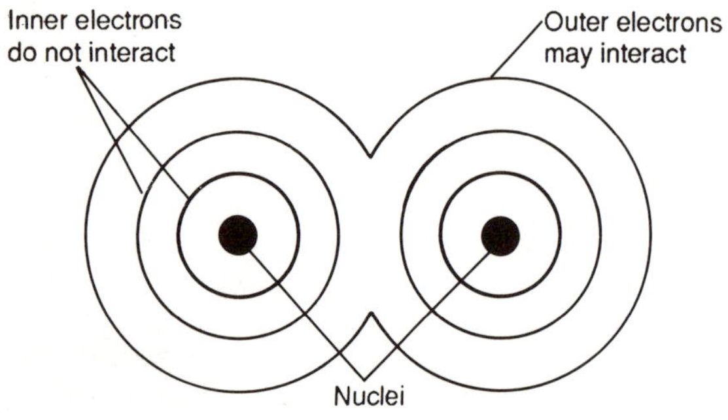

Figure 2.5 *Interaction between atoms*

2.4 Periodic Table of the Elements

This is a table of the elements arranged in order of increasing atomic number in such a way that:

1. Elements with atoms having the same number of electrons in the outermost electron shell fall into vertical columns called **groups**.
2. Elements with atoms which have the same number of shells occupied by electrons fall into horizontal rows called **periods**.

It is observed that elements in the same group of the Periodic Table have similar properties and this indicates that the behaviour of elements is determined largely by the number of electrons which they have in the outermost electron shell. These outermost electrons are often called **valency electrons** and so we may say that the behaviour of elements is determined largely by the number of their valency electrons. You will notice that the Periodic Table used in this book has its largest groups designated as IA, IIA, . . . These groups are often called the main groups of the Periodic Table and they include most of the elements with which we will be concerned. The number of valency electrons possessed by an element in any one of the main groups is simply equal to the number of the group. Thus all members of Group IVA have four valency electrons, all members of Group VIA have six and so on. Some groups of the Periodic Table are referred to by well-established names. For example, Group VIIA is the **halogens**, Group IA is the **alkali metals** and Group IIA is the **alkaline earth metals**.

The group of elements on the far right of the Periodic Table is of particular significance. This group is known as the **inert gas** or **noble gas** group because its members are very unreactive. Due to this low reactivity they were the very last set of elements discovered and, prior to the discovery of argon in 1895, their existence had not even been suspected. The next member of the inert gas group to be discovered, also in 1895, was helium. Next came krypton, then xenon, which were both discovered in 1898. The relative atomic mass values for these gases were determined and showed clearly that they belonged in the Periodic Table between the halogens of Group VIIA and the alkali metals of Group IA. The other member of the group is radon which is a radioactive gas formed as a result of the decay of certain radioactive atoms. It was discovered in 1900.

The inert gases have practical importance. Neon, argon, krypton and xenon are used in electric lights of various sorts. Helium is used in airships and in the production of artificial breathing atmospheres for divers. The inert gases are also important for theoretical reasons because they are the only atoms which prefer to exist by themselves. This is taken to indicate that the number of electrons which any inert gas has is an inherently stable number and this stability is used as the basis of a simple theory which accounts for the ratios in which atoms combine, and for some of the properties which their compounds exhibit. The theory will be described later in this chapter.

The elements on the left of the Periodic Table are nearly all solids which readily conduct heat and electricity. Elements having these properties are known as **metals**. The elements on the right of the Periodic Table are usually poor conductors of heat and electricity and many of them are gases. Elements with these properties are known as **non-metals**. As one moves across the Periodic Table from left to right, the nature of the elements change markedly from metallic elements on the left to non-metallic elements on the right. As one proceeds down the Periodic Table there is a trend from non-metallic at the top towards metallic at the bottom but this is much less pronounced than the change which occurs across the table.

There is no sharp line which can be drawn through the Periodic Table to separate metals from non-metals. In the version of the table which is used in this book a zig-zag line is drawn starting at position 5 and ending at position 85. Most of the elements found in the Periodic Table along this line have properties characteristic of both metals and non-metals and are often called **metalloids**. Some examples are silicon, germanium, arsenic and antimony. Of these, silicon and germanium have great commercial importance because of their use in the manufacture of transistors, solar cells and computer chips. As one moves away from this zig-zag line towards the bottom left of the table the elements become more metallic. Above the line and towards the right of the table they become more non-metallic.

The items of information available from the Periodic Table used in this book include group number, period number, atomic number and relative atomic mass. For the element phosphorus these are:

group number	VA
period number	3
atomic number	15
relative atomic mass	30.97

You should have no difficulty using the Periodic Table at the front of the book to determine these values for any other element.

2.5 Atomic Organisation: Molecular and Non-molecular Structures

Atoms of the inert gases are capable of existing by themselves and they usually do. A sample of helium gas consists of single helium atoms which are quite independent of each other. In this respect the inert gases are exceptional because no other atoms are capable of existing by themselves under normal conditions.

Even in the case of the uncombined elements, where there is only one type of atom present, all atoms, other than those of the inert gases, join with each other to form characteristic structures. It is possible to determine the positions which atoms occupy, relative to one another, in substances and this type of study, applied to many different substances, has shown that atoms form two quite different types of structure. These are called **molecular** and **non-molecular** structures.

2.5.1 *Molecular Organisation of Atoms*

Many materials have their atoms organised into small, independent groups called **molecules**. Among the chemical elements, molecular structures are displayed by the elements towards the right-hand side of the Periodic Table (the non-metallic elements). For example, the element oxygen exists as molecules which contain two atoms joined together. These molecules are represented by the formula O_2. Some other elements which exist as simple molecules are listed in Table 2.5 together with their melting points and boiling points.

Molecular substances have their atoms tightly held within molecules but each molecule is only held weakly to the other molecules around it. *This is why molecular substances have low melting points and boiling points.* These processes (melting and boiling) separate molecules from each other without affecting the arrangement of atoms within the molecules themselves.

Table 2.5 *Melting points and boiling points for some molecular elements*

Element	Molecular formula	Melting point (°C)	Boiling point (°C)
nitrogen	N_2	–210	–196
phosphorus	P_4	44	280
sulphur	S_8	119	445
chlorine	Cl_2	–101	–35
bromine	Br_2	–7	58

2.5.2 *Non-molecular Structures*

In some substances the atoms are not organised into molecules but, instead, are organised into vast lattice structures. These are called non-molecular substances and this type of structure is typical of the elements on the left of the Periodic Table (the metallic elements).

Some very well known properties of metals are: good electrical conductivity, high melting point and high boiling point. Metals are good conductors of electricity because their valency electrons are only held loosely to the nucleus. This loose hold allows them to form a 'sea' of electrons which 'bathes' all atoms in the lattice. When different points on the metal's surface are made to have different electrical potentials (by connection to a battery or some other electrical supply) the 'sea' of electrons begins to drift in a particular direction and we say that the metal is conducting electricity.

The sea of electrons existing within metal lattices also affects their melting points and boiling points because the electrons exert strong forces of attraction on all the metal atoms in the lattice. Furthermore, there are no molecules which may be readily separated from each other, and if a metal is to melt then *all the forces acting between all its atoms must be overcome*. This ensures that most metals have high melting points and boiling points.

2.5.3 *Molecular and Non-molecular Compounds*

Compounds are combinations of different elements and so contain more than one type of atom. However, it is still found that the atoms in compounds organise into either molecular or non-molecular structures. The likelihood of a compound having one particular type of structure, rather than the other, may be predicted from the positions which its constituent atoms occupy in the Periodic Table. When the elements are widely separated in the table, the structure will usually be non-molecular. When the elements in a compound are all close together and from the right-hand side of the table, the structure will usually be molecular. There are some exceptions to the second part of this generalisation. Compounds formed by the combination of silicon with oxygen are non-molecular even though silicon and oxygen are both located on the right-hand side of the Periodic Table. These compounds are rarely encountered in discussions of the function of living creatures and so we do not need to consider them in any detail. Another exception must be made for the element hydrogen. Being the element of lowest atomic number this is usually written into the Periodic Table in the top, left-hand corner but it has the properties of a typical non-metal, that is, of an element usually found on the right-hand side of the Periodic Table. Consistent with this, its combination with elements from the right-hand side of the table always produces molecular compounds.

The important differences between the arrangements of atoms in molecular and non-molecular structures are illustrated in Figure 2.6. The element carbon is used as an example of a non-molecular substance and the compound water (in its solid state, ice) as an example of a molecular substance.

Molecular and non-molecular substances (both elements and compounds) display marked differences in melting points, boiling points, solubility in water, electrical conductivity and odour. These differences are summarised in Table 2.6. and the significance of some of the properties are discussed briefly below.

Melting Point and Boiling Point. These are determined by heating a sample of the substance and noting the temperature at which it changes from a solid to a liquid (melting point) and then the temperature at which

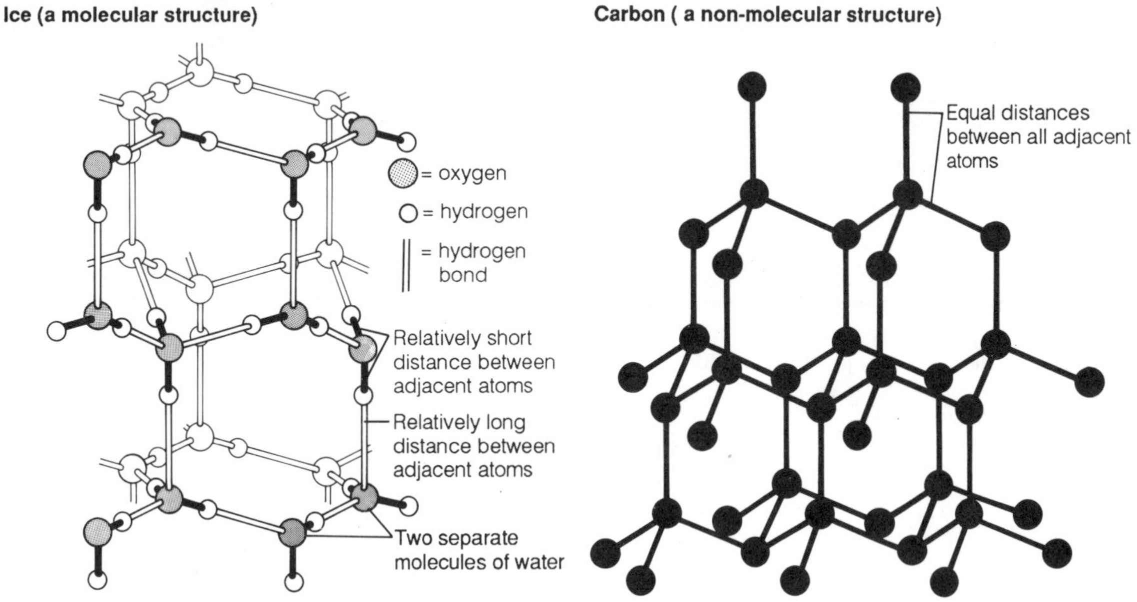

Figure 2.6 *Molecular and non-molecular structures*

the liquid changes to a gas (boiling point). At the melting point, the substance changes from one state (solid) where its particles are held in fixed positions with respect to each other, to another state (liquid) where they are able to move about from place to place within the substance. At the boiling point the substance changes to a state (gas) where its particles have completely escaped from the liquid and move freely about in the atmosphere. Because melting and boiling correspond to separation of the particles of a substance from the others around them, *melting points, and particularly boiling points, provide a measure of the strength of the forces which operate between the particles.* Thus, the forces operating between the particles of non-molecular compounds must be strong while those operating between the particles of molecular compounds must be weak.

Electrical Conductivity. This can be determined by placing two electrical conductors (electrodes) in contact with a sample. One of them is connected to the positive side of an electrical supply and the other to the negative side. If the substance in contact with the electrodes is a conductor of electricity then an electrical current will flow between the electrodes. This flow of electricity can be detected using a meter known as an **ammeter**, which measures **electric current**. When a substance conducts electricity this means that it contains electrically charged particles which are free to move. Thus, non-molecular compounds, when molten or dissolved in water, must contain, or produce, charged particles which are free to move. Molecular compounds usually do not.

Odour. If a substance has an odour then its particles must be escaping into the atmosphere, because we only smell substances which are present in the air making contact with our olfactory nerves. These are located inside the head at the back of the nose. If the particles of a substance escape readily into the atmosphere then there must be relatively weak forces operating between them. It is important to realise that there are substances to which our olfactory nerves do not respond (water is an example). Thus, we may say that a strong odour is good evidence that a substance is molecular in structure, but the absence of an odour tells us nothing about the structure of a substance.

2.6 Chemical Bonds

So far, we have been mainly concerned with the ways in which atoms are organised, but very little has been said about the forces which must act between atoms in order to allow these organisations to exist. These forces are electrical in nature and are called **chemical bonds**.

Table 2.6 *Comparison of the properties of molecular and non-molecular compounds*

Non-molecular compounds	Molecular compounds
Solids with high melting points and boiling points.	Gases, liquids or solids with low melting points and boiling points.
Often soluble in water and insoluble in organic liquids.	Often insoluble in water but soluble in organic liquids.
When heated sufficiently to cause melting the molten substance conducts an electric current and in the process is decomposed into its constituent elements. All these compounds also conduct electricity when dissolved in water.	In pure form do not conduct electricity, although some conduct when dissolved in water.
No odour if pure.	May have an odour.
Examples NaCl (sodium chloride) MgO (magnesium oxide) $Ca(NO_3)_2$ (calcium nitrate)	*Examples* $CHCl_3$ (chloroform) $C_4H_{10}O$ (ether) C_2H_6O (alcohol) SO_2 (sulphur dioxide)

On the one hand, it is not surprising that chemical bonds are electrical in nature because we have seen that atoms contain electrically charged particles in the form of protons (positive) and electrons (negative). On the other hand, we have so far considered atoms to be electrically neutral due to their having equal numbers of these oppositely charged particles. However, this is only the case for atoms which are isolated from each other. When atoms come into contact it turns out that electrons can be transferred, or shared between them, in ways which produce unbalanced charges. These unbalanced charges are responsible for the forces of attraction which hold atoms in place within molecules and within non-molecular structures.

2.6.1 *Chemical Bonds in Non-molecular Compounds*

Since virtually all the non-molecular compounds present in the human body are formed by the combination of elements which are widely separated in the Periodic Table we shall only consider non-molecular compounds of this type. In these compounds atoms interact by transfer of electrons from one atom to another. The electron transfer takes place between the outside portions of the electron clouds of the atoms involved. It is always the atom further to the left in the table (the metal) which loses electrons and the atom further to the right (the non-metal) which gains them. The effect of this transfer is to change neutral atoms into ions. The metal atom becomes a positive ion (cation) and the non-metal atom a negative ion (anion). These oppositely charged ions exert strong forces of attraction on each other which hold them tightly together in a vast lattice. The forces are called **ionic bonds** and, quite often, the word 'ionic' is incorporated into the name of non-molecular compounds which are then referred to as **ionic, non-molecular compounds**. This is a reminder that there are two aspects to the structure of materials: the bonding between atoms and the way in which atoms are organised.

2.6.2 *Predicting the Charges on Ions in Ionic Compounds*

A question which arises naturally at this point is: 'How *many* electrons are transferred between atoms when they interact and form ionic bonds?' In order to answer this question we must attach special significance to the observation that atoms of the inert gases do not interact with each other, or with atoms of other elements. This is taken to indicate that the number of electrons which any inert gas has is an inherently stable number that other atoms will attempt to achieve. These stable numbers, and the corresponding inert gases, are listed in Table 2.7.

Table 2.7 *Inert gases and stable electron numbers*

Inert gas	Symbol	Stable electron number
Helium	He	2
Neon	Ne	10
Argon	Ar	18
Krypton	Kr	36
Xenon	Xe	54
Radon	Rn	86

Using the Periodic Table, one may quickly determine the number of electrons which a particular atom has. For example, atoms of the element sodium have 11 electrons (see Figure 2.7) which is one more than the stable number of 10 possessed by atoms of neon. The simplest way in which a sodium atom may achieve a stable number of electrons is for it to lose one electron and form an ion with a single, positive charge.

11	Atomic Number
Sodium	Name
Na	Symbol
22.99	Relative Atomic Mass
2, 8, 1	Electron structure

Figure 2.7 *Sodium 'cell' from the Periodic Table*

$$\underset{\substack{\text{sodium atom} \\ \text{11 electrons}}}{Na} \xrightarrow{\text{loss of 1 electron}} \underset{\substack{\text{sodium ion} \\ \text{10 electrons}}}{Na^+}$$

As an example of an element from the other side of the Periodic Table, let us consider chlorine. From the Periodic Table we can see that it has 17 electrons, which is one less than the stable number of 18 possessed by argon. On the same basis as before we would expect atoms of chlorine to gain one electron each and form ions with a single, negative charge.

$$\underset{\substack{\text{chlorine atom} \\ \text{17 electrons}}}{Cl} \xrightarrow{\text{gain of 1 electron}} \underset{\substack{\text{chloride ion} \\ \text{18 electrons}}}{Cl^-}$$

The transfer of electrons between sodium and chlorine atoms is illustrated in Figure 2.8.

2.6.3 *Accounting for the Properties of Ionic, Non-molecular Compounds*

The compound formed when the two elements sodium and chlorine combine is a typical ionic compound called sodium chloride (table salt). We are now in a position to account for some of its properties.

The melting point of sodium chloride is 801 °C and this high melting point is due partly to the strength of the ionic bonds which operate between its oppositely charged ions, and partly to its non-molecular nature. It will only melt when *all* the forces acting between *all*

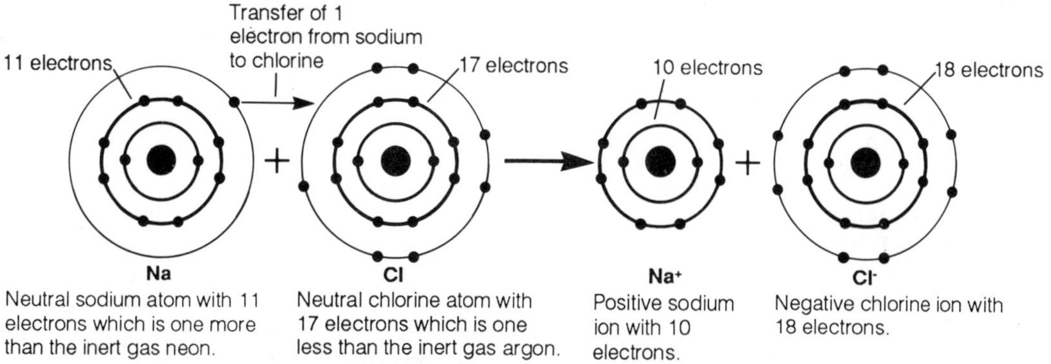
Transfer of 1 electron from sodium to chlorine
11 electrons
17 electrons
10 electrons
18 electrons
Na
Neutral sodium atom with 11 electrons which is one more than the inert gas neon.
Cl
Neutral chlorine atom with 17 electrons which is one less than the inert gas argon.
Na+
Positive sodium ion with 10 electrons.
Cl-
Negative chlorine ion with 18 electrons.

Figure 2.8 *Transfer of electrons between atoms*

the ions within the substance have been overcome. There are no molecules of sodium chloride which can be separated easily from each other.

The ability of sodium chloride to conduct electricity when molten, or dissolved in water, is due to the ions of which it is composed. In molten sodium chloride, and in its aqueous solution, these ions are free to move so allowing the conduction of electricity.

One of the most familiar characteristics of a chemical compound is its formula. This states the ratio in which its different atoms are present. Sodium chloride has the formula NaCl because it contains sodium and chlorine atoms in the ratio 1:1. This ratio arises because each sodium atom loses one electron in combining with other atoms while each chlorine atom gains one electron. When they combine with each other they must do so in equal numbers. Otherwise the substance formed would contain an excess of either positive or negative electrical charge and we know from our everyday experience of chemical materials that they are electrically neutral.

The formula of any ionic compound containing one particular type of atom will be dependent on the identity of the other atoms which are present, but this formula can always be accounted for in terms of the numbers of electrons which the atoms lose or gain when they combine. These numbers, in turn, can usually be predicted by reference to the positions which the atoms occupy in the Periodic Table. You should now attempt Exercise 2.1 which requires you to predict the formulae for compounds formed by the combination of particular pairs of elements. You will probably need to refer to the Periodic Table on the front inside cover.

Exercise 2.1
Predict the formulae for the ionic, non-molecular compounds formed by combination of the following pairs of elements:
(a) Na, O (b) Mg, O (c) Ca, Cl (d) K, S

2.6.4 *Chemical Bonds in Molecular Compounds*

Molecular compounds are formed when atoms on the right of the Periodic Table combine with each other, or with hydrogen. In molecular compounds the elements combining are too similar in their natures to allow one completely to lose electrons while the other completely gains them. Instead, they *share* electrons. The electrons involved are still only those at the outside of the electron cloud. The shared electrons exert a force of attraction on the nucleus of each atom involved. This force of attraction holds the two atoms in position on either side of the shared electrons and is known as a **covalent bond**. The situation is represented in Figure 2.9.

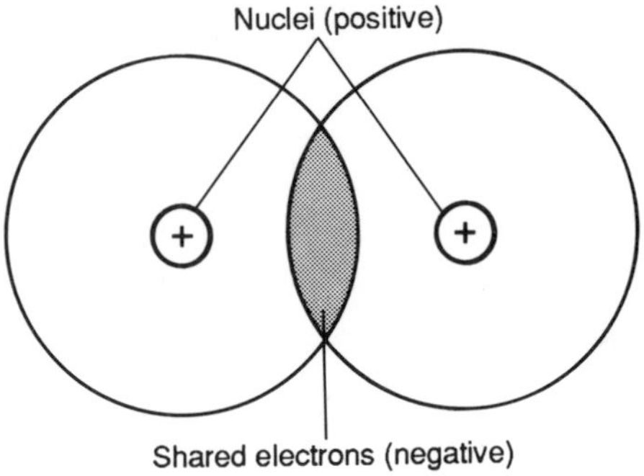

Figure 2.9 *Sharing of electrons. The covalent bond*

When atoms share one electron each, the covalent bond formed is called a **single covalent bond**, when they share two electrons each it becomes a **double covalent bond** and when they share three electrons each it becomes a **triple covalent bond**. The number of electrons which atoms share when they form covalent bonds may be predicted from their positions in the Periodic Table. This is done in much the same way as it was for the electron transfers which take place as ionic bonds form.

Different atoms have different attractions for electrons and so when electrons are shared between different atoms the sharing is unequal. In this situation the covalent bond is said to be **polarised** and is referred to as a **polar covalent bond**. This terminology is used because the word 'polarise' means to divide into two opposite groups: an issue which polarises public opinion is one which forces people to adopt one or another of two quite different opinions. When a polar covalent bond forms one atom involved in the bond becomes slightly negative (this is the atom having the greater attraction for electrons) and the other becomes slightly positive (this is the atom having the lesser attraction for electrons).

A simple example of a polar covalent bond is the single covalent bond which operates between hydrogen and oxygen atoms in molecules of water. Oxygen has a greater attraction for electrons than hydrogen and so, in the water molecule, the oxygen atom is slightly negative while the hydrogen atom is slightly positive. It is important to realise that the electrical charges which are present on the atoms in a polar covalent bond are only **fractional charges**, they are much smaller than the charges existing on ions. These fractional charges are often represented using the symbols δ+ and δ– (see Figure 2.11).

When the atoms involved in a covalent bond are identical to one another the sharing of electrons between them is equal and the bond is called a **non-polar bond**. The bonds which exist between atoms in the molecules of elements such as oxygen (O_2), nitrogen (N_2) and phosphorus (P_4) are non-polar bonds.

Let us now consider, in some detail, the combination of hydrogen with oxygen to form water. Hydrogen has one electron, which is one less than the stable number of two possessed by the inert gas helium. Oxygen has eight electrons, which is two less than the stable number of ten possessed by neon. Oxygen can, in a sense, achieve the stable number of ten electrons if it shares two of its own electrons with one electron from each of two hydrogen atoms. At the same time each of these two hydrogen atoms achieves a stable number of two electrons. This is illustrated in Figure 2.10.

You may have noticed something a bit strange about the way that we have counted electrons in this example. We said that oxygen shares two of its electrons and ends up with a stable number of ten, while each hydrogen atom shares its electron and ends up with a stable number of two. This adds up to a total of fourteen electrons when we really have only ten made up of eight from the oxygen atom and one each from the two hydrogen atoms. The apparent discrepancy arises because each shared electron is counted as belonging to both atoms involved in the sharing. If an accountant were to do this sort of thing with money he would end up in jail! In chemistry, it is allowed because it does no one any harm and it gives us the ability to make reliable predictions about the ways in which atoms combine.

The number of electrons which an atom shares when it forms covalent bonds with other atoms is known as the **valency** or **covalency** of the atom. In Exercise 2.2 you are asked to predict a likely valency for atoms of several different elements.

Exercise 2.2

Predict a likely valency for atoms of the following elements:

(a) chlorine (b) carbon (c) nitrogen
(d) phosphorus (e) sulphur (f) bromine

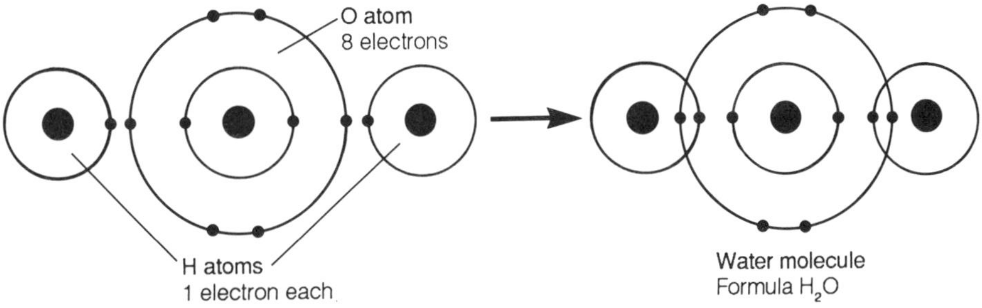

Figure 2.10 *The water molecule and covalent bond formation*

2.6.5 *Accounting for the Properties of Covalent, Molecular Compounds*

We are now in a position to account for some of the properties which are displayed by covalent, molecular compounds. They have relatively low melting and boiling points because their molecules are electrically neutral and exist as discrete units. Being electrically neutral the molecules do not exert strong forces on each other and therefore can be easily separated.

It is often thought that the low melting point of covalent, molecular compounds is proof that covalent bonds are weak. This is *not* true and it is very important to realise that the melting of covalent, molecular compounds does not involve the breaking of any covalent bonds. These bonds hold atoms together *within* molecules but do not operate *between* molecules. Covalent bonds are very strong. In order to break the covalent bonds which hold oxygen and hydrogen atoms together within water molecules the temperature must be raised many hundreds of degrees above its boiling point.

Covalent, molecular compounds do not usually conduct electricity because they do not contain electrically charged particles. Some conduct electricity when dissolved in water and this is because they undergo a chemical reaction with the water to produce ions. This is discussed in more detail in Section 7.2.

The formula of a covalent, molecular compound formed by the combination of two elements can usually be predicted from a knowledge of the number of electrons which atoms of its constituent elements share when they combine. The ratio in which the atoms combine must be such that the number of electrons shared by atoms of one type is always equal to the number shared by atoms of the other type. For example, if atom A shares four electrons and combines with atom B which shares one, then the compound formed will have the formula AB_4. This is because four atoms of B are required in order to use up the four electrons available from each atom of A. In Exercise 2.3 you are asked to predict the formulae for the compounds which form by combination of certain pairs of elements.

Exercise 2.3

Predict the formulae for the compounds formed by combination of each of the following pairs of elements:

(a) C, H (b) H, S (c) C, O
(d) C, Cl (e) N, H (f) O, F

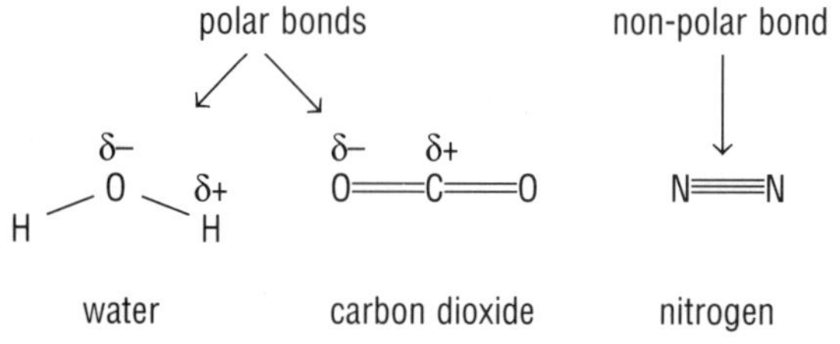

Figure 2.11 *Representation of polar and non-polar covalent bonds*

2.6.6 *Representation of Bonding Within Molecules*

The covalent bonds within molecules are usually represented by straight lines drawn between the atoms participating in the bond. For each pair of shared electrons one line is drawn and so a single covalent bond is represented by one line, a double covalent bond by two lines and a triple covalent bond by three lines. Some examples of this type of representation are shown in Figure 2.11 where the polarity of bonds is also indicated.

In some texts you will encounter slightly different representations of the water molecule, for example the representation shown in Figure 2.12. The additional lines associated with the oxygen atom represent additional pairs of electrons at the outside of its electron cloud. The lines are restricted to the oxygen atom because the electrons are not involved in bonds with the hydrogen atoms. Such pairs of electrons are called **non-bonding electrons** which is a rather sensible name for them.

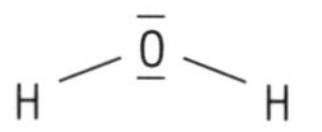

Figure 2.12 *Representation of the water molecule, showing non-bonding electron pairs*

You may be wondering why the atoms in a water molecule do not lie along a straight line. The explanation is that electron pairs repel each other and, in a water molecule, there are four separate pairs of electrons at the outside of the oxygen atom's electron cloud. These four electron pairs adopt positions in space which minimise the repulsion between them and the shape formed is roughly tetrahedral around the central oxygen atom. This is shown in Figure 2.13. With this arrangement the two hydrogen atoms and the

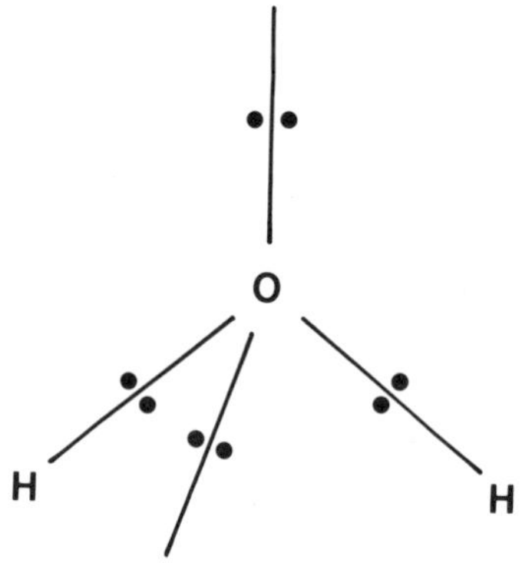

Figure 2.13 *Distribution of electron pairs in a water molecule*

oxygen atom form the V-shape which is usually drawn for a water molecule.

The carbon dioxide molecule has a simple straight-line shape because the central carbon atom has only two separate sets of electrons (each consisting of four electrons) at the outside of its electron cloud. Repulsion between these two sets of electrons is at a minimum when they are on exactly opposite sides of the carbon atom. Considerations of this sort determine the shapes of all molecules.

Exercise 2.4

Draw representations of the covalent bonding within molecules formed by combination of the following elements. There is no need to indicate the shape of the molecule.

(a) C, H (b) H, S (c) C, O (d) C, Cl (e) N, H

2.6.7 *Exceptions to the Rule*

Our discussion of the structure and bonding in chemical substances is now complete, except for an acknowledgement that not all common substances behave in complete accord with the simple ideas which have been set out above. For example, the element sulphur forms substances in which its atoms share more electrons than is needed for them to obtain the same number as the inert gas argon. Two examples are: sulphur dioxide, SO_2, and sulphuric acid, H_2SO_4. The covalent bonds holding atoms together in molecules of these two substances are represented in Figure 2.14.

Sulphur is not unique in this respect and the ability

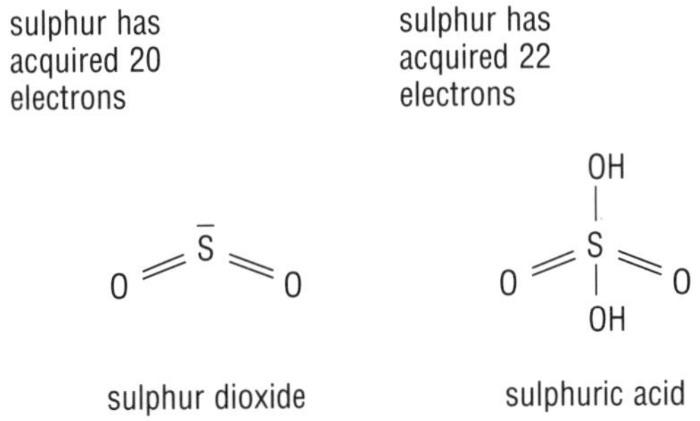

Figure 2.14 *Bonding in sulphur dioxide and sulphuric acid*

to acquire, through sharing, more electrons than the corresponding inert gas atom is a characteristic of many elements found on the right of the Periodic Table in Period 3 and below. Even so, the ideas which have been set out above explain a great deal of the behaviour displayed by the most common elements found in living tissue.

A summary of the main points made so far in this chapter is set out in Figure 2.15.

2.7 Chemical Elements in the Human Body

There are 24 chemical elements which the human body requires in order to function properly. These are known as the **essential elements** and they are listed in Table 2.8. Information concerning the relative amounts of these elements is also presented in Table 2.8 and you will notice that this depends on whether the amount is expressed in terms of numbers of atoms or mass. For example, hydrogen accounts for 63% of all the atoms present in the body and, in this sense, is the most abundant element. However, it only accounts for 9.4% of the body's mass and, in this sense, is less abundant than either carbon or oxygen.

2.7.1 *No Life Without Carbon*

Whichever way the relative amounts of the essential elements are expressed the four most abundant account for more than 94% of the body's material. These are the elements carbon (C), hydrogen (H), nitrogen (N) and oxygen (O). Of these, the most important is carbon even though it accounts for less of the body's mass than oxygen and fewer of the atoms present in the body than either oxygen or hydrogen. The importance of carbon becomes apparent when a comparison is made between the number of compounds which can be obtained from the set of the three elements hydrogen, nitrogen and oxygen and the number which can be obtained from the set of four elements consisting of these same three plus carbon. From the hydrogen, nitrogen, oxygen set the number of compounds obtainable is less than 100. Once carbon is added to this set the number becomes many thousands and it far exceeds the number of compounds formed by any other set of four elements which does not include carbon.

Clearly, there must be something very special about carbon enabling it to form this vast number of different compounds. This is the ability of its atoms to form covalent bonds with each other and so create long

Atoms, Ions and Molecules

Atoms

(Atomic number, isotope mass number, element)

Interaction of two or more of the 90 different atoms which occur naturally.

Molecules

Interaction by **sharing** of electrons between atoms on the right of the Periodic Table.

Molecular covalent compounds

Atoms are organised into small groups called molecules. The atoms within molecules are held tightly together by covalent bonds but since the molecules are electrically neutral overall only weak forces operate between molecules. These compounds have relatively low melting points, do not usually conduct electricity and are usually soluble in organic liquids but not in water. They *may* have noticeable odours.

Ions

Interaction by electron **transfer** between atoms widely separated in the Periodic Table.

Ionic, non-molecular compounds

Consist of oppositely charged particles called ions. These exert strong forces of attraction on each other which cause them to organise themselves into large lattice structures. These compounds have high melting points, usually dissolve in water but not in organic liquids, and conduct electricity when molten or dissolved in water. They have no odour.

Figure 2.15 *A summary of relationships between atoms, ions, molecules, elements and compounds*

chains which may branch at many points and which may include cyclic arrangements. In Chapter 13, 'Organic Compounds, the Basis of Life', there are many examples of structural formulae for organic compounds which illustrate all these possibilities.

The study of carbon compounds constitutes one of the main branches of chemistry, called **organic chemistry**. This name goes back to the start of the nineteenth century when it referred to the chemical compounds produced by living things. It is a name which conveys the sense of living or being derived from life. All the compounds found within living things, or which were excreted by living things, were shown to contain carbon and at first it was considered that these carbon compounds were fundamentally different from compounds found in the non-living world. It was thought that they formed within living things as a result of the action of some vital force and would therefore not be capable of formation in the non-living world. This idea was soon proven wrong when the organic compound **urea**, which is an important component of urine, was made from entirely non-living materials.

By the middle of the nineteenth century it had become accepted that there was no fundamental difference between the compounds produced by living creatures and those found in the non-living world, or produced in a laboratory. The term 'organic chemistry' came to represent the study of all compounds of carbon regardless of their origin and this is the case today. However, there is an important branch of chemistry devoted to the study of the behaviour of chemical compounds within living things and this is known as **biochemistry**.

More will be said about organic chemistry in a separate chapter. For the time being it is sufficient to know that this field of study deals with an enormous number of compounds, nearly all of which contain carbon combined with one or more of the elements hydrogen, nitrogen and oxygen. As far as we can tell,

Table 2.8 *Percentages of the essential elements making up the human body*

Element	Relative amount present in the human body: Percentage of the total number of atoms	Percentage of the total mass
Bulk elements		
hydrogen	63	10
oxygen	26	63
carbon	9	18
nitrogen	1	3
Macrominerals		
calcium		2.4
phosphorus		1.0
potassium, sulphur, chlorine, sodium, magnesium	$\leqslant$1	$\leqslant$1
Trace elements		
iron, cobalt, copper, chromium, fluorine, iodine, molybdenum, silicon, selenium, tin, vanadium, zinc, manganese	$\leqslant$0.01	$\leqslant$0.01

$\leqslant$ means 'less than or equal to'.

carbon is the only element capable of forming the vast number of different compounds needed to perform all the complex functions of life.

2.7.2 *Everlasting Atoms and Natural Cycles*

Nearly every atom present in your body was present on earth when it formed from a cloud of interstellar dust about 4.5 billion (4.5×10^9) years ago. At that time the earth was a most inhospitable place. The temperature at its surface was about 1500 °C compared to –10–40 °C which is the case for most parts of the world today. The atmosphere contained no uncombined (elemental) oxygen, whereas today it consists of about 20% oxygen. Over a period of about 1.5 billion years the earth cooled and the composition of its atmosphere began to change. During this period the first forms of life appeared and the process of evolution began. This process has created the vast array of living things found on earth today. Human beings are among its most recent products, having appeared a mere 130 000 years ago.

It is not only the case that the atoms of your body have always been present on earth. They have also been part of the bodies of countless thousands of other creatures which have lived before you, and they will be part of countless thousands yet to come. Most atoms are truly everlasting and atoms of the essential elements cycle constantly between different living creatures and between the living and non-living worlds. This insight into the nature of the relationship between the earth and the living things on it is expressed in the following words taken from Genesis 3:19: 'You shall gain your bread by the sweat of your brow until you return to the ground; for from it you were taken. Dust you are, to dust you shall return'.

For the two elements carbon and oxygen there is a close relationship between the cycling processes and this is represented in Figure 2.16. Most of the carbon present on earth is in the form of carbonate minerals which account for 99.75% of the element. Carbon in this form is effectively unavailable for use by living things because carbonates are insoluble in water and non-volatile (they do not form a vapour). Once they have been laid down in the earth's crust they remain there forever. The cycling of carbon involves the remaining 0.25%. This is the carbon present as carbon dioxide (CO_2) in the atmosphere, carbon dioxide dissolved in the oceans, rivers and lakes of the earth, carbon in coal and oil deposits and carbon present in all living things. The distribution of carbon among these four pools is as follows:

CO_2 in the atmosphere	3%
CO_2 in the oceans	70%
living matter	3%
coal and oil	24%

Oxygen is by far the most abundant element on earth and most of it is in the form of insoluble, non-volatile compounds, for example the silicate minerals which make up a significant proportion of the earth's crust. Like the carbon contained in the carbonate minerals, this oxygen is largely unavailable for use by living things. The natural cycling of oxygen involves the free element, which comprises 20% of the atmosphere, and the element in combined form as carbon dioxide, water and the organic compounds found in living matter.

The close relationship between the cycling of carbon and oxygen reflects the operation of two processes known as **photosynthesis** and **respiration**. Photosynthesis is a process carried out by plants and some microorganisms. It depends on the complex organic compound **chlorophyll** which these things contain. Chlorophyll enables the plant, or microorganism, to capture the energy in sunlight and use it to convert carbon dioxide and water into the complex organic compound **glucose** ($C_6H_{12}O_6$) and oxygen. The glucose becomes part of the plant and is then used by it to produce many other compounds. The oxygen is released into the atmosphere. Respiration is the reverse of photosynthesis and involves the combination of glucose, or other complex organic compounds, with oxygen to form carbon dioxide and water. In this process energy is released. These two processes may be represented as follows:

Photosynthesis

$$6CO_2 + 6H_2O + \text{energy as sunlight} \xrightarrow{\text{chlorophyll}} C_6H_{12}O_6 + 6O_2$$

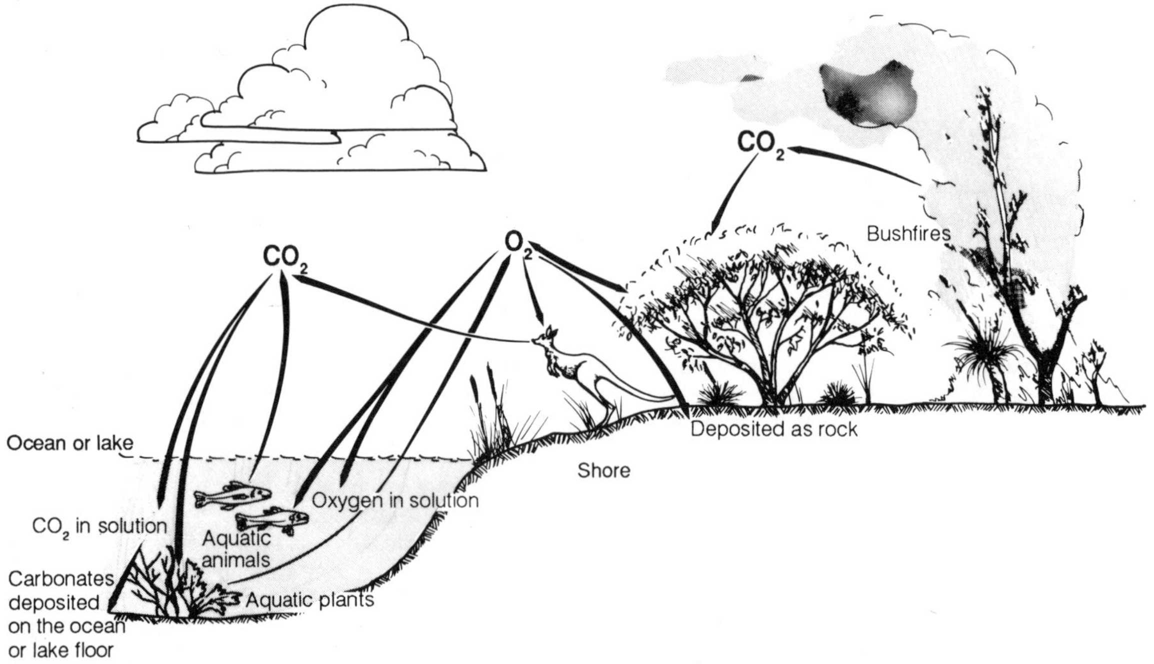

Figure 2.16 *Oxygen–carbon cycle*

Respiration

$$C_6H_{12}O_6 + 6O_2 \longrightarrow 6CO_2 + 6H_2O + \text{energy as heat}$$

It is important to be aware that nearly all living things are involved in the process of respiration. It is through respiration that the energy needed to maintain the life processes becomes available. Photosynthesis, however, is restricted to living things, particularly plants, which contain chlorophyll. Through their photosynthetic activity these plants capture energy from the sun and store it in the form of complex organic chemicals. Respiration makes this energy available to the plants and then to the animals which eat them. It would be possible for plant life to exist without animal life because photosynthesis produces the oxygen which the plant needs for respiration. Animals, however, could not exist without plants because they have no independent means of obtaining the complex organic compounds needed for respiration, or for producing the oxygen which the process also requires.

The essential element nitrogen cycles in quite a different way from carbon and oxygen. The uncombined element comprises about 80% of the atmosphere but very few living things can make use of it in this form. This is in contrast to oxygen which is used in its uncombined form by nearly all plants and animals.

In order to make use of atmospheric nitrogen most living things depend on it first being converted into some combined form such as ammonia (NH_3), the nitrite ion (NO_2^-) or the nitrate ion (NO_3^-). This conversion is known as **nitrogen fixation**. In nature the most important method of nitrogen fixation involves the action of certain microorganisms found in the soil. These often depend upon higher plants for their supplies of nutrient. For example, the class of plants known as the **legumes**, which includes peas, beans, clover and alfalfa, have nitrogen-fixing bacteria which live in close association with their roots. These bacteria convert atmospheric nitrogen into ammonia which is then absorbed by the plant roots and converted into a class of complex organic compounds known as the **amino acids**. Other methods of natural nitrogen fixation are: fixation caused by lightning and fixation caused by the action of the sun's radiation on atmospheric nitrogen. The nitrogen cycle is completed by bacteria known as **denitrifying bacteria** which are capable of producing elemental nitrogen from its fixed forms.

Nitrogen cycles much more slowly than either carbon or oxygen. This is seen by comparing the times taken for one half the available atoms of carbon, oxygen and nitrogen to complete the cycle of movement from the atmosphere into living matter and back to the atmosphere. For carbon this is 100 years, for oxygen 3000 years, but for nitrogen 10^8 years. The slow natural fixation of nitrogen has been supplemented by humans through the practice of planting huge crops of legumes and through the use of an industrial process known as the **Haber Process**. In this process nitrogen and hydrogen are made to react at high temperatures and pressures in the presence of a suitable catalyst (an agent which alters the rate of a chemical process without being permanently altered itself). The product, **ammonia** (NH_3), is then used to manufacture a range of ionic nitrogen compounds for use as fertilisers. These compounds are added to the soil to replace the fixed nitrogen used up as crops are grown and harvested. These activities add about 10% to the amount of nitrogen which is fixed each year and they have had a dramatic impact on the productivity of modern agriculture. Interestingly, but not surprisingly, the Haber Process, which was developed in 1913, was first used to make explosives rather than fertilisers. Without the Haber Process Germany could not have sustained its war effort in the conflict of 1914–18.

2.7.3 *Disturbances in Natural Cycles*

Few people would want to argue against the view that the increase in agricultural productivity made possible by our modern understanding of the nitrogen cycle is a positive thing. However, it is important for us to be aware that even this obviously beneficial development has had some undesirable side effects. For example, in some areas the use of nitrogen fertilisers has led to an excess of nitrate in the soil. All nitrates are soluble and are therefore subject to being washed, by rainfall, into lakes and rivers. If the nitrate levels become too high these bodies of water suffer the effects of **eutrophication**. This occurs when the excess nutrient allows the growth of large numbers of plants and algae. As these organisms die and then decay the concentration of oxygen in the water is depleted to such an extent that it cannot support the normal range of aquatic life. For several centuries this was the case with the lower section of the Thames River in the United Kingdom. In recent times, however, considerable progress has been made in correcting the situation and fish are returning to this part of the Thames.

There have also been cases where infants have suffered nitrite (NO_2^-) poisoning as a result of high levels of nitrate (NO_3^-) present in drinking water. This occurs because bacteria capable of converting nitrate into nitrite may be present in the stomach of an infant. If there is enough nitrate passing through the infant's stomach then a level of nitrite sufficient to cause severe poisoning may be formed. Adults are not usually vulnerable to this sort of poisoning because the contents of an adult's stomach are too acidic to allow the offending bacteria to survive. These two examples illustrate a general truth which is now well known but often ignored: many living things, including human beings, can suffer significant ill-effects when quite minor changes occur in the chemical composition of their surroundings. This is discussed in more detail in Chapter 15, 'Commercial Chemicals and Human Health'.

2.7.4 *Macrominerals and Trace Elements*

The essential elements, other than carbon, hydrogen, nitrogen and oxygen, fall into two groups according to the amounts of them found in the body. Members of the more abundant group are called **macrominerals** and they are required in quantities which range from 0.4 to several grams per day. For each of the macrominerals a number of important roles in body function have been defined.

The element **calcium** is important in the formation of bones and teeth, and 99% of the body's calcium is found in these structures. The remaining 1% is found in soft tissues and body fluids. Calcium affects the contraction of muscles, including the heart, the transmission of nerve impulses and the clotting of blood. It exists in the body as doubly charged positive ions, Ca^{2+}, and another of its functions is to regulate the movement of other positive ions within the body. The main source of calcium in our diets is dairy products.

Phosphorus is also important for the formation of bones and teeth, and 90% of the body's phosphorus is used for this purpose. It is present in teeth and bone in the form of negative phosphate ions, PO_4^{3-}. Other negative ions of phosphorus are important in controlling the acidity of the blood. Covalent, molecular compounds containing phosphorus are important for the supply of energy to cells and the element is also present in many of the complex organic molecules needed for normal cell function. Phosphorus is present in most of the foods that we eat and it is very rare for a person to suffer from any condition caused by an inadequate supply of the element.

The **trace elements** are those listed in Table 2.8 as making up less than about 0.01% of the body's mass and they are required in quantities of less than 0.4 g per day. There are 13 trace elements. Three are non-metals (fluorine, iodine and selenium), one is a metalloid (silicon) and the remainder are metals. The functions performed by some trace elements have not been clearly defined. Silicon, for example, is thought to play some role in bone development but its exact function is unknown.

On the other hand, iron and cobalt are known to be essential components of **haemoglobin** and **vitamin B_{12}** respectively. Haemoglobin is a protein found in the blood and it is responsible for the transport of oxygen to all tissues. Vitamin B_{12} plays a role in the formation of red blood cells. Another trace element having a function which is well understood is iodine. This element is a component of the hormone **thyroxine** which is produced in the thyroid gland. Thyroxine controls the rate at which the body utilises food.

2.7.5 *Deficiency and Toxicity Diseases*

There are some common diseases associated with the levels of certain macrominerals and trace elements present in the body. When the disease is caused by a lower than normal level of the element it is called a **deficiency disease** and when it is caused by a higher than normal level the term **toxicity disease** may be used. **Anaemia** and **goiter** are two examples of a deficiency disease and **Wilson's Disease** is an example of a toxicity disease.

Anaemia. This condition occurs when the level of iron in the body is abnormally low. Its main symptoms are general body weariness and apathy. Anaemia is most common among infants at about six months of age and women in the age group 30–50 years. Its cause may be an iron-deficient diet or an abnormally high rate of loss of iron from the body as may occur during menstruation.

Goiter. This condition occurs when the level of iodine in the body is abnormally low. The most obvious symptom of the disease is an enlarged thyroid gland. Under normal conditions this gland is a small structure located in the neck. In a person suffering from goiter the gland may enlarge to such an extent that it becomes visible as a pronounced swelling of the throat.

Both anemia and goiter can be treated by adjustments in diet to ensure that appropriate amounts of iron or iodine are available.

Wilson's Disease. In this condition the essential element copper builds up to a high level in the body due to its being excreted at a reduced rate. This reduced excretion rate is caused by a genetic abnormality. The excess copper builds up in liver, kidney and brain tissue. If left untreated Wilson's disease leads to mental illness and then death. It can be controlled to some extent by administration of medicines which attach to the copper atoms and promote their excretion in urine.

Bibliography

Bloomfield, Molly M. *Chemistry and the Living Organism* (second edition). John Wiley and Sons, New York, 1980.

McTigue, P. T. (ed.). *Chemistry, Key to the Earth.* Melbourne University Press, Melbourne, 1979.

Questions

1. Which of the following statements about atoms is *false*?
   - J. They are mostly empty space.
   - K. Nearly all their mass is concentrated in the nucleus.
   - L. In a neutral atom protons and electrons are equal in number.
   - M. The nucleus contains equal numbers of protons and neutrons.
2. In which of the following sequences are particles listed in order of increasing size from left to right?
   - J. electron, atom, proton, molecule
   - K. molecule, atom, proton, electron
   - L. atom, proton, electron, molecule
   - M. electron, proton, atom, molecule
3. Which of the following is the name of a sub-atomic particle?
   - J. anion
   - K. cation
   - L. molecule
   - M. neutron
4. Two atoms have the same mass number but different atomic numbers. Which of the following statements concerning these atoms is *true*?
   - J. Each has the same number of neutrons in its nucleus.
   - K. They are isotopes.
   - L. They are atoms of different elements.
   - M. Each has the same number of protons in its nucleus.
5. The element occupying Group VA and Period 4 of the Periodic Table has atomic number
   - J. 33
   - K. 34
   - L. 51
   - M. 52
6. Some atoms of iodine, I, contain 53 protons and 78 neutrons in their nuclei. A correct symbol for these atoms would be:
   - J. $^{131}_{53}I$
   - K. $^{78}_{53}I$
   - L. $^{131}_{78}I$
   - M. $^{53}_{78}I$
7. Which of the following atoms normally forms ions having a single, positive charge?
   - J. Mg
   - K. S
   - L. Cl
   - M. K
8. Which of the following statements concerning isotopes is *false*?
   - J. They contain the same number of protons in their atoms.
   - K. They contain the same number of electrons in their atoms.
   - L. They contain the same number of neutrons in their atoms.
   - M. They have very similar chemical properties.
9. The element nitrogen exists as molecules, N_2. Which of the following representations of the bonding in a molecule of nitrogen is correct?
   - J. N^+N^-
   - K. N–N
   - L. N=N
   - M. N≡N
10. Which of the following properties is least likely to be possessed by a covalent, molecular substance?
    - J. strong odour
    - K. high solubility in water
    - L. melting point above 400 °C
    - M. low electrical conductivity
11. The diagrams below display the covalent bonds present in a series of simple molecules. In which case is the diagram *incorrect*?
    - J. carbon dioxide, O–C–O
    - K. carbon tetrachloride, Cl–C–Cl (with Cl above and Cl below C, each joined to C by a single bond)
    - L. ammonia, H–N–H (with H below N, joined to N by a single bond)

M. water, H–O–H

12. Describe, as fully as you can, the information which is conveyed by the following symbols:

$^{4}_{2}He$ $^{18}_{8}O$ $^{23}_{11}Na$ $^{40}_{19}K$ $^{56}_{26}Fe$

13. A pure compound, which exists as a solid, has a strong odour. Is it more likely to be an ionic compound or a covalent, molecular compound? Explain your answer.

14. Water is a very poor conductor of electricity and yet it is considered hazardous to work with electrical equipment using wet hands or while standing on a wet floor. What makes water a hazardous substance in these circumstances?

15. Comment on the following statement: water melts at a low temperature and therefore the forces holding hydrogen and oxygen atoms together in its molecules must be weak.

16. A substance is a white solid which has no odour and dissolves readily in water. The solution which it forms does not conduct electricity. On the basis of this information state whether you think the compound is ionic or covalent, molecular. Give your reasoning.

17. For each of the covalent, molecular compounds whose formula is written below, draw a diagram which shows the bonds operating between atoms within each molecule.

(a) CS_2 (b) SCl_2
(c) CF_4 (d) NCl_3

18. What is it about the element carbon which makes it so important for living things?

19. In what forms do the elements carbon, oxygen and nitrogen cycle between the living and non-living worlds?

CHAPTER 3

Learning to Speak Chemistry

In Section 1.4, 'The Language and Literature of Science', we described some of the important features of scientific language. We were concerned then with features which applied to all branches of science. In this chapter we will deal with the special features of the language used in chemistry. The basic components of this language are the symbols for the chemical elements and these have already been discussed in Section 2.3.2. A complete set of the symbols for the elements may be found in the Periodic Table inside the front cover. The language of chemistry consists of:

1. the symbols for the chemical elements;
2. a set of rules which govern the ways in which the atomic symbols may be written out in a sequence to create a chemical formula for a pure substance;
3. a set of rules which govern the ways in which the formulae for pure substances may be used to create chemical equations.

Do not be intimidated by the symbolic nature of chemical language. It involves nothing more complicated than simple arithmetic. As has already been pointed out in Section 1.4, quite complicated mathematical relationships are usually capable of expression as fairly simple sentences. This is also the case with relationships involving chemical symbols. There are additional words needed to express these relationships and they are: the names of the chemical elements, combinations and modifications of those names and other terms such as ion, molecule, compound and so on.

Of course, it is not necessary for a nurse to be a fluent speaker or writer of chemistry. Our aim in this book is only to provide an insight into the basis of chemical language. This insight should allow you to be more confident when handling chemical materials and make it easier for you to decide when you have the correct chemical for a particular purpose. Last, but by no means least, a modest understanding of the language of chemistry will make a very big difference in your ability to follow discussions in a wide range of scientific fields.

In this chapter we provide a brief survey of the language used in chemistry. Even so, you may find it a bit daunting, particularly if you have not studied chemistry before. You should not regard the contents of the chapter as something that you need to remember. Instead, you should just be satisfied that it contains the means of understanding what is meant by such terms as molecular formula, empirical formula, mole and equilibrium, and the means of interpreting the symbols, formulae and names used to describe pure substances and their reactions. It is a chapter that you can return to as often as the need arises.

Learning Objectives

At the completion of this chapter you should be able to:

1. Use the chemical formula for a compound to determine the elements which it contains and the ratio in which their atoms are present.
2. Explain the meanings of the terms empirical formula, molecular formula and structural formula.
3. Describe, in a general way, the origins of common names and systematic names for compounds.
4. Use the rules set out in the chapter to decide the name of an inorganic compound given its formula and vice versa. *You should not expect to be able to remember these rules.*
5. Write chemical equations given the correct formulae for the substances involved in the equation.
6. Explain what is meant when chemical reactions are described as having an equilibrium nature.
7. Explain the basis on which chemical reactions are usually classified.
8. Define the terms relative atomic mass, Avogadro constant, relative formula mass and molar mass.
9. Give a definition for the mole and, from the chemical formula for any pure substance, calculate the mass of one mole of the substance.

3.1 Symbols and Formulae

3.1.1 *Elements and Atomic Symbols*

For many centuries the chemical elements, and other substances, were represented by diagrammatic symbols. The symbols used for iron and copper are shown in Figure 3.1. They are the same as those we use today for male and female. The connection between this use for the symbols and their ancient use as symbols for iron and copper is that iron was a very hard metal while copper was, in comparison, soft and yielding. These are characteristics which many people, even today, attribute to men and women respectively. In contrast to this the modern symbols do not attempt to be descriptive of the properties of the elements and are simply shorthand ways of writing their names.

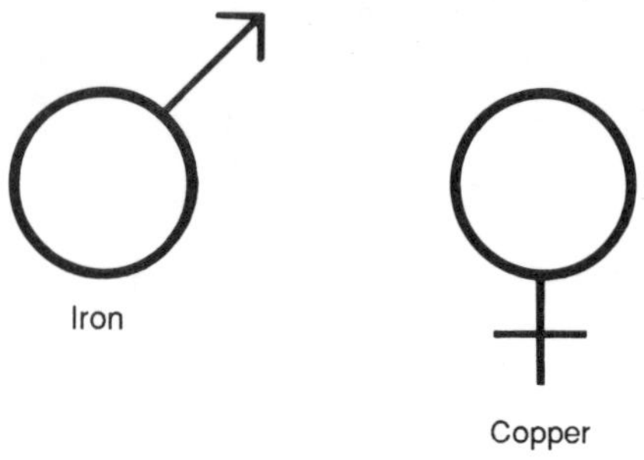

Figure 3.1 *Ancient symbols for iron and copper*

The modern names and symbols for a number of common elements are presented in Table 3.1. No atomic symbol contains more than two letters and the first, or only, letter of the symbol is always upper case while the second letter is always lower case. Remember this whenever you encounter symbols: CL is not the correct symbol for chlorine, and CO is the formula for the compound carbon monoxide, not the symbol for the element cobalt, which must be written as Co.

Table 3.1 *Names and symbols for some chemical elements*

Element	Symbol	Element	Symbol
hydrogen	H	sulphur	S
carbon	C	chlorine	Cl
nitrogen	N	potassium	K
oxygen	O	calcium	Ca
sodium	Na	iron	Fe
magnesium	Mg	copper	Cu
aluminium	Al	bromine	Br
phosphorus	P	iodine	I

Strictly speaking, each atomic symbol represents a single atom of the element. However, the only elements which exist predominantly as single atoms under normal conditions are the inert gases. A few of the other elements exist as molecules containing a small number of atoms joined together and this is the case with H, N, O, P, S, Cl, Br and I. The remaining elements exist as non-molecular materials in which billions of atoms are organised into lattice structures.

The molecular elements are usually represented in a way which makes clear the composition of their molecules. This was done in Table 2.5 by using the appropriate number as a subscript at the right-hand side of the symbol. Thus, from the representation of phosphorus as P_4 we may conclude that it exists as molecules in which four atoms are joined together.

It is quite a simple matter to represent molecules of elements in this way. We only have to deal with one symbol and one number. Even so, it is important to keep in mind that the meaning of a number which accompanies a chemical symbol is dependent on the position which the number occupies in relation to the symbol. For example:

> ^{2}H stands for one atom of the hydrogen isotope of mass number 2, whereas H_2 stands for one molecule of the element hydrogen;
> 2 O stands for two separate atoms of oxygen, but O_2 stands for one molecule of the element oxygen.

For most of the elements listed in Table 3.1 the symbol is obviously derived straight from the element's English name. However, this is not true in all cases. For example, potassium has the symbol K, rather than P or Po, which are the symbols for phosphorus and polonium respectively.The symbol for potassium is derived from the arabic word for the element which is kalium. In many other cases the symbol for an element is derived from its latin name and some examples are presented in Table 3.2.

The non-English names for chemical elements are quite commonly used in medicine. When the concentration of potassium in blood plasma rises above the normal range the condition is called **hyperkalemia**. **Hypokalemia** is the term used for plasma potassium concentrations which are less than normal. In the case of sodium the corresponding conditions are called **hypernatremia** and **hyponatremia**. Another example of the use of these Latin names is the term **plumbism** which is often used to describe cases of lead poisoning. The trade of plumbing owes its name to the fact that, in its early days, it involved the extensive use of metallic lead.

Table 3.2 *Atomic symbols derived from the Latin*

Element	Symbol	Latin name
gold	Au	aurum
copper	Cu	cuprum
mercury	Hg	hydrargyrum
sodium	Na	natrium
lead	Pb	plumbum
tin	Sn	stannum

3.1.2 *Chemical Formulae for Compounds*

Chemical compounds consist of two or more elements joined together so that their atoms are present in fixed ratios. A compound always has properties which are quite different from those of the elements of which it is composed. The chemical formula for a compound must show which elements are present and the ratio of their atoms. We have already made some use of chemical formulae in Chapter 2 and some additional examples are presented in Table 3.3.

Some of the formulae appearing in Table 3.3 are more elaborate than those which we have encountered previously. Nevertheless, any chemical formula, no

Table 3.3 *Chemical formulae for some compounds*

Compound	Formula	Elements present	Ratio of atoms
water	H_2O	H, O	2 : 1
sodium chloride (common salt)	$NaCl$		
carbon dioxide	CO_2		
hydrogen peroxide	H_2O_2		
alcohol	C_2H_6O		
calcium carbonate (limestone)	$CaCO_3$		
calcium phosphate	$Ca_3(PO_4)_2$		
copper sulphate	$CuSO_4.5H_2O$		

matter how elaborate, can be interpreted quite easily. It is only necessary to remember that the significance of a number appearing in a formula depends, in a commonsense way, on its location within the formula, and on what is written immediately to its left. The following rules apply:

1. Any number written as a subscript specifies the number of atoms of the element immediately to its left in the formula. Such a number says nothing about the numbers of atoms of elements appearing elsewhere in the formula. For example, in the formula Na_2CO_3 (sodium carbonate) the 2 means two atoms of sodium and the 3 means three atoms of oxygen.

2. Where a number written as a subscript has a bracket immediately to its left then the number applies to all the elements appearing within the brackets. If there are numbers within the brackets then those numbers are interpreted in accord with rule 1 and multiplied by the number outside the brackets to determine the total number of atoms of each type which are represented in the formula. For example, the formula $Ca(NO_3)_2$ (calcium nitrate) tells us that atoms calcium (Ca), nitrogen (N) and oxygen (O) are present in the ratio of 1 : 2 : 6.

3. When a number appears within a formula on the same level as the symbols for the elements then it applies to all the elements which appear on its right in the formula. Such numbers are usually encountered when chemical equations are being used. They appear at the start of formulae and are called coefficients. There are, however, some cases in which one of these numbers appears within the formula, and an example (copper sulphate) is given in Table 3.3.

Exercise 3.1
The best way to become familiar with the rules which govern the meaning of chemical formulae is to practice their use. See if you can complete Table 3.3.

The formula for hydrogen peroxide deserves some comment. It could be written as HO instead of H_2O_2 and it would still be correct because it does specify the types of atom present in the substance and their ratio (the ratio 1:1 is the same as the ratio 2:2). In the language of chemistry these two formulae are distinguished from each other by saying that HO is the **empirical formula** for hydrogen peroxide while H_2O_2 is its **molecular formula**. In an empirical formula the ratio of atoms is stated as the simplest possible whole number ratio. A molecular formula specifies the actual number of atoms of each type present in each molecule of the substance. Very often the two formulae will be the same, but when they are different, as is the case with hydrogen peroxide, it is the molecular formula which is more commonly used.

3.1.3 *Symbols and Formulae for Ions*

The rules set out above apply to ions as well as molecules. In addition, though, ions have a net electric charge and so their formulae must show the sign and magnitude of the charge (as well as the types of atoms present and their ratio). This is done by using a superscript written to the right of the formula. This superscript consists of a number which represents the size of the charge and a sign which indicates whether the charge is positive or negative. The formulae for a number of common ions are presented in Table 3.4.

Exercise 3.2
Complete Table 3.4.

3.1.4 *Structural Formulae*

So far, the chemical formulae which we have used only provide information about the types of atoms

Table 3.4 *Formulae for some common ions*

Ion	Formula	Charge	Elements present	Ratio of atoms
hydroxide ion	HO^-	–1		
bicarbonate ion	HCO_3^-			
phosphate ion	PO_4^{3-}			
sodium ion	Na^+			
calcium ion	Ca^{2+}			
ammonium ion	NH_4^+			

present in a compound and their ratio. This may not be sufficient to distinguish between different compounds. In Table 3.3 the formula C_2H_6O was given for a compound called alcohol. There is another compound with the same formula which is called dimethyl ether. These two compounds are markedly different in their behaviour and this raises the question of how two compounds containing atoms of the same type, joined in the same ratio, may be different? The answer is that in molecules of these two compounds the atoms are joined to each other in different sequences. These different sequences are shown in Figure 3.2. When the formula of a compound is written out as illustrated in Figure 3.2, or in any manner which makes clear the way in which each atom is joined to the other atoms in one of its molecules, we refer to this as a **structural formula** for the compound.

alcohol dimethyl ether

Figure 3.2 *Structural formulae for alcohol and dimethyl ether*

A structural formula is much more informative than a simple empirical or molecular formula. For this reason structural formulae are used very frequently, and they are quite indispensable for discussions of the nature of important biological molecules. However, structural formulae do have the important disadvantage that they cannot be easily incorporated into normal text. Usually, they must be set apart from it as was done with the formulae for alcohol and dimethyl ether in Figure 3.2.

3.2 Names for Chemical Compounds: Chemical Nomenclature

3.2.1 *Names and Formulae*

You will be well aware that chemical compounds have names as well as formulae. For example, unless you are a very unusual person, you would have heard the substance glucose referred to by that name long before you encountered its formula, $C_6H_{12}O_6$. You probably also talked about water using that name well before learning that the substance has the formula H_2O.

In most cases the name used for a compound is related to its formula in such a way that, knowing the name, one may work out the formula and vice versa. Such a name is known as a systematic name. In other cases, though, the name used for a compound has no relationship to its formula. Such names are called common names and an example is water.

The common names of chemical compounds, and the rules for the formulation of their systematic names, make up an elaborate system. It is not appropriate in a book such as this to attempt to provide a full account of this system. We shall have to be satisfied with a description detailing only its main features. In this chapter we begin with a discussion of common names and go on to describe the systematic methods used for the naming of simple, **inorganic** compounds. This will cover most of the compounds referred to in the next several chapters. The method used for the naming of organic compounds is outlined in Chapter 13, 'Organic Compounds, the Basis of Life'. This method is useful in understanding the relationships which exist between the members of many families of medicines (many medicines are organic compounds).

Common names. These names do not provide much information about the elements present in a compound or the ratio of their atoms. Some examples are given in Table 3.5.

Table 3.5 *Common names and formulae for compounds*

Common name	Formula
water	H_2O
ammonia	NH_3
caustic soda	NaOH
salt	NaCl
limestone	$CaCO_3$
cinnabar	HgO
formic acid	CH_2O_2
acetic acid	$C_2H_4O_2$

Common names form a link between chemical language and ordinary language. Although the names have little meaning as far as the composition of a compound is concerned they often do have a meaning in terms of its source, or its behaviour. This may be illustrated using examples from Table 3.5. The name 'caustic soda' comes from the word 'caustic', meaning a substance that burns or corrodes tissue, and 'soda', meaning a compound of sodium. Thus, its meaning is: a compound of sodium which has a corrosive or burning effect on tissue. The name 'formic acid' is derived from the latin word for ant which is '*formica*'. Formic acid is found in the secretions produced by ants and other insects and it is responsible for much of the pain and damage to tissue caused by their bites.

Common names will always be an important part of the language of chemistry but they have the great practical disadvantage that each name must be remembered separately along with the corresponding formula. The use of common names must therefore be restricted to a relatively small number of compounds in widespread use. But there are millions of different chemical compounds already known and thousands more are discovered each year. Ideally, scientists should be able to talk and write to one another about any one of these compounds and be confident that all parties to the communication are quite clear about the compound's identity. This ideal has been substantially achieved by the adoption of systematic methods for the naming of chemical compounds. The rules used to formulate these names have been devised and authorised by an organisation called the International Union of Pure and Applied Chemistry (IUPAC). They ensure that once a systematic name for a chemical has been correctly written it can be used to work out the elements present, the ratio of their atoms and the manner in which the atoms are joined to each other in the compound.

The methods for naming compounds outlined in the sections immediately below and elsewhere in this book are generally consistent with the IUPAC rules. However, there are some differences in specific cases where substances have common names, or alternative systematic names, which are firmly entrenched.

3.2.2 *Systematic Names for Inorganic Compounds*

Any compound which does not contain the element carbon is an inorganic compound. There are a few additional compounds which are considered to be inorganic even though they do contain carbon, and some examples are calcium carbonate, $CaCO_3$, carbon dioxide, CO_2, and sodium bicarbonate, $NaHCO_3$.

Compounds Formed by the Combination of a Metal with a Non-metal. Systematic names for inorganic compounds always have two parts. For the simplest case of an inorganic compound consisting of only two elements (such compounds are called **binary** compounds) the two parts of the name correspond to these two elements. In the case of any simple ionic compound, where one element will be a metal and the other a non-metal, the name of the metal is written first. The second part of the name consists of a stem derived from the name of the non-metal and the suffix 'ide'. Thus,

KBr has the name potassium bromide,

from the metal — from the non-metal — suffix

$CaCl_2$ has the name calcium chloride.

You may be wondering why $CaCl_2$ does not have the name calcium dichloride to show that it has two chlorine atoms in its formula. The reason for this is that calcium always forms ions with two positive charges and so it can only form one compound with chlorine. Whenever this is the case it is considered unnecessary to specify the number of atoms of any particular type which are present in the formula. It is assumed that the reader will know this or be able to work it out.

There are some metals which may form more than one ion and in these cases it is necessary to provide something in the name which will allow the reader to decide which one is meant. There are two methods commonly used to do this. One of these methods makes use of roman numerals to indicate the charge on the metal ion. The other method differentiates between metal ions of different charge by means of the suffixes 'ic' and 'ous'. These suffixes are added to a stem obtained from the name of the metal atom. The suffix 'ic' is used for the ion of higher charge and 'ous' for the ion of lower charge. Both systems are illustrated by the examples presented in Table 3.6.

The use of suffixes is much less satisfactory than the use of roman numerals. For example, a suffix does not reveal the actual charge on the ion and this must simply be remembered. Thus, one must remember that the ferric ion has a charge of 3+ but the cupric ion has a charge of 2+. In addition to this there is the fact that, in some cases, the name used for the metal is derived from its usual name but in others it is derived from the latin name. For these reasons it is almost certain that the use of suffixes for metal ions of different charge will give way entirely to the use of roman numerals. In the meantime, however, both types of systematic name are quite likely to be encountered.

Compounds Formed by the Combination of Two Different Non-metals. These compounds are relatively few in number and the most frequently encountered system for naming them makes use of the Greek prefixes **mono** (one), **di** (two), **tri** (three), **tetra** (four), **penta** (five) and so on. The part of the name written first is that corresponding to the element further to the left and lower in the periodic table. It consists of the Greek prefix standing for the number of atoms of that element appearing in the formula, and the name of the element. However, the prefix mono is omitted when there is only one atom of this element appearing in the formula.

The second part of the name is obtained by adding the appropriate greek prefix to a stem derived from the name of the other element and then adding the suffix 'ide' to this. Some examples of names and formulae which illustrate this system of naming are presented in Table 3.7.

Table 3.7 *Formulae and systematic names for compounds of non-metals*

Formula	Name
CO_2	carbon dioxide
CO	carbon monoxide
SO_3	sulphur trioxide
N_2O_4	dinitrogen tetraoxide
P_2S_5	diphosphorus pentasulphide

Compounds of a Metal Joined with Two or More Non-metals. Most of the commonly encountered compounds in this category are ionic compounds in which the positive ion is a simple metal ion. The negative ion usually consists of several atoms joined together by covalent bonds but having a net, negative charge (such ions are often called **polyatomic anions**). Formulae and names for some of the more common ions of this type are given in Table 3.8. You will notice that all the ions listed have names which end in either 'ate' or 'ite'. These endings are used for the names of all polyatomic anions containing oxygen. The atoms other than oxygen which are present usually determine the first part of the name. The endings 'ate' and 'ite' are used to distinguish between anions in which the same type of atom is joined to oxygen but in a different ratio. The name of the ion with the higher proportion of oxygen present ends in 'ate' and the name of the other ends in 'ite'.

In Table 3.8 the names bicarbonate and bisulphate have been given as alternatives to hydrogencarbonate and hydrogensulphate respectively. These alternatives are very commonly encountered and the name bicarbonate is used more frequently than hydrogencarbonate even though it is less systematic.

The methods used to name inorganic compounds which contain polyatomic anions are exactly the same as those used to name binary ionic compounds. When the metal forms only one type of ion, the first part of the name is simply the name of the metal and the second part of the name is the name of the polyatomic anion. Thus: the compound $NaNO_3$ has the name sodium nitrate, and the compound $MgCO_3$ has the name magnesium carbonate.

Table 3.6 *Formulae, systematic names for inorganic compounds in which the charge on the metal ion is variable*

Formula	Systematic name, roman numerals	Systematic name, suffixes, 'ic', 'ous'	Charge on metal ion
$FeCl_2$	iron(II) chloride	ferrous chloride	2+
$FeCl_3$	iron(III) chloride	ferric chloride	3+
Cu_2O	copper(I) oxide	cuprous oxide	1+
CuO	copper(II) oxide	cupric oxide	2+
$CrBr_2$	chromium(II) bromide	chromous bromide	2+
$CrBr_3$	chromium(III) bromide	chromic bromide	3+

Table 3.8 *Formulae and names for polyatomic anions*

Formula	Name
CO_3^{2-}	carbonate
HCO_3^-	hydrogencarbonate (bicarbonate)
NO_2^-	nitrite
NO_3^-	nitrate
PO_4^{3-}	phosphate
HPO_4^{2-}	monohydrogenphosphate
$H_2PO_4^-$	dihydrogenphosphate
MnO_4^-	permanganate
$C_2O_4^{2-}$	oxalate
SO_3^{2-}	sulphite
SO_4^{2-}	sulphate
HSO_4^-	hydrogensulphate (bisulphate)

When the metal can form ions which have different charges then the different possibilities are distinguished using roman numerals or the suffixes 'ic', 'ous'. Some examples have been presented in Table 3.9 and you can compare them with the names for binary compounds which appear in Table 3.6 to verify that the names have been formulated in the same general way.

Table 3.9 *Formulae, systematic names for compounds containing polyatomic anions and metal ions of variable charge*

Formula	Systematic name, roman numerals	Systematic name, suffixes 'ic', 'ous'
$FeSO_3$	iron(II) sulphite	ferrous sulphite
$Fe_2(SO_4)_3$	iron(III) sulphate	ferric sulphate
$CuNO_2$	copper(I) nitrite	cuprous nitrite
$Cu(NO_3)_2$	copper(II) nitrate	cupric nitrate
$Cr_3(PO_4)_2$	chromium(II) phosphate	chromous phosphate
$Cr(H_2PO_4)_3$	chromium(III) dihydrogenphosphate	chromic dihydrogenphosphate

3.3 Chemical Equations

A chemical equation is a shorthand method used to describe chemical changes (changes in which new compounds are formed). As an example, let us consider the burning of carbon. In words, this chemical change could be described as the combination of carbon with oxygen to form carbon dioxide. As a chemical equation it would be written:

$$\underset{\text{carbon}}{C} + \underset{\text{oxygen}}{O_2} \longrightarrow \underset{\text{carbon dioxide}}{CO_2}$$

In a chemical equation the materials appearing to the left of the arrow are called **reactants** and the materials appearing to the right are called **products**. So, carbon and oxygen are reactants while carbon dioxide is the product.

You may be wondering why the term 'equation' has been used to describe this type of symbolic statement since equations usually include an equals sign. As a matter of fact, you will occasionally find a writer who does use an equals sign, instead of an arrow, but this is normally avoided because the two sides of the equation are not literally equal. A mixture of carbon and oxygen (the reactants) is not the same as carbon dioxide (the product).

However, there is one important respect in which the reactants are always equal to the products. During chemical reactions atoms are never created or destroyed and so the number of atoms of a particular type present in the reactant materials will always equal the number of atoms of that type present in the products. To reflect this, a chemical equation should have the same total number of atoms of each type appearing on both of its sides. Such an equation is said to be **balanced**. The equation above is balanced and writing it in the balanced form simply involved writing the correct formula/symbol for each substance involved. However, writing a balanced equation is often not as easy as this. Consider, for example, the reaction of oxygen with hydrogen to form water.

$$\underset{\text{hydrogen}}{H_2} + \underset{\text{oxygen}}{O_2} \longrightarrow \underset{\text{water}}{H_2O}$$

This is not a balanced equation because there are two atoms of oxygen to the left of the arrow and only one to the right. A balanced form of the equation would be:

$$2H_2 + O_2 \longrightarrow 2H_2O$$

A novice chemistry student will often try to balance the equation by writing:

$$H_2 + O_2 \longrightarrow H_2O_2$$

This is quite wrong! Although the equation has been balanced it now describes a different reaction in which the product is hydrogen peroxide (H_2O_2) and not water. Obtaining a balanced equation involves the following steps:

1. Write the correct formula/symbol for each of the substances involved in the reaction, making sure that reactants and products are placed on the correct side of the equation.
2. Adjust the coefficient for each formula/symbol until the number of atoms of each type appearing on both sides of the equation is the same. For many equations this step can be done by inspection.

Exercise 3.3

In the table below you are provided with names and formulae for the reactants and products involved in several different reactions. See if you can write balanced equations for these reactions.

Reactants	Products	Balanced equations
1.		
carbon dioxide, CO_2	glucose, $C_6H_{12}O_6$	
water, H_2O	oxygen, O_2	
2.		
urea, CON_2H_4	ammonia, NH_3	
water, H_2O	carbon dioxide, CO_2	
3.		
calcium hydroxide, $Ca(OH)_2$	calcium chloride, $CaCl_2$	
hydrogen chloride, HCl	water, H_2O	

3.4 Types of Chemical Reaction

In chemical reactions, atoms rearrange themselves to form new substances, and chemical reactions may be classified according to the type of atom rearrangement which occurs. In this book the main types of reaction with which we shall be concerned as we discuss the body's chemical activity are: precipitation, oxidation–reduction, acid–base, hydrolysis and conjugation. Each of these reaction types is described below, but only in brief terms. More detail is provided, as necessary, in later chapters where there is some discussion of the role played in body function by reactions of that particular type.

Precipitation reactions. The word precipitate is used in ordinary language to describe a rapid change in circumstances: 'by working hard over many years he was able to accumulate great wealth, but the stock-market crash of October 1987 served to precipitate his ruin'. In chemistry the word precipitate is also used to describe a rapid change in circumstances. It refers to the formation of insoluble material from a solution. One or more components of the solution changes from being dispersed throughout the solution to being part of a solid or liquid which has separated from the solution. A precipitation reaction is one in which ions in a solution combine to form an insoluble ionic compound which separates from the solution. These reactions often occur very rapidly. An example is the formation of calcium oxalate which takes place when a solution containing oxalate ions is mixed with a solution containing calcium ions.

This reaction is put to use in the treatment of poisoning by oxalate compounds. A person who has swallowed one of these compounds may be given a preparation of calcium which causes precipitation of the oxalate thereby removing it from solution and preventing its absorption into the circulation. The precipitate of calcium oxalate is then removed from the stomach by vomiting or by **gastric lavage**. This is a technique in which a solution is introduced into the stomach via a tube inserted through the mouth (or nose) and eosophagus. After the solution has had an opportunity to mix with the contents of the stomach the mixture formed is withdrawn through the tube. In the equation for the formation of calcium oxalate, an arrow, pointing downwards, appears alongside the formula of calcium oxalate. This is a common method used to indicate that a substance has precipitated from solution.

$$C_2O^{2-}_{4aq} \quad + \quad Ca^{2+}_{aq} \longrightarrow CaC_2O_4 \downarrow$$

oxalate ion   calcium ion   calcium oxalate

An arrow alongside a formula and pointing upwards indicates that the substance is a gas which escapes from the reaction mixture as it forms. Thus:

$$2Na \; + 2H_2O \longrightarrow 2NaOH \; + \; H_2 \uparrow$$

sodium   water   sodium hydroxide   hydrogen

If you look back at the equation for the formation of calcium oxalate you will notice that the ions on the left-hand side of the equation have the subscript 'aq' written alongside. This subscript stands for 'aquo' meaning water and it has been written alongside the formulae of the ions present in solution to emphasise that when an ion is dissolved in water it attracts nearby water molecules and becomes associated with them. As each ion moves about in the solution these water molecules are carried with it.

Acid–Base Reactions. With this class of reaction the rearrangement of atoms which occurs is a transfer of an H^+ particle from one molecule or ion to another. The molecule or ion which loses the H^+ is called the acid and that which gains the H^+ is called the base. An acid can only act as an acid and give up an H^+ particle if a base is present which can accept it. This is why we use the term acid–base reaction rather than talk separately about acid reactions and base reactions.

Oxidation–Reduction Reactions. This class of reaction may be defined in a number of ways. We shall define it in terms of loss or gain of the atoms oxygen or hydrogen. Oxidation is combination with oxygen or loss of hydrogen. Reduction is loss of oxygen or combination with hydrogen. Just as an acid can only react as an acid when a base is present, so oxidation and reduction can only occur together and we usually talk about oxidation–reduction reactions rather than separate oxidation reactions and reduction reactions. An example is the reaction of the cyanide ion with the permanganate ion.

$$5CN^-_{aq} \quad + \quad 2MnO^-_{4aq} \quad + \quad 6H_3O^+_{aq} \longrightarrow$$

cyanide ion   permanganate ion   hydronium ion

$$5CNO^-_{aq} \; + \; 2Mn^{2+}_{aq} \; + \; 9H_2O$$

cyanate ion   manganese (II) ion

This is another reaction which can be used in the treatment of poisoning. Cyanide compounds are very toxic and when a person has swallowed a cyanide compound they can be given a dilute solution of potassium permanganate. This causes the above oxidation–reduction reaction to occur in the stomach. The toxic cyanide is oxidised to the much less toxic cyanate and the permanganate is reduced to manganese(II) ions. Unfortunately, cyanide compounds are often so toxic that death occurs well before this action, or any other, can be taken.

Hydrolysis Reactions. This class of reaction always has water as one of the reagents. The prefix 'hydro' means water and this accounts for the first part of the name. In hydrolysis reactions the water reacts with some other molecule, breaking it into two or more parts. The biological term for the breaking of a large structure into smaller components is 'lysis' and this accounts for the second part of the name. Hydrolysis reactions are very important, and very common, in biological systems. An example is the conversion of maltose into glucose.

$$C_{12}H_{22}O_{11} \; + \; H_2O \longrightarrow C_6H_{12}O_6 + C_6H_{12}O_6$$

maltose   water   glucose

Conjugation reactions. These are reactions in which molecules join with each other to form a larger molecule. In ordinary language the words conjugal and conjugate are used to convey a sense of two things or two people being joined together, and so the term conjugation reaction is another illustration of the fact that scientific language has grown out of ordinary language. Many drugs entering the body undergo conjugation reactions in which they join with molecules already present in tissues. This process is particularly common in the liver and an example is the conjugation of paracetamol with glucuronic acid. An equation for this particular conjugation reaction could be written as:

$$C_8H_9NO_2 \quad + \quad C_6H_{10}O_7 \longrightarrow$$

paracetamol   glucuronic acid

$$C_8H_8NO_2{-}C_6H_9O_6 \; + \; H_2O$$

paracetamol glucuronide   water

If you compare this equation with the one written for the hydrolysis of maltose you will notice that the conjugation reaction is an hydrolysis reaction in reverse.

3.5 The Mole: Fundamental Unit for Amount of Chemical

In everyday transactions we measure the amounts of substances in units such as the kilogram (kg) for mass or the litre (l) for volume. We have many devices which we can use to perform these measurements and a knowledge of the amount of substance in kilograms or litres is sufficient for most everyday purposes. We are all quite happy to pay for our petrol by the litre, our meat by the kilogram and so on. We all know that recipes for the preparation of food specify the quantities of the ingredients in these same units or others which are closely related to them.

However, for many scientific purposes measurement of the amount of chemical as so many kilograms or litres is not appropriate. The reason for this is that matter consists of particles (atoms, molecules or ions) and the changes which matter undergo are changes in which these particles interact with each other. These changes are controlled by the *numbers* of particles which are involved and the mass which those particles have or the volume which they occupy are much less important.

In science, then, we need a way of knowing how many particles there are in a sample of a substance. Unfortunately, for all substances which are not gases we have no way of directly measuring the number of particles which are present in a sample. This brings us to the mole.

3.5.1 *Avogadro's Number and a Definition for the Mole*

What is a mole? It is not a gangster's girlfriend (that is spelt 'moll') and it is not a high-ranking official in the British Ministry of Defence. *A mole is an amount of substance which contains a fixed number of chemical units*. The fixed number is 6×10^{23} and it is called the 'Avogadro Constant' or 'Avogadro's Number' in honour of the Italian scientist, Amadeo Avogadro (1776–1856), who was the first person to understand clearly the difference between atoms and molecules. Avogadro's number is the number of atoms present in exactly 12 g of the carbon isotope, $^{12}_{6}C$. It also turns out to be the number of atoms present in a sample of any element which has a mass, in grams, equal to the element's relative atomic mass. This property indicates the average mass of atoms of the element compared to that of other atoms. For example, the relative atomic mass of oxygen is sixteen and that of hydrogen is about one. These values indicate that an oxygen atom has a mass about sixteen times as great as the mass of a hydrogen atom.

The term 'chemical units' used in the definition of the mole means the set of atoms represented by the formula of the substance. A chemical unit may be an atom, a molecule, an ion or a collection of ions.

It is worth saying something about the magnitude of Avogadro's number. It may not appear to be very large when it is written as 6×10^{23} and a better impression of its size is obtained by writing it as 600 000 000 000 000 000 000 000. The magnitude of Avogadro's number is well beyond direct human experience. If you have been to the Melbourne Cricket Ground on the Victorian Football League's grand final day you have some direct experience of the number 10^5 (one hundred thousand) because that is the number of people who attend that sporting fixture and most of them can be seen from many parts of the ground. If you have been in Rome at Easter time you may have some direct experience of the number 10^6 (one million) because that many people have sometimes assembled to hear the Pope's Easter message. Our commonsense tells us that 10^5 and 10^6 are large numbers but they are tiny in comparison to Avogadro's number which is so big that we can only imagine it.

3.5.2 *Obtaining a Mole of a Pure Substance*

It is one thing to say that a mole is a sample of substance which contains 6×10^{23} chemical units and another thing altogether actually to obtain such a sample. However, there is a simple procedure which can be followed to obtain a mole of any pure substance *provided that its formula is known*. This procedure makes use of relative atomic mass values and it relies on the fact that in a sample of any element which has a mass in grams equal to its relative atomic mass, Avogadro's number of atoms are present.

Let us take water as an example. This has the formula H_2O and a mole of water is a sample which contains 6×10^{23} water molecules (these are the chemical units referred to in the definition of the mole).

Each water molecule contains two hydrogen atoms and one oxygen atom. Therefore, a mole of water may be said to consist of 12×10^{23} hydrogen atoms and 6×10^{23} oxygen atoms which just happen to be joined to each other to form water molecules.

The relative atomic mass of hydrogen is 1.008 and this is the mass, in grams, of 6×10^{23} hydrogen atoms.

Our mole of water contains twice this many hydrogen atoms and so the mass of hydrogen present in the water will be 2.016 g. Using the same reasoning and 16.000 as the relative atomic mass of oxygen we find that our mole of water contains 16.000 g of oxygen. Thus the total mass of a mole of water is 2.016 + 16.000 = 18.016 g. This is a number of grams which we have simply obtained by adding the relative atomic mass values for all the atoms appearing in the formula of water. The same line of reasoning is applicable to any pure substance for which the formula is known and so can be used to calculate the mass of one mole. From now on we shall refer to the sum of the relative atomic mass values for all atoms appearing in a formula as the **relative formula mass** of the substance. We are now in a position to define the mole in a way which makes it much easier to handle:

> A mole of any substance is a sample which has a mass, in grams, equal to the relative formula mass of the substance.

The usefulness of this definition of the mole is illustrated by two examples set out below.

A mole of aspirin

1. The formula of aspirin is $C_9H_8O_4$.
2. The relative atomic mass values for the elements present in aspirin are: C, 12.011; H, 1.008; O, 16.000.
3. The relative formula mass for aspirin is the sum of all these relative atomic mass values: $9 \times 12.011 + 8 \times 1.008 + 4 \times 16.000 = 180.163$.
4. A mole of aspirin has a mass of 180.163 g. Rounded off to four significant figures this becomes 180.2 g.

A mole of calcium chloride

1. The formula of calcium chloride is $CaCl_2$.
2. The relative atomic mass values for the elements present in calcium chloride are: Ca, 40.08; Cl, 35.45.
3. The relative formula mass for calcium chloride is the sum of these relative atomic mass values: $40.08 + 2 \times 35.45 = 110.98$.
4. A mole of calcium chloride has a mass of 110.98 g (111.0 g to four significant figures).

If we refer to the mass of a mole of any substance as its **molar mass** then the relationship between the mass of a sample of any pure substance and the number of moles which it contains is:

$$\text{number of moles} = \frac{\text{mass in grams}}{\text{molar mass}}$$

This relationship can be used to change a number of moles into a number of grams and vice versa. For example:

0.600 mole of aspirin, how many grams?

$$\text{number of moles} = \frac{\text{mass in grams}}{\text{molar mass}}$$
$$0.600 = \frac{\text{mass in grams}}{180.2}$$
$$0.600 \times 180.2 = \text{mass in grams}$$
$$\text{mass in grams} = 108 \text{ (three significant figs)}$$

200.0 grams of calcium chloride, how many moles?

$$\text{number of moles} = \frac{\text{mass in grams}}{\text{molar mass}}$$
$$\text{number of moles} = \frac{200.0}{111.0}$$
$$= 1.802 \text{ (four significant figs)}$$

In later chapters of this book extensive use is made of the mole and other units closely related to it. You should simply regard the mole as being another unit, besides kilogram and litre, which is used to measure the amount of substance. It has the advantage of providing information about the number of atoms, molecules or ions that are present in the sample. As a nurse there is no need for you to be able to perform extensive calculations using the mole but you should understand the general nature of the unit and the reasons for its use. In this section we have attempted to make the general nature of the mole clear and in later chapters where the unit is used you should develop an appreciation of its importance.

3.6 The Equilibrium Nature of Chemical Reactions

In the previous section we talked about chemical reactions as processes in which certain pure substances (reactants) changed into different pure substances (products). However, this change is usually a two-way change and once the products of a reaction are present in significant quantity they begin to re-form the reactants. Let us consider, as an example, the reaction which takes place when hydrogen gas (H_2) and iodine gas (I_2) are heated together. They form a new substance, hydrogen iodide (HI). The hydrogen and iodine are reactants, hydrogen iodide is the product. The reaction could be represented as:

$$\underset{\text{hydrogen}}{H_2} + \underset{\text{iodine}}{I_2} \longrightarrow \underset{\text{hydrogen iodide}}{2HI}$$

However, the reaction does not continue until all the reactants are gone. After a while, a situation is reached where there are significant quantities of the two reactants **and** the product present in the reaction mixture. Furthermore, these quantities stay the same indefinitely (provided the reaction system is not changed by altering the temperature or by addition of extra substance). It is as if the reaction has stopped. However, it can be shown that the hydrogen and iodine are still combining to form hydrogen iodide. The reason their quantities remain the same is that the hydrogen iodide is also reacting to re-form them. This process could be represented as:

$$2HI \longrightarrow H_2 + I_2$$

When the hydrogen and iodine are first mixed their quantities are relatively high and they react at a relatively fast rate to form hydrogen iodide. This immediately begins to react and re-form the hydrogen and iodine. In the early stages of the reaction, though, the quantity of hydrogen iodide is very low and so its rate of reaction is low. During this period there is a net conversion of reactants into product. However, as time goes by, the quantities of the reactants decline and their rate of conversion into products also declines. During the same time the quantity of the product increases and its rate of conversion into reactants also increases. Eventually the rates of the two opposing processes become the same and beyond that point there is no further change in the quantity of any of the substances involved in the reaction. All of this is displayed, in graphical form, in Figure 3.3. In the situation portrayed in Figure 3.3 equal numbers of moles of hydrogen and iodine have been mixed to begin with.

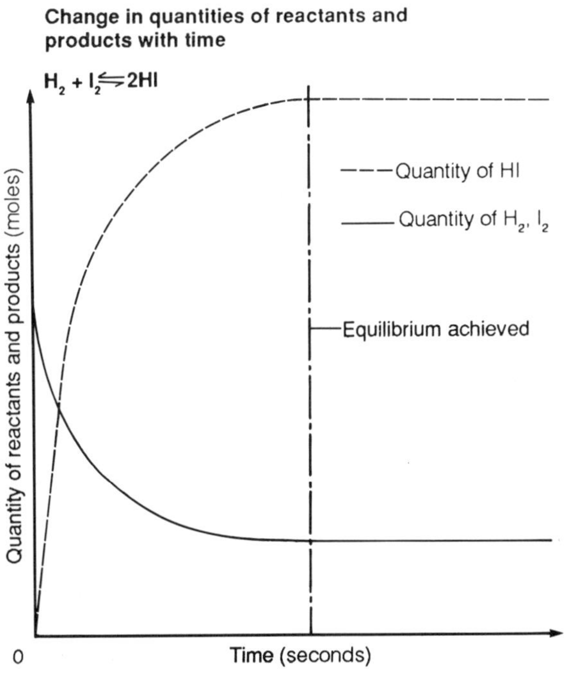

Figure 3.3 *Variation in concentrations of reactants and products with time*

This behaviour is described by saying that the reaction has reached **equilibrium** and, provided that no reactant or product escapes from the system in which a reaction is occurring, every chemical process eventually reaches an equilibrium position. In some cases the amounts of *reactants* left when equilibrium is reached are so small that the equilibrium aspect of the reaction can be ignored. There are other reactions where the amounts of *products* present at equilibrium are so small that the reaction is regarded as having not taken place.

The question which arises now is: 'How can we indicate that a reaction reaches an equilibrium position'? The common method used is to draw two arrows between the reactants and products and use their lengths to show whether, at equilibrium, there are greater quantities of reactants or products present. From Figure 3.3 you can see that when hydrogen and iodine reach equilibrium with hydrogen iodide more than half the reactants are used up. We would say that this equilibrium *favours the formation of products* and represent it as:

$$H_2 + I_2 \xrightleftharpoons[\leftarrow]{\longrightarrow} 2HI$$

This method of representation will be used from now on wherever the equilibrium nature of a reaction needs to be emphasised.

Bibliography

The Association for Science Education. *Chemical Nomenclature, Symbols and Terminology.* The Association for Science Education, Hatfield, England, 1972.

Petrucci, R. H. *General Chemistry, Principles and Modern Applications* (third edition). Macmillan Publishing Company, New York, 1982.

Questions

1. Ethane is a compound which has a formula C_2H_6. Is this an empirical formula or a molecular formula? Explain your answer. Draw a structural formula for ethane.
2. What is the identity of the elements and the ratio of their atoms in each of the following compounds?
   (a) $CHCl_3$ (b) $NaHCO_3$
   (c) CON_2H_4 (d) $Cu(NO_3)_2$
   (e) H_3PO_4 (f) CH_3CO_2H
3. Refer to Section 3.2.2 and write systematic names which correspond to the following formulae.
   (a) NO_2 (b) CrO
   (c) Cr_2O_3 (d) Na_2CO_3
   (e) K_2HPO_4 (f) $NaMnO_4$
4. Refer to Section 3.2.2 and write formulae which correspond to the following systematic names.
   (a) potassium phosphate
   (b) sodium oxalate
   (c) phosphorus pentachloride
   (d) diphosphorus trioxide
   (e) carbon monoxide
   (f) manganese(II) chloride
5. Balance the following equations
   (a) $N_2 + H_2 \longrightarrow NH_3$
   (b) $CH_4 + O_2 \longrightarrow CO_2 + H_2O$
6. Calculate the mass of one mole of each of the following compounds.
   (a) paracetamol, $C_8H_9NO_2$
   (b) calcium hydroxide, $Ca(OH)_2$
   (c) Ammonium chloride, NH_4Cl
   (d) benzoic acid, $C_7H_6O_2$

CHAPTER 4

Biomechanics

Mechanics refers to the study of how things move and what causes them to move. Biomechanics, more specifically, is the study of the motions produced by the body's musculoskeletal system. Scientists have successfully described the causes of motion in terms of 'forces' so this chapter will invest some time in developing an understanding of what force is. Having defined a force we will introduce the concepts that are essential to the understanding of mechanics. These include mass, weight, inertia, friction, gravity, work, speed, distance, time, vectors and scalars. We will demonstrate how these concepts are drawn together by Newton's laws and are used to describe the actions of simple machines. Upon this foundation, we will be able to build an understanding of the forces produced by the muscles of the body, the interaction of the muscles and the skeleton as a system of levers and of hospital traction systems.

Learning Objectives

At the completion of this chapter you should be able to:

1. Explain the concept of force.
2. Define the terms force, mass, weight, gravity, centre of gravity, base of support and work.
3. Know the symbols and units for the quantities called force, mass, weight and work.
4. Describe some situations in terms of Newton's laws of motion.
5. Understand that force is a quantity with a direction.
6. Understand the forces of friction and tension.
7. Identify the location of the fulcrum, the load and the effort for some body levers.
8. Apply a knowledge of levers, pulleys and muscle tension to the action of muscles on bones and to traction systems.
9. Explain correct lifting technique in terms of levers, force, centre of gravity and base of support.

4.1 The Concept of Force

The concept of force arose out of the desire to explain the way things moved. For the first natural philosophers, explaining why the sun, moon and known planets moved in the regular way they did was a considerable problem. The sun moved across the sky each day without fail and without slowing down. On the other hand, objects on earth only moved when considerable effort was used on them. It seemed that 'heavenly bodies' could somehow keep moving without obvious propulsion, but objects on the earth soon stopped if the cause of their motion was removed. For a long time it was believed that what happened in the 'perfect' heavens, the abode of the Gods, was somehow fundamentally different from what could occur on the 'imperfect' earth, where the base creatures called humans existed.

4.1.1 *Aristotle's Contribution*

Aristotle was one of the most famous of the Greek philosophers and educators and one of the first recognised 'scientists'. For the 2000 years from his time (about 340 BC), Aristotle's notion that 'a moving body comes to a standstill when the force which pushes it along no longer acts to push it' was believed. This statement in fact describes our everyday experience, that balls eventually stop rolling, that bicycles come to a stop sometime after pedalling ceases and that cars need to have the 'accelerator' pedal depressed if they are to continue moving without slowing down. Thus it is not surprising that Aristotle's views held sway for so long, or that present-day students of physics still need the falseness of Aristotle's statement explained to them.

Aristotelians (those holding to Aristotle's teaching) further believed that a constant force was needed to keep things moving at a constant speed and that an increasing force was needed for acceleration.

Thus it was Aristotle who introduced the idea that the natural state of objects was to remain motionless and that *a force was that influence* that produced motion. This statement about force, inadequate though it is, can serve as the starting point for the development of our understanding of what a force is.

Aristotle's ideas produced what today seem like bizarre explanations of the continued motions of the sun and moon, of puffs of smoke and of other observed phenomena within the experience of Aristotle's students. The planets were drawn across the sky by heavenly chariots and followed by teams of angels beating their wings. The continued flight of an arrow, long after it had left the propulsive force of the bow string behind was due to the movement of the air as it closed in behind the arrow after it had passed. Galileo Galilei (1564–1642) challenged many of the Aristotelian ideas about motion and gravity, pronouncing that it was better to say 'I know it not' rather than to invent extravagent explanations.

4.1.2 *Galileo's Contribution*

Galileo stopped asking 'what keeps things moving' and instead asked 'what causes moving objects to stop?'. He also conducted experiments (something that Aristotle had not done) with polished, perfectly spherical balls rolling down tilted smooth tracks. Galileo had the correct notion that contact between the ball and track produced friction and reduced the motion, so he took steps to eliminate the friction and so test his notion. He timed the ball's movement with a 'water clock' (accurate mechanical clocks were not yet available). From his experiments Galileo was able to conclude that the balls eventually came to a standstill because of frictional forces between the ball and track and between the ball and the air.

If the frictional forces could be removed, the ball would go on forever. The sun and moon go on forever because they encounter no friction. Galileo asserted that a stationary body stays that way and that a moving body goes on moving in a straight line if there is no other force acting on it. This assertion is known as Galileo's law of inertia. Later Newton restated it as his first law of motion. It was left to Newton also to explain why the sun and moon *did not* move in a straight line but continually circulated around the earth.

Thus Galileo introduced the idea that *a force was what caused motion to start, to stop or to alter in direction.* For Galileo, the 'natural state' of an object was to maintain constant its magnitude and direction of speed. Whether the speed had a zero or non-zero value, a force was necessary to alter it. He had used gravity, acting on rolling spheres, as a convenient force in his investigation of motion and its cause.

4.1.3 *Newton's Contribution*

The study of gravity (the first of the fundamental forces to be extensively investigated) was considerably extended by Isaac Newton. So much so that his name is synonymous with gravitation and indeed is the name of the unit of force.

Newton found it desirable to describe the observed motions and interactions of moving bodies in terms of the three fundamental quantities of mass, length, and time. From these and a set of principles that gave a consistent account of his observations, Newton introduced a fourth quantity, called force, and defined it in his second law, force = mass × acceleration. For Newton, *a force was the result of an action.*

In the period 1665 to 1667, Newton devoted much thought to his theories of light and of gravitation and planetary motion. He was able, through calculation, to prove that the force that caused objects to fall towards the earth was the same as the force which caused the moon to 'fall' towards the earth. By 1684 Newton had proved, using the mathematical technique of calculus which he had devised for the purpose, that the force between the sun and planets operated according to an 'inverse square' law. That is, if the distance between objects increased, the gravitational force between them *decreased* by a factor equal to one divided by the distance multiplied by the distance ($1/d^2$). Newton had shown that this must be the case in order to produce the observed elliptical orbits of the planets. He had taken the step of identifying the attractive force that operated in the heavens between the sun and planets with the attraction of the earth for the moon and of the earth for every object on it. Newton had proposed the concept of **universal gravitation** whereby every body in the universe attracts every other body. This put paid to the notion that the 'perfect' heavens were subject to different laws from those which applied on the 'imperfect' earth.

Newton did not go on to describe the precise nature of gravity. It could be argued that, according to Newton, the angels had changed their position and were now beating their wings at the moon in the direction of the earth. He purposely refrained from saying what we believe today, that gravity was due to some (undefinable) property inherent in physical objects. He had described gravity but would not hazard an opinion of what it was.

It is difficult to imagine an action which exerts an influence over an object some distance away, as the earth does on the moon, but this is just what happens. We know that a door will close when our hand makes contact with it and pushes it, and we think we know why it closes (because we push it!). On an atomic scale, when our hand makes 'contact' with the door, the electrons in the atoms of our hand are very close to the electrons in the atoms of the door (less than one atomic radius away). Electrons all carry a negative electrical charge and so will repel each other. It is this repulsion between the electrons of adjacent atoms that causes the door to swing away from our hand. However, the notion of 'action at a distance', that is, acting without contact, is difficult to fathom. Nevertheless, two objects will gravitationally attract each other, even over immense distances, without physical 'contact'. They will do this, not for some easily explicable reason, not because of the angels, but because they just do.

Scientists can cope with this strange state of affairs because it is not necessary to understand what something is to describe and explain what it *does*. The search for greater understanding is a continuing one and our 'understanding' of gravity goes further than has been described above. Field theory and particle exchange theory are two attempts to understand gravity (and other forces) more completely, but these theories will not be described here.

Including gravity, there are four 'basic interactions' in nature that can produce forces (although some people hope to show the equivalence of some of them and hence reduce the number). These are:

1. **Gravitational interactions** which involve attraction between masses. This interaction may be said to hold the universe together.
2. **Electromagnetic interactions** which involve attraction and repulsion between moving charges and between stationary charges. This interaction may be said to hold molecules together, hold electrons to their atoms, cause objects to bounce off each other and indeed to cause the door to shut when we push it.
3. **Strong nuclear interactions** which involve attraction between particles in the nucleus of an atom. This interaction may be said to hold the nucleus together.
4. **Weak nuclear interactions** which are involved 'inside' the protons and neutrons of the nucleus. This interaction is not well understood.

A scientist describes movement in terms of the forces produced by magnets, electrically charged objects, objects with mass and by the material within the nucleus of an atom. All known forces are produced from one of these sources. We will consider in more detail the force produced by an object's mass, that is, the force of gravity.

4.2 The Definition of a Force

The word 'force' is in common and varied use in conversational language. It has the sense of a capacity to produce change. In scientific usage, force is given precise meaning. An unbalanced force (see Section 4.2.1) is acting when an object is:

1. made to move or to stop;
2. made to move faster or slower;
3. made to change its direction of motion;
4. deformed.

The magnitude of a force is stated in multiples of the unit called the 'newton' and given the symbol N. One newton is the weight of a mass of 100 g. The weight of nine Australian twenty cent coins is (to within 0.4%) one newton.

4.2.1 *The Concept of an Unbalanced Force*

It is commonplace for an object to be subjected to several forces at the same time without any motion occurring. For example, the chair that you are sitting in experiences a gravitational force attracting it downwards to the earth. It is prevented from sinking into the floor by the upwards force of the floor. The chair is also forced down by your weight. Furthermore, by putting your feet on the floor and pushing, you are exerting a sideways force on the chair, but the chair probably does not move because of the friction force between the chair and floor. Thus despite all of these forces, the chair remains motionless. The reason that no motion is occurring is that each force is balanced by another force which acts in the opposite direction so that the total force is zero.

Only when forces are not balanced, that is when there is a net force in a particular direction, will motion be produced (in the direction of the net or unbalanced force). Note that the forces that are acting on the chair are noticeable because they will produce temporary deformations in the floor, upholstery of the chair and on your body.

4.2.2 *Newton's Second Law*

Newton's second law is also used to define a force. Since an unbalanced force produces changes in motion, the quantity of force may be determined from the amount of change in the motion that is produced. A change in motion, be it an increase in speed, a decrease in speed or only a change in the direction of travel, is called an **acceleration** (a deceleration is more correctly known as a negative acceleration). Newton's second law says that amount of force is proportional to the mass of the accelerated object and to the acceleration produced. Thus:

Force (in newtons) = mass (in kilograms) × acceleration (in m/s^2)

Specific types of forces may be known by their own names. Examples of these are: a 'tension' is a pulling or stretching force (in a muscle, for example); a 'shear' is a force applied at an angle other than 90° or 180° (when slouching in a chair, your bottom applies a shearing force to the seat of the chair); a 'compression' is a squashing force; 'friction' is the force acting between any two surfaces in contact; 'gravity' is the force of attraction that holds all objects to the earth. Since force is a directional quantity, that is, a force acts in a certain direction, it is a **vector quantity**. Vector quantities should be stated with both a magnitude and a direction, for example a bulldozer may exert a force of 50 000 N south, on a mound of soil.

4.3 The Distinction Between Inertia, Mass And Weight

The meanings of these three words in scientific use are more precise and not as broad as when used in ordinary conversation.

4.3.1 *Inertia*

Inertia is an idea. It is the tendency of an object to remain stationary, or to continue moving with constant speed and direction despite forces acting on the object. A laden semi-trailer truck has a lot of inertia because it is difficult to set in motion and difficult to stop. A bowling ball has more inertia than a tennis ball. A bed with a patient in it has more inertia, because it has more mass, than the same bed without a patient. Inertia is not a directly measurable quantity so has no units; however, mass is a measure of inertia and vice versa. In fact if it is not possible to weigh an object, a measure of the amount of mass in the object can be obtained from its inertia. For example, a balloon resting on a horizontal 'frictionless' surface (such as polished steel) is easily set in motion by a swift kick. On the other hand, a bowling ball would be set in motion with difficulty (and pain). Thus the bowling ball has more inertia than the balloon and from this fact we can surmise that it has more mass as well.

Newton's First Law (Galileo's Law of Inertia). Newton's first law may be stated as follows:

> All objects will remain at rest, or continue with constant speed in a straight line, unless an 'unbalanced' force acts upon them.

Newton's first law may be summarised as follows:

if $F = 0$, then, *change in* $v = 0$

F stands for unbalanced force and v stands for velocity.

The Distinction Between Speed and Velocity. Velocity and speed are similar because they both measure the rate at which a number of metres is travelled and hence have the same units (metres per second). They differ because speed is the rate at which the number of metres *along the path taken* (regardless of any bends it may have) is travelled. Velocity disregards the length of the actual path and just measures the rate at which the distance *along a straight line* joining the starting point to the finishing point is travelled (see Figure 4.1).

Velocity is a vector quantity, so is always stated with a magnitude and the direction of the finishing point from the starting point of the motion. The practical difference between speed and velocity may be highlighted by considering a racing car on a circular track. If the car maintains a speed of 100 km/h around the track, its speed is said to be constant. However, its velocity is continually changing because the *direction of its motion* is continually changing. At the end of the 'race' the average speed of the car can be said to have been 100 km/h, but the average velocity was zero. Despite the car travelling many times around the track, the distance that separates the place where the race started and where the race finished was zero, hence average velocity (but not speed) is zero.

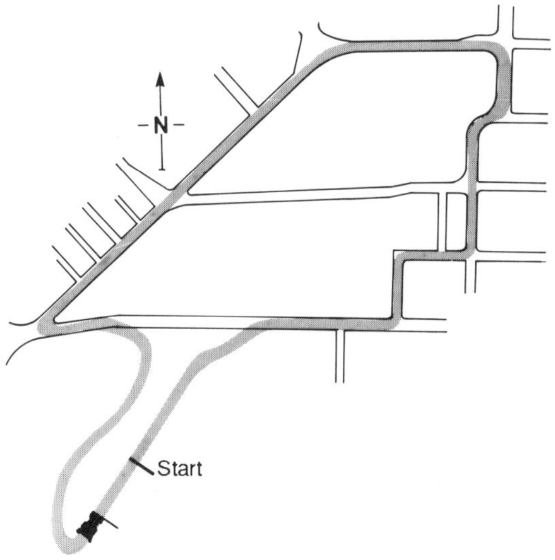

Figure 4.1 *A racer travelling from the start of the Adelaide Grand Prix track to the start of pit straight has travelled a distance of about 3.8 km in about 80 s. The average speed is 141 km/h. The average velocity, however, is only about 4 km/h south-east* (see Errata)

To illustrate the effect of inertia consider 'Simon', a person sitting in a stationary car at a traffic light. When another vehicle runs into the back of the stationary car, Simon will be forced forward (suddenly) by the car seat pushing against his back as the moving vehicle hits his car. However, Simon's head will remain 'at rest' in accordance with Newton's first law, causing hyperextension, until the forward motion of Simon's body and the elasticity of his neck 'snaps' his head forward. The resulting hyperextension and hyperflexion of Simon's neck produces a 'whiplash' injury. Such injury can be greatly reduced if a head rest is fitted to the car seat. In this case the head rest would push against Simon's head (and its inertia), causing it to move forward at the same speed as the rest of his body thus preventing hyperextension of the neck.

Now we will apply Newton's first law to a car driver driving along a straight country road. Suppose that the driver dozes off and the car drifts off the road and drives into a large tree trunk by the side of the road. The car will come to a sudden stop. The *driver* will continue with constant speed in a straight line into the steering wheel and windscreen (due to inertia) unless stopped (slightly less suddenly) by a seat belt. Unfortunately, the driver's *head* will continue forward anyway, as it is not restrained by the seat belt, and the neck undergoes hyperflexion, again causing a whiplash injury.

4.3.2 *Mass*

Mass is a fundamental quantity. It is the amount of matter contained in an object and is measured in units of kilograms. Mass is a **scalar quantity**; it needs only a magnitude to be completely defined, and no direction is involved. Mass is also a measure of inertia, in that the greater is the mass of an object, the greater is its inertia.

Our concept of mass has had to be modified somewhat in the light of Albert Einstein's theory of relativity. From before Newton's time, mass was thought to be an unchanging quantity. That is, we disregard the growth that occurs in living things, the extra weight that materials have when they are wet and restrict ourselves to inanimate objects. Thus the mass of a stone does not alter unless a piece is chipped off. Even then, if all the fragments of stone are kept together, their combined mass is still the same as that of the original stone.

However, relativity theory shows us that the mass of an inanimate object can change: it increases (ever so slightly) as its speed increases. A 100 kg mass travelling at 1500 km/h would experience a mass increase of much less than a microgram. In fact the mass increase is not significant unless the speed involved exceeds about one tenth of the speed of light. It is possible to accelerate sub-atomic particles to 'relativistic' speeds (that is, close to the speed of light), but macroscopic objects have never been made to move faster than about 60 000 km/h. Light travels almost twenty thousand times faster than this, so the relativistic increase in mass remains the preserve of the research physicist, and need not concern us any further.

Einstein showed that mass is another form of energy, and that the two are related by the square of the number 3.00×10^8 m/s (the speed of light). Thus when mass and energy interconvert, energy (in J) = change in mass (in kg) × (speed of light)^2.

$$E = m \times c^2$$

The conversion of mass to energy and vice versa occurs in nuclear reactions and will be discussed in Chapter 14.

4.3.3 *Weight*

Weight is a force, and is thus a vector quantity (its direction is always towards the centre of the earth). The unit of weight is the newton (N). Weight is the force that a body exerts on the supporting floor (or chair or rope or bathroom scales) due to the gravitational attraction of the earth. By this definition you would weigh more in a lift that is accelerating upwards, because the floor is pushing harder on your feet. If the lift accelerates downwards, you weigh less because the supporting force of the floor is less (you can try this by standing on a bathroom scales in a lift). The force of weight is balanced by the force exerted by the supporting surface and so only produces an acceleration if there is no support. Hence a skydiver in free fall accelerates towards the earth because of the gravitational force between her and the earth and because of the absence of any supporting force.

The 'weightlessness' experienced by an astronaut orbiting the earth is not due to the absence of gravitational force (it is still there), but due to the absence of a supporting force. The astronaut and his capsule are 'falling' towards the earth. An 80 kg astronaut orbiting at 40 000 km above the earth would be subject to a gravitational force of 15 N, which is about 2% of that on earth.

CAON (nee Stone). — Jemma Loria, born (easily) on August 10, at F.M.C., weighing 37.7 newtons. Janet and Martin both doing well.

Figure 4.2 *How much did the baby weigh? Weight is a force so is measured in newtons (N). The kilogram (kg) is the unit of mass*

For our purposes the three words, mass, weight and inertia, even though they have different meanings, may be used almost interchangeably, because mass is a measure of inertia and mass and weight are directly proportional. For example, in conversational use we state the 'weight' of an object in kilograms instead of (the strictly correct unit) newtons (see Figure 4.2). Thus a nurse who 'weighs' 60 kg, actually has a *mass* of 60 kg and in fact *weighs* $60 \times 9.8 = 588$ N. Since the 'conversion factor' between mass and weight is constant on earth at 9.8 m/s^2 (to two sig. figs), we tend to accept the two terms as almost synonymous. The conversion factor is different for other places (for example, on the moon).

4.3.4 *Acceleration and Newton's Second Law*

Newton's second law relates the mass (m) of an object to its weight (F), by multiplying mass by the acceleration (a) that is produced by the force of gravity. It may be stated as the equation

$$F = m \times a$$

In the example above of the nurse's weight, a is 9.8 m/s^2, the acceleration due to the earth's gravity.

Acceleration is the term given to the *rate* at which speed or velocity changes. Recall that speed and velocity are themselves rates of change, so that acceleration is the rate of change of a rate of change. In part this explains the stutter-like unit of acceleration, the 'metre per second per second' (m/s^2).

Newton's second law may be used to understand why a moving human body is damaged if it crashes into something. The act of colliding while in motion implies that the velocity, and the speed, of motion will change. That is, an acceleration will occur. Given that the mass of an individual's body is constant during the collision, Newton's second law tells us that the force exerted on the body (and hence the injury produced) is proportional to the acceleration. So to decrease the injury we should attempt to decrease the acceleration. Acceleration may be calculated by subtracting the velocity before the collision (v_1) from the velocity after the collision (v_2) and dividing the answer by the time (t) it took for the change to occur. In symbols,

$$a = \frac{v_2 - v_1}{t}$$

The easiest way to minimise the acceleration is to maximise the time over which the velocity is changing. Vehicle designers achieve this by padding the dashboard so that a head striking the dashboard is brought to a stop as gradually as possible while the padding is squashed. Someone leaping from a bench to the ground 'breaks their fall' by bending at the ankles, knees and hips and using muscle tension to slow their limbs. Thus allowing their vertical speed to decrease gradually to zero and avoiding large forces on their bones.

The body has very sensitive detectors of acceleration in the inner ear: the **utricle** for straight-line acceleration and the three **semi-circular canals** for detecting changes in the direction of motion and in the rate of rotation (angular accelerations). The 'sense of acceleration' is not usually listed as one of the human senses, nevertheless the stimulation of this sense by the large and changing accelerations produced by snow skiing, fairground rides, car racing, playground equipment and so on produces a (much sought after) pleasurable feeling. The good health of our utricles and semi-circular canals is vital for proper functioning. Walking is difficult with an impairment to our sense of acceleration. Furthermore, dizziness, sea sickness and motion sickness result from the over-stimulation of our acceleration-detecting organs.

4.4 Gravity and Centre of Gravity

Gravity has a beneficial effect on our bodies. Gravitational force acting on the skeleton as it supports the weight of the body causes healthy bones to strengthen (if they were weak) or ensures that bones maintain their strength. Prolonged bed rest removes most of the body's weight from the skeleton and causes the loss of bone mineral. The bones recover when normal activity is resumed. Athletes in training have stronger bones (that is, of greater diameter) than non-athletes because the skeleton responds to the extra stress on the athlete's weight-bearing bones by laying down more bone.

Gravity will cause liquids to move to the lowest possible level. Thus if we require a liquid to flow under the influence of gravity alone, from one container (A) to another (B), B must be lower than A. Hence drainage bags must be placed at a position lower than the patient, and containers used to hold liquids for intravenous entry, blood transfusion and so on must be above the level of the patient. Since blood is a liquid, the circulation of blood is affected by the vertical position of body parts. Thus elevating limbs will decrease the blood supply to them because the heart is working against gravity. Conversely, lowering the head of people who feel faint will increase the blood flow to the head.

The force of gravity acts on every part of an object. However, there exists a point in (or near) an object called the 'centre of gravity' or centre of mass (see Figure 4.3a, b). For a symmetrical object like a sphere, a cube or a cylinder, the centre of mass lies at the geometrical centre of the object. The centre of mass of non-symmetrical rigid objects may be found by hanging them up. When any object is suspended by a cord attached to a single point on the object, it assumes an orientation in which it is in equilibrium (that is, it

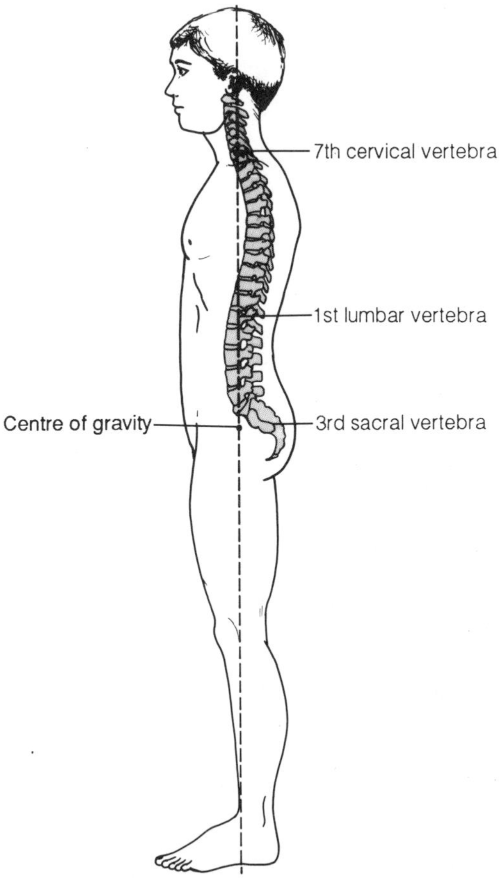

Figure 4.3a *The centre of gravity of a standing person is located on the vertical line joining the seventh cervical vertebrae and the first lumbar vertebrae, at about the level of the third sacral vertebrae*

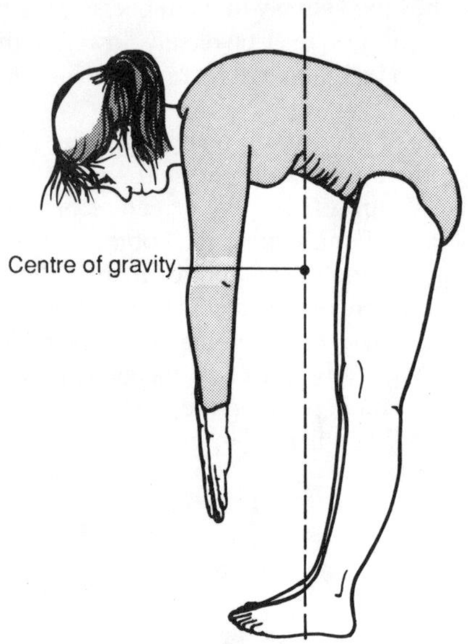

Figure 4.3b *The centre of gravity can be moved to outside the body by bending over to touch the toes*

hangs motionless). When motionless, the line of the cord may be imagined to extend through the object. By hanging the object from several different points and continuing the line of the cord through the object each time, all such lines are found to intersect at one point, the centre of mass. An interesting phenomenon regarding the centre of mass is that this point would move in a parabolic path if the object was thrown, and move in a straight line if the object was dropped, despite any tumbling motion that the object may perform.

The human body in the anatomical (standing) position has its centre of gravity approximately located behind the naval at about the third sacral vertebra, but

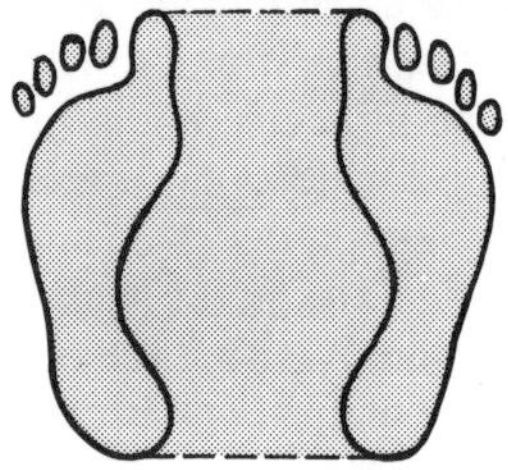

Figure 4.4a *The base of support is the area bounded by the feet*

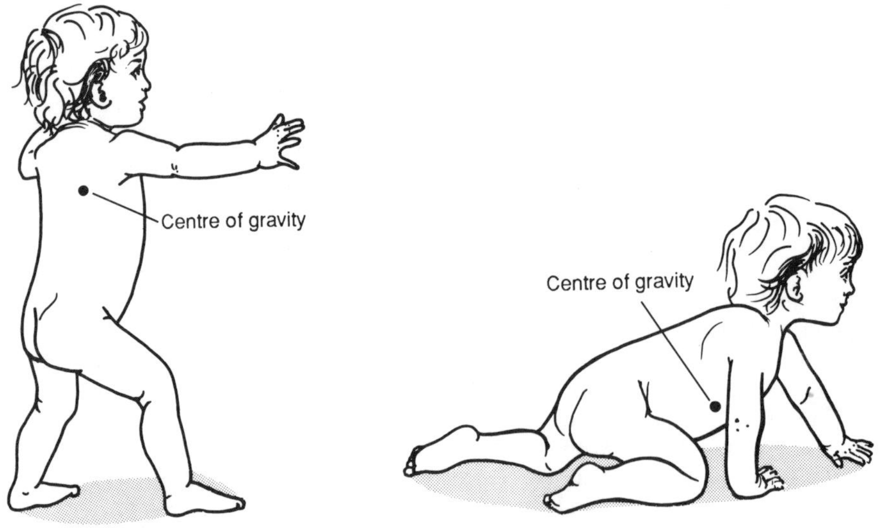

Figure 4.4b *A crawling baby is more stable than one learning to walk because in the crawling position, the baby's centre of gravity is closer to the ground and its base of support covers a greater area*

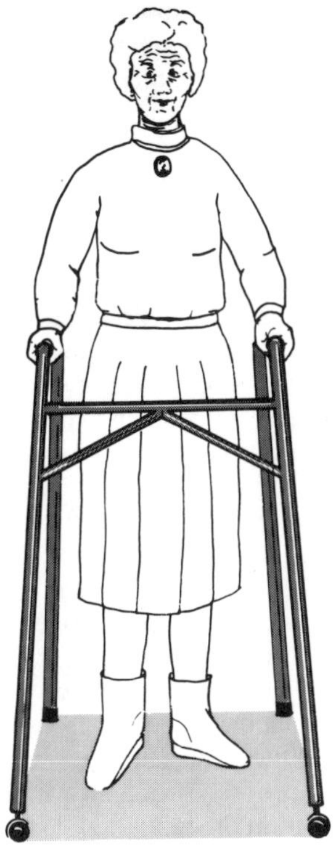

Figure 4.4c *A walking frame provides a large base of support. This increases stability because it is easier to keep the centre of gravity within its bounds. Also, the frame takes some of the weight-bearing duty away from weak leg muscles*

it varies with different body shapes (for example, the extensive paunch that some men allow to develop would shift it forward). Correct posture maintains the centre of gravity in the most comfortable position and reduces muscular fatigue because muscles do not have to work against a greater than necessary gravitational load. For example, the 'physiologically efficient' standing posture for the human body when viewed from the side has the line joining the centre of the earth and the body's centre of gravity bisecting the transverse axis of the hip joint and the knee joint and piercing the seventh cervical vertebrae (see Figure 4.3a).

The position of the body's centre of gravity may be changed (and even shifted to outside of the body) by moving the arms and legs and by bending at the waist. The practical importance of the centre of gravity is that its position (relative to the base of support) determines whether an object is stable, or a human body is balanced. A stable object is one that does not fall over if pushed slightly; it merely 'rocks' back to position. A person maintains their balance by ensuring that the imaginary line joining their centre of gravity and the centre of the earth always passes through their **base of support** (the area bounded by their feet; see Figure 4.4a). This is achieved by shifting the feet. Devices such as walking sticks, crutches and walking frames not only take away some of the force experienced by the weight-bearing bones and joints, but also extend the base of support so that weak muscles do not need to strain as much to maintain balance.

When a heavy box is being carried in front of the body, the centre of gravity of the combined mass of the box and body must be kept above the base of support. To achieve this we tend to lean backwards so that the weight of our upper body balances the extra weight of the box. This is easiest to do when the box is held as close as possible to the body. Holding a heavy weight away from your body often leads to a strained back. When helping a patient to walk, the assistance provided should be used to keep their centre of gravity over their base of support. Otherwise the nurse may not be able to exert a force large enough, without muscle strain, to prevent the patient from falling.

4.5 The Force of Friction

When your car accelerates from a traffic light, it does so because the engine and drive mechanism exerts a turning force on the wheels. When your foot is removed from the accelerator pedal the car slows down. From our definition of force, there must be a force producing this decrease in motion. **Friction** is the name of the retarding force which decreases motion and is operating whenever two surfaces are in contact with each other. There is friction between our blood and the vessels that it passes through, between our internal organs as they move against each other and between muscle fibres as they slide over each other.

The amount of friction present is proportional to the strength of the force pressing the two surfaces together. If two surfaces in contact are stationary, we say that 'static friction' is operating, whereas when surfaces are sliding over each other, the lesser force of 'sliding friction' is operating. The origin of friction is the electromagnetic forces between the particles in the atoms of the opposing surfaces. Friction may be reduced by making the surfaces as smooth as possible and by using lubricants, but is never eliminated (see Figure 4.5).

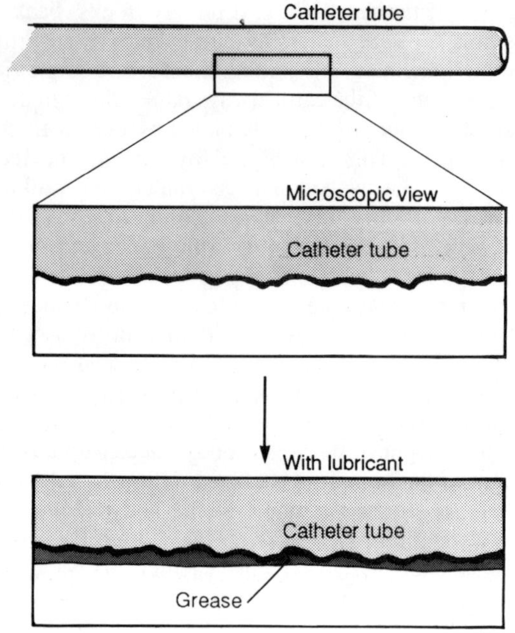

Figure 4.5 *Even smooth looking tubes have surface irregularities when looked at microscopically. These will result in friction and damage to the cells of tissues over which the tube passes. Friction is reduced by using lubricants*

Friction may be desirable. For example, the friction between the soles of our shoes and the ground enables us to walk, friction between car tyres and the road enables the car to speed up, slow down and turn corners. Friction within our muscles when we exercise, and between blood and the blood vessels, produces a considerable amount of heat so is a significant factor in maintaining a constant body temperature. Where friction is desirable it may be increased by choosing surfaces that produce a large amount of friction, for example rubber tyres on wheels and bitumen on roads, good soles on sport shoes, rubber caps on the tips of crutches, a towel between instruments and the tray they rest on.

Friction also produces some bad effects. It causes moving parts in any device to eventually wear out. It causes chafing of skin and blisters. Where friction is undesirable it may be reduced by the use of lubricants (greases and oils). Frictional forces between liquids are less than those between solids so liquid oils and greases will decrease friction. The internal organs of the body are continually moving over each other as we breathe, as our heart beats and as our posture changes. Friction between these moving surfaces is reduced because of the fluids and mucus that cover our organs.

The insertion of gastric tubes, catheters, etc. is aided by the use of lubricants to prevent friction 'burns' to the patient's membranes. It is easier still if the tubes are inserted in one smooth continuous motion. In this case static friction is avoided and only the lesser sliding friction need be overcome.

The ease of movement of the human body is due in large part to the lack of friction in the weight-bearing joints of the hips, knees and ankles (except in people with arthritis). The 'coefficient of friction' (a number assigned to the ease with which two surfaces in contact move over each other) of a healthy knee joint is only 0.01. This is lower than the friction coefficient encountered in ice skating. For comparison some coefficients are 0.03 for steel on ice, 0.06 for steel on lubricated steel and about 0.7 for car tyres on the road. As the cartilage-capped ends of bone move over each other in a knee joint, they are lubricated by synovial fluid. Synovial fluid is an extremely good lubricant, better than any manufactured oil. Its viscosity decreases as the stress on the joint increases, which means that its lubricating properties actually improve as more weight is placed on the joint.

Newton's Third Law. Newton's third law may be stated

> When an object exerts a force F_1 on another, the second object exerts an equal force F_2 on the first object, but in the opposite direction.

It may be summarised as: $F_1 = -F_2$ (the negative sign indicates an opposite direction).

Often, 'action' is used to describe the first object's force, and 'reaction' the second object's force. Newton's third law may be applied to friction. Friction is often the reaction force that opposes the action. The muscular act of walking exerts a force on the ground in the backwards direction (the action) and friction between the foot and the ground provides the reaction force on the foot in the forwards direction. Since the earth is more massive than a human, the human is moved forward while the earth does not move back.

4.6 Force and Vectors

All measurable quantities are one of two types, either **scalar** or **vector**. A scalar quantity (and some examples are time, length, volume, concentration, mass, pressure, density, energy, temperature) is completely defined by magnitude only. For example, a temperature is stated as 30 °C, time as 3.15 pm. It makes no sense to say 30 °C 'to the left', or 3.15 pm northeast, because direction is not appropriate to temperature or time. A vector quantity (such as force, velocity, acceleration, displacement, momentum) requires a direction to be stated, as well as a magnitude, in order to be completely defined. Thus a traction force of 30 N in the direction parallel to the femur's long axis and from hip to knee may aid bone repair but 30 N perpendicular to the femur would not.

The addition of scalar quantities (to each other) is a simple arithmetic problem, for example 30 minutes + 80 minutes = 110 minutes; that is, the magnitudes of scalar quantities are summed. However, to add vector quantities is a more difficult geometrical problem (or an even harder algebraic one!). A diagram, drawn to scale, must be used in order to take account of the direction of the vectors. Furthermore, only vectors of the same type may be added. That is, forces are added to forces, an acceleration may be added to another acceleration but not to a force or anything else.

A vector may be represented by a length of straight line, drawn to scale, marked with an arrowhead symbol.

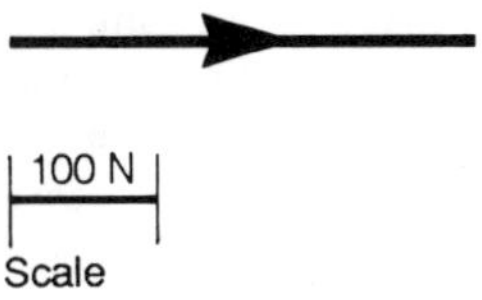

Figure 4.6 *Representation of a vector, in this case 320 N to the right*

The orientation of the line and the arrowhead indicate the direction of the vector, and the length of the line represents the magnitude of the vector. Thus, using a scale where 1 cm of length is equivalent to 100 N, the vector drawn as an arrow of length 3.2 cm in Figure 4.6 represents 320 N to the right.

When vectors are added using a scale diagram, the lines representing the vectors are arranged so that the tail of the second vector touches the head of the previous vector (see Figure 4.7b). The resulting vector is the line that joins the tail of the first vector to the head of the second vector (the head to tail rule). In this example the resulting force is 490 N in the direction shown.

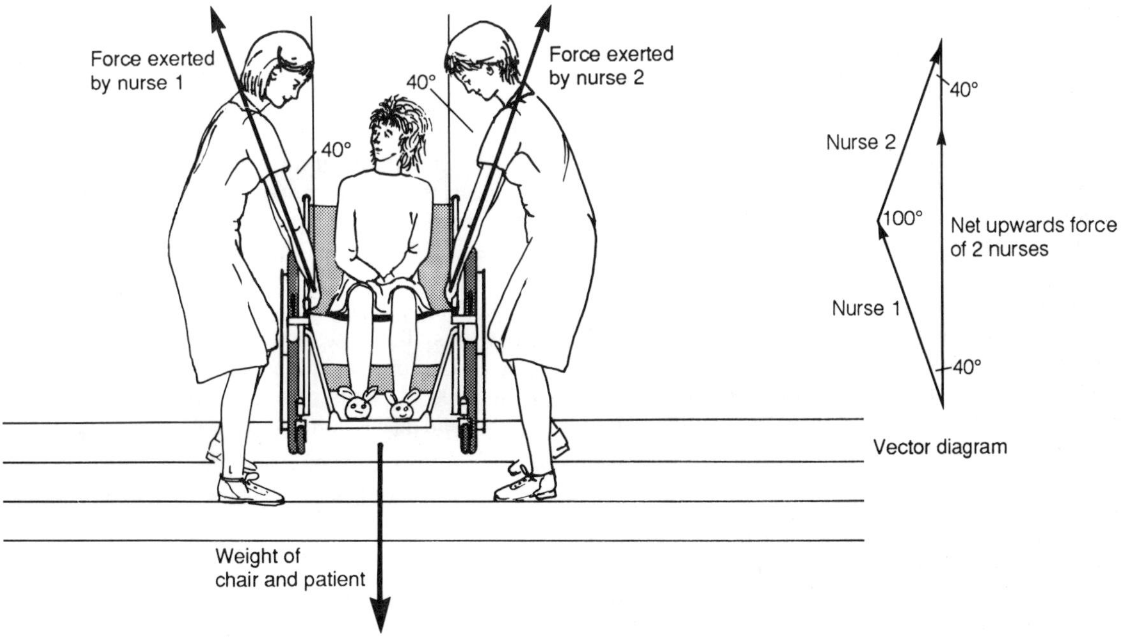

Figure 4.7 *Two nurses lifting a wheelchair and patient down some steps each exert 260 N of force in the direction of their arms. By vector addition, the resultant force on the wheelchair is vertical and of magnitude 490 N* (see Errata)

Consider two nurses helping each other carry a patient in a wheelchair down a short flight of steps. Suppose each nurse exerts a force of 260 N on the wheelchair in a direction that is upwards and 20° from the vertical (see Figure 4.7). The **resultant** force from their combined effort is neither of magnitude 260 N (or even 520 N) nor in the direction of effort of either nurse. The resultant force vector is found by **vector addition** using the 'head to tail' rule and then completing the triangle. The resultant force is 490 N upwards (therefore the patient and wheelchair have a combined mass of 50 kg).

4.7 Vectors Applied to Muscle Action

For many movements in the human body, several muscles will contract together to produce the resulting movement. An example is the action of nodding 'yes' with the head. This movement is achieved by the combined action of the sternocleidomastoid muscles on each side of the neck contracting together. However, if the muscle on only one side contracts, the head will be turned to the side. Another example of vector addition of muscle forces is the action of the hamstrings (biceps femoris, semitendinosus and semimembranosus). When all three muscle groups contract together, the leg flexes, and the resultant force on the lower leg is straight up. However, the tension in each individual muscle is not in a vertical direction (see Figure 4.8).

Thus if one of the team of muscles that work together to produce an action is damaged, the whole movement may be compromised. This is because the damaged muscle could not exert its normal force and the resultant force of the other muscles in the team would not be in the normal direction or be of normal magnitude. In the case of the hamstrings the resultant force would no longer be straight up. Hence it may be necessary to immobilise a whole group of muscles to allow one of them to heal.

We can use vector addition to calculate the force on the spine in a bad lifting position, where the vertebral column is used as a lever. Suppose a nurse was going to lift a child weighing 300 N, and the weight of the nurse's upper body was also 300 N, concentrated at the shoulders (as the centre of gravity of the upper body in the position shown is between the shoulders). A simplified view of the force vectors involved in the poor lifting position is shown in Figure 4.9. When the back is leant forward so that the spine makes an angle of 20° to the horizontal, the angle between the spine and the erector spinae muscle (the sacrospinalis) — as determined from skeletal measurements — is about 11°. The *magnitude* of the forces in the erector spinae and the spine are unknown, but the *direction* of the forces must be along the erector spinae and along the spine and at the angles indicated in the Figure 4.9. A vector diagram can be drawn from this information and the length of the vectors measured and converted to newtons via the scale. It can be seen that both the spine and the erector spinae are subjected to a force of about 3000 N. Thus in a bad lifting position every vertebra and disc is compressed with a force equivalent to the weight of three very large men. Small wonder that muscles strain, vertebrae crush and discs slip when weights are lifted incorrectly.

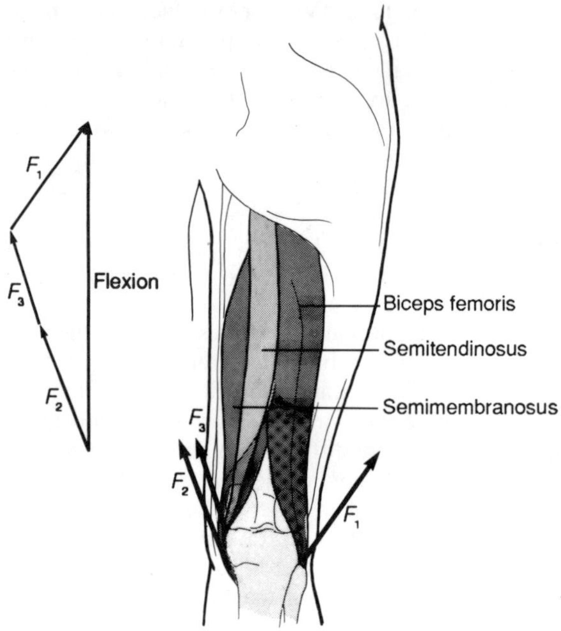

Figure 4.8 *The hamstrings flex the leg. The direction of the force that they exert via their tendons on the point of insertion is shown. The vector sum of their forces achieves flexion*

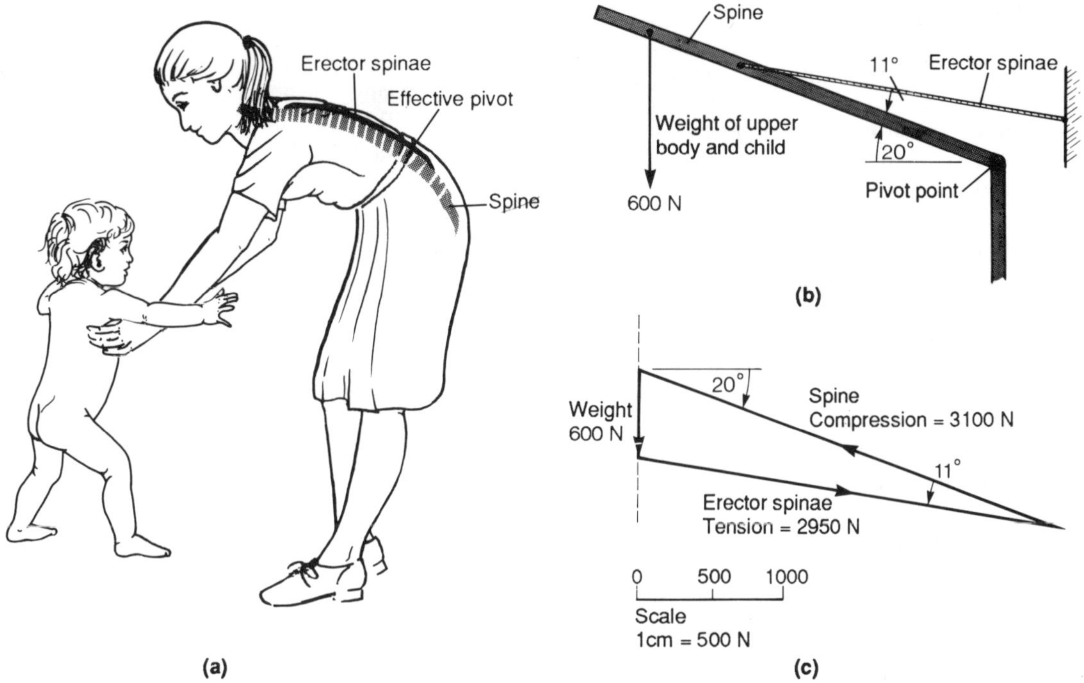

Figure 4.9 *(a) The body in a poor lifting position. (b) An idealised mechanical model of the situation. (c) The vector diagram that uses the directions of the forces to estimate the magnitude of the forces involved*

4.8 Work and Simple Machines

The word 'work' is another that has a conversational meaning that is far broader than its scientific meaning. Scientifically speaking, work occurs only when a force causes a displacement. Thus if no force is exerted, or if a force is exerted but *no movement is produced*, then work has not occurred. Even though a weightlifter strains to hold a barbell steady above her head, no work is done on the barbell while it is motionless (Figure 4.10). Of course she feels tired because of the physiological changes occurring in her muscles. However, the energy she is using up is *not being transferred to the barbell*, hence she does no work on the barbell. Another definition of work is the amount of energy that is transferred from one object to another.

Simple 'machines' such as levers, wedges (or ramps), the wheel and axle, pulleys and screws allow us to perform work more easily. A haemostat is an example of a lever, a wheelchair ramp is a wedge, patients in wheelchairs propel themselves by using a wheel and axle, and traction systems use pulleys to harness the force of gravity and change its direction.

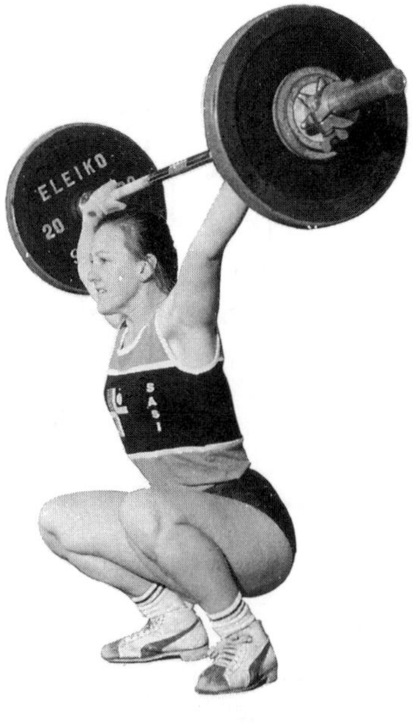

Figure 4.10 *Even though a weightlifter strains to hold a barbell above her head, no work is done on the barbell while it is motionless*

4.9 Pulleys

A pulley is a wheel with a groove around the rim (much like the wheel on a bicycle when the tyre and tube are removed) that is free to turn on an axle (see Figure 4.11). A cord sitting in the groove causes the wheel to turn when the cord is pulled. The pulley changes the direction of the tension due to the cord by changing the direction of the cord. Pulleys are useful in traction systems where the force on a limb must be applied from a specified direction. If the wheel turns freely on the axle and the cord is not frayed and does not stick in the groove, the tension in the cord is transmitted around the pulley undiminished. If a pulley is not moved backwards or forwards as its cord is pulled, it is called a **fixed pulley**. Those pulleys that do move are termed **movable pulleys** (turning on its axis does not count as movement).

A pulley can serve two functions.

1. It can change the direction of the cords, and thus the direction of the force exerted by the cords. Both fixed pulleys and movable pulleys perform this function.

2. Movable pulleys, in addition, provide a **mechanical advantage**. That is, they multiply the effect of an applied force (to twice its value in the case of a single movable pulley).

Some bones perform the function of fixed pulleys in that they change the direction of the force produced by a muscle. When a tendon passes over a bone such as a knee cap or a knuckle, it has its direction changed and hence the direction of the tension force of the muscle which pulls on the tendon is also changed in direction.

4.10 Body Levers

4.10.1 *Levers*

A lever is any bar or rod (or bone!), bent or straight, arranged in such a way that it can pivot about a point (the **fulcrum**). Since one of the primary functions of many bones in the body is to act as levers to transmit the forces produced by muscles, a study of levers can give a better understanding of muscle action. By pivoting about the fulcra of the body (the movable joints), some resistance force (for example, the weight of a limb) can be overcome by applying an effort force (that is, the pull of a muscle). Muscles can only change

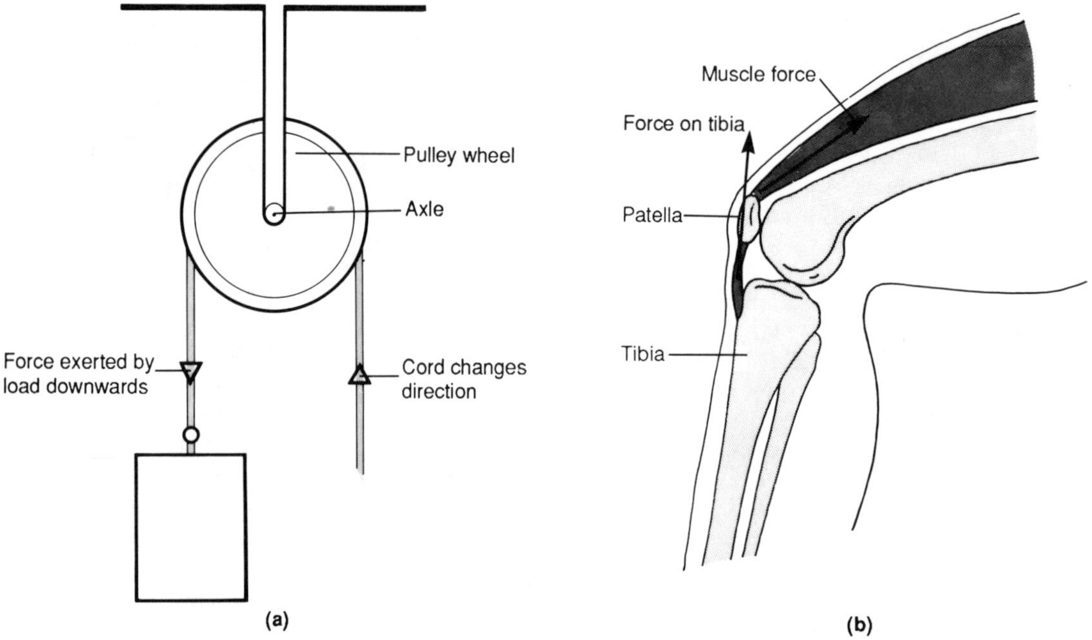

Figure 4.11 *(a) A single fixed pulley changes the direction of the applied force. (b) The kneecap, by changing the direction of the force of the quadriceps muscle, is acting as a fixed pulley*

their length (by contracting) by about 20%. Bones, by acting as levers, magnify the motions of muscles. Thus a relatively short muscular contraction in the arm may be translated into a movement of more than one metre by the hand.

For any particular lever, the fulcrum (*F*), resistance (or load) force (*R*) and effort force (*E*) may be arranged in one of the three ways shown in Figure 4.12. The three types of levers are usually called 'first-class', 'second-class' and 'third-class levers'. Examples of first-class lever actions in the body are the flexion and extension of the hand, the whole arm and the whole leg. Performing 'situps' involves a second-class lever system (the effort is the tension in the rectus abdominus muscle and the fulcrum is the buttocks), while third-class levers are very common in the movements of the arms and legs.

The **perpendicular** distance between the fulcrum and the line of action of the effort force is called the 'effort arm' (see Figure 4.13). The perpendicular distance between the fulcrum and the line of action of the load force is called the 'load arm'. For second-class levers the effort arm is always longer than the load arm, while for third-class levers the reverse is true. First-class levers have a variable relationship between the two 'arms'.

1. Fulcrum between the two forces — *R F E* — e.g. nodding 'yes' with your head
2. Resistance between fulcrum and effort — *F R E* — e.g. raising feet from flat to tiptoe
3. Effort between fulcrum and resistance — *F E R* — e.g. bicep action in flexion of the forearm

Figure 4.12 *Types of levers: (1) first-class lever; (2) second-class lever; (3) third-class lever*

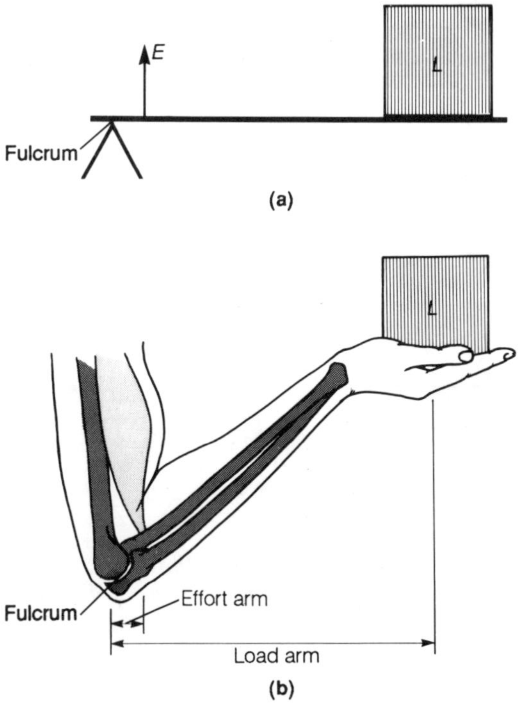

Figure 4.13 *The effort arm is the horizontal component of the distance between the effort and the fulcrum. The load arm is the horizontal component of the distance between the load and the fulcrum*

4.10.2 *Mechanical Advantage and Velocity Ratio*

Generally speaking, hand tools such as spanners, crowbars, tin openers, hammers and so on, are used to provide a mechanical advantage (sometimes called leverage) in that a small muscular effort can be multiplied to produce a much larger force that acts on the load (or resistance).

$$\text{mechanical advantage} = \frac{\text{load}}{\text{effort}}$$

Although this sounds as if we are getting more out than we put in, this is not so. The trade-off is that the load moves only a small distance while the effort must be exerted through a larger distance. Thus while the end of the spanner may turn through 20 cm, the nut only turns through a few millimetres. The term used to describe this disparity in distance moved by the load and the distance over which the effort must act is the **velocity ratio**.

$$\text{velocity ratio} = \frac{\text{distance moved by the effort}}{\text{distance moved by the load}}$$

Thus hand tools achieve a large mechanical advantage by allowing the velocity ratio to be large. The human body is the reverse of the situation with hand tools in that a large mechanical advantage is sacrificed in order to achieve as low a velocity ratio as possible (less than one). Our muscles (the effort force) are limited in the distance over which they can contract (to 20% of their relaxed length), yet we wish our limbs (the load force) to have a very wide range of movement. That is, our bodies require a low value for the velocity ratio. This can only be achieved if the mechanical advantage of our body levers is kept low.

The basic physics of levers shows us that a lever cannot magnify *both* motion and force at the same time. If motion is magnified then force is reduced; if force is magnified then it can be achieved only over small distances. So when changing the wheel on a car, we use a jack to magnify the force of our muscles and so lift the car. However, the force of our muscles must be made to act over a large distance as we crank the jack again and again. The benefit that we derive from our efforts is that the massive force of the car is moved upwards by a few centimetres, enabling us to change the wheel.

4.10.3 *Efficiency*

Efficiency refers to the proportion of the energy, expended on a simple machine (such as a lever), that is transferred to the load. One way of calculating efficiency as a percentage is to divide the mechanical advantage by the velocity ratio (and then multiply by 100). If efficiency was 100% then mechanical advantage would equal the velocity ratio. However, some energy is always converted to heat and sound so efficiency can never be 100% and the mechanical advantage must always be less than the velocity ratio.

The efficiency of our muscles is considerably less than 100%, so the mechanical advantage of our muscles must be *less than* the velocity ratio. Recall that the velocity ratio between our muscles and our limbs is much less than one, so mechanical advantage is even less than that.

Looking back at the formula for mechanical advantage, a low value means that the effort is much greater than the load. Most of the bones in our bodies act as third-class levers. Thus they are an inefficient type of lever because the mechanical advantage is always considerably less than one. A mechanical advantage of one would mean that a force of 100 N (say) could lift a load of the same weight. Mechanical advantage is less than one whenever the muscle insertion (the effort) is closer to the joint than the centre of gravity of the object being lifted (the load). A consequence of this is that *the tension force generated in the muscles operating third-class levers is much greater than the weight being shifted.* For example: to hold a 5 kg block (which has a weight of about 50 N) in the palm of your hand as shown in Figure 4.14, the tension in your bicep would be in the vicinity of 500 N (and the mechanical advantage would be about $\frac{50}{500} = 0.1$).

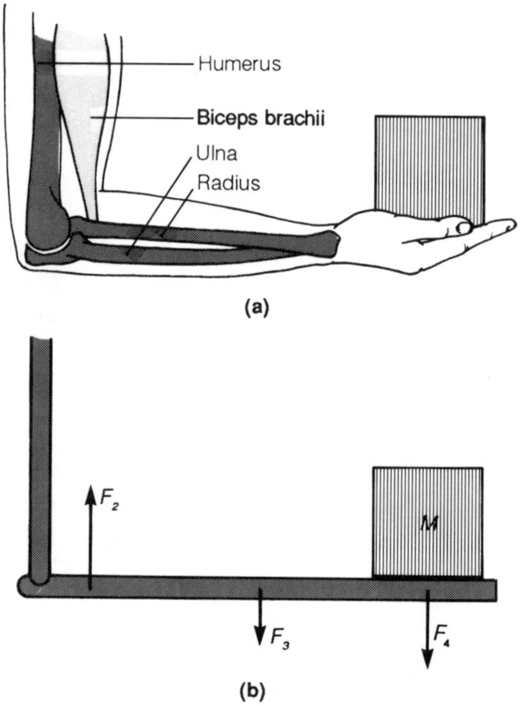

Figure 4.14 *The effort force of the biceps brachii (F_2) is much greater than the load forces (F_3 and F_4) because the effort is so close to the fulcrum*

This example is not an isolated one. All tensions in muscles and tendons and the forces in the joints are several times as large as the load applied from outside. The large stresses that are generated in the body during vigorous activity can easily damage it if the body is not in good physical condition. A consequence of the very large forces that are generated in the muscles of athletes is that they are easily strained if abused. Consider a sportsman exerting large forces in his leg muscles as he dodges and weaves while sprinting. If a sharp blow is struck to a muscle, joint or tendon while the muscle is under tension, the extra force of the blow may be enough to snap the tendon, tear the muscle or to pull off a piece of bone as the tendon is displaced.

Despite the relative inefficiency of the third-class lever systems of the body, our musculoskeletal system can easily generate the necessary forces that are required for movement and can cope with the normal stresses that result. The benefit to us of having muscle insertions so close to their joints is that the range of movement available to our limbs is very large. Our third-class levers translate the short (a few centimetres) muscular contractions in our muscles to quite long (more than a metre) movements of the extremities of our limbs.

4.11 Correct Lifting Technique

About three out of four Australians suffer back disorders at least once during their lives, and two thirds of all workers' compensated back injuries are caused by lifting (National Occupational Health and Safety Commission figures for 1986–87). Nurses are more prone to back disorders than any other injury. They account for 52% of all injuries in the nursing profession.

A person stooping, that is, bending at the waist, to pick up something from ground level is using their vertebral column as a third-class lever. Consequently the tension force in the back muscles will be much greater than the weight force of the object being lifted. The tension in back muscles is passed to the vertebrae as a compressive force. The muscular tension force is the 'action' (in Newton's third law) while the compression force in the spine is the 'reaction' force. If this reaction force is great enough a 'disc' may be crushed or the vertebrae displaced sideways, both of which may produce chronic back pain.

To lift a heavy object from the floor, correct lifting technique should be used. That is, spread the feet comfortably apart so that the base of support is extended, stand as close to the object to be lifted as is practicable, even place the feet on either side of the object if possible. This will ensure that the combined centre of gravity of the object and lifter is over the base of support and that the distances between the object's centre of gravity and the fulcra of the body (that is, the load arms) are minimised. Bend at the knees and not at the waist so that the large thigh muscles and not the weaker back muscles exert the effort force. This also ensures that the rigid leg bones, and not the flexible vertebral column, are used as levers.

4.12 Traction

When a limb is painful as a result of inflammation of a joint or a fracture of one of the bones, the controlling muscles go into spasm. Since the antagonistic muscles around a fractured bone are not all equally powerful, the stronger muscles in spasm can cause apposition of the bone fragments to be lost. If a fracture is allowed to heal with the bone ends improperly positioned, a malunion occurs and deformity may result. In turn deformity may impair the function of the limb.

4.12.1 *Traction and Counter-traction*

Traction, the act of drawing out or pulling on a limb, can overcome the deforming force of the muscles in spasm and thereby relieve pain and allow the limb to rest in the best functional position while the fracture heals. The traction force required to pull against the muscles in spasm may be supplied by gravity acting on weights that are hanging from cords that are in turn attached to the limb. Alternatively the force may be supplied by stretching the limb against an appliance or splint.

To understand the use of traction, a knowledge of pulleys, vector addition of tension forces and Newton's first and third laws is required. Newton's third law may be stated as:

> When one object exerts a force on a second object, the second object exerts an equal but oppositely directed force on the first object.

Traction is the original force and counter-traction is the equal but opposite force. Without these two opposing forces being equally balanced, the patient would be set in motion (he or she would slide along the bed) in the direction of the stronger force (in accord with Newton's first law).

4.12.2 *Fixed Traction and Sliding Traction*

There are two forms of traction, **fixed traction** and **sliding traction**. Fixed traction does not involve hanging weights. A tension is applied between (say) the lower leg by pulling on it with cords and counter-traction is applied to a part of the body (say, the ischial tuberosity below the pelvis) by pushing on it. Note that there are two forces, a push and a pull and between the points where the forces are applied, the leg is 'stretched' to the normal length. An appliance such as a Thomas splint applies the forces to the fixed points at each end of the leg. As counter-traction is not dependent upon gravity, the apparatus is self-contained, and the patient may be lifted or moved without risk of displacement of the fracture.

Sliding traction is also called **balanced traction** or **suspended traction**. Traction is supplied by the force of gravity acting on masses which hang from cords that pass over pulleys, and eventually attach to the limb at one or more places. The resultant magnitude and direction of the traction force on the limb is determined by adding the tension force in these cords, using the vector method of 'head to tail'. The counter-traction force is supplied by the opposing pull of the patient's muscles, friction between the patient and the bed, and gravity acting on the patient's body. The help of gravity is enlisted to provide counter-traction by tilting the bed so that the patient would tend to slide away from the traction force, if the cord was cut (see Figure 4.15).

Both fixed traction and sliding traction may be used together on a particular patient. Newton's second law allows us to calculate the magnitude of the gravitational force that produces the traction:

$$\text{gravitational force (in N)} = \text{hanging mass (in kg)} \times 9.8$$

The gravitational force is the same as the tension acting in the cords, provided that the pulleys rotate freely. The traction force acting on a limb will be in a different direction to the gravitational force producing it, because of the pulley. The direction of the traction force acting on the limb may be in a different direction to the ropes and can actually be greater than the gravitational force acting on the hanging masses if a movable pulley is used (see Hamilton-Russell traction below).

Traction relies on getting a good grip on the patient. If the traction force is applied to the skin by the friction produced by an adhesive strapping, it is called **skin traction**. If the traction force is applied directly to the bone by a pin inserted in the bone it is called **skeletal traction**. Such a surgically made, direct mechanical connection to the bone allows larger traction forces than are possible with skin traction.

4.12.3 *Examples of Traction*

Buck's extension (popularised by Buck (1861) during the American Civil War) is a sliding traction applied to the skin and is also known as 'straight leg' traction

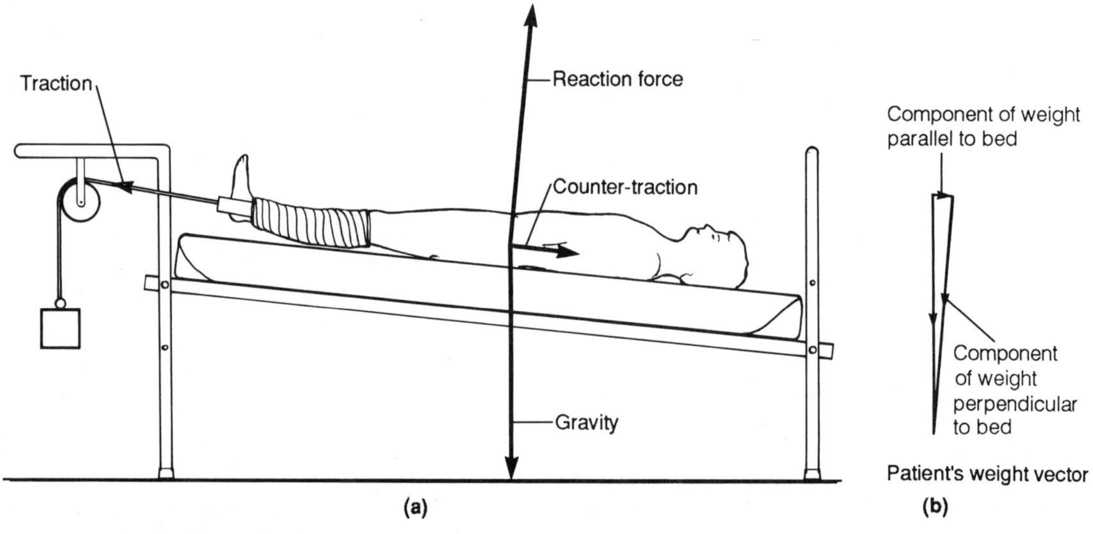

Figure 4.15 *Straight leg traction (Buck's extension)*

or Pugh traction (see Figure 4.15). The traction force is supplied by the weight (mass in kg ×9.8) hanging at the end of the bed which exerts tension in the rope. This tension is redirected by the fixed pulley so that it is parallel to the bed.

Counter-traction is supplied by the *component of the patient's weight that is parallel to the bed* (plus tension in the patient's muscles and friction between the patient and the bed). Note that the bed is tilted; this allows the patient's weight (which is directed towards the centre of the earth) to be resolved into two **component vectors**. These component vectors are at right angles to each other, one being directed parallel to the bed and the other perpendicular to the bed (see vector triangle in Figure 4.15). Notice that the 'counter-traction vector' is short compared to the more lengthy 'patient's weight vector'. This is to be expected, since the counter-traction force need only equal the traction force of about 30 N (a 3 kg mass) whereas the patient's weight may be 700 N. The greater the traction mass used, the higher the end of the bed must be raised (about 5 cm per kg), as raising the bed will increase the parallel component of the patient's weight. This parallel component is the counter-traction force.

Bryant's traction (gallows traction) is a type of suspended skin traction (see Figure 4.16). The pulleys change the direction of the gravitational pull on the cords from a downwards direction to upwards. It is used on small children who have a fractured femur because their body weights are not sufficient to provide the necessary counter-traction that is required if the traction cords were pulling horizontally. By positioning their legs vertically, almost the whole body weight of the child is used for counter-traction, rather than just friction between the child and the bed.

Hamilton-Russell traction is a form of traction that employs fixed pulleys (numbered 1, 2 and 4 in Figure 4.17) to redirect the cords and a movable pulley (numbered 3), attached to the foot, to magnify the force. Hence the resultant force, R, is the vector sum of the forces F_1, F_2 and F_3, each of which is the tension acting in the cord attached to the leg. The resultant force is actually greater than the tension in the cord, that is, more than the hanging mass × 9.8. Its

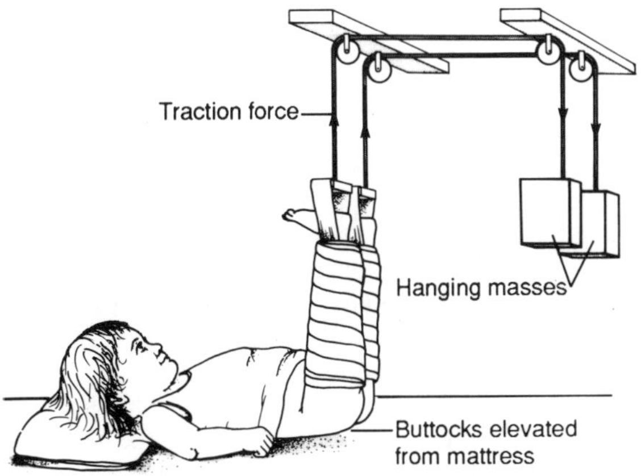

Figure 4.16 *Bryant's traction for reducing a fracture of the femur in small children. Notice that the fixed pulleys used produce an upwards force on the legs*

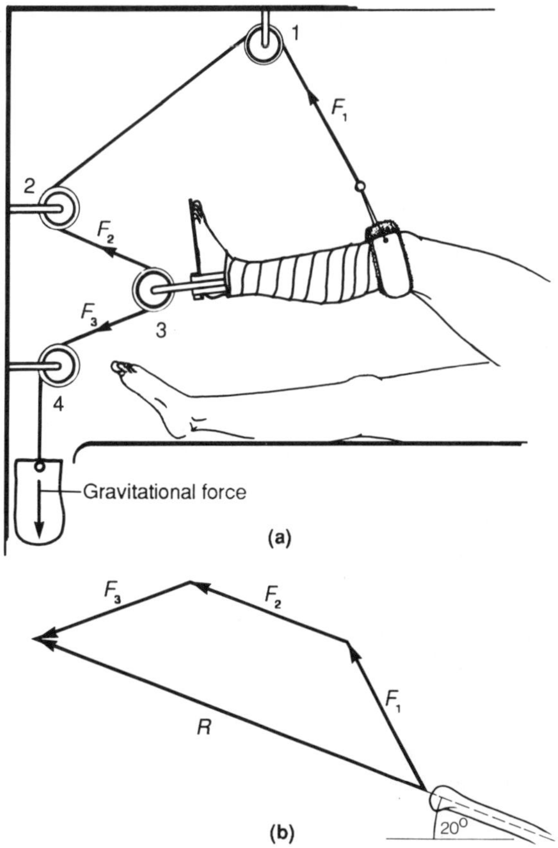

Figure 4.17 *Hamilton-Russell traction for fractures of the femur. Notice that the length of the vector representing the traction force on the femur (R), is the resultant of the vector sum of the three equal forces exerted by the cords that are attached to the leg*

magnitude and direction may be determined from the vector diagram. Notice that the resultant force is in the direction of the femur.

The traction mass needed to 'reduce' (correctly align the fractured bone) or maintain reduction of a fracture depends upon the site of the fracture, age and weight of patient, power of his or her muscles, muscle damage and friction in the system. The actual mass is determined by trial and observing the behaviour of the fracture. If a multiple pulley system is used, the mechanical advantage of the system must be known, so that the correct mass is applied. In the Hamilton-Russell above, a 4 kg mass (39.2 N weight) exerts a force of 98 N (equivalent to a 10 kg mass), thus the mechanical advantage is 10 divided by 4 (that is, 2.5).

Bibliography

Strait, L.A. and Inman, V.T. 'Sample illustrations of physical principles selected from physiology and medicine', *American Journal of Physiology*, **15**, 375–382, 1947.

Questions

1. Choose the one correct statement.
   J. The unit of weight is the kilogram.
   K. The unit of mass is the newton.
   L. Weight is a force.
   M. Inertia is mass multiplied by 9.8.

2. Which of the following is not an example of a force?
   J. tension
   K. friction
   L. inertia
   M. weight

3. If the imaginary line joining a person's centre of gravity to the centre of the earth passes through the person's base of support, we say that the person is
   J. unstable
   K. balanced
   L. using their back as a lever
   M. not doing any work

4. Which one of the following describes what could happen to an object when a balanced force is acting on it?
   J. The object starts to move.
   K. The object changes its direction but not its speed.
   L. The object changes its shape.
   M. Nothing happens.

5. In the schematic diagram of an arm, rod 1 represents the humerus and rod 2 the radius and ulna. *M* is a block being supported by the 'hand'. The positions indicated by *p*, *q*, *r* and *s* are the locations of the
   J. effort (*p*), centre of mass of the radius and ulna (*q*), fulcrum (*r*) and load (*s*)
   K. fulcrum (*p*), effort (*q*), centre of mass of radius and ulna (*r*) and load (*s*)
   L. centre of mass of radius and ulna (*p*), effort (*q*), load (*r*) and fulcrum (*s*)
   M. fulcrum (*p*), centre of mass of radius and ulna (*q*), effort (*r*) and load (*s*)

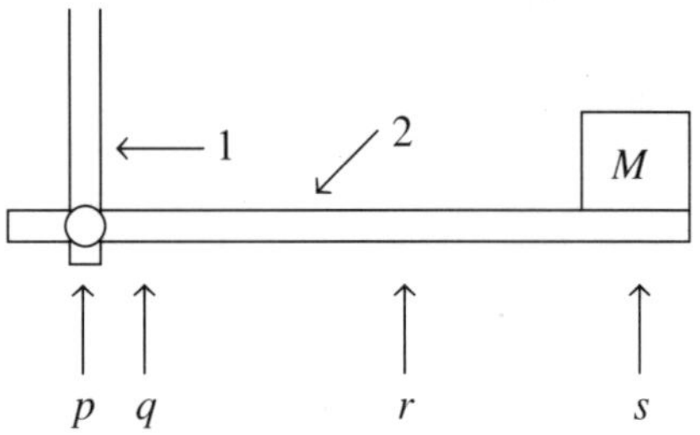

6. The lines below represent levers. The fulcrum (or pivot) is at *F*, the load is at *L* and the effort of a muscle is at *E*. Which lever could not represent one found in the human body?
   J. *E* ... *F* *L*
   K. *L* ... *F* ... *E*
   L. *F* *E* ... *L*
   M. *E* ... *L* ... *F*

7. In which of the following cases is the greatest amount of work being done on the object that is experiencing the force?
   J. 10 000 N is exerted on a wall for 30 s.
   K. 2000 N is used to raise an object by a height of 10 m.
   L. 5000 N is used to push an object a distance of 4 m.
   M. 1000 N is used to pull an object over 50 m.

8. What is the aim of 'correct lifting technique'?
   J. To maintain balance by keeping the centre of gravity over the base of support.
   K. To avoid working with heavy loads that are on the ground.
   L. To use the bones and muscles of the leg.
   M. To keep the back straight while using it as a lever.

9. The best definition of the *weight* of an object is the
    - J. force of attraction between the earth and the object
    - K. tendency of a body to maintain its state of motion
    - L. amount of matter contained in the body
    - M. mass of the object multiplied by its acceleration
10. The third-class lever systems of the human musculoskeletal system are inefficient because
    - J. third-class lever systems are the least efficient
    - K. the muscle insertion is closer to the joint than the load is
    - L. muscles can contract only by about 20% of their relaxed length
    - M. the force of muscle tension is less than the weight of the load
11. The meaning of 'work' in the scientific sense is
    - J. an artist's completed painting
    - K. the amount of energy transferred between objects
    - L. the functions performed during the course of paid employment
    - M. sustained physical or mental activity

CHAPTER 5
Energy

Our bodies use energy derived from food to operate and maintain their various organs, to keep a constant body temperature and to do external work. We have seen in Chapter 4 that energy changes are associated with the operation of forces. In the body, forces are always operating. For example, muscles are continually in action to pump blood, to maintain posture, to breathe, to move the contents of the digestive tract and to produce body movements. Thus our bodies are continually using energy (or more correctly, changing it from one form to another) in order to function. Furthermore, energy changes (and therefore forces) are also involved in the chemical reactions that are occurring in our bodies. Chemical changes can be thought of as involving the electrical forces that bind atoms together into molecules. Some of these chemical changes release the energy that our body needs for normal functioning.

In this chapter we will develop our understanding of the concept of energy and of energy conservation. Then we will consider how the body gains energy and how it uses and loses energy. Along the way we will quantify the amount of energy that our bodies use and investigate how the concept of heat is related to energy.

Learning Objectives

At the completion of this chapter you should be able to:

1. Define energy and name some of the forms of energy.
2. Know the principle of conservation of energy and give examples of it.
3. Distinguish between energy, work and power and know their units.
4. Understand how the energy values assigned to foods are arrived at.
5. Be familiar with metabolic rate and basal metabolic rate.
6. Use kinetic theory to understand temperature.
7. Describe the relationship between temperature, heat and energy.
8. Understand that heat moves by conduction, convection and radiation and apply these to heat therapy.
9. Explain how the body loses heat by sweating and how we can regulate the amount of heat lost from the body.
10. Understand melting and evaporation in terms of the energy of the particles.

5.1 The Concept of Energy

Energy is a familiar concept and one that is used in everyday living. We use electrical energy, gas and wood to cook our food or to run household appliances so we know that the burning of fuels is associated with producing electrical energy, heat and light. On some occasions we feel energetic while at other times we feel tired so we habitually associate energy with our bodies and our state of wellbeing. We are familiar with the debate about 'the energy crisis' and renewable and non-renewable energy resources, so we know that energy is stored in some things and that energy can be unleashed by certain processes. We are charged by the gas supply companies for the number of megajoules of energy we consume, and by the electrical authorities for the number of kilowatt-hours of power we use. This implies to us that energy is measurable and something that we use up. More correctly we change the forms of energy we pay for into other forms that are more useful to us. We might naively think that such a familiar concept and one as practical as energy should be easy to define, but let us try.

It is easy to see energy 'in action', but to define it simply presents a problem because energy is intangible. Rather than being a concrete object, energy is a combination of interactions and physical properties. Energy comes in many forms but is only evident when it changes form. Energy is known by many names depending on the interaction with which it is associated. Thus we have 'translational kinetic energy' in objects that are moving and 'rotational kinetic energy' in spinning objects. 'Potential energy' is stored in objects that have been raised in height (gravitational potential energy), in objects that have been compressed or stretched against their internal forces (elastic potential energy) and in the bonding between atoms (chemical potential energy). Electrically charged objects possess electrical potential energy when near each other. Within the atom we talk about the 'nuclear binding energy' that holds the atom together and the 'mass energy' of which the particles within atoms are made. Sound, heat and electromagnetic radiation are further manifestations or forms of energy.

5.1.1 *Towards a Definition for Energy*

The concept of energy is closely related to the concepts of force and work. We have defined force in Chapter 4. So we will use this definition to define work and in turn, use our work definition to define energy.

We have seen that an unbalanced force is an action (or an interaction) that causes a deformation or a change in the motion of the object on which it acts. Thus our muscles exert a force on our body when we suddenly stop walking, or when we move our arms, or when we expand our thoracic cavity during inspiration. When a force causes the object on which it acts to move or deform, then we say that 'work has been done on that object'. Two things enter into every case where work is done:

1. the exertion of a force;
2. the movement of something by that force.

Thus a clerk asleep at his desk is doing no work (in the physics sense) on his surroundings because no conscious forces are being exerted by his muscles. Furthermore, the shopper holding a 5 kg bag of groceries in each hand while waiting at the bus stop, is doing no work on the bags because they are not moving. When the shopper eventually boards the bus, the shopper's muscles cause the bags to move forwards and upwards, so work is done on the bags to lift them into the bus.

The amount of work done can be calculated, for the simplest case of a constant (unchanging) force that produces movement in a straight line, by the formula

$$\text{work} = \text{force} \times \text{distance} \ (W = F \times s)$$

Since force has units of newtons and distance has units of metres, the unit of work is the 'newton metre' but this cumbersome sounding unit is renamed the **joule**.

Having defined work in terms of force and motion (and previously having defined a force in terms of its effect on objects), we can now base our definition of energy on work. When work is done on an object, something is given (transferred) to the object. *This 'something' is energy.*

We know from experience that given certain circumstances, objects can do work. For example, a crane can lift a demolition ball over an old building and then allow it to drop. The act of stopping the falling ball will cause part of the building to collapse. That is, work has been done on the building. When water flows downhill through a pipe to push against the blades of a rotor, it causes a turbine to spin, that is, work is done on the turbine. By burning fuel, water can be made to boil to generate steam, which can be used to operate the piston of a steam engine and so cause work to be done. A wound spring can cause a clockwork mechanism to turn an assembly of gears and levers and so do work. *We call this capacity for doing work 'energy'.*

The energy of a body is measured by the work it can do. Conversely the energy possessed by an object is the amount of work that had to be done on it to bring the object to its current speed or position or condition.

To put it as simply as possible, we will ignore any energy that is converted to heat, sound or light and say that the increase in energy of an object is the amount of 'useful' work that was done on the object. In the case of the demolition ball, the useful work done on it is equal to the gravitational potential energy it gained by being lifted by the crane. In lifting the ball the crane also expended a lot of energy doing work that was not useful. This 'wasted' energy produced a lot of noise, movement of the crane and heat in the engine. The decrease in energy of an object is the amount of work done (both useful and useless) by the object on its surroundings. The ratio of the useful work done to the total energy used is called the efficiency of the change.

work = the increase (or decrease) in energy of an object

The relationship of energy to work is similar to the relationship between having cash and spending it. Cash is the energy and spending it is the work. Efficiency then can be likened to the money paid for an item compared to that item's cost in another shop. Because of this close relationship between energy and work, it should not be surprising that energy and work have the same unit, the joule.

5.1.2 *The Different Forms of Energy*

The nature of the circumstances mentioned above that resulted in work being performed by the various objects were quite different. These differences make it convenient to distinguish different forms of energy. Despite the mental struggling to define what energy is, there are many formulae that may conveniently be used for calculating the amount of energy present, as long as the situation is not complicated.

The energy that an object possesses by virtue of its movement is called **kinetic energy**. In simple cases, kinetic energy can be calculated by using the following equation:

$$\text{kinetic energy} = \frac{1}{2} \times m \times v^2$$

where m stands for mass (in kg) and v stands for speed (in m/s). Thus a 70 kg jogger running at 3 m/s has 315 J of kinetic energy. A 1200 kg car moving at 60 km/h (16.7 m/s) would have 167 000 J of kinetic energy. To stop the jogger would require 315 J of work, while to stop the car requires 167 000 J of work.

The energy possessed by an object by virtue of its height above some ground level is called **gravitational potential energy**. In simple cases it may be calculated using the following equation:

$$\text{gravitational potential energy} = m \times g \times h$$

where m is mass (in kg), g is 9.8 m/s^2, and h is height (in metres). Thus a 60 kg jogger who runs up a two-metre-high flight of steps has increased her gravitational potential energy by 1176 J. To lift two bags each containing 5 kg of groceries from the ground to carrying height (40 cm above ground) would require 39 J of work and would transfer 39 J of gravitational potential energy to the groceries.

The energy possessed by an object because of its mass is called **mass energy**. The energy released in a nuclear reaction can be calculated from the famous equation discovered by Einstein:

$$\text{mass energy} = m \times c^2$$

where the mass consumed, m, is in kg and c is the speed of light (3×10^8 m/s). There are two nuclear reactors in Australia, the HIFAR reactor and MOATA, both at Lucas Heights near Sydney. At maximum power, HIFAR can produce 10 MW of heat (10 000 000 J each second). To produce this much energy for one hour would require the consumption of 0.4 mg of mass (assuming 100% efficiency). About 2.6 thousand million times as much coal (that is, 1050 kg) would produce about the same amount of heat as it is burned.

The energy stored in a stretched rubber cord or a steel spring is called **elastic potential energy**. It may be estimated using the following equation:

$$\text{elastic potential energy} = \frac{1}{2} \times k \times d^2$$

where d is the length (in metres) by which the cord or spring has been extended from its relaxed length, and k (the spring constant) is a number peculiar to individual elastic objects. k depends on the springiness of the object. In New Zealand, near Queenstown, the practice of 'bungy jumping' is popular among some people. A long (and strong) rubber cord (the bungy) is attached to the 'jumper' before they throw themselves from a tall bridge crossing a river. We will consider the energy changes that occur to 'Mark' as he jumps.

Before the jump, Mark (a 70 kg devotee), is standing on the bridge, 43 m above the water and his body is in possession of 29 500 J of gravitational potential energy.

On falling 15 m Mark will have 10 300 J of translational kinetic energy and be travelling at 17 m/s (62 km/h). Mark, by now quite exhilarated, will have 19 200 J of gravitational potential energy left (because the sum of kinetic and gravitational energies must be 29 500 J). At this point the rubber cord will begin to stretch and (hopefully) gradually reduce Mark's speed to zero. When fully extended, the bungy is about 35 m long and Mark would have a speed of zero and be just above the river surface. The stretched bungy will have just less than 29 500 J of elastic potential energy stored in it (some of Mark's original gravitational potential energy would be converted to heat in the bungy and to sound). These figures allow us to calculate k for the rubber bungy to be about 148 J/m^2. As you can imagine, such calculations are essential to ensure the safety of the jump.

Light (one of the forms of electromagnetic radiation — see Section 12.6) is composed of a huge number of separate packets of energy that are called photons. The energy carried by each photon depends on the frequency of the photon and may be determined from the following relationship:

$$\text{electromagnetic energy} = h \times f$$

where f is the frequency of the radiation and h is the number 6.63×10^{-34} Js. A photon of visible light carries about 3×10^{-19} J of energy. Even this small amount of energy, carried by 100 or so photons, is sufficient to produce the changes in our retina that give us the sensation of vision. Much more energy is carried by a gamma ray photon, which may have several million times the amount of energy of a visible light photon.

The amount of electrical energy that an appliance 'consumes' may be determined from its electrical resistance (R), the current flowing through it (I) and the potential difference applied to it (V). In fact, any two of these three quantities are sufficient if the time (in seconds) for which the current flows is also known. Thus, if V is in volts, I in amperes and R is in ohms the number of joules of electrical energy consumed can be calculated from the following equation:

$$\text{electrical energy} = V \times I \times \text{time} = I^2 \times R \times \text{time} = \frac{V^2 \times \text{time}}{R}$$

5.2 The Conservation of Energy

Macroscopic and non-living objects may be said to possess **mechanical energy** in the form of kinetic energy and potential energy (and internal energy, but more about this one later!). The kinetic energy of a body may be interpreted as its ability to do work by virtue of its motion. If an object is in motion it has kinetic energy. Potential energy represents a form of stored energy that can be fully recovered and converted to kinetic energy. The total mechanical energy of a system must remain the same, regardless of how the parts of the system may interact or are arranged.

We may generalise a law from our experience to include all forms of energy. It is known as the **principle of conservation of energy** (first stated clearly in 1847 by Hermann von Helmholtz):

> Energy may be transformed from one kind to another, but it cannot be created nor destroyed.

In other words *the total amount of energy (kinetic plus potential plus internal energy plus other forms) does not change, it is constant.*

In science, 'conservation' is a term used to signify that the total remains the same. However, in general conversational usage 'conservation of energy' refers to the 'wise use of resources'. In this book conservation of energy refers to the principle expressed above.

Whenever energy 'appears' in forms that were not previously present, then energy transformations have occurred to give rise to the changed form of energy. Despite the transformations, the total amount of energy in the universe is believed to be constant.

Often in history the principle seemed to fail, for example when the discoveries of radioactivity, X-rays and the neutrino were made. Furthermore, the explanations for the high temperatures in the earth's interior, the radiation of energy from a 'black body' and the energy source of the sun all defied human imagination for a time. In fact the energy source for the astronomical objects called 'quasars' (quasi-stellar objects) is still unknown. Each apparent failure of the principle stimulated the search for reasons. Experimentalists searched for phenomena besides motion that accompany the forces that act between objects. Such phenomena have always been found and energy conservation has never been known to fail. Scientists are so confident of the validity of the principle of energy conservation that they confidently look forward to the future explanation of quasars and eagerly await the new insights that it will bring.

5.2.1 *Energy Transformations and the Sun*

Let us consider a chain of energy transformations, which begins with the sun. The sun is so massive that the gravitational force of attraction it produces is large enough to accelerate the hydrogen nuclei of which it is largely composed to speeds which allow them to fuse with each other when they collide. Different elements with heavier nuclei are produced by the fusion of hydrogen nuclei and some of the mass of the original hydrogen nuclei is transformed into kinetic energy. The continually accelerating and fast-moving charged particles in the sun produce electromagnetic radiation which carries energy into space in all directions.

The earth intercepts a small amount of the sun's energy output. Some of it is scattered by the atmosphere, some of it warms the earth and some of it is absorbed by green plants. These plants use their captured energy to photosynthesise and so produce food for humans and grazing animals (or fuel for our industry). We ingest energy in the form of plant and animal tissue (or materials refined from them) and we store it in our bodies. As it is required, this stored energy is used to maintain our internal functions, and to contract our muscles. Some of the energy we derive from our diet is used to warm our clothes and the air near our skin and so is lost to our surroundings. The earth re-radiates some of its energy (that ultimately came from the sun) back into space and so is able to cool. As long as the amount of energy that the earth receives is matched by the amount of energy the earth re-radiates, the planet remains an hospitable environment.

5.2.2 *Conservation of Energy in the Human Body*

We can apply the principle of energy conservation to the human body. Suppose that no food or drink is ingested (it would increase chemical potential energy and internal energy), no faeces or urine is excreted (they would carry internal energy away), and the surroundings are shaded from the sun and at a lower temperature than the body (otherwise the body would gain energy by radiation). In the body, energy may be stored in the chemical bonds in body fat, glycogen and adenosine tri-phosphate (ATP), and as body heat. Then any change in the energy that is stored in the body must be due to the loss of body heat and to the work done by the body on the surroundings. That is, the loss of one form of energy from the body is matched by the increase in the amount of another form of energy outside the body. Conservation of energy in the body can be written as an equation.

$$\underset{\text{the change in stored energy}}{\Delta U} = \underset{\text{heat lost from the body}}{\Delta Q} + \underset{\text{work done by the body}}{W}$$

In order to verify the principle for the human body it was necessary to construct a calorimeter which was large enough to accommodate a man for several days in reasonable comfort. Such a calorimeter was constructed by Atwater and Benedict in 1895 and used for human experiments over the next 15 years. The chamber was surrounded by five separate walls to prevent any gain or loss of heat and fitted with devices to cool and ventilate it. The temperature difference between the air inflow and the outflow was measured as was its water vapour and carbon dioxide content. The amount of heat withdrawn by the cooling system, the energy value of the food handed in and of the excreta handed out were all measured. The man was also weighed.

The average of 12 experiments over 41 days showed that the daily energy input for the subject was 9500 kJ and was within 0.3% of the daily energy output. When the subject was required to perform work, the average of 20 experiments over 66 days showed that the daily energy input was 17 500 kJ. Again this was within 0.3% of the energy output. Because the energy input was (within acceptable experimental error) equal to the energy output, we can say that the principle of conservation of energy holds for human metabolism. The efficiency of the 'human machine' was also calculated to be about 25%. This means that if a man is to perform a known number of joules of work, it is necessary to supply him with extra energy equal to four times the amount of work to be done.

5.3 The Units of Energy

About 1840 in Britain, James Joule demonstrated that when mechanical energy was used to turn paddles that stirred water, the temperature of the water was raised. That is, he demonstrated that mechanical energy could be transferred to water and appear as a rise in temperature. In other words he showed that *heat was just another form of energy* (quite an achievement at the time). For his ingenuity and influence the metric unit of energy, the **joule** (J), is named in his honour.

It takes 4187 J of energy to raise the temperature of one kilogram of water (which has a volume of one litre) by one degree Celsius. In comparison, a one kilogram mass that has been lifted vertically through 427 m (higher than a building of 100 stories) has gained 4187 J of gravitational potential energy. A one kilogram mass moving at 91.5 m/s (330 km/h) has 4187 J of kinetic energy. Clearly water has the ability to absorb a large amount of internal energy, without a major change in its temperature. Only one other substance (hydrogen gas) produces a smaller temperature rise as it absorbs internal energy.

As energy is converted from one form to another, we say 'work is done'. Since work is the same thing as energy change, work has the same unit as energy. For example, 4187 J of work was done on the one kilogram mass to raise it 427 m. The speeding one kilogram mass would do 4187 J of work in coming to rest. *Work is equivalent to the amount of energy being converted from one form to another*. However, if energy, stored as chemical potential energy, is released by oxidation and/or combustion we say 'heat is given out' rather than work is done.

Power refers to how *quickly* energy is converted from one form to another (or how fast work is done, or how much heat is produced in a set time). Thus power is distinct from work and energy and is measured in joules per second. This unit is renamed the **watt** (W) in honour of James Watt who (in the 1770s) made major improvements to the steam engines of his day. He in fact suggested the 'horsepower' as a unit of power. One horsepower is the rate of work that can be performed by 'an honest horse' and is approximately equal to 746 W (or 0.746 kW).

NUTRITION INFORMATION
Servings per package: 24. Serving size: 30 g (2 biscuits)

	Per Serving	Per 100 g	2 BISCUITS WITH 1/2 CUP (125 ml) WHOLE MILK	SO GOOD
ENERGY (kJ)	410	1380	750	735
PROTEIN (g)	3.7	12.4	7.8	7.9
FAT (g)	0.8	2.7	5.5	5
CARBOHYDRATE				
TOTAL (g)	19.3	64.3	25	25.2
SUGARS (g)	0.7	2.3	6.4	2.7
SODIUM (mg)	80	270	153	149
POTASSIUM (mg)	105	350	297	280

In accordance with the regulations set out in the Australian Food Standards Code, the following information refers to the quantity of 60 g (4 biscuits) alone, and with 1 cup (250 ml) of whole milk or So Good Non-Dairy Drink.

60 g OF SANITARIUM WEET-BIX CONTAINS

* D. A. = Daily Allowance

	ALONE		WITH 1 CUP (250 ml) WHOLE MILK		SO GOOD	
	By Weight (mg)	% D. A.*	By Weight (mg)	% D. A.*	By Weight (mg)	% D. A.*
THIAMINE	0.55	50	0.65	59	0.66	60
RIBOFLAVIN	0.8	50	1.22	76	1.22	76
NIACIN	5.5	50	5.75	52	6.63	60
IRON	5.0	50	5.25	52	6.25	62

INGREDIENTS: WHOLE WHEAT, RAW SUGAR, SALT, MALT EXTRACT, VITAMINS (NIACIN, THIAMINE, RIBOFLAVIN), MINERAL (IRON). NO ARTIFICIAL FLAVOURINGS OR COLOURINGS.

*Weet-Bix is a Trademark of Sanitarium Health Food Company.

Figure 5.1 *A nutrition information label. Notice that the energy value per 100 g is given in kilojoules*

5.4 Food Energy

Since the joule is a relatively small quantity of energy, the energy value of foods are usually quoted in kilojoules (thousands of joules) or megajoules (millions of joules) (see Figure 5.1). Lavoisier suggested (in 1784) that food is **oxidised**. This means that oxygen is consumed during the process of metabolism of food in the body. In oxidation by combustion (burning), heat is released. In the oxidation process within the body, heat is also released, as energy of metabolism. An approximation of the nutritional energy available from a food may be obtained by burning the food in pure oxygen inside a device called a **calorimeter** (see Figure 5.2). Food is burnt in the oxidation chamber and the energy produced is transferred as heat to the water surrounding the chamber.

Applying the principle of conservation of energy, the energy given off during combustion must equal the heat energy gained by the calorimeter (as long as care is taken to correct for the loss of heat to the surroundings). From the measurement of calorimeter temperature before and after combustion the equation

$$Q = sm\,\Delta T$$

may be used to calculate energy released, where Q = energy released (in kJ), s = specific heat of water (0.004187 kJ/g/°C), m = mass of water (in g) and ΔT = temperature change of water in calorimeter (in °C).

Foods are highly variable in their carbohydrate, fat and protein contents. Thus any kilojoule value that appears in published tables, such as Table 5.1, can only be a guide. As such, it may not correspond to the energy value of a particular sample. Nevertheless, in the hands of experienced health professionals, these tables are a valuable resource.

5.5 Basal Metabolic Rate

When completely at rest, a human body typically consumes energy at the rate of 170 kJ per hour per square metre of body surface. The rate of energy consumption increases approximately in proportion to the body surface area. The dependence on area arises because the body loses heat through its outer surface. Hence the rate at which the body loses heat is a function of body surface area. A 'typical' man (70 to 80 kg) has

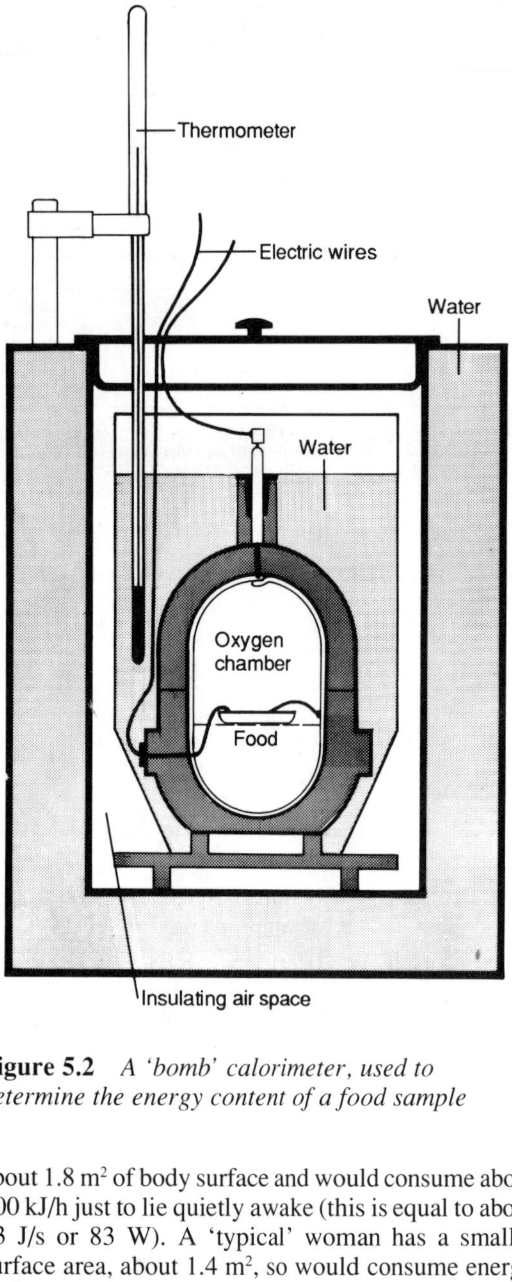

Figure 5.2 *A 'bomb' calorimeter, used to determine the energy content of a food sample*

about 1.8 m^2 of body surface and would consume about 300 kJ/h just to lie quietly awake (this is equal to about 83 J/s or 83 W). A 'typical' woman has a smaller surface area, about 1.4 m^2, so would consume energy at the rate of about 66 W.

Body surface area may be easily determined (with the aid of a calculator) from the following empirical formula:

$$\text{area (in square metres)} = (\text{mass}^{0.425}) \times (\text{height}^{0.725}) \times 0.007184$$

where mass is in kilograms and height is in centimetres and both are raised to the fractional power indicated.

Any body activity requires energy. To achieve the minimum rate of energy usage (a state we may call 'absolute rest'), as many unessential activities as possible must be eliminated. Fasting for about 12 hours will eliminate digestive activity. Lying down for 30 minutes after a period of several hours without strenuous activity, having had an adequate night's sleep, being in a calm and relaxed frame of mind and being in a room of comfortable temperature all help to reduce metabolic activity to a minimum. The rate of energy utilisation during 'absolute rest', but while awake, is called the **basal metabolic rate** (BMR) and is expressed in units of kilojoules per square metre of body area per hour. It is the minimum energy required to perform essential functions such as breathing, pumping blood through the arteries and maintaining body temperature. BMR can be measured directly by placing the subject inside a respiration calorimeter, as described in Section 5.2.2.

BMR may be measured indirectly (and far more easily) by measuring the oxygen consumption of a person when completely rested. About 20.9 kJ of energy is produced for each litre of oxygen consumed and about 0.24 l/min is consumed by a 70 kg male while asleep (consumption rises to about 0.6 l/min when sitting and listening attentively). Since metabolic rate is dependent on, among other things, thyroid hormone secretion, the determination of BMR can be used to assess thyroid function. When corrections are made for age, weight and sex, 85% of healthy persons have been found to have a BMR within 10% of the average.

Patients with extensive burns to their body have a higher BMR than normal (up to twice as high) so need a higher-energy diet than other bedridden patients. Patients with cancer or recovering from surgery also have higher metabolic rates in order to recover or cope with their condition and may need a diet higher in protein.

5.6 The Energy Consumed by Physical Activities

The food energy used in performing various physical activities may be estimated by measuring oxygen consumption (in litres per minute) during the activity. The technique is based on the fact that the ultimate origin of most of the heat released by the body is from the chemical reactions between oxygen and food. About 20.9 kJ of energy are released per litre of oxygen consumed. Note that the energy consumed while performing an activity will vary between individuals

Table 5.1 *Food kilojoule table*

Food		Mass (g)	Energy content (kJ, approx.)
orange juice	250 ml		430
whole milk	250 ml		650
skim milk	250 ml		340
beer (2–3% alc.)	250 ml		290
beer (3.5–4.5% alc.)	250 ml		430
dry wine	250 ml		580
spirits	250 ml		2420
lemonade	250 ml		460
wholemeal bread	3 slices	90	930
white bread	4 slices	90	940
crumpets	2	108	820
rice boiled		100	450
macaroni boiled		100	500
dried dates		100	1200
dried apricots		100	1120
sultanas, raisins		100	1170
carrots (raw)		100	150
celery (raw)		100	100
lettuce		100	100
tomato		100	90
cabbage		100	110
beef, rump steak (lean) grilled		100	840
lamb loin chops (lean) grilled		100	320
pork chops grilled		100	1825
chicken breast (boned)		100	830
fish crumbed and fried		100	1060
sausage		100	1290
salami		100	1680
apple		100	220
banana		100	320
grapes		100	280
strawberries		100	160
watermelon		100	120
cheddar cheese		100	1700
butter		100	2900
margarine		100	2900
cooking oil		100	2500
chocolate		100	2300

because of height, mass and sex differences. Table 5.2 lists the approximate energy consumed by some activities.

To sleep all day would require about 7200 kJ. To sleep for 7 hours and 'walk fast' for 17 hours would require about 27 600 kJ. Your daily energy requirement probably lies between these two extremes. For example, 7 hours sleep (2100 kJ), 2 hours of moderate activity (3000 kJ), 10 hours of light activity (7000 kJ) and 5 hours of resting activities (3000 kJ) would require an intake of about 15 100 kJ. Many of you would require less than this much energy as your level of activity would be less or your body size smaller than 'average'.

We may apply the input and output of energy to the 'problem' of trying to lose weight. For each 30 000 kJ you eat above your requirements, your body stores about one kilogram of fat. To lose half a kilogram of body fat per week would require your daily energy output to be 2000 kJ more than the energy value of the food you eat each day. This can be achieved by walking fast for an hour and twenty minutes *every* day or by reducing the energy content of your diet (or a combination of both). Clearly it is easier to eat less of the foods with very high energy values. Nevertheless extravagent claims for miracle diets continue to appear in newspapers. Figure 5.3 is typical of such advertisements.

Table 5.2 *The energy cost (for adults) of different aerobic activities*

Activity type	Examples
resting activities (using 5–10 kJ/min)	sleeping, lying quietly awake, sitting relaxed at rest, standing relaxed
light activity (using 10–20 kJ/min)	light gardening, slow walking, household work with modern appliances, golf, painting, gymnastic exercises
moderate activity (using 20–30 kJ/min)	ballroom dancing, tennis, swimming, cycling, fast walking (120 steps/minute), general labouring with pick and shovel
strenuous activity (using 30–40 kJ/min)	skipping, jogging, climbing stairs, running, playing football/soccer/hockey
very strenuous activity (using 40+ kJ/min)	fast swimming, hill climbing, cross-country running

5.7 Heat, a Form of Energy

Until the start of the nineteenth century heat was thought to be a physical substance called 'caloric' which transferred or flowed like water between objects at different temperatures. Benjamin Thomson (an American who later became Count Rumford of Bavaria) showed in 1798 that heat was not a material substance. Instead it was an observable property produced as a result of mechanical work being done. Nevertheless we still describe many common temperature changes as the transfer of 'something' from one body at a higher temperature to another at a lower temperature. This 'something' we call **heat**. A common definition is *heat is that which is transferred between a system and its surroundings as a result of temperature differences only.* James Joule arrived at the true nature of heat in 1840 when he succeeded in measuring the amount of heat produced by a known amount of work. We now understand that heat is a form of energy rather than a substance.

5.8 Temperature and Kinetic Theory

Heat and temperature are not the same thing, even though in everyday language they are used synonomously. Try repeating the experiment of John Locke in 1690. Put your right hand in 'hot' water and your left in 'cold' water. Then put both hands in water of intermediate 'hotness'. Your right hand will feel the water to be 'cold' while your left finds it 'warmer'. A steel ruler lying alongside a plastic ruler will feel 'colder' than the plastic one even though both rulers are at the same temperature. Clearly our judgement of temperature can be misleading. The human sensations of 'hot' and 'cold' depend on the local skin temperature, the temperature of the object being touched and whether the object is a good or poor conductor of heat.

"Here is an unbelievable secret for losing weight"

A scientific discovery allowed me to lose 49 kilograms in less than a year while I was eating 6 times a day.

Now you can lose weight while you eat everything you want (even a whole chicken for dinner). No pills to take. No exercise routine.

Famed Spanish singer Julio Eetalote lost 2 kilos per week by eating 6 times a day – one of which is a whole chicken.

Julio's book, co-written with expert dietitian Valerie Thinska, tells you:
1. Which foods form fat when eaten together at the same meal and therefore must be avoided.
2. Which foods do not form fat when eaten together and therefore can be eaten at any time.

His secret: complementary foods

You eat all you want and as much as you want. Just be sure not to eat certain foods together during the one meal. For example: you can eat as much beef as you want with as many vegetables as you like. But you can't eat French fries or milk.

Other secrets

In the book Julio Eetalote also tells you:
* Why you must drink lots of water.
* The incredible benefits of certain vegetables for your health.
* Mouth-watering recipes that let you eat like royalty while you lose weight.

Figure 5.3 *This simulated newspaper advertisement is not dissimilar to some that appear in the daily press. The real ad cannot appear for copyright reasons*

The atomic view of matter is that any piece of matter is composed of an almost inconceivably large number of particles. In solids the particles are more or less rooted to a particular place relative to the neighbouring particles, but are able to vibrate in their fixed position. Since the particles vibrate, they are in motion (albeit of very limited extent). This means that the particles have kinetic energy. Kinetic theory (see also Section 10.7) relates the temperature of an object to the average kinetic energy of the particles that make up the object. Thus the faster the motion of the constituent particles, the higher the temperature. In fact the average speed of oxygen and nitrogen molecules in air at a temperature of 20 °C is close to 500 m/s (some molecules will have lesser speeds and some will have much greater speeds).

In solids, particles are fixed in place alongside their neighbours by chemical bonds (that is, electric forces). Nevertheless, these particles can vibrate around their average position with an amplitude (maximum displacement) of about 10^{-11} m. As the temperature of the solid increases so does the amplitude of the vibration of the particles. Since all the particles are increasing their vibration as temperature rises, they take up more space, that is, solids *expand when heated* because the vibration of the particles causes them to occupy more space.

If a solid is heated, its temperature rises (that is, its particles increase their kinetic energy by vibrating faster) until melting begins. At this point temperature remains constant while the heat energy being added is used to break the bonds that hold the particles of the solid in place. When the bonds are broken, the particles move independently of one another and in random directions. The solid has melted when most of the bonds are broken and the material is said to be in the liquid state. With further heating, the temperature of the liquid rises (that is, its particles increase their kinetic energy by moving with higher speed) until boiling begins. At this point temperature remains constant while the heat energy being added is used to sever completely the weak bonds that hold liquid particles in the vicinity of one another. When this is achieved, the particles are moving at high speed, in random directions, as gas particles. Note that during boiling the temperature remains constant, even though heat energy is continually being added, until all the liquid has become gas. The temperature of the gas then begins to rise if more heat energy is applied. We can now distinguish between heat and temperature:

> Temperature is a measure of the average random translational kinetic energy of the particles of a substance.

> Heat is the energy that transfers from an object at a higher temperature to one at a lower temperature.

Thermal energy is a term used in an attempt to avoid the ambiguous conversational usage of 'hot' and 'cold'. The human sensation of hot and cold may depend on the temperature difference between two objects, on the temperature difference between our skin and an object, and on the ability of the material to conduct heat. The thermal energy of an object is the sum of the kinetic energies involved in the random translational, rotational and vibrational motion of all the particles in the object. Thus 200 g of steel at 20 °C has more thermal energy than 100 g of steel at the same temperature. Despite the particles in each sample of steel having the same average kinetic energy, there are twice as many particles in 200 g, so their total energy must add up to be more than the total for 100 g. The 100 g of steel at 20 °C has more thermal energy than 100 g of steel at 10 °C even though the number of particles is the same, because the particles at 20 °C have a higher average kinetic energy than those at 10 °C.

Internal energy includes another form of energy in addition to the three kinetic energies that make up the thermal energy of an object. Internal energy is the sum of the thermal energy of an object and the work done on the object. In the case of melting ice, work must be done on the ice (that is, energy added to it) to overcome the bonding forces that hold the water molecules rigidly in place in the ice crystal. This work does not add to the kinetic energy of the water molecules, so the thermal energy does not increase, but the extra energy is added to the total energy present, that is, the internal energy.

Thus one litre of water at 0 °C has more internal energy than the same number of molecules of ice at 0 °C because work has been done to break the bonds between molecules. In this case the water and ice have the same temperature and so have the same thermal energy. On the other hand, one litre of water at 20 °C has more internal energy than one litre of water at 10° C because the molecules at the higher temperature have a higher average kinetic energy and so possess more thermal energy.

5.9 Temperature Measurement

To measure temperature we use a property of substances that depends in a uniform manner upon temperature. For example, mercury expands uniformly when heated and Kircher (in 1643) used this fact to construct the first mercury thermometer. In a clinical (or fever) thermometer, the mercury expands more than the glass surrounding it and thus produces an increase in the level of liquid in the capillary. The expansion of the liquid in a thermometer is not large; mercury increases in volume by only 1.82% in going from 0 °C to 100 °C. In order to show this expansion, thermometers are designed so that the mercury is forced to rise from the bulb into a tube of very small diameter (called a capillary tube). The smaller the diameter of the capillary, the greater is the sensitivity of the thermometer. A clinical thermometer, which needs to show fractions of a degree, requires a capillary of less than 0.1 mm in diameter (see Figure 5.4). Such a thin line would be difficult to see were it not for the magnifying effect of the glass front. The visibility of the mercury thread is further enhanced by being set against a white background.

A clinical thermometer is a 'maximum reading' thermometer. This means it will continue to display the maximum temperature that it has reached even after being removed from the patient. The capillary tube has a constriction in it that mercury is able to push through as it expands up the thermometer. When

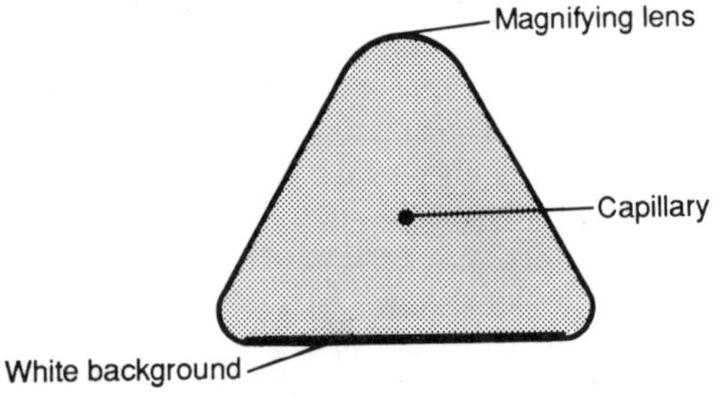

Figure 5.4 *A cross-section through a clinical thermometer (10 times the actual size)*

mercury contracts, the thin column of mercury breaks at the constriction leaving its level unchanged in the thermometer.

The Swede Anders Celsius (in 1742) proposed the temperature scale we use today based on 100 degrees. For reference points he used the temperature of an ice and water mixture (he nominated this temperature to be 0 °C) and the temperature of the steam above boiling water (this temperature Celsius designated as 100 °C). The Celsius thermometer is then marked with 100 equal intervals between these two reference marks. In 1854 William Thomson (who later became Lord Kelvin) proposed a thermodynamic temperature scale, also called the absolute temperature scale. Kinetic theory and thermodynamic theory both predict the existence of an 'absolute zero' of temperature where the kinetic energy of particles is at a minimum.

On the Kelvin scale, 0 K is the absolute zero; temperatures below this do not exist. To convert from degrees celsius to kelvins, simply add 273.15 to the celsius reading. Note that one kelvin degree is the same-sized interval as one celsius degree, so that 0 K = –273.15 °C and 273.15 K = 0 °C and 373.15 K = 100 °C. Note also that the absolute zero of tempera–ture has defied all attempts to reach it experimentally but that it is possible to come very close. Liquid helium boils at 4.2 K (–268.95 °C), but in very low pressures, helium can be made to boil even closer to zero kelvin.

5.10 The Transmission of Heat

Energy, in the form of heat, can transfer between non-living objects at different temperatures by three distinct processes: conduction, convection and radiation. In almost all cases, the three processes operate together. An automobile's cooling system has a liquid circulating through the motor (a forced convection movement) which gains heat from the motor by conduction. The high-temperature liquid then loses its heat when it moves into the fluted metal parts of the 'radiator'. The radiator in turn loses its heat by convection to the stream of air that moves over it (thus a truer descriptive name for a car's radiator would be 'convector'). When a car stops and its bonnet is lifted, the radiative heat loss from the motor is immediately obvious.

Evaporative heat loss is a mechanism by which heat may be transferred away from objects that can be wetted. An example of this is the canvas water-bag which was common before 'eskys' became widely available. The water-bag keeps its contents cool by continually evaporating water from the canvas. This mechanism for losing heat will be described in greater detail in Section 5.11.3.

5.10.1 *Conduction*

When two objects at different temperatures are touching, the one at the higher temperature will pass heat to the one at lower temperature. The particles of the object at the higher temperature are, on average, moving faster than the particles of the object at lower temperature. Each particle passes heat to the particle next to it *by contact*. The faster-moving particles of the high-temperature object collide with the slower-moving particles of the low-temperature object (and vice versa!). The result will be an *increase* in speed (and kinetic energy) for the slower-moving particles and a *decrease* in speed (and kinetic energy) for the faster-moving particles. The process of transfer of kinetic energy will continue until the particles of both objects have the same average kinetic energy. At that point, the objects will be at the same temperature.

When heat is transmitted through a solid body in this way the process is called conduction. 'Cold' hands can be 'warmed up' if they are tucked under someone's jumper and placed on their bare skin. The 'warm' skin underneath the jumper is at a higher temperature than the skin of the hands, so heat will flow into the hands. The hands and skin are 'in contact' so the heat transfer is by conduction. A hot-water bottle in bed also transfers heat by conduction.

Substances differ quite markedly in the ease with which they allow heat conduction to occur (see Table 5.3). Generally speaking gases are poor conductors of heat compared to liquids and solids (gases have thermal conductivities of less than one mW/cm/K). Water has a conductivity of 59 mW/cm/K. Most good conductors are metals or metal alloys.

Because metals conduct heat well, they 'feel cold' when in contact with our skin. They can withdraw heat rapidly from us, and its loss produces the sensation of 'coldness' even though the metal is at room temperature. When you touch a very cold metal object, heat energy transfers from your hand to the metal. Since metal is a good conductor of heat, energy will move from that part of the metal being touched by your hand to all other parts of the metal. Heat will continue to flow out of your hand (and the metal will continue to 'feel cold') until the whole object is at the same temperature as the skin on your hand. Vaso-constriction will probably allow the temperature of your skin to drop to below the value it was before

Table 5.3 *Thermal conductivity* (k) *of some common substance*

Substance	k (mW/cm/K)
air	0.25
clothing	0.4
human body fat	2
water	5.9
bricks/mortar/concrete	8
steel	400
aluminium	2100
copper	3900
silver	4200

contacting the metal, so this will reduce the rate at which heat is lost from the hand.

If your hand touches a very cold but poorly conducting object, like wood or clothing, only the area in contact with your hand will gain heat. Only that area of contact will rise in temperature until it is at the same temperature as the hand. Because the object is made of poorly conducting material, it does not allow the heat to be transferred to other parts of the object. Consequently the hand does not lose as much heat. That part of the poor conductor in contact with the hand reaches hand temperature sooner. At this temperature, the poor conductor no longer 'feels cold'.

To avoid discomfort for the patient, a nurse should warm the bed pans and other metal objects (like the bell of a stethoscope) from room temperature to skin temperature before placing them in contact with the patient's body.

Heat transfer by conduction can be reduced by wrapping the object to be isolated from heat in an insulating substance (a poor conductor). The fat of the subcutaneous tissues is a heat insulator for the body because fat conducts heat at about one third of the rate of other tissue. Each millimetre of fat insulates to the extent that a person can feel comfortable in a 1.5 °C lower temperature. Body fat alone is not a sufficient insulator for humans, so clothes which are made from insulating materials are usually worn.

'Ice-packs' placed in contact with the body help control swelling after sprains, bruises and muscle strains by 'applying cold'. In fact 'withdrawing heat' is a better description of what they do. The difference in temperature causes heat to flow from the body to the ice pack which in turn causes vasoconstriction. With less blood moving into the damaged area, less swelling can occur. If the ice is wrapped in a wet towel, heat transfer by conduction is facilitated because the wet towel makes good contact with the skin (by excluding air). Furthermore, while the ice is melting, the wet towel is kept at almost 0 °C because the heat that transfers to the wet towel is used to break the bonds between the water molecules in ice, rather than to increase the random kinetic energy of water molecules. If the temperature of the ice pack is allowed to increase until it is at the same temperature as the skin, there is no longer a temperature difference, so no more heat will flow from the body. In this situation the average vibrational kinetic energy of the particles in the ice pack is the same as that of the particles in the skin.

5.10.2 *Convection*

When the material through which heat is flowing is not a solid, the particles of the material are free to move. This means that as well as heat moving away from the higher-temperature object by conduction, the particles themselves can move away. This movement of fluid that has gained heat is called convection.

The particles of a fluid in the vicinity of a source of heat move faster as energy is transferred to them. They occupy more space as they move further apart. This causes the fluid to expand. The expansion decreases the density of the fluid in the vicinity of the heat source and the warmed and less dense fluid rises through the surrounding fluid, allowing fluid of greater density (and lower temperature) to take its place. This replacement fluid also will gain heat, expand and rise. The cyclic flow of heated particles from one place to another at a lower temperature is called a **convection current** and allows heat to be transferred by convection (see Figure 5.5).

Clothing our bodies with poorly conducting materials such as wool (which has a conductivity of 0.4), cotton and synthetic fabrics, prevents heat loss by conduction, but also allows air to be trapped close to the body. This trapped air is heated by the body but is largely prevented from forming convection currents by the clothing, and so is prevented from transferring heat away. The warm layer of air provides further insulation against heat loss. A slow loss of heat does take place since small convection currents are set up in the air occupying the minute spaces or pores in the material. Such heat loss may be reduced by wearing an extra layer of clothing or by wearing a relatively non-porous material like plastic or leather.

A breeze can hasten the loss of heat by convection because the heated molecules are moved away from the body faster. This may be achieved by opening windows or by using electric fans. Sitting in a bath of water at a temperature lower than body temperature will transfer heat from the person both by conduction and convection (as will jumping into a swimming pool!).

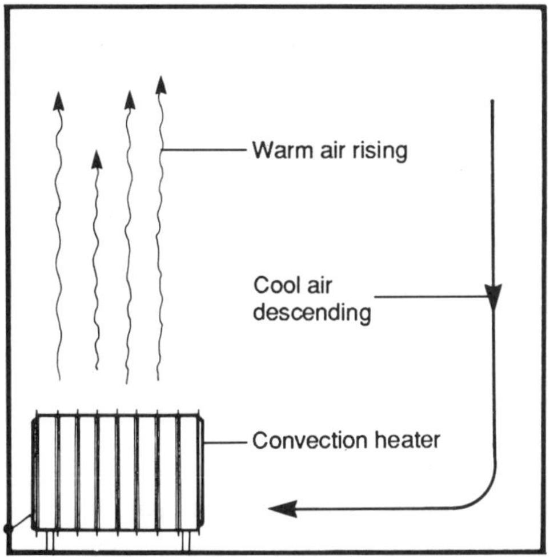

Figure 5.5 *A convection heater warms a room by promoting the vertical movement of air according to its density (and temperature)*

5.10.3 *Radiation*

All objects, regardless of their temperature, emit electromagnetic radiation of a frequency that depends on the temperature. If the temperature of an object is sufficiently high ('red hot' or 'white hot') some of the radiation is visible. However, at body temperature, the radiation is infrared (IR) which is not visible. Thus the human body emits radiation that is characteristic of its temperature and absorbs the radiation emitted by its surroundings. If the temperature of the body is higher than its surroundings (as it usually is), the body experiences a net loss of heat through radiation. About half of the human body's heat loss is through radiation. Most of the infrared rays emanating from the body have wavelengths of between 5 and 20×10^{-6} m.

An image may be formed from the body's infrared emission. A **thermogram** is a body surface temperature 'map'. It can be made by measuring the amount of radiation emitted from the naked body once the skin has adapted to room temperature. The thermogram can then be displayed on a cathode ray tube. Since radiated energy, W, is proportional to the fourth power of temperature T ($W \propto T^4$), areas of elevated temperature (such as malignant tumours) may be distinguished from areas of lower temperature (regions of higher temperature appear lighter).

Infrared radiation is sometimes called 'thermal radiation' or 'heat radiation' because it produces the sensation of warmth when it is absorbed by us. Strictly speaking infrared radiation is electromagnetic energy which, on absorption by the electrically charged particles in our body, causes them to vibrate faster. We notice this vibration as the sensation of warmth.

5.11 Heat Loss from the Body

5.11.1 *Conductive, Convective and Radiative Loss*

In normal circumstances the human body loses most of its heat through convection and radiation. The amount of heat lost by convection depends on the temperature difference between skin and air, on the area of exposed skin and on the amount of time that the skin is exposed. Since clothes are almost transparent to the radiation emitted by the body, the amount of heat lost as radiation (in a given time) depends on the temperature difference between the skin and the surrounding objects, and on the surface area of the body.

$$\text{convective heat loss} = K_c \times \text{exposed area} \times \text{temperature difference}$$

$$\text{radiative heat loss} = K_r \times \text{body area} \times \text{temperature difference}$$

K_c (which depends on the speed of movement of air) and K_r are numbers (termed 'constants' which need not concern us here). Since rate of heat loss depends on the *difference* in temperature, human behaviour on hot days has a significant effect on heat loss. If the surroundings are at a higher temperature than the skin, heat will flow into the body. We can seek out environments with temperatures lower than skin temperature such as in and near water, in the shade, underground and in air-conditioned rooms. In this way, the temperature difference between skin and air and between skin and the surroundings can be maximised. In turn, this will maximise our heat loss to the environment. Heat loss is further promoted if extra skin area is exposed by wearing summer clothing (or by not wearing it!). Furthermore, by keeping muscular activity as low as possible, the amount of heat that our body generates is minimised.

Conductive heat loss is not a major consideration for the human body, because we are usually have clothes between us and the objects we contact. However, we can transfer heat by conduction by applying 'hot' packs, 'cold' packs or by immersing the body in water. To some extent the food and drink we consume is also involved in conductive heat transfer.

5.11.2 *Heat Loss, Body Mass and Surface Area*

The rate at which the body *produces* heat from metabolic processes depends on the *mass* of the body. However, the rate at which the body *loses* heat depends on the *surface area* of the body. The relationship between these two rates can be expressed as the ratio of surface area to body mass, SA:BM. We will compare the surface area to body mass ratio for a baby with that for an adult.

Baby		Adult	
mass	3 kg	mass	70 kg
area	2400 cm^2	area	18 000 cm^2

The surface area to body mass ratio may be calculated as follows:

$$\text{baby's SA:BM} = \frac{2400}{3} = \frac{800}{1} \text{ or } 800 : 1$$

$$\text{adult's SA:BM} = \frac{18\,000}{70} = \frac{260}{1} \text{ or } 260 : 1$$

Thus each kilogram of baby has an area of 800 cm^2 from which to lose heat, whereas each kilogram of adult has an area of 260 cm^2 from which heat is lost. Hence babies will lose heat more rapidly than adults. Clearly, the baby requires a higher food energy intake per kilogram to replace the energy that it loses and so maintain its temperature than does an adult. Heat losses from babies are greatly reduced by their 'baby fat' and by wrapping them in multiple layers of clothes.

One of the particular problems of the premature infant is its inability to maintain a normal body temperature. Their temperature tends to approach that of their surroundings. If their surroundings are maintained at normal body temperature, as happens in an incubator, the infants' heat loss can be managed.

An obese person has a lower surface area to body mass ratio than a thin person. Consequently the obese body shape is less efficient at losing heat on a warm summer day. On the other hand, the obese shape is more suited to retaining heat in a cold winter climate.

5.11.3 *Evaporative Heat Loss*

A basic premise of kinetic theory tells us that the particles of a gas or liquid are in continual motion and that their individual speeds can be any value from zero to extremely fast. The temperature of the fluid is a measure of the **average speed** of the particles. Whatever the temperature is, there will be particles with less speed and some particles with much higher speed than the average that determines the temperature. Even at very low temperatures there are still a few particles whose speeds are very high. It is these particles that possess speeds many times the average that we will consider now.

In order for evaporation to occur, some particles must have enough speed to break away from the attraction of their neighbours at the surface of the liquid and escape into the atmosphere. From kinetic theory we know that there are always some particles with sufficient speed to escape, no matter at what temperature the liquid is. The higher is the temperature, then the more particles there will be that have a speed that is in excess of the escape speed and evaporation will proceed faster.

The consequence to a liquid of losing those particles with the fastest speeds is that the particles that are left behind will have a lower average speed. The escaping fast particles take with them more than an average particle's share of the kinetic energy. This means that the particles that have not evaporated have less average kinetic energy than before. A lower average kinetic energy means that the temperature of the remaining liquid is less than before evaporation occurred. Thus the consequence of evaporation is that the temperature of the object from which evaporation has occurred, is decreased. Evaporation causes cooling.

The human body has two major avenues of evaporative heat loss. These are respiratory heat loss and the evaporation of sweat. We lose about 10–15% of our heat with the water vapour that we exhale. Exhaled water vapour has been evaporated from the alveoli. In order to evaporate, water molecules on the alveoli need to have enough kinetic energy to escape from the liquid state and become gas. This leaves the remaining water molecules with a lower average kinetic energy and hence (albeit momentarily) at a lower temperature. Because of the temperature difference, heat will flow from the alveoli to the water. The continual transfer of heat energy from the blood to the water molecules on the alveoli prevents their kinetic energy from falling despite the loss by evaporation of those water molecules with the highest kinetic energy (speed). Consequently, water evaporates continuously from the alveoli and is breathed out. In this way, heat is continuously flowing from the blood to the outside atmosphere.

Consider the evaporation of sweat from our bodies. For the water molecules in perspiration to become vapour, they need considerable kinetic energy in order to break away from each other. The fastest moving molecules will be continually evaporating and hence decreasing the temperature of those left behind. However, those left behind are continuously having their temperature restored, by conduction, to the temperature of the skin. This enables additional water molecules to evaporate. Thus heat energy flows from the skin to the water molecules and the water molecules carry this energy with them as kinetic energy when they evaporate. So on becoming vapour, the water molecules have gained kinetic energy from the skin, which leaves the skin at a lower temperature. This *transfer of energy* from skin to water molecules is a flow of heat which cools the body.

A healthy unacclimatised person may produce a maximum of around 700 ml of sweat per hour. After exposure to several weeks of hot weather, the person progressively sweats more profusely until sweat production is as much as one and a half to two litres per hour. In this way, evaporative heat loss may double. To ensure that perspiration is available for evaporation, liquid must be drunk to replace that being perspired. If the atmosphere is saturated with water vapour (that is, humidity is 100%), perspiration cannot evaporate so the effectiveness of this heat loss mechanism is decreased.

Loss of heat through evaporation is involved when a patient with an elevated temperature is sponged with tepid water because the water evaporates (since tepid water is at a lower temperature than the skin, it will 'cool' the body by conduction as well). Evaporative cooling is more dramatic if a breeze moves over the wet area, or a volatile liquid such as isopropyl alcohol is mixed with the water.

5.12 Melting and Boiling

If heat and temperature were the same thing (or even proportional to each other) the graph of heat added to a substance against the consequent rise in temperature would look like the graph in Figure 5.6a below. However, it looks like the graph in Figure 5.6b. Notice that it takes only 2 J of energy to raise the temperature of one gram of ice by 1 °C, but that it takes 330 J of energy to melt one gram of ice that is at 0 °C. Note also that it takes 4.2 J of energy to raise the temperature of one gram of water by 1 °C, but that it takes 2260 J of energy to vaporise one gram of water that is at 100 °C. Clearly a great deal of energy is required to produce a change of state in water and while the change of state is occurring, no rise in temperature is possible.

The addition of heat to solid substances will cause them first to melt (liquefy) and then eventually to boil

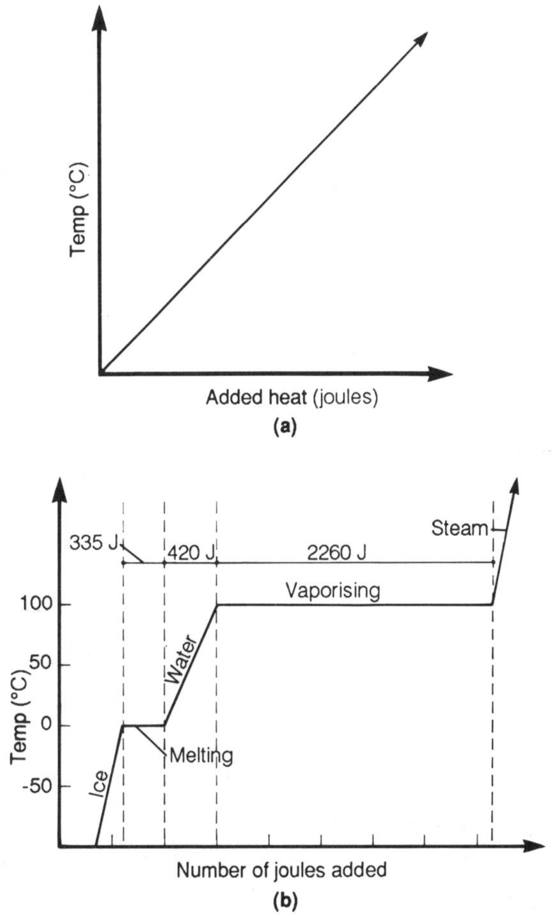

Figure 5.6 *The energy added to one gram of water and the changes of state that it produces. See text for explanation of (a) and (b)*

(vaporise). During the time taken to melt a solid completely or cause a liquid to boil to dryness, the heat being added does not cause a rise in temperature. Rather, the heat energy added is used to break the bonds between particles and appears as increased kinetic and potential energy of the particles. After melting, particles are free to move about and they do so independently of each other. During vaporisation the particles gain further kinetic energy and rise above the liquid, thus increasing their distance from each other. Hence the particles of a gas take up more space than they did as a liquid.

Because the heat energy that causes melting or vaporisation does not manifest itself as a rise in temperature (but is used to break bonds between particles), it is called the **latent heat of fusion** and **latent heat of vaporisation** respectively. The word 'latent' means concealed or disguised.

Earlier we mentioned ice packs as a means of reducing swelling. Ice is more effective than cold water alone because the temperature of cold water will rise as it gains heat from the skin; this decreases the temperature difference between the skin and water and so the rate of heat flow will also decrease. On the other hand, ice that is melting will remain at 0 °C, despite gaining heat from the body. In this case the body's heat energy is used to melt the ice and until all the ice has melted, a temperature rise is not possible. The maintenance of the temperature gradient between the ice pack and skin ensures effective cooling and vasoconstriction.

Evaporative heat loss was mentioned in Section 5.11.3. Now respiratory heat loss (and the cooling effect that perspiration has) may be understood in terms of latent heat of vaporisation. The air we exhale is at 37 °C and is saturated with water vapour whereas the inhaled air was unsaturated and (usually) at a lower temperature. The exhaled water vapour takes with it the latent heat of vaporisation that is supplied to the water molecules by the blood in the alveolar capillaries. It is continually used to raise the average kinetic energy of the water molecules and so replace the kinetic energy carried away by the evaporating molecules. Furthermore some body cooling is due to the loss of the heat that was used to raise the temperature of the inhaled air to 37 °C. Consequently, the body loses heat from the lungs and nasal passages. If it is desirable to reduce the respiratory heat loss from a patient on a ventilator, the air forced into the lungs may be preheated and saturated with water vapour (humidified).

5.13 Heat Therapy

Two primary therapeutic effects take place in a heated area of the body: there is an increase in metabolism because reactions proceed faster at higher temperature (resulting in vasodilation); and as a result there is an increase in blood flow as blood moves in to remove heat from the area. Both are beneficial to damaged tissue. Some physical methods of producing heat in the body (apart from vigorous rubbing!) are conductive heating, infrared or radiant heating, and diathermy (see below).

The conductive method relies on heat transferring from the object of higher temperature to the body. The total heat transferred will depend upon the area of contact, the temperature difference, the time of contact and the thermal conductivity of the materials (the efficiency with which heat is transferred from particle to particle within a substance via collisions). Hot baths, hot packs, electric heating pads and occasionally hot paraffin applied to the skin heat the body by conduction. Conductive heat transfer leads to local surface heating (since circulating blood prevents deeper tissues from heating), and is used in treating rheumatoid arthritis, neuritis, sprains and strains, contusions, sinusitis and back pain.

Infrared radiation is another means used for surface heating of the body. The energy from infrared radiation produces the sensation of warmth we feel when exposed to the sun or an open fire. Artificial sources of infrared rays are glowing metal radiators and incandescent lamps. The range of wavelengths used for heating is from 8×10^{-7} m (which is very 'near' infrared) to 4×10^{-5} m (far infrared). Infrared rays penetrate to a depth of 3 mm and increase the surface temperature. Excessive exposure causes erythema (reddening) and sometimes oedema (swelling). Very prolonged exposure causes browning or hardening of the skin. Radiative heating is used for the same conditions as conductive heating, but is considered more effective because the heat can penetrate more deeply.

Ultrasonic waves are used for deep heating of body tissue. They produce a rapid vibratory motion of the particles in tissues, as do audible sound waves, but the ultrasound frequencies that are used for heating are much higher (about one megahertz) than audible sound. As the ultrasonic waves move through the body, the particles in their path oscillate back and forth. The increase in kinetic energy of the particles constitutes a temperature rise in the tissue. Ultrasound deposits its energy in the deeper muscles and tissues of the body while causing little temperature rise in the soft surface tissue layers. It is the most effective heater of bones and joints because they absorb ultrasound energy more effectively than does soft tissue. This makes ultrasound helpful in the treatment of joint disease and stiffness.

If the frequency is high enough, alternating electric current produces heat in the body without appreciable electric shock. The process is called **diathermy**. In short-wave diathermy, frequencies of 30 MHz cause ions in the tissue to move back and forth (oscillate) at the same frequency. In this way they gain kinetic energy and then lose it in collisions with neighbouring particles. Microwave diathermy uses higher frequencies and deposits its energy in tissues with high water content, so selectively heats muscle rather than fat.

Table 5.4 *The temperature of various sites in the body*

Body site	Temperature (°C)
mouth	36.7
axillae	36.1
rectum	37.3
liver	37.8*
skin (clothed)	30 to 34*

* Values taken from Best and Taylor, *The Physiological Basis for Medical Practice* (seventh edition). Williams and Wilkins, Baltimore, 1961.

5.14 Heat and Rate of Chemical Reactions

In general, chemical reactions proceed faster at higher temperatures. A 1 °C rise in body temperature will increase the basal metabolic rate by between 4 and 13%. A fall in body temperature to below normal may mean the reactions do not proceed fast enough to sustain life. In order to preserve biological tissues such as blood, sperm, ova, bone marrow and food low temperatures are used to prevent their decay. Whole blood mixed with anticoagulant can be stored for about 21 days at 4 °C. Since about 1% of blood cells break (haemolyse) each day, the blood is not usable after this time. Whole blood can be preserved for much longer if rapidly frozen and stored in liquid nitrogen at a temperature of –196 °C (77 K).

5.15 The Physics of Heat Stroke

The body uses a number of systems to maintain a more or less constant body temperature. This occurs despite the variation in the rate of heat production in the body that physical activity causes, and the variation in the temperature of the environment. Normal body temperature is about 37 °C. However, this varies with:

- time of day (the range may be 1.7 °C between the low at about 3 am and the high at 3 to 5 pm);
- age (temperature declines with age);
- menstrual cycle (temperature drops just before ovulation);
- exercise (heavy exercise raises temperature);
- location in the body (see Table 5.4).

If body temperature is to remain constant, the principle of conservation of energy tells us that the rate of heat energy generation within the body, plus the energy flows into the body (from direct solar radiation, radiation from objects in the environment, conduction from the air and input from hot foods), must equal the sum of all the energy flows from the body. These include radiation, convection and conduction as well as respiratory, evaporative and excretory heat losses.

The importance of losing heat from the body can be appreciated in the light of the knowledge that cell growth stops above about 40.6 °C and that permanent damage to the brain may result from body temperatures above 42 °C. The normal setting of the body's 'thermostat' (located in the hypothalamus) is 37.1 °C. If body temperature falls below this, the body automatically reacts by shivering, producing 'goose bumps' and decreasing peripheral circulation. In addition humans can consciously decide to put on extra clothes for extra insulation, move into the sunlight, drink a hot beverage or increase muscular activity. By shivering and other muscular activity, the body uses its chemical energy stores to do work and so raise its power output to a level that is above its power losses. This excess results in heat being stored in the body so its temperature rises. If the body temperature rises above the point set by the hypothalamus, then the body begins to sweat and to increase peripheral circulation.

Let us consider how the body loses heat. Heat is lost through the surface of the body, so before heat can be lost to the environment it must be brought to the skin surface by blood moving in the peripheral circulation. The rate at which heat is lost depends on the characteristics of the environment including temperature, relative humidity (the ratio of the amount of water vapour in the air to the amount that would produce saturation at that temperature) and the extent of air movement. We will consider three environments that produce different heat stresses on the body.

First, consider a day when the shade temperature is pleasantly below body temperature (as it usually is), and a person (wearing clothes) is engaged in activities that do not 'raise a sweat'. Then the person will lose heat through the mechanisms listed in Table 5.5. Respiratory heat loss is the energy carried away with the expired water vapour from the lungs and consists of the kinetic energy acquired by water molecules evaporating from the lungs (the latent heat of vaporisation of water). Even when the sweat glands are not producing perspiration, there is some evaporation of water from the skin because the skin is not impermeable to water. **Insensible perspiration** is the water loss through the skin due simply to the diffusion of water from the tissues below the skin to the outside of the skin. Insensible perspiration stops if the water concentration gradient is removed, that is, if the skin is wet. The five heat-loss mechanisms listed in Table 5.5 are easily sufficient to cope with the body's need to lose heat in an undemanding environment.

Table 5.5 *Major avenues for the loss of body heat*

Mechanism	Heat loss
radiation	50%
convection	25%
respiratory loss	14%
insensible perspiration	7%
conduction	almost 0% (with clothes on)

Second, consider another situation where the temperature is above 34 °C in the shade (approximate skin temperature), such as a hot but dry summer day. Then the evaporation of sweat is the only effective means of losing heat from the body. For the evaporation of water at 40 °C, the latent heat of vaporisation is 2.4×10^3 J/g. In other words 2400 J of heat is lost by the body for each millilitre of sweat that evaporates from the skin. Note that if the perspiration drips off the body or is wiped off, then it can not remove heat by evaporating. The specific heat of the different body tissues varies but an average value can be 3.6×10^3 J/kg/°C. This means that 3600 J of energy would raise the temperature of one kilogram of average tissue by one degree centigrade.

A 70 kg person reclining on a lounge in the shade is producing heat due to basal metabolic activity at the rate of about 75 W (75 J/s). In one hour the metabolic heat generated is 270 000 J (see the calculation below):

$$\begin{aligned} \text{energy} &= \text{thermal power} \times \text{time} \\ &= 75\ \text{W} \times 3600\ \text{s} \\ &= 270\ 000\ \text{J} \end{aligned}$$

This is equivalent to about 3860 J per kilogram of body mass. This amount of heat would raise the body temperature by about 1 °C during the hour if it wasn't for the evaporation of perspiration. To dissipate 270 kJ of heat would require the evaporation of 111 ml of sweat.

$$\text{ml of sweat} = \frac{270\ 000}{2400} = 111\ \text{ml}$$

As the person's level of activity increases then so does the need to dissipate heat. The body is about 20% efficient at converting its chemical energy into work (physical activity); the remaining 80% of energy becomes heat. If the activity is performed in the sunshine then the heat input to the body from direct solar radiation must also be dissipated by the evaporation of sweat. Table 5.6 lists the rate of heat generation for several levels of activity, the body's rate of temperature rise if no heat is lost, and the volume of water that must evaporate (in the absence of other heat-loss mechanisms) from the skin to dissipate the heat produced.

It is rare for a normal unacclimatised person to produce more than about 700 ml of sweat per hour, so someone unused to strenous activity is not able to produce enough sweat to dissipate the heat that they generate. Instead the heat remains in their body and produces a rise in body temperature. If the strenuous activity is maintained for a lengthy period then heat stroke is inevitable. An acclimatised person can produce more perspiration, up to one and a half to two litres per hour. However, some of the sweat drips from the body or is absorbed on clothing and so does not contribute to heat loss. Hence more perspiration must be produced than actually evaporates from the skin in order for the evaporation rates in Table 5.6 to be reached. Two hours of activity in the sun can result in more than 4% of body weight being lost through perspiration. Thus even trained athletes and manual labourers are at risk of heat stroke if they exercise strenuously on a hot day.

In order to maintain a high rate of perspiration, water must be drunk to replace that perspired, otherwise dehydration will occur and perspiration will stop. Dry skin is a symptom of severe heat stroke. Dehydration

Table 5.6 *Rate of heat energy production (thermal power) in the human body* at different levels of activity*

	Thermal power (W)	Rate of temp. rise (°C/hour)	Evaporation (ml/hour)
basal metabolism	75	1	111
moderate activity	300	4	450
very strenuous activity (in the sun)	1000	13	1460

*The body has a mass of 70 kg and specific gravity of 3600 J/kg/°C.

also decreases blood volume and increases blood viscosity. The decrease in blood volume causes a drop in blood pressure and consequent increase in heart rate. Increased viscosity means that the heart will have to expend more energy to pump the same volume of blood and so adds to its stress. A 70 kg marathon runner could lose three and a half litres of sweat in two hours if no water is drunk. Such loss is 5% of body weight and would result in collapse with dehydration exhaustion. Not surprisingly then, well-organised marathons have many drinking points and are conducted in the coolest part of the day.

The third and most stressful environment is one where the temperature is above 34 °C and the air is saturated with water vapour. In this situation the body has a problem trying to lose the heat it produces. Perspiration will not evaporate, so the most effective heat loss mechanism is disabled. Some work environments approximate this heat stress environment. In these cases metabolic heat production (from work) will have to be minimised by having adequate rest breaks, and heat loss will need to be enhanced by acclimatising the workers over two to three weeks, ensuring adequate air movement, providing cool environment retreats and providing plenty of drinking water.

Potentially stressful environments are provided by hot spa tubs and humid saunas. Spas and humid saunas disable the bodies evaporative heat loss mechanism. Furthermore, since the temperature is above body temperature, heat flows into and is stored in the body. In addition to gaining heat from the environment, basal metabolic heat production continues and can not be lost to the environment. As body temperature rises, peripheral circulation increases in order to bring blood close to the skin to facilitate heat loss. However, instead of losing heat by this response, the blood is heated by the environment. The heating causes a further increase in body temperature which signals a further dilation of the blood vessels. A cycle of positive feedback is set up which causes maximal peripheral dilation and the body temperature to rise. The increase in peripheral circulation causes a drop in blood pressure, an increase in cardiac output and a reduction in blood flow to other parts of the body.

The regulatory systems of the body attempt to maintain blood flow (and hence oxygen) to the brain. If this is not possible, the person may become dizzy and disorientated and lose the ability to decide to get out of the spa. The situation will become life threatening if allowed to continue. Sensible safety guidelines for the use of hot tubs are to maintain their temperature no higher than 39–40 °C and to stay in the tub for no more than 20 minutes at a time. These precautions should ensure that the body does not overheat. Given these parameters, we can calculate the expected rise in body temperature for someone submerged up to the neck. We assume a thermal conductivity of 0.3 for the epidermis (it is 0.56 for water), an epidermal layer 0.5 mm thick, a body surface area of 1.8 m^2 and a temperature difference of 3 °C between the body and the spa water.

$$\begin{aligned}\text{rate of heat flow} &= \text{thermal conductivity of skin} \\ &\quad \times \text{surface area of body} \\ &\quad \times \text{temperature gradient} \\ &= 0.3\ \text{J/s/m/°C} \times 1.8\ \text{m}^2 \times \frac{3\ \text{°C}}{0.0005\ \text{m}} \\ &= 320\ \text{W}\end{aligned}$$

To this heat inflow must be added the basal rate of metabolic heat production, 75 W, which cannot be lost to the environment. An inflow of almost 400 W would cause a 70 kg person's body to rise in temperature by about 2 °C in 20 minutes. Getting out after this time will ensure that heat stroke does not occur.

The best heat-loss mechanism in the case of a hot tub or humid sauna is to get out of them, so people who are not thinking clearly due to medication, alcohol or other drugs should not use them. As a consequence of the decreased systemic blood flow, pregnant women should not use spas or saunas because of the risk of impaired blood flow to the foetus, causing it brain damage.

Bibliography

Bartlett, A. A. and Braun, T. J. 'Death in a hot tub: the physics of heat stroke', *American Journal of Physics*, **51**(2), p. 128, table I, 1983.

Benedict, F. G. and Carpenter, T. M. *Respiration Calorimeters for Studying the Respiratory Exchange and Energy Transformations of Man.* Carnegie Institute of Washington. Publication No. 123, 1910.

Best, C. H. and Taylor, N. B. *The Physiological Basis for Medical Practice* (seventh edition). Williams and Wilkins, Baltimore, 1961.

Questions

1. The particular energy value ascribed to a food is a measure of its
   J. translational kinetic energy
   K. gravitational potential energy
   L. chemical potential energy
   M. average kinetic energy per molecule
2. A clinical (or fever) thermometer differs from a standard thermometer in that it
   J. contains mercury
   K. is a maximum reading thermometer
   L. measures temperature in kelvins
   M. contains a capillary tube
3. The evaporation of perspiration from our bodies cools our skin because the evaporated water carries with it the
   J. latent heat of vaporisation
   K. heat lost by radiation
   L. latent heat of fusion
   M. heat lost by convection
4. When a material that is a poor conductor of heat is wrapped around a hot object it prevents the loss of heat from that object because:
   J. The particles of the poor conductor easily transfer the kinetic energy of their vibrations to their neighbours.
   K. Water vapour is prevented from escaping to the air.
   L. It reflects radiated heat back into the hot object.
   M. Air trapped within the poor conductor prevents convection currents from occurring.
5. Heat is a
   J. measure of the temperature of an object
   K. transfer of energy by convection currents
   L. measure of the average translational kinetic energy of the particles
   M. form of energy transfer along a temperature gradient
6. Which one of the following statements does not accurately describe energy?
   J. Energy can be created but not destroyed.
   K. The total amount of all types of energy remains constant.
   L. The energy gained by an object is the amount of work done on the object.
   M. Energy is the heat given out when oxidation occurs.
7. Kinetic theory allows us to understand that the temperature of an object is a measure of the
   J. heat that it contains
   K. average kinetic energy of its particles
   L. hotness or coldness of it
   M. number of degrees kelvin it is
8. To convert 30 °C into degrees kelvin you must
   J. add 212
   K. subtract 212
   L. add 273
   M. subtract 273
9. In order to lose body weight, diet and exercise must be organised so that the energy value of the food intake is
   J. less than the energy used daily
   K. more than the energy used daily
   L. equal to the daily energy use
   M. greater than the daily exercise
10. Which of the statements about heat is true? Heat is
   J. one of the forms of infrared radiation
   K. transmitted through a solid object by convection currents
   L. a measure of the temperature of an object
   M. the flow of energy from one body to another at a lower temperature
11. On a normal winter day, the human body loses most of its heat through
   J. convection
   K. conduction
   L. radiation
   M. evaporation

12. A cold pack, applied to reduce swelling, is more effective if it contains melting ice at 0 °C rather than cold water at 0 °C. This is because

   J. melting ice is colder than the cold water
   K. ice has a higher latent heat of vaporisation
   L. melting ice remains at 0 °C until it has all melted
   M. ice cools by conduction whereas water cools by convection

13. When the label on a packaged food item states that 100 g contains 650 kJ of energy, it means that

   J. the human body is able to extract 650 kJ of heat and useful work by digesting the food
   K. 650 kJ of energy was consumed in growing or producing or making the food
   L. 650 kJ of heat energy is released when 100 g of the food is burned in an atmosphere of pure oxygen
   M. ultimately your body will be able to perform 650 kJ of work for every 100 g of the food that you eat

14. Which one of the following statements best describes what is meant by the 'principle of conservation of energy'?

   J. Internal energy is the sum of kinetic energy, thermal energy and potential energy.
   K. Energy may be transformed from one form into another, but it cannot be created or destroyed.
   L. Kinetic energy is gradually transformed into potential energy and vice versa.
   M. The earth has a finite amount of energy and modern society must learn to use less of it and to use it more efficiently.

15. A person's metabolic rate is defined as the rate

   J. of energy utilisation by their body
   K. of energy utilisation by their body during 'absolute rest'
   L. at which they consume oxygen
   M. at which they produce heat

CHAPTER 6

Water, the Essential Liquid

Among all the simple compounds found on earth there is none more important than water. As far as we can tell, it is essential for the existence of all forms of life. A human being can survive for many weeks on a severely restricted food supply, but it is not possible to survive for an extended period on much less than the normal supply of water. In the human body the activity of every cell takes place in a watery environment and water is essential for the processes of digestion, circulation, respiration, excretion and the regulation of body temperature. Depending on age and gender, the human body consists of 60–75% water and a person may only lose 0–5% of this without noticeable effect. Loss of 10–15% will normally cause considerable distress and when the percentage loss reaches 20% life is threatened.

This chapter commences with an outline of the availability of water and a description of some of its properties which have particular significance for living things. It goes on to explain these properties in terms of the nature of the water molecule.

Learning Objectives

At the completion of this chapter you should be able to:

1. Explain what is meant when water is described as 'a common but extraordinary substance'.
2. Describe how hydrogen bonds arise and state some important differences between hydrogen bonds and covalent bonds.
3. Account for some important properties of water in terms of hydrogen bonds.
4. Predict whether or not a substance is likely to dissolve in water given information about its bonding and structure.
5. Explain the action of soaps and detergents in terms of the nature of their particles.
6. Discuss the significance which the thermal and solvent properties of water have for body function.

6.1 Availability of Water

Earth has often been described as the water planet. This is an apt description because water is easily the most abundant simple compound found on earth. It covers about 70% of the planet's surface and often to a depth of thousands of metres. There is so much water on earth that if it was shared equally among all the people alive today each would receive more than enough to fill a small reservoir.

Unfortunately, nearly all this water is unsuitable for drinking, and the availability of fresh water is a critical factor determining the viability of all human societies, even those which may be quite advanced in their technological development. This is not too surprising because technologically advanced societies always have a very high consumption of fresh water. When all industrial, agricultural and domestic uses are taken into account the consumption of fresh water in developed countries, such as Australia and the United States, is several million litres for each person each year. This may be compared with a volume of a few thousand litres each year which is sufficient for the needs of an Aborigine living a traditional life style in one of the arid regions of Australia. Something else which illustrates our dependence on water is the fact that about 80% of all sickness in the world is caused by contamination of fresh water supplies. Of course, this is not the situation applying today in Australia, or in the other technologically advanced countries of the world, but we should not take the present availability of fresh water for granted. It may not always be there in whatever quantities we require.

Water is such a familiar substance that we are inclined to regard it as being very ordinary. But water has some quite extraordinary properties which not only set it apart from all other compounds but also explain why it is so important to living things. We shall now give detailed consideration to some of these.

6.2 Properties of Water

6.2.1 *Thermal Properties*

The thermal properties of a substance are those properties which enable us to predict the changes in temperature and physical state which it will undergo as it gains or loses heat energy. For example, the melting point of a substance is a property which allows us to predict the temperature at which the substance will change from a solid to a liquid as heat energy is supplied to it. The latent heat of fusion of a substance is a property which allows us to determine the quantity of heat energy that we will need to supply in order to change a given amount of solid into its liquid form. Corresponding to these two properties are the properties of boiling point and latent heat of vaporisation which apply when the liquid form of a substance changes into a gas. As melting and boiling occur there is no change in temperature as long as some solid (in the case of melting) or liquid (in the case of boiling) remains. All the heat energy flowing into a substance in these situations goes to cause the change of state and none of it is available to cause a temperature change until the change of state is complete. All changes of state involve a change in the positions which the particles of the substance involved occupy relative to one another. As we have seen in Chapter 5, energy associated with position is called potential energy and so in a change of state heat energy is converted to potential energy (or vice versa depending on the direction of the change). The term 'latent heat' deserves a comment. The word 'latent' means 'hidden' or 'disguised' and the heat which accompanies a change of state can be regarded as being hidden or disguised because it flows into or out of a substance without causing a change in temperature of that substance.

The most insulting thing that you can say about a person's cooking skill is that 'They even burn the soup'. Food burns when its temperature is raised high enough to cause its molecules to begin decomposing and forming carbon which appears as a black powder. This cannot happen to soup until all its water content has been boiled away, because, as long as there is some water present, the temperature of the soup will not rise above the boiling point of water, which is 100 °C, a temperature too low to cause burning. Since soup is mainly water it takes a very careless and incompetent cook to burn it.

Yet another thermal property is **specific heat** (sometimes called specific heat capacity). This property tells us how much heat is required to change the temperature of a certain quantity of substance by a given amount.

In Tables 6.1 and 6.2 these thermal properties of water are compared with those of other compounds. In every case the value for water is the largest of all those listed.

Table 6.1 *Melting points and boiling points of water and related compounds*

	Water (H_2O)	Hydrogen sulphide (H_2S)	Ammonia (NH_3)	Phosphine (PH_3)
melting point (°C)	0	–86	–78	–134
boiling point (°C)	100	–61	–33	–87

Table 6.2 *Latent heats and specific heats for water and some other common liquids*

	Water (H_2O)	Alcohol (C_2H_6O)	Chloroform ($CHCl_3$)	Ether ($C_4H_{10}O$)
latent heat of fusion (J/g)	334	109	74	98
latent heat of vaporisation (J/g)	2280	917	264	376
specific heat (J/g/ °C)	4.18	2.45	0.97	2.32

The consistently high values for the thermal properties of water are very significant. For example, the high specific heat of water makes it an excellent heat 'sink'. This means that any body of water must lose or gain a relatively large amount of heat in order for its temperature to change by a given amount. Alternatively, one could say that the loss or gain of a given amount of heat will cause a smaller temperature change when water is involved rather than some other substance. This is illustrated in the calculation below.

Heat Absorption by Water and Ether

1. Specific heat of water = 4.18 kJ/kg/°C
   Specific heat of ether = 2.32 kJ/kg/°C

In Section 5.4 we saw that, for an object undergoing a temperature change:

$$\text{energy} = \text{mass} \times \text{temperature change} \times \text{specific heat}$$

This expression may be rearranged to give:

$$\text{temperature change} = \frac{\text{energy}}{\text{mass} \times \text{specific heat}}$$

2. The quantity of heat energy needed to change the temperature of 50 kg of water by 5 °C is:

$$\begin{aligned}\text{heat} &= 50 \times 5 \times 4.18\\ &= 1045 \text{ kJ}\end{aligned}$$

The quantity of heat needed to change the temperature of 50 kg of ether by 5 °C is:

$$\begin{aligned}\text{heat} &= 50 \times 5 \times 2.32\\ &= 580 \text{ kJ}\end{aligned}$$

3. The temperature increase which occurs when 1000 kJ of heat is absorbed by 50 kg of water is:

$$\begin{aligned}\text{temperature increase} &= \frac{1000}{50 \times 4.18}\\ &= 4.8\ °\text{C}\end{aligned}$$

The temperature increase which occurs when 1000 kJ of heat is absorbed by 50 kg of ether is:

$$\begin{aligned}\text{temperature increase} &= \frac{1000}{50 \times 2.32}\\ &= 8.6\ °\text{C}\end{aligned}$$

Have you ever noticed that when hot food is served with gravy it is the gravy that remains hot for the longest period of time? The reason for this is that gravy has a large water content and, because of the high specific heat of water, it must lose more heat than the rest of the food on the plate in order to drop in temperature by the same amount. This larger heat loss takes longer to occur. The high specific heat of water produces important effects on a much bigger scale than this. It has a dramatic effect on weather conditions all over the earth and this may be illustrated by reference to the great ocean currents of the world. One of these is the Gulf Stream which rises off the coast of Mexico and flows north to Norway. Along the way, the water of the Gulf Stream falls in temperature by about 20 °C as it transfers heat to the cooler regions it encounters. Its rate of flow is such that the Gulf Stream transfers northward, in every 12 hours, as much heat as can be obtained by burning all the coal that is mined throughout the world each year. This massive transfer of heat energy from a warm part of the world to a much colder region has a large effect on the weather there. The United Kingdom and Norway are two countries which, due to the influence of the Gulf Stream, enjoy climates far more temperate than would otherwise be the case.

The very large latent heat of vaporisation of water is even more important in influencing climate than its specific heat. This is because water evaporates at a significant rate even when its temperature is well below the boiling point. We know this from our everyday experience. For example, when it rains, quite large quantities of water accumulate in pools on waterproof surfaces such as bitumen or concrete. The water cannot soak through these surfaces and yet it disappears quite quickly as it evaporates and disperses into the atmosphere. This is not boiling and the rate at which the water is changing to a vapour is much less under these conditions than at the boiling point. Nevertheless, the process still requires the absorption of heat and about the same amount per gram of water that is required for boiling. This heat is supplied by the sun, by contact with the surface on which the water is lying and by the water's own heat energy. It is stored in the water vapour and carried by air currents to whatever destination the vapour eventually reaches. Large-scale air currents carry enormous quantities of water vapour from the warmer regions of the world to regions which are colder. But the amount of water vapour which air can hold decreases as the temperature decreases, and so, in these cold regions, much of the water vapour is deposited as rain and snow. As this occurs the heat energy stored within it is released, delivering a large quantity of heat to these cold regions of the world and making them less cold than they would otherwise be.

The latent heat of vaporisation of water is important in the maintenance of a constant body temperature. As water evaporates from the external surface of the body and from the lungs it absorbs heat. This is the only means which we have of keeping the body at its normal temperature when the temperature of the surroundings is higher. Some spectacular evidence of the efficiency of this cooling mechanism is provided by two accounts from the scientific literature written in 1775 by Charles Blagden ('Experiments and observations in an heated room', *Philosophical Transactions of the Royal Society of London*, 65, pages 111–123 and 484–494).

Blagden described experiments conducted by himself and several other men, including Joseph Banks who had, a few years earlier, accompanied Captain James Cook on his voyage of discovery to Australia. Blagden, Banks and these other men went into a room which had been heated to a temperature of over 120 °C! They took with them: a piece of raw steak, a dog (placed in a basket so that its feet would not be burned by contact with the hot floor), a container of water in which the water surface was covered by oil and another container of water in which the surface was free. While the men and the dog remained in the room the steak was cooked and the water with its surface covered by oil (but not the other water) began to boil. The men and the dog then emerged from the room none the worse for their experience. They were protected from the extreme temperature by the cooling effect of water evaporating from the skin (men) and lungs (men and dog).

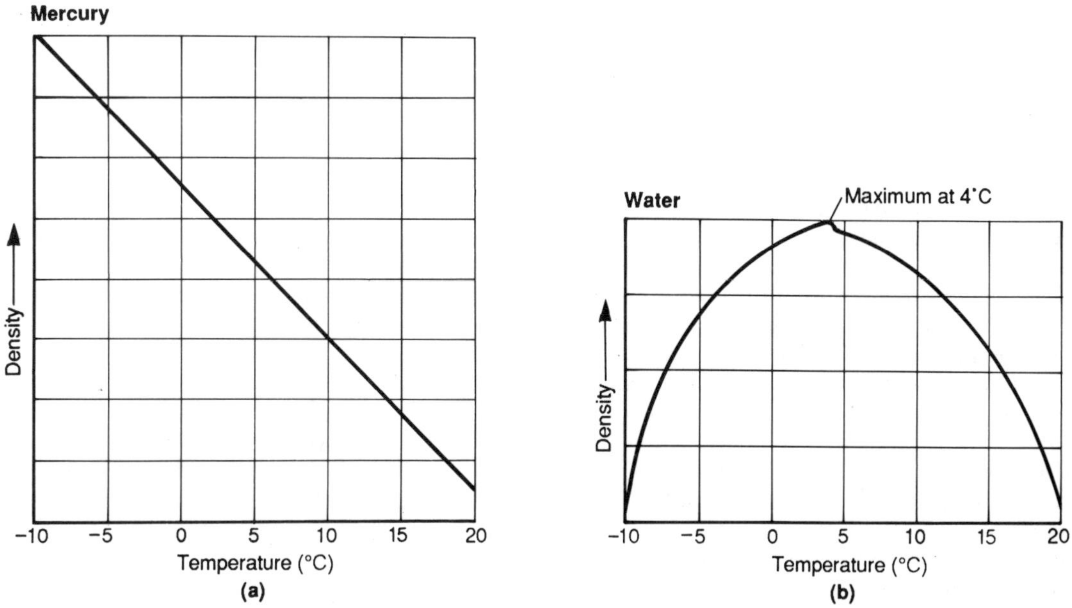

Figure 6.1 *Graphs which show the change in density, with temperature, for (a) mercury and (b) water*

6.2.2 *Expansion on Freezing*

Water is the only compound which expands when it freezes. As it is cooled towards its freezing point of 0 °C it behaves as other substances do and contracts until the temperature reaches 4 °C. It then begins to expand. As it freezes at 0 °C it expands by about 10%. This fact is well known to many people who have left their glass bottles of liquid refreshment for too long in the freezing compartment of a refrigerator! The bottles burst as a result of the very large forces exerted against their walls, from the inside, when the water freezes and expands. Such an event is usually just a nuisance but the expansion of water as it freezes is a highly significant property in other situations.

The Partial Freezing of Lakes, Rivers and Oceans. In many parts of the world the onset of winter sees air temperature fall quickly to 0 °C and below. In these places the surface layers of lakes, oceans and rivers are cooled through contact with this cold air. As the surface water cools towards 4 °C it becomes more dense and sinks, displacing warmer water, from below, towards the surface. In turn, this water is cooled, becomes more dense, and sinks. In this way a cycle is established which sees water come repeatedly to the surface to be cooled before it sinks back into the depths. This continues until the temperature of the surface layer reaches 4 °C. Cooling below this temperature causes a decrease in density, rather than an increase, and so the colder water stays at the surface until it freezes at 0 °C. The layer of ice formed in this way insulates the water below from the cold air and the rate of further cooling decreases. The ice layer does continue to increase in thickness but at a reduced rate and, provided that the body of water is reasonably deep, it will not freeze completely and so will be able to support life throughout the winter season.

If water behaved as nearly all other substances do, and became more dense when it froze, the ice formed initially on the surface of a body of water would sink to the bottom. This would expose more water to the cooling effect of the cold winter air with the result that the bottom layer of ice would increase steadily in thickness. Shallower bodies of water would freeze solid and, on the bottoms of much deeper ones, a thick ice layer would form. In many parts of the world today air temperatures are sufficiently low all year round to ensure that such ice layers would be permanent, and would simply increase in thickness during winter and decrease during summer. In such a circumstance many existing life forms could not exist. Furthermore, life itself probably began in the shallow seas and lakes of the earth. If the bottoms of those shallow seas and lakes had been permanently covered by ice, they would have provided a much less hospitable environment for the development of life than was the case. So, we may speculate that this simple property of water has had a profound effect on the development of life on earth, even to the point of making it possible.

Frostbite. Sometimes the expansion of water on freezing is not advantageous. This is well illustrated by the example of **frostbite**, a condition which occurs when parts of the body suffer prolonged exposure to wind and cold. Fingers, toes and prominent parts of the face are particularly susceptible.

The body's first response to cold is an increased blood supply to the affected areas. However, when severe cold persists for a very long period the blood supply to the cold, surface regions is reduced in order to conserve heat. Once this happens, those parts of the body affected will begin to cool. If the conditions are severe enough then the fluid bathing cells of the affected tissues (**extracellular fluid**) will begin to freeze. This is frostbite.

As frostbite occurs, ice crystals form in extracellular fluid and as they do they exert forces of compression on cells, causing many of them to rupture and die. In serious cases of frostbite the damage to tissues can be severe enough to require amputation of hands and feet.

6.2.3 *Surface Tension of Water*

When water drips slowly from a tap it forms drops which are almost perfectly spherical; some insects can move about on the surface of water without sinking; it is even possible to lay a razor blade on the surface of water and see it 'float' even though it is made from steel, which is much more dense than water and, therefore, should sink (see Section 7.6 for a discussion of density).

All these observations are the result of **surface tension**, a property which all liquids possess. Surface tension is a force which acts within the liquid surface causing it to contract and behave like a tightly stretched 'skin'. In the case of water the force of surface tension is able to support an object made out of quite dense material provided that the object has a shape which ensures that there is no part of the surface which experiences too large a force. Surface tension is also responsible for the spherical shape of water drops because it leads them to assume a shape with the smallest possible surface area and this is a sphere.

All liquids have a surface tension and some relative values for this property are presented in Table 6.3. Water has been arbitrarily assigned the value of 1.0 to allow easy comparison with the other liquids listed.

Table 6.3 *Relative surface tensions for water and other liquids (temperature = 20 °C)*

Liquid	Relative surface tension
water	1.00
ethyl alcohol	0.31
diethyl ether	0.23
carbon tetrachloride	0.37
benzene	0.40
mercury	6.70
chloroform	0.37
ethyl acetate	0.36
sulphuric acid	0.75

Surface tension is very important in determining the behaviour of water whenever it comes in contact with the surface of another material. For example, water in contact with clean glass or metal will spread to form a thin film and make good contact, but on a plastic surface, or a greasy surface, it forms droplets and the contact achieved is poor. These effects can be explained by taking account of the nature of the surface involved and the nature of the forces responsible for surface tension. This is discussed in more detail in Section 6.6 which deals with the action of soaps and detergents.

6.2.4 *The Solvent Power of Water*

Water is capable of dissolving a very large number of different compounds including many from each of the two main classes of compound (ionic, non-molecular compounds and covalent, molecular compounds). This is in contrast to most other liquids which are only capable of dissolving a restricted range of covalent, molecular compounds. Because of its ability to dissolve a wide range of compounds, water is often called the **universal solvent**. Its high solvent power is very important for the effective functioning of all organisms.

Every cell in a living organism must receive nutrients from the outside world and must remove the waste products of its own metabolic activity to the outside world. These nutrients and waste products include both ionic, non-molecular and covalent, molecular compounds. The processes which move them in and out of a living organism depend upon the materials being soluble in the fluids which fill, and circulate around, cells. Water is the ideal material to have as the major component of these fluids because of its abundance and its ability to dissolve a wide variety of different compounds.

In the preceding paragraphs a range of important properties of water have been described and you should, by now, be convinced that ordinary water is quite an extraordinary substance. There are so many ways in which water stands out from other substances that one is left suspecting that this must be due to some single property of the substance upon which all the others depend. This idea is taken up in the next section.

6.3 Polarity of the Water Molecule

The most important factor in determining the behaviour of water is the polarity of its molecules and this is a property which depends upon two things: the shape of the molecule and the polarity of the covalent bonds within it. In Section 2.6.6 we saw that water molecules are V-shaped rather than straight, and it was explained that this was due to repulsion between the four pairs of electrons which are arranged on the outside of the electron cloud of the oxygen atom. Covalent bond polarity was discussed in Section 2.6.4 and this term refers to the fact that atoms differ in the attraction which they have for electrons. The atom with the greater attraction for electrons receives a bigger share of the electrons involved in the bond and so acquires a fractional negative charge. The other atom acquires a fractional positive charge of equal magnitude. This is shown in Figure 6.2.

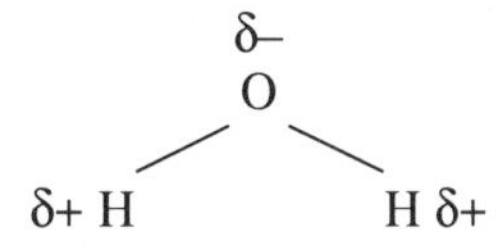

Figure 6.2 *Shape and polarity of the water molecule*

The polarity of the oxygen–hydrogen bond, combined with the V-shape of the water molecule, results in the molecule having two differently charged ends. One of these (the hydrogen end) is positively charged and the other (the oxygen end) is negatively charged. Such a molecule is said to be **polar**. It is most important to realise two things about polar molecules. They do not have a net electrical charge as ions do, because the fractional negative charge which exists in one section of the molecule is balanced by an equal positive charge existing in another section of the same molecule. The other thing to realise is that the bonds in a molecule may be polar without the molecule itself being polar. This is so in the case of carbon dioxide the molecular structure of which is shown in Figure 6.3.

$$\delta-\ \mathrm{O}{=}\overset{\delta+}{\mathrm{C}}{=}\mathrm{O}\ \delta-$$

Figure 6.3 *Carbon dioxide, polar bonds in a non-polar molecule*

The attraction of oxygen atoms for electrons is greater than that of carbon and so the carbon–oxygen bond is quite polar. However, the carbon dioxide molecule is completely symmetrical and its two ends are identical. Therefore, the molecule itself is not polar and this is the case for all perfectly symmetrical molecules regardless of the polarity of the bonds which exist within them.

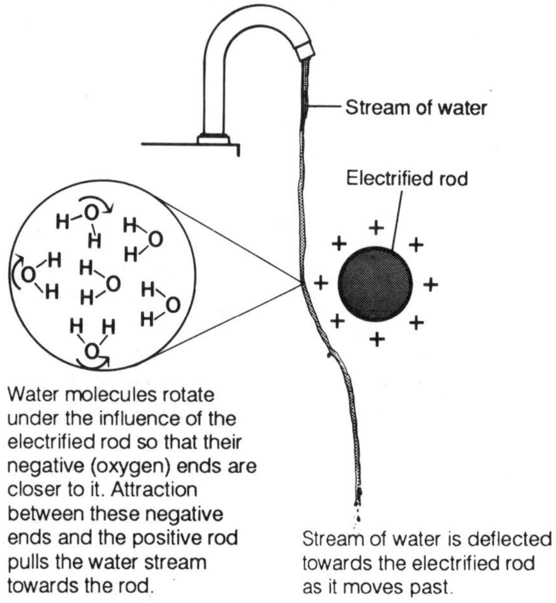

Figure 6.4 *Confirming the polarity of water molecules. Deflection of a water stream by a charged object*

A simple experiment which demonstrates the polarity of water molecules may be conducted using a piece of plastic (a comb will do) and a narrow stream of water from a slow-running tap. The plastic must be rubbed vigorously with a piece of woollen cloth and then brought close to the stream of water. As it passes by the plastic the water stream is deflected as shown in Figure 6.4. This behaviour may be explained as follows: rubbing the plastic causes it to acquire an electrical charge. When it is then brought close to the water stream it exerts a force of attraction on the ends of the water molecules which have the opposite charge. The force of attraction causes the molecules to rotate and orient themselves so that this end is closer to the plastic. It then pulls the water molecules towards the plastic causing the deflection observed.

6.4 Forces Between Water Molecules: the Hydrogen Bond

In Chapter 2, detailed consideration was given to the forces which hold atoms together *within* molecules, that is, covalent bonds. A little bit of careful thought makes it clear that forces must also operate *between* molecules. Otherwise, it would not be possible to obtain molecular compounds in liquid or solid form, and it is well known that many molecular substances exist as liquids or solids under normal conditions.

In the case of substances which have polar molecules, the forces operating between the molecules are electrical forces of attraction between the oppositely

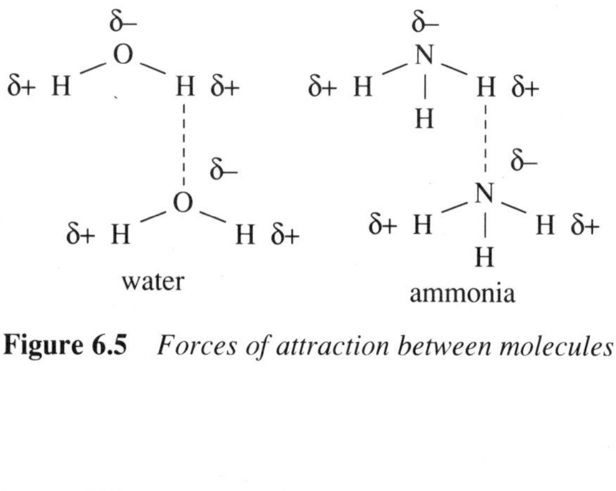

Figure 6.5 *Forces of attraction between molecules*

charged ends of different molecules. This is illustrated, for the two cases of ammonia and water, in Figure 6.5.

The force of attraction which operates between separate water or ammonia molecules will also operate between any molecules which contain the sets of atoms –OH and –NH. Wherever such sets of atoms are located within molecules they will constitute polar sections of the molecule and be capable of exerting forces of attraction on the corresponding sections of other molecules nearby. This is shown in Figure 6.6.

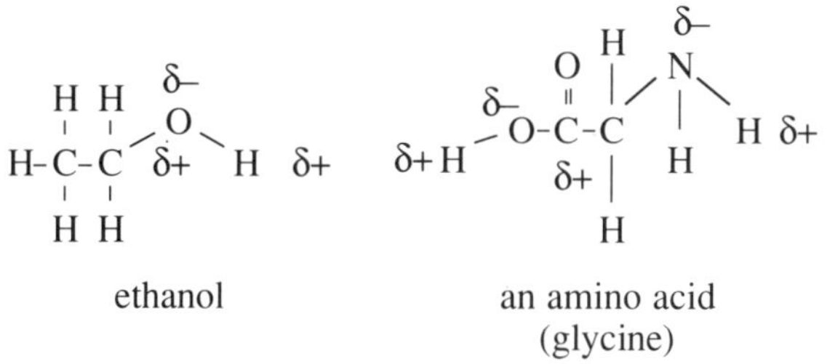

Figure 6.6 *Polarity of ethanol and amino acid molecules*

All polar molecules have forces of attraction operating between their oppositely charged ends, but, in the cases of water, ammonia and other substances which contain –OH or –NH groups of atoms, the forces are unusually strong compared to those operating between polar molecules which do not contain these groups. Due to their unusually large strength, and because the –OH and –NH groups of atoms are very commonly encountered in molecules, these forces are given the special name of 'hydrogen bond'. The hydrogen bond may be defined as the force of attraction which operates between –OH and –NH groups of atoms in separate molecules or between these groups of atoms occupying different positions within the same molecule.

In the next section we shall see that hydrogen bonds account for much of the unusual behaviour of water and then, in Chapter 13, 'Organic Compounds, the Basis of Life', they will be used to account for some important properties of proteins and nucleic acids. Right now, though, it is important for you to be clear that, while hydrogen bonds are strong in comparison to other bonds operating between molecules, they are still very weak in comparison to the covalent bonds which hold atoms together within molecules. Covalent bonds determine the chemical properties of materials. When they are broken, new materials, with different properties, are formed.

Hydrogen bonds influence mainly physical properties and they break during physical changes such as melting, boiling or dissolving. Their breakage does not alter the chemical nature of the substance involved. For example, the chemical nature of ice is the same as that of liquid water which is the same as that of water vapour. As water is made to change from any one of these states to another, there is no effect whatsoever on the covalent bonds which hold oxygen and hydrogen atoms together within the water molecules. Only the hydrogen bonds acting between the molecules are disrupted.

6.5 Hydrogen Bonds and the Properties of Water

6.5.1 *Thermal Properties*

The relatively high melting point and high boiling point of water simply reflect the fact that the hydrogen bonds which hold water molecules together are stronger than the bonds acting between the molecules of most other molecular substances. This also accounts for water's large latent heats of fusion and vaporisation.

The large heat capacity of water is due to the fact that, in the liquid state, hydrogen bonds hold clusters of water molecules together. In effect, liquid water retains some of the characteristics of its solid form and, as it is heated, a lot of the heat is used to completely break up these clusters of molecules.

6.5.2 *Expansion on Freezing*

Water expands on freezing because, at the freezing point, water molecules adopt positions such that each molecule of water is surrounded tetrahedrally by four others to which it is joined by hydrogen bonds. In this arrangement there is a great deal of empty space which is the reason for the density of ice being less than that of water (see Figure 6.7).

6.5.3 *Surface Tension*

Surface tension is due to the fact that the set of attractive forces experienced by molecules at the surface of a liquid is different from that experienced by molecules in the interior (see Figure 6.8). Those in the interior experience attractive forces around them in all

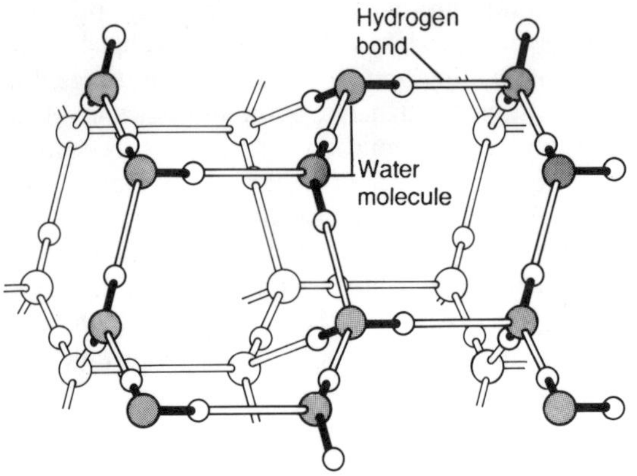

Figure 6.7 *The open structure of ice*

directions and the net effect of these forces is zero. Molecules at the surface experience more attractive forces tending to pull them inwards than outwards and so there is a net force inwards.

The high surface tension of water simply reflects the fact that the forces of attraction acting between water molecules (hydrogen bonds) are much stronger than those which act between molecules of most other substances. However, mercury is one example of a liquid which has a higher surface tension than water (see Table 6.2). Mercury is a metal and its particles have forces operating between them which are much stronger than hydrogen bonds. On this basis it is not surprising that the surface tension of mercury should be so high.

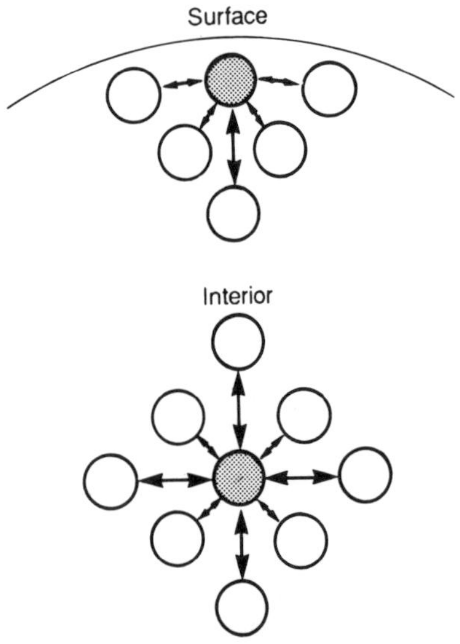

Figure 6.8 *The basis of surface tension*

6.5.4 *Solvent Power*

Solution formation is a very ordinary experience and we encounter it every day as we do such things as sugar our coffee, make a jelly, prepare a salt solution for gargling with and so on. However, there are some aspects of the formation of a solution which are quite remarkable. For example, we saw in Chapter 2 that ionic compounds have very high melting points. In order to separate the ions in an ionic substance from each other, by heating, it is often necessary to raise the temperature of the substance to 600 or 700 °C. And yet these same compounds will often dissolve readily in water at room temperature and in this way their ions are also separated from each other. How is it possible to achieve by the simple, mild act of mixing with water what otherwise requires a temperature of many hundreds of degrees centigrade? In order to answer this question it is first of all necessary to consider the solution process in general terms.

Solutions form when two or more substances are mixed, with their particles becoming uniformly and permanently distributed among each other. When one of the substances is present in much greater proportion than any other it is called the solvent and the other substances are called solutes. The solution process is represented in Figure 6.9.

In order for a solution to form the forces acting between the particles of the separate substances must be overcome to some extent at least. Consider the case of sodium chloride dissolving in water. Before the sodium chloride is mixed with the water, its Na^+ and Cl^- particles are held together by ionic bonds. In order for the material to dissolve these ionic bonds must be completely overcome. In this same situation water molecules, before being mixed with the sodium chloride, are held together by the hydrogen bonds acting between their molecules and these bonds must also be overcome, to some extent, as the solution forms. Of course, the effect on the hydrogen bonds of water is much less than the effect on the ionic bonds of sodium chloride, because water is the major component of the system. At any instant there will always be many water molecules in the system which are in direct contact mainly with other water molecules, and so continue in a condition very similar to the one which was operating before the solution formed. Even

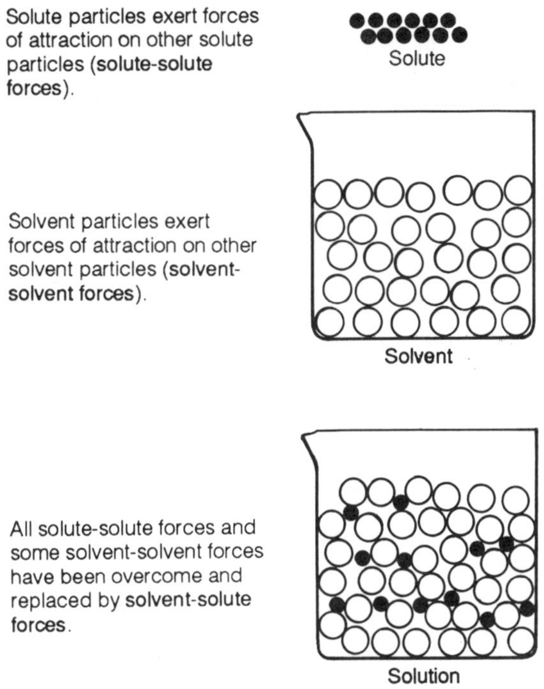
Solute particles exert forces of attraction on other solute particles (**solute-solute forces**).
Solute
Solvent particles exert forces of attraction on other solvent particles (**solvent-solvent forces**).
Solvent
All solute-solute forces and some solvent-solvent forces have been overcome and replaced by **solvent-solute forces**.
Solution

Figure 6.9 *The solution process*

so, in many situations, solutions are prevented from forming because of the disruption which would be caused to the attractive forces between water molecules.

In the world of large objects, such as tables and chairs, motor vehicles, people and so on, we know that a force can only be overcome by applying a larger force. Thus, all these objects experience the force of gravity which normally holds them on the earth's surface. Each will only move away from the earth's surface if a lifting force larger than the force of gravity is applied to it. In the world of atoms and molecules it is also the case that forces are only overcome by the action of larger forces. A solution will only form when the solvent and solute particles are capable of exerting forces of attraction on each other which are comparable in strength to those acting within unmixed samples of solute and solvent.

Solubility of Ionic Compounds. Ions located at the outside of an ionic crystal are not completely surrounded by other ions and so are held in position less securely than others located in the body of the crystal. Water is able to dissolve many ionic compounds because the charged ends of the polar water molecules can exert forces of attraction on ions. The hydrogen end of the molecule (which is positive) attracts negative ions, and the oxygen end (which is negative) attracts positive ions. These forces of attraction are sufficient to pull ions away from the outside of the crystal and into the solution. Once the ion has separated from the crystal it becomes surrounded by water molecules, each one of which exerts forces of attraction upon it. While each of these forces is relatively weak their total effect is considerable. In addition, the water molecules prevent oppositely charged ions from coming close to each other so that it is not possible for them to exert forces on each other of the same magnitude as they do within an ionic crystal. All of this is illustrated in Figure 6.10.

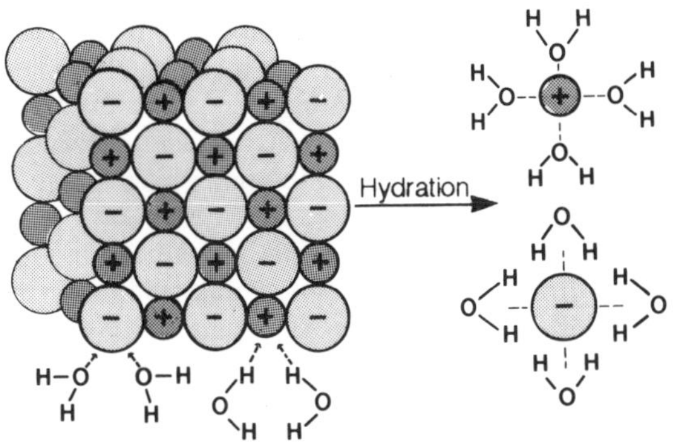
Hydration

Figure 6.10 *An ionic compound dissolving in water*

Ionic compounds will not dissolve in non-polar liquids such as oil or fat because the molecules of those liquids, being non-polar, cannot exert forces of attraction on the ions to pull them away from the crystal.

Solubility of Covalent, Molecular Compounds. Covalent, molecular compounds display quite a different pattern of solubility from ionic compounds. Nevertheless, it is a pattern which may be explained in similar terms. Many covalent, molecular compounds will not dissolve in water and these compounds have molecules of low polarity. They do not mix readily with water because, in order to do so, their molecules would have to force their way in among the water molecules and so disrupt the forces of attraction (hydrogen bonds) operating between water molecules. Being of low polarity themselves they are not capable of exerting forces of attraction on the water molecules to replace the hydrogen bonds disrupted and so solution formation does not occur. These same compounds will, however, readily form solutions with low polarity solvents. This is because, as mixing occurs, the forces of attraction which their molecules exert on the solvent molecules are of about the same strength as those which act between the solvent molecules themselves.

Let us turn now to the covalent, molecular compounds which dissolve readily in water. This is a very important group of compounds. It includes glucose and most of the amino acids. These compounds are essential for the nourishment of tissues and they must be transported, in the blood, from the gastrointestinal tract to all parts of the body. This group of water-soluble, covalent, molecular compounds also includes the toxic compound, **urea**, which forms as a result of the chemical activity occurring constantly in all cells. Urea must be transported in the blood from all tissues of the body to the kidneys where it can be eliminated from the body by excretion in urine. Since the blood consists mainly of water these vital transport processes are only effective because the compounds involved are soluble in water.

Covalent, molecular compounds which dissolve readily in water are always composed of polar molecules. In many cases this polarity is due to the presence, within the molecules, of –OH and –NH groups of atoms. These groups allow the molecules to participate in hydrogen bond formation. When the compounds dissolve in water the hydrogen bonds which act between their molecules must be overcome, as must some of the hydrogen bonds acting between water molecules. The solution process occurs only because the dissolving molecules are able to compensate for this disruption by forming hydrogen bonds with water molecules.

Covalent, molecular compounds, which dissolve readily in water, will not usually dissolve in solvents of low polarity. Their molecules, being polar, exert forces of attraction on each other far stronger than any which could be exerted upon them by molecules of a non-polar solvent.

All this discussion of the factors affecting solubility is summarised by the phrase 'like dissolves like'. Polar solutes will dissolve in water but not in non-polar solvents. Solutes which are non-polar will dissolve in non-polar solvents but not in water. The solubility of ionic compounds also obeys this simple rule because ionic compounds may be considered as being extreme cases of polarity.

The solubility behaviour of chemical materials has considerable biological significance. It has already been pointed out that solubility in water is essential for the transport of nutrients and toxins from one part of the body to another via the bloodstream. In addition, there is the important fact that each cell in the body consists of a membrane composed largely of low polarity, fatty material which separates the aqueous contents of the cell from another aqueous solution surrounding it. Life can continue only for as long as a wide range of chemical substances continue to move between the aqueous environments inside and outside the cell across the fatty membrane which separates them. This movement is governed, to a large extent, by solubility considerations of the sort which have just been discussed.

6.6 Soaps, Detergents and Solubility: Getting the Best of Both Worlds

Most of our washing and cleaning is done using water, and yet a lot of the material which we wash off our bodies, our clothes and eating utensils is oil or grease, which we know is not soluble in water. Of course, we also know that water alone is not effective as a washing agent and must have soap or detergent mixed with it. What is it then, about soaps and detergents, which gives them the capacity to render oil and grease soluble in water?

Most soaps and detergents consist of particles which have an ionic 'head' attached to a long, non-polar 'tail'. Thus, they have a dual nature and the ionic head of a soap or detergent particle makes it compatible with water but not with oil or grease. On the other hand, the non-polar tail of the particle makes it compatible with grease or oil but not with water. Such a particle would appear to have a fundamental problem because its two distinctly different parts are joined firmly together and where one goes so must the other. The effect of all this is that whenever a soap or detergent is added to water it accumulates at the surface where it can achieve some contact with air as well as water. In this way it satisfies, as best it can, the conflicting demands of its two different natures. At the surface of the water the ionic heads of its particles can still interact strongly with water by projecting into the bulk of the liquid. At the same time the non-polar tails of the particles can minimise their interaction with water by projecting towards the surface and the water–air interface.

When water which contains soap or detergent is brought into contact with objects contaminated with oil and grease then the soap or detergent will accumulate at the interface between these materials and the water, as well as at the water–air interface. In this way the dual nature of the soap or detergent is satisfied completely because the non-polar tails of the soap or detergent particles can dissolve in the grease or oil and still have their ionic heads projecting into the water. The effect of this is that the oil or grease is broken into a large number of small lumps, each having many soap or detergent particles attached to its surface in such a way that their ionic heads project into the surrounding water. The electrical charges on these ionic heads ensure that the small grease particles repel each other and this prevents them from coalescing to form larger lumps. This action of dispersing a large lump of material is known as **emulsification**. Once grease or oil has been emulsified it can be separated from any surface simply by draining and rinsing. Thus, soaps and detergents work, not so much by making oil and grease soluble in water, but by breaking it into small lumps and dispersing it throughout the washing water. The dual nature of soap or detergent particles and their mode of action are represented in Figure 6.11.

The Wetting Action of Water. Another important factor which influences the cleansing effect of water is its wetting action. This is its ability to spread out and form a thin film on a surface thereby ensuring efficient contact. On clean metal and glass, water has a good wetting action but on many plastics, and on greasy surfaces, its wetting action is poor. This behaviour can be explained in terms of surface tension, and the natures of the different surfaces.

The surface tension of water, which arises from the forces of attraction acting between water molecules, produces a tendency for water to form into drops rather than spread out into a thin film. However, if water is placed on a surface which contains particles capable of exerting forces of attraction on water molecules, then this tendency will be overcome, to some degree, and the water will spread out. This is the case with metal and glass surfaces. Metals contain positively charged ions and negatively charged electrons. Glass contains positive and negative ions. These charged particles can exert quite strong forces of attraction on water molecules, overcoming the surface tension effect and drawing the water out into a thin film across the surface. Many, but not all, plastics and greases contain no charged particles of any sort, and often consist of molecules which have very low polarities. These molecules are not capable of exerting any significant forces of attraction on water molecules, and so water is not able to wet the surface of such materials effectively.

The ability of soaps and detergents to reduce the surface tension of water has a dramatic effect on its wetting action. Water which contains soap or detergent will be able to wet effectively just about any surface, and this is another way in which the cleansing action of water is enhanced by the presence of these materials.

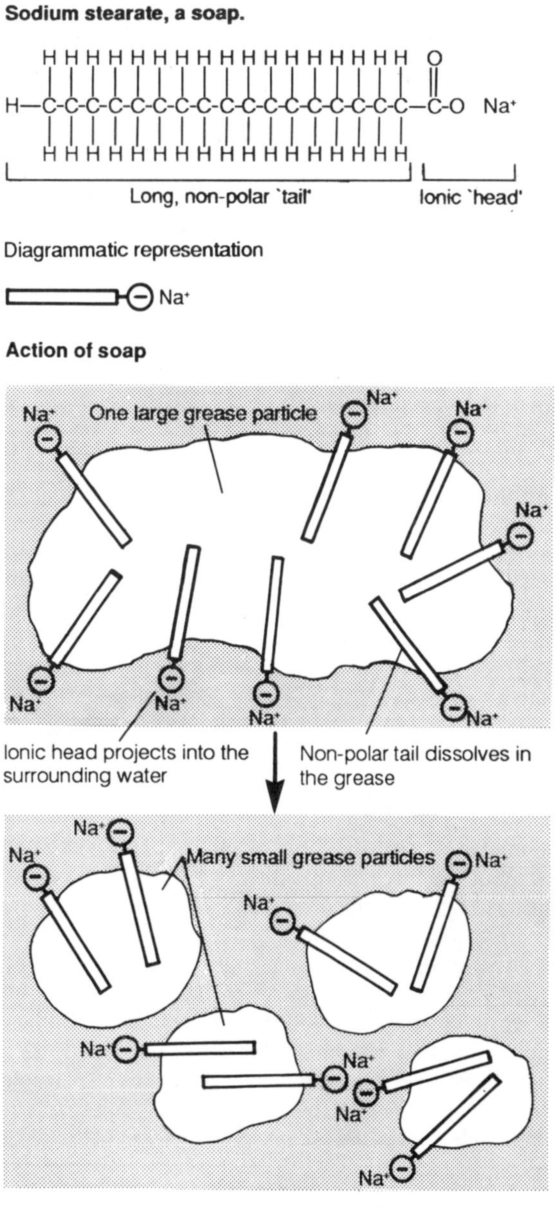

Figure 6.11 *Mode of action of soaps and detergents*

The extent of contact between water and metal surfaces is an important factor in determining the rate at which the metal corrodes. The greater the contact, the greater the rate of corrosion. Corrosion of metal surfaces is usually undesirable and we often go to a lot of trouble to prevent it happening. This is why people polish their motor vehicles. In this process a thin layer of non-polar material, in the form of polish, is applied to the metal surface of the car. When water falls onto the surface of the car it makes contact with this layer. The forces of attraction between the molecules of polish and water molecules are weak and the much greater surface tension of the water (due to hydrogen bonding between water molecules) causes it to form drops rather than spread out in a film as it would do if the polish was not present. Some drops tend to run off the vehicle and out of contact with the metal. The water in the remaining drops is in poor contact with the metal and so its corrosive action is kept at a minimum.

Surface Tension and Capillarity. A capillary tube is a tube usually made out of glass and having a very small internal diameter. When a clean capillary tube is dipped into water, the water wets the glass surface and is drawn up into the tube. This effect is called **capillarity** and it is due to the combined effects of surface tension and the attraction which glass is able to exert on water molecules. The attraction between glass and water molecules is stronger than the forces of attraction which exist between water molecules themselves (hydrogen bonds) and this causes water to rise up the tube and form a curved surface, which is called a **meniscus**. The force of surface tension (due to hydrogen bonds between water molecules) acting within the meniscus causes it to contract (much like a trampoline mat contracts as the trampolinist bounces upwards), lifting water up the tube as it does so. Water continues to rise in the capillary tube until the combined effect of the force of attraction between the glass and the water, and surface tension, which is pulling the water upwards, is balanced by the downward force of gravity acting on the water column in the tube. The smaller the internal diameter of the tube the greater the distance the water will rise inside it. In a capillary tube of internal diameter 0.5 mm the water will rise a distance of 5 cm. The operation of the forces responsible for capillarity is illustrated in Figure 6.12. These forces are acting on water which is very close to the wall of the capillary tube.

Capillary tubes are used for blood sampling. The technique involves pricking the skin and squeezing out a drop of blood. The capillary tube is then placed in the blood drop and blood is drawn into it by capillarity. In this way, samples of about 3 μl may be obtained for blood testing.

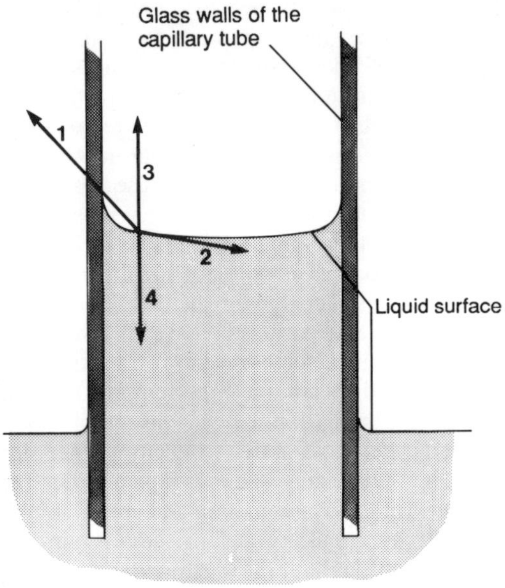

Figure 6.12 *Forces responsible for capillarity. 1, the force of attraction between water and glass; 2 the force of surface tension; 3 the resultant force of 1 and 2; 4, the force of gravity, equal and opposite to 3*

Surfactants in the Body. Because of their ability to reduce surface tension, and their tendency to accumulate at surfaces, soaps and detergents are often called 'surfactants' — surface-active agents. Surfactants play some important roles in the body. **Bile**, which is produced in the gall-bladder, contains some very effective surfactants in the form of compounds known as **bile salts**. When food reaches the intestine, bile is released to mix with it. This emulsifies the fatty component of the food and aids its digestion.

A surfactant is also present in the lungs. Its role is to reduce the surface tension of the film of moisture which covers the surface of the lungs. This makes it easier to expand the lungs during breathing. In infants born before about 28 weeks gestation this surfactant may be absent, making it very difficult for the child to breathe. In this situation the action taken is to insert a tube through the child's trachea and maintain a positive pressure within the lungs. This prevents the alveoli from collapsing completely and makes breathing much easier.

Some medications must be sprayed, as an aqueous mixture, onto the membranes of the throat. The effectiveness of these medications depends on the extent of contact between the medication and the membranes. Since the membranes are composed largely of lipid (see Section 13.11), which has a low polarity, there is a tendency for the medication to form droplets and this would reduce the extent of contact achieved. In order to improve the contact which the medication makes with the membranes a surfactant is included in the aqueous spray mixture. The surfactant reduces the surface tension of the mixture and allows it spread out in a film over the membrane surface.

Bibliography

Blagden, C. 'Experiments and observations in an heated room', *Philosophical Transactions of the Royal Society of London*, **65**, pp. 111–123 and 484–494, 1775.

McIntyre, A. K. (ed.). *Water: Planets, Plants and People*. Australian Academy of Science, Canberra, 1978.

McTigue, P. (ed.). *Chemistry, Key to the Earth*. Melbourne University Press, Melbourne, 1979.

Timberlake, Karen. *Chemistry* (third edition). Harper and Row, New York, 1983.

Questions

1. Which of the following substances would you expect to be most soluble in water?
   - J. KCl
   - K. $C_{10}H_8$
   - L. CCl_4
   - M. CH_2Cl_2

2. Which of the following covalent, molecular compounds would you expect to be most soluble in water?
   - J. $CHCl_3$
   - K. CCl_4
   - L. H–N(H)–CH_2–C(=O)–OH
   - M. CH_3CH_2–O–CH_2CH_3

3. Which of the following properties of water is most affected by the addition of soap?
   - J. melting point
   - K. boiling point
   - L. molecular shape
   - M. surface tension

4. Which of the following statements concerning hydrogen bonds is *false*?
   - J. They operate between water molecules.
   - K. They are weak in comparison to covalent bonds.
   - L. They are unaffected by melting and boiling.
   - M. They operate between water molecules containing –OH or –NH_2 groups.

5. Which of the following changes undergone by one gram of water involves the most heat energy?
   - J. from ice at 0 °C to water at 50 °C
   - K. from water at 50 °C to water at 100 °C
   - L. from water at 0 °C to water at 100 °C
   - M. from water at 100 °C to steam at 100 °C

Latent heat of fusion of water = 334 J/g; latent heat of vaporisation of water = 2280 J/g; specific heat of water = 4.18 J/g/°C.

6. Human beings have a capacity to maintain their body temperature constant at 37 °C even when the surroundings are at a much different temperature. What properties of water assist in this and in what way?

7. A sample of ice is taken from the freezing compartment of a refrigerator and heated. Its temperature is measured at regular time intervals and a graph constructed using the temperature–time values. The graph is shown below. Interpret it as fully as you can.

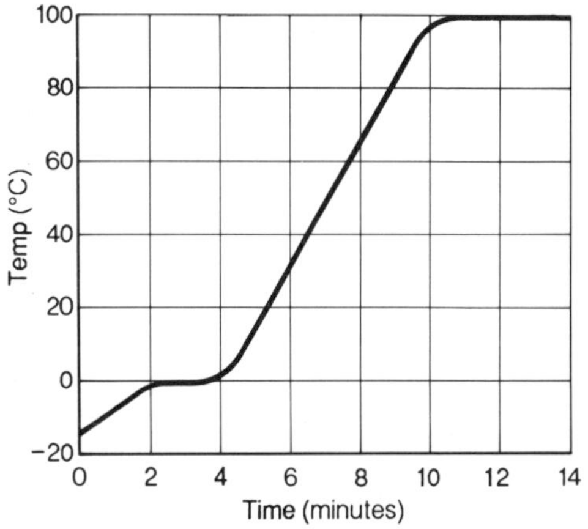

8. Water dissolves a wider variety of substances than any other common liquid. Why is this important for the effective functioning of the human body?

9. On a hot day a person may lose 2 l of water by evaporation from the skin and lungs. Calculate the quantity of heat which is lost as this water evaporates. The latent heat of vaporisation of water is 2280 J/g.

10. Assume that the person in Question 10 has a mass of 70 kg and that human tissue has a specific heat of

4 J/g/°C. If all the heat lost as the 2 l of water evaporated from this person's skin and lungs had been retained by the body calculate the increase in body temperature that it would have caused.

11. When water is sprayed onto a freshly polished car it forms many separate droplets on the car's surface but when it is sprayed onto a car which has not been polished it forms a film over the surface. Explain this.

CHAPTER 7

Aqueous Mixtures

In Chapter 6, 'Water, the Essential Liquid', the emphasis of the discussion was on the properties of pure water. In this book, though, our aim is to develop an understanding of the role which water plays in the human body where it is usually present as the major component of some mixture containing a wide variety of other compounds. A mixture in which water is the dominant component is usually referred to as an aqueous mixture and in this chapter we consider some important properties of this type of mixture. We shall see that some of the properties of an aqueous mixture are very similar to those of pure water. This is so for melting point, boiling point and density. However, we shall also see that some components of an aqueous mixture can cause it to acquire properties which are quite different from those of pure water. Some properties for which this is the case are: electrical conductivity, surface tension and acid–base nature.

This chapter begins with a brief description of three classes of aqueous mixture: mechanical suspensions, colloidal suspensions and solutions. It goes on to consider aqueous solutions in more detail and, in particular, their acid–base nature.

Learning Objectives

At the completion of this chapter you should be able to:

1. Describe several different classes of aqueous mixture and give examples of each.
2. Define the terms electrolyte, non-electrolyte, ionisation, dissociation, saturated solution and unsaturated solution.
3. Define the common units used for the measurement of concentration and perform calculations involving solution concentrations.
4. Describe the effects of changes in temperature and pressure on the solubilities of solids and gases.
5. Define the terms density and specific gravity and describe the effects of increasing the solution concentration on density, melting point and boiling point.
6. Explain the meaning of the terms acid, base, salt, neutralisation and pH.
7. Distinguish between the pairs of terms strong/weak and concentrated/dilute.
8. Nominate the normal pH range for several different body fluids and describe some clinical uses for acids, bases and salts.
9. Predict whether a particular salt will form a neutral, acidic or basic solution when it dissolves in water.
10. Describe the main features of buffer solutions and explain their action.

7.1 Classes of Aqueous Mixture

7.1.1 *Mechanical Suspensions*

This is the simplest type of aqueous mixture. Its formation only involves the dispersal of material throughout the water. Any finely divided solid can be made to form a mechanical suspension with water simply by shaking the two together. A mechanical suspension will begin to separate into its components as soon as shaking stops. Muddy water is a mechanical suspension of soil in water. If it is left to stand the soil particles will separate from the water. If it is passed through an ordinary filter made out of paper or cloth then the soil will be retained by the filter and the water will pass through. All mechanical suspensions behave in this way because the particles dispersed through the water are relatively large (more than 100 nm in diameter). This prevents them from passing through the small pores of an ordinary filter and ensures that they have sufficient mass to drift through the liquid to either the top or bottom surface according to whether the material is more or less dense than water.

The properties of mechanical suspensions are used in large-scale water purification. Water which contains suspended solids is run into large holding tanks or ponds where it remains undisturbed long enough for a large proportion of the suspended material to settle out. The settling-out process is usually accelerated by the addition of compounds such as aluminium sulphate [$Al_2(SO_4)_3$] or iron(III) sulphate [$Fe_2(SO_4)_3$]. These form flocculent precipitates which settle rapidly, carrying the suspended soil particles with them as they go.

7.1.2 *Colloidal Suspensions*

In a colloidal suspension the particles are smaller (1–100 nm in diameter) than in a mechanical suspension but still larger than most single atoms, ions or molecules. They consist either of a large number of small molecules or ions collected together, or of a single, very large molecule such as a protein (see Section 13.8).

If a colloidal suspension is allowed to stand undisturbed then the separation of its components will only occur very slowly or not at all. In some cases this is entirely due to the buffeting which the colloidal particles get from the molecules surrounding them. This keeps all the particles constantly on the move and prevents them from combining with each other to form larger particles which would settle out. In other cases the colloidal particles have an electric charge which causes them to repel each other and this also helps to keep the particles suspended for a long period of time. The small size of colloidal particles allows them to pass through ordinary filters such as cloth or paper. However, they are too large to pass through biological membranes even though some of these membranes do allow the passage of water and other small molecules such as urea ($C_2H_4N_2O$) or glucose ($C_6H_{12}O_6$). Membranes having this property are called **semi-permeable membranes**.

A simple test used to recognise a colloidal suspension is the Tyndall Effect, which is seen when a beam of light is shone through the suspension (see Figure 7.1). The colloidal particles scatter the light and this makes the beam visible from the side as it travels through the suspension. Thus, although the particles are not seen directly their presence is revealed by this scattering of light.

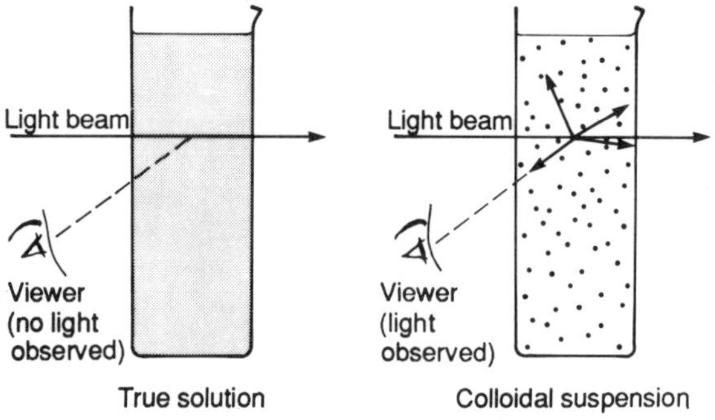

Figure 7.1 *The Tyndall Effect*

A very familiar example of the Tyndall Effect is the scattering of sunlight which is seen when the sunlight enters a darkened room. In this situation scattering is caused by dust particles which are present as a colloidal suspension in the air. Dusty air is just one familiar material which is a colloidal suspension. Others are: **fog**, a colloidal suspension of water in air; **mayonnaise**, a colloidal suspension of vegetable oil in water; **blood plasma**, a colloidal suspension of protein in water.

The terms 'dispersed phase' and 'dispersion medium' are often used in discussions of colloidal mixtures. They correspond respectively to the terms solute and solvent which were introduced in Section 6.5.4. The dispersed phase is the substance existing as colloid-sized particles and distributed through the other substance which is called the dispersion medium. There are also a number of additional terms which are commonly used to describe different types of colloidal mixture.

Foam. This is a colloidal mixture in which a large volume of gas is dispersed through a much smaller volume of liquid or solid. Shaving cream and whipped cream (gas dispersed in liquid) and styrofoam (gas dispersed in solid) are examples of foams.

Emulsion. This is a colloidal mixture in which one liquid is dispersed in another and an example is mayonnaise which is vegetable oil dispersed in water.

Gels. These are colloidal mixtures which set to a solid or semi-solid state and the most familiar example is jelly which is eaten as a sweet.

Sol. This term refers to a diverse set of colloidal mixtures and may be used to describe any colloidal mixture in which a solid is dispersed through a gas, a liquid or another solid. It may also be used to describe colloids in which a liquid is dispersed through a gas. The name of a sol often includes a prefix which indicates the identity of the dispersion medium. Thus sols which consist of substances dispersed in air are called **aerosols** and those which consist of substances dispersed in water are called **hydrosols**. Examples of sols include fog (an aerosol) and blood plasma (a hydrosol).

7.1.3 *Solutions*

This third category of aqueous mixture is the most important and a description of the process by which solutions form was given in Section 6.5.4. The fundamental difference between a solution and a colloidal suspension is that in a solution all components of the mixture are present almost exclusively as relatively small, individual ions or molecules. The particles in a solution are smaller than those found in a colloidal suspension and, as a result, they pass readily through all ordinary filters and, in many cases, through biological membranes. Furthermore, the particles in a solution are too small to produce a Tyndall Effect and this provides the simplest way of distinguishing between a solution and a colloidal suspension.

The main features of the three different classes of aqueous mixture are listed in Table 7.1.

Table 7.1 *Distinguishing characteristics of mechanical suspensions, colloidal suspensions and solutions*

	Mechanical suspensions	Colloidal suspensions	Solutions
type of particle present	individually visible lumps of material	collections of atoms, ions or molecules; one single large molecule	single atoms, ions or molecules
particle size	>100 nm	1–100 nm	<1 nm
effect of ordinary filters	dispersed material is separated	no separation of dispersed material	no separation of dissolved material
effect of semi-permeable membranes	dispersed material is separated	dispersed material is separated	no separation of dissolved material
Tyndall Effect	positive	positive	negative
settling rate	dispersed material settles quickly	dispersed material settles slowly or not at all	dissolved material does not settle at all

7.1.4 *Blood as an Aqueous Mixture*

One of the most common clinical procedures is the taking of a blood sample for laboratory analysis. This is done routinely during all comprehensive physical examinations, even those which are being carried out on people who appear to be quite healthy. It is also a routine part of the diagnosis of many diseases. The manipulations to which blood samples are subjected in the clinical laboratory provide a good opportunity to illustrate much of what has been said above about the three classes of aqueous mixture.

Blood as a Mechanical Suspension. A blood sample is usually subjected to centrifugation soon after it arrives at the clinical laboratory. In this technique the sample is placed in a centrifuge and spun rapidly. The cells present in the blood experience a strong 'force' (centrifugal force) which 'pushes' them to the outside of the circle through which the sample has been made to spin. This separates them from the blood plasma in which they were previously dispersed (see Figure 7.2b). This behaviour shows that the cells are mechanically suspended in the plasma. As a matter of fact, the cells present in blood will begin to settle as soon as blood is removed from the body and allowed to stand undisturbed. Centrifugation simply accelerates this process. Inside the body the agitation caused by the pumping action of the heart is sufficient to keep the cells suspended throughout the plasma as blood travels through the vessels of the circulatory system.

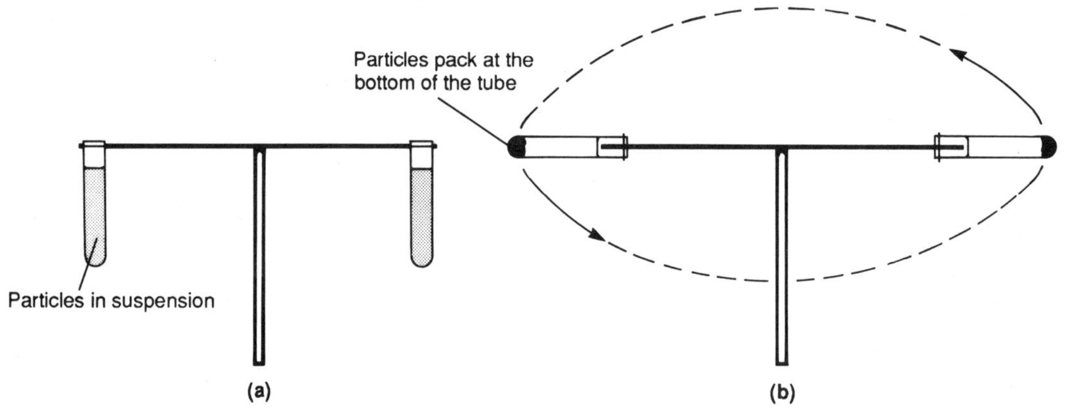

Figure 7.2 *The action of a centrifuge*

Blood as a Colloidal Suspension. In some procedures it is necessary to have samples in which the protein component of blood has been separated from the cells and from most of the dissolved material. These samples are obtained from blood by first removing the cells by centrifugation. The clear plasma obtained is then placed inside a container made entirely, or partly, of a semi-permeable membrane. This container is then placed in a stream of running water. After a while it is found that the material other than water remaining inside the container consists almost entirely of protein. This behaviour is consistent with the protein being present in the blood in colloidal form. If it had been present as a mechanical suspension then it would have been removed from the blood by centrifugation. It remains inside the semi-permeable container because colloidal particles are not able to pass across semi-permeable membranes.

This technique, in which the components of a mixture are separated from each other by passage through a semi-permeable membrane, is known as **dialysis** and is discussed in considerable detail in Chapter 9, 'Aqueous Solutions in the Body'.

Blood as a Solution. There are many components of blood which are capable of passing across semi-permeable membranes. These are simple solutes and their presence in blood makes it a solution as well as a mechanical suspension and a colloidal suspension. It is quite common for the concentrations of some of the solutes in blood to be determined, for example sodium, potassium and chloride ions (ionic solutes) and glucose, urea and cholesterol (molecular, covalent solutes).

7.1.5 *Aqueous Mixtures Used as Medications*

It is very rare for medicines to be used in the form of pure compounds. They are nearly always mixed with other substances. These other substances often have no direct therapeutic effect but they contribute to the efficacy of the medicine in other ways. For example, most medicines administered in the form of tablets (the most common of all methods of administration) have been mixed with a substance called a binder, which increases the ability of medicine particles to stick to one another. This assists in the formation of tablets of uniform mass and increases their hardness so that they are not subject to disintegration as they bang against one another in the bottle prior to use. Some commonly used binders include gelatin and glucose.

While the tablet is the most common form in which medicines are administered there are many which are prepared as aqueous mixtures. This form of medicine, being liquid, is the most versatile as far as delivery of the medicine to target tissues is concerned. Aqueous mixtures may be ingested, injected, inhaled or applied directly to surfaces on the outside or inside of the body.

Mechanical Suspensions. Most lotions, magmas and milks are mechanical suspensions. A lotion is a mixture designed for external application to the body and one of the best known examples is calamine lotion, a mechanical suspension of zinc oxide (ZnO) in water. Calamine lotion is used to obtain relief from sunburn, insect bites and similar discomforts. Magmas and milks are mechanical suspensions in water which may be taken internally. Two common examples are 'Kaomagma' and 'Mylanta'. Kaomagma is a suspension of aluminium hydroxide [$Al(OH)_3$] and it is used as a treatment for diarrhoea. Mylanta is a suspension of aluminium hydroxide and magnesium hydroxide [$Mg(OH)_2$]. It is used as an antacid and anti-flatulent. These medications, being just mechanical suspensions, are likely to settle on standing and they should always be clearly labelled 'Shake Well Before Use'. Most mechanical suspensions used as medications contain ingredients which increase the time taken for the suspended material to settle as well as other ingredients which ensure that the settled material is easily re-dispersed on shaking. The hormone insulin, which is used for the control of *diabetes mellitus*, may be combined with zinc to form a substance which is then dispersed in water as a mechanical suspension. This suspension is administered by subcutaneous injection and cannot be administered intravenously. The vials containing the preparation must be agitated before use to ensure that the insulin is uniformly distributed within the dispersion medium.

Colloidal Suspensions. There are many medications which are colloidal suspensions in water, but in most cases it is not the medicine itself which is colloidally dispersed. Usually the medicine is dissolved or mechanically dispersed in a colloidal suspension of some inert substance such as acacia gum (often called Gum Arabic) or agar. Acacia gum is exuded by the stem and branches of the acacia tree and agar is extracted from algae. These otherwise inert colloids are used to give the medication some desirable physical property. For example, the colloid may thicken the preparation and help keep some mechanically suspended material from settling out of the mixture. An example of a medication which is a simple colloidal suspension in water is kaolin which is used to treat the diarrhoea caused by food poisoning.

Solutions. This is a particularly convenient form in which to have a medicine and many more medicines would be prepared as solutions were it not for two things. Medicines in solution are much less stable than their solid forms which means that they generally have a shorter shelf life when in solution. The other reason is that many medicines are insoluble in all the liquids that people can safely consume or otherwise be in direct contact with.

Aqueous solutions are used for antiseptic washing of the skin, as gargles and mouthwashes, as douches and as enemas. All these uses mainly involve the ingredients of the solution producing an effect only on the tissues with which the solution makes direct contact. Other aqueous solutions are swallowed and the medicines present in the solutions exert their effects after having been absorbed into the circulation and carried to many different parts of the body. Two terms used to describe aqueous solutions in this category are 'elixir' and 'syrup'.

An elixir is a solution in which the solvent is a mixture of water and alcohol with the alcohol being present to increase the solubility of the drug. The alcohol content of an elixir may be as high as 23% (v/v) which is comparable to the alcohol content of champagne and much higher than that of beers and table wines. A syrup does not contain alcohol but it does contain a high concentration of sucrose. This gives it a sweet taste which is useful in masking the bitter or otherwise unpleasant tastes possessed by many medicines. The taste of a syrup or elixir may also be enhanced by the presence of flavouring agents such as caramel or peppermint.

7.2 Electrolytes and Non-electrolytes

Pure water is a poor conductor of electricity and yet we are constantly reminded that water increases the danger of electrocution. We are told, and quite rightly so, that we should not operate electrical equipment while our hands are wet or while we are standing on a damp surface. The danger which we face in these situations is due to the fact that water on a person's hands or on the floor is not pure. It is a solution and it contains dissolved materials which form free-moving ions in the solution. This makes the solution a conductor of electricity and increases the danger of electrocution. It does not take much dissolved material to produce a dramatic increase in the electrical conductivity of a solution. Sodium chloride is present on the skin and this explains why water in contact with the hands is a good conductor of electricity.

Any substance which produces ions when it dissolves in water is known as an **electrolyte**. If the substance exists in solution entirely as ions it is called a **strong electrolyte**. If it exists in solution partially as ions but predominantly as molecules it is called a **weak electrolyte**. All ionic compounds are strong electrolytes. Examples are sodium chloride, potassium bromide and calcium chloride. These compounds are strong electrolytes because they are composed of ions and when they dissolve in water the ions are released into the solution in a process known as **dissociation**. Once an appreciable amount of any one of them has dissolved the solution will be a good conductor. Some ionic compounds, however, are not very soluble in water and even though they are strong electrolytes, according to the definition which we have used, they cannot produce solutions which are good conductors of electricity.

There are also some molecular, covalent compounds which are strong electrolytes, for example hydrogen chloride (HCl), hydrogen sulphate (H_2SO_4, usually called concentrated sulphuric acid) and hydrogen nitrate (HNO_3, usually called concentrated nitric acid). These compounds, when pure, exist entirely as molecules and they contain no ions. However, when they are mixed with water they react with it and all their molecules are converted into ions in a process known as ionisation.

Some equations for the dissociation and ionisation of strong electrolytes are written below.

Dissociation

$$NaCl \longrightarrow Na^+_{aq} + Cl^-_{aq}$$

sodium chloride → sodium ion + chloride ion

$$KOH \longrightarrow K^+_{aq} + OH^-_{aq}$$

potassium hydroxide → potassium ion + hydroxide ion

Ionisation

$$HCl + H_2O \longrightarrow H_3O^+_{aq} + Cl^-_{aq}$$

hydrogen chloride → hydronium ion + chloride ion

$$HNO_3 + H_2O \longrightarrow H_3O^+ + NO^-_{3aq}$$

concentrated nitric acid → nitrate ion

Weak electrolytes are always covalent, molecular compounds and they form ions in solution by the process of ionisation in the same way as the covalent, molecular compounds that are strong electrolytes do. However, only a small proportion of molecules are converted into ions. Some equations for the ionisation of weak electrolytes are written below.

$$NH_3 + H_2O \rightleftarrows NH^+_{4aq} + OH^-_{aq}$$

ammonia → ammonium ion + hydroxide ion

$$H_2CO_3 + H_2O \rightleftarrows H_3O^+_{aq} \quad HCO^-_{3aq}$$

carbonic acid → hydronium ion, bicarbonate ion

Notice that in these equations for the ionisation of weak electrolytes two arrows appear in the equation and this is to emphasise that the processes are equilibrium processes which favour the reactants (see Section 3.6).

There are many compounds that do not produce ions when they dissolve in water and these are called **non-electrolytes.** They are always covalent, molecular compounds and two examples are sucrose ($C_{12}H_{22}O_{11}$, table sugar) and alcohol (C_2H_6O).

The term electrolyte is commonly encountered in discussions of blood plasma, gastrointestinal fluid, saliva and other body fluids. In these situations it usually refers to a single ion such as the sodium ion, Na^+, chloride ion, Cl^-, or calcium ion, Ca^{2+}. The amounts of such ions present in body fluids can provide important clues about a person's state of health and they are very commonly determined in the clinical situation.

7.3 Concentration of Solutions

7.3.1 *Percentage Concentration*

There are many ways of describing the concentration of a solution but all of them turn out to be statements about the relative amounts of solute and solvent which are present in the solution. For example, it is very common to encounter the term 'percentage concentration (w/v)' which is defined as: the mass of solute dissolved in 100 ml of solution. Thus a 5% (w/v) solution is one which contains 5 g of solute dissolved in each 100 ml portion of solution. The mathematical expression for percentage concentration (w/v) is:

$$\text{percentage concentration (w/v)} = \frac{\text{mass of solute in g}}{\text{volume of solution in ml}} \times 100$$

The abbreviation '(w/v)' which accompanies percentage concentration defined in this way stands for the phrase 'weight for volume' and is used to provide information about the way in which the relative amounts of solute and solution have been measured (solute as a weight (mass) and solution as a volume). Percentage concentrations may also be designated as '(w/w)', if the amounts of solute and solution have both been determined as weights (masses) or as '(v/v)' if they have both been determined as a volume. Percentage concentration (v/v) is only used for solutions of liquids in liquids. It is used for alcoholic beverages and is closely related to the rather archaic proof spirit scale. On this scale an alcoholic beverage might be described as being '90 proof' and this means that it has a percentage concentration (v/v) of alcohol of 45. Thus concentration on the proof spirit scale is simply double the percentage concentration (v/v).

The term 'proof spirit' has its origins in seventeenth-century England. When whiskey was bought and sold in those days the method used to ensure that it had not been diluted with water was to pour a sample onto gun powder and light it. If the gun powder would still ignite this was taken as 'proof' that the whiskey was full strength and the transaction would then proceed. Hence the term 'proof spirit'.

7.3.2 *Concentration Expressed in Moles per Litre: Molarity*

The mole is the fundamental unit for measurement of the amount of substance and so, in science, concentrations expressed in terms of moles are usually preferred. The most commonly used concentration term of this type is moles per litre. It is calculated using the expression:

$$\text{concentration in moles per litre} = \frac{\text{number of moles}}{\text{solution volume (l)}}$$

When it comes to preparing a solution which contains a certain number of moles per litre we must first work out the corresponding number of grams because we have no means of directly measuring moles. The relationship between the number of moles of a pure substance in a sample and the mass of the sample is:

$$\text{number of moles} = \frac{\text{mass in grams}}{\text{molar mass}}$$

If we now substitute this expression for number of moles in the expression for concentration in moles per litre we obtain:

$$\text{concentration in moles per litre} = \frac{\text{mass in grams}}{\text{molar mass} \times \text{solution volume (l)}}$$

In the SI system of units the symbol for the mole is mol and so the SI unit for concentration expressed in moles per litre is mol/l. A concentration expressed in mol/l is often called the molarity of the solution and given the symbol M. Thus, a solution having a concentration of 1.5 moles per litre may be represented as 1.5 mol/l or 1.5 M. Yet another way used to represent concentration in moles per litre is to enclose the formula of the dissolved substance in brackets and write an expression such as

$$[NaCl] = 1.5$$

which means 'the concentration of the substance of formula NaCl (sodium chloride) is 1.5 mol/l'.

7.4 Concentration Calculations

There are a number of ways in which a nurse might have to make use of a knowledge of concentration and these will now be described using percentage concentration (w/v) as the example. This is the type of concentration most commonly encountered by nurses but, in any case, it is a simple matter to apply the same approach to situations involving concentrations expressed in different ways.

7.4.1 *Preparing a Solution of Known Concentration*

Let us suppose that 500 ml of 2% (w/v) disinfectant solution is required for disinfecting equipment. The disinfectant is in the form of a powder. We need to work out how many grams of the disinfectant powder are needed. We can determine this in two ways.

Using a verbal definition of percentage concentration (w/v): Percentage concentration (w/v) is the number of grams of solute present in every 100 ml of solution. We require a 2% disinfectant solution and so we require a solution that contains 2 g of powder in every 100 ml of solution. We require 500 ml of solution and so we need 5 × 2 = 10 g of disinfectant powder.

Using the mathematical expression for percentage concentration (w/v):

$$\text{percentage concentration (w/v)} = \frac{\text{mass in grams}}{\text{solution volume (ml)}} \times 100$$

$$2 = \frac{\text{mass in grams}}{500} \times 100$$

$$\text{mass in grams} = \frac{2 \times 500}{100}$$

$$= 10$$

Now that we know how many grams of disinfectant powder we must use we would obtain our solution by dissolving the 10 g in a volume of water rather less than 500 ml. We would then transfer this solution to a vessel (volumetric flask or graduated beaker or measuring cylinder) graduated in some way which would allow us to increase the volume of the solution to 500 ml by the addition of water. We would use some water to rinse all traces of disinfectant from the container in which it was first dissolved and add this to the vessel prior to making the solution up to 500 ml in volume.

The final solution of disinfectant must be shaken thoroughly before use to ensure that it is of uniform concentration throughout. All these manipulations are illustrated in Figure 7.3.

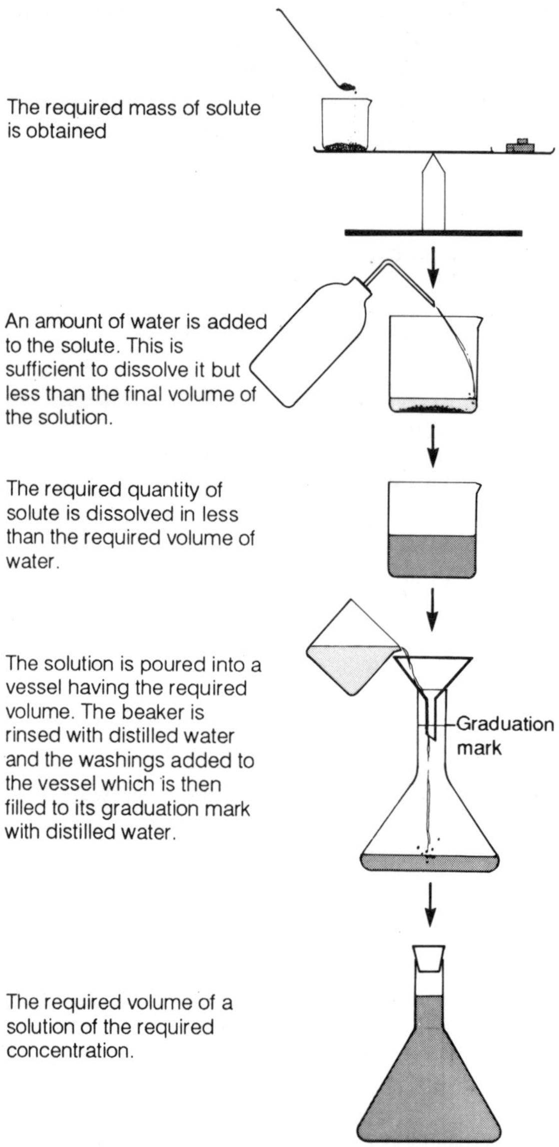

The required mass of solute is obtained
An amount of water is added to the solute. This is sufficient to dissolve it but less than the final volume of the solution.
The required quantity of solute is dissolved in less than the required volume of water.
The solution is poured into a vessel having the required volume. The beaker is rinsed with distilled water and the washings added to the vessel which is then filled to its graduation mark with distilled water.
Graduation mark
The required volume of a solution of the required concentration.

Figure 7.3 *Steps in the preparation of a solution of known concentration*

7.4.2 *Calculating the Volume of Solution which Contains a Specified Mass of Solute*

Suppose a person is undergoing a glucose tolerance test as part of the process of diagnosing *diabetes mellitus*. If this person is given 70 g of glucose dissolved in 250 ml of solution what is the concentration of the solution?

Using the verbal definition of percentage concentration (w/v): The solution of glucose contains 70 g of glucose in 250 ml of solution. The amount present in 100 ml would be 70 × 100/250 = 28 g. The percentage concentration (w/v) is, therefore, 28.

Using the mathematical expression for percentage concentration (w/v):

$$\text{percentage concentration (w/v)} = \frac{\text{mass in grams}}{\text{solution volume (ml)}} \times 100$$
$$= \frac{70}{250} \times 100$$
$$= 28$$

7.4.3 *Dilution of a Solution from One Concentration to Another*

It is quite often the case that a solution of one concentration is available and a solution of another concentration is required. For example, hydrochloric acid is sold in the form of a 36% (w/v) solution but when it is used for the treatment of **hypochlorhydria** (insufficient hydrochloric acid in gastric juice) it is diluted to about 10% (w/v) by the addition of distilled water. The dose of acid to be administered is specified as a volume of this diluted acid and this volume is mixed with a relatively large volume of water before it is drunk.

How can we decide what volume of the 36% (w/v) solution and distilled water must be mixed in order to obtain a solution which is 10% (w/v)? Let us call the concentration and volume of solution before dilution C_1 and V_1 respectively and the concentration and volume after dilution C_2 and V_2. Now, in all situations where a solution is diluted by the addition of the pure solvent (in this case, pure water) the following points apply.

1. For the solution before dilution,

$$C_1 = \frac{\text{mass of solute}}{V_1} \times 100$$

from which it follows that

$$\text{mass of solute} = \frac{C_1 \times V_1}{100}$$

It is important to realise that V_1 refers to the portion of the more concentrated solution which is to be mixed with water and not to the total volume of that solution which happens to be available.

2. After the solution has been diluted by the addition of pure water,

$$C_2 = \frac{\text{mass of solute}}{V_2} \times 100$$

from which it follows that

$$\text{mass of solute} = \frac{C_2 \times V_2}{100}$$

3. The mass of solute is the same after dilution as it was before because only pure solvent has been added. Therefore we may write,

$$\frac{C_1 \times V_1}{100} = \frac{C_2 \times V_2}{100}$$

and then

$$C_1 \times V_1 = C_2 \times V_2$$

In this way we have shown that in any dilution process the concentrations and volumes before and after the dilution are related by the expression

$$\begin{matrix}\text{concentration}\\ \text{before}\end{matrix} \times \begin{matrix}\text{volume}\\ \text{before}\end{matrix} = \begin{matrix}\text{concentration}\\ \text{after}\end{matrix} \times \begin{matrix}\text{volume}\\ \text{after}\end{matrix}$$

This expression is valid no matter what concentration units are used.

Now we can return to the problem of deciding how to go about obtaining a 10% (w/v) solution of hydrochloric acid by dilution of a 36% (w/v) solution. We must, of course, decide how much of the diluted solution we require. Let us suppose we need 800 ml. This is the volume after dilution and we can now substitute values in our expression,

$$\begin{matrix}\text{concentration}\\ \text{before}\end{matrix} \times \begin{matrix}\text{volume}\\ \text{before}\end{matrix} = \begin{matrix}\text{concentration}\\ \text{after}\end{matrix} \times \begin{matrix}\text{volume}\\ \text{after}\end{matrix}$$

and obtain

$$36 \times \text{volume before} = 10 \times 800$$

from which it follows that

$$\text{volume before} = \frac{10 \times 800}{36}$$
$$= 222 \text{ ml}$$

Thus, to obtain 800 ml of a 10% (w/v) hydrochloric acid solution we must take 222 ml of 36% (w/v) solution and add enough distilled water to increase the volume to 800 ml.

7.5 Limits to Solubility

There is usually a limit to the amount of solute that will dissolve in a solution and this is what is meant by the term 'solubility'. The solubility of a substance is the maximum amount of the substance which can be dissolved in a given amount of solution at that temperature. For example, the solubility of sodium chloride in water is 363 g/l of solution at 25 °C. Once this quantity of sodium chloride has dissolved in a litre of solution at 25 °C no more will dissolve. If more sodium chloride is added it will simply sit on the bottom of the container and remain undissolved indefinitely.

A solution which contains the maximum amount of a dissolved substance is also said to be saturated with that substance while a solution which contains less than the maximum amount is said to be unsaturated.

A common commercial method used to obtain large quantities of sodium chloride depends upon the formation of a saturated solution of sodium chloride from sea water. This method illustrates quite nicely the relationship between solution concentration and solution saturation. It involves allowing sea water to run into large, shallow ponds which can be isolated from the sea.

In sea water the concentration of sodium chloride is about 28 g/l. Its solubility in water is 363 g/l at 25 °C and so sea water is nowhere near saturated with sodium chloride. The next most abundant substance dissolved in sea water is magnesium chloride ($MgCl_2$) and its concentration is about 5 g/l which is also very much less than its solubility of 572 g/l at 25 °C. Once sea water has been run into shallow ponds shut off from the sea, evaporation of water commences and the concentrations of all the substances dissolved in the sea water begin to increase.

When 90% of the water has evaporated the concentrations will have increased by a factor of 10. The concentration of sodium chloride will be 280 g/l and the concentration of magnesium chloride will be 50 g/l. Now the concentration of sodium chloride is quite close to its solubility and the solution is getting close to being saturated with sodium chloride. The concentration of magnesium chloride is still far below its solubility.

Once enough water has evaporated for the concentration of sodium chloride to reach its solubility the compound will begin to precipitate from the solution. Magnesium chloride, and most of the other compounds which are present in sea water, remain dissolved long after a large amount of sodium chloride has deposited and so this very simple method provides sodium chloride of high purity.

7.5.1 *The Effects of Temperature and Pressure on Solubility*

The solubilities of most solids are not significantly altered as the pressure acting on the solution changes but they usually do alter with temperature and, in nearly all cases, the solubility increases as the temperature increases. The exact relationship between temperature and solubility for a number of compounds is shown in Figure 7.4. You can see that the magnitude of the effect which temperature change has on solubility varies greatly from one compound to another.

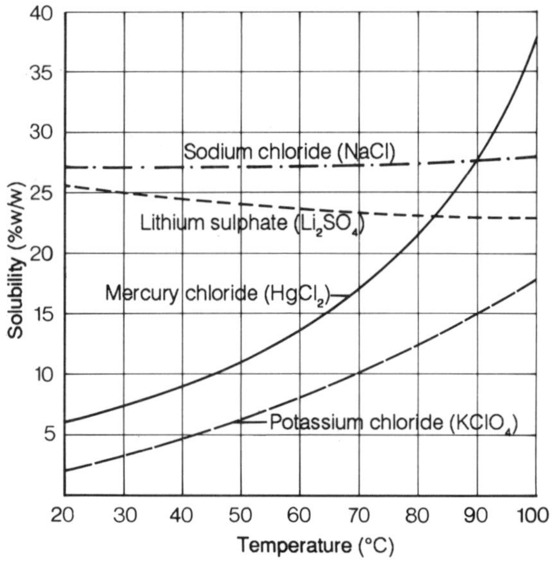

Figure 7.4 *Variation of solubility with temperature* (see Errata)

The change in solubility with temperature is not a matter of much significance as far as solutions inside the body are concerned because body temperature remains constant at about 37 °C. It is, however, partly responsible for the fact that the urine of a healthy person is clear when it is first eliminated from the body but becomes cloudy on standing. Urine leaves the body at 37 °C at which temperature all its components are dissolved. As it stands outside the body it cools to room temperature and the solubilities of its dissolved components become less. In some instances the concentration of a dissolved compound may exceed its solubility at the lower temperature and, if this is the case, the compound will precipitate from the urine causing it to become cloudy.

The solubility of a gas in a liquid is markedly affected by both temperature and pressure. It increases as the pressure of the gas in contact with the liquid increases but decreases as the temperature of the liquid increases. This is illustrated by the familiar behaviour of carbonated beverages such as Coca-Cola and beer. These beverages are packed inside bottles and cans in contact with a gas which consists mainly of carbon dioxide. The pressure of this gas is higher than atmospheric pressure. The high proportion of carbon dioxide in the gas mixture and the relatively high pressure cause a large amount of carbon dioxide to dissolve. When the container is opened the beverage is brought into contact with the atmosphere which contains less than 1% carbon dioxide. This reduces the solubility of carbon dioxide to a value well below the concentration which is present in the beverage. The excess carbon dioxide quickly leaves the solution producing the well-known effervescent effect which helps make carbonated beverages so popular.

When a warm container of carbonated beverage is opened the effervescence may be much greater than that obtained with a cold container. This is because gas solubility decreases with increasing temperature and more carbon dioxide must leave the solution in order to reduce its concentration to the same value as its solubility. The larger quantity of carbon dioxide leaving the solution may produce such a large effervescent effect as to make the beverage difficult to pour and less pleasing to drink. This is part of the reason why carbonated beverages are usually consumed cold, although the lower temperature is by itself a factor affecting the pleasure which the beverage provides.

The relationship between the pressure of a gas and its solubility plays an important role in understanding the processes which operate to ensure that the human body has an adequate supply of oxygen and is able to rid itself of excess carbon dioxide. Furthermore, there are situations encountered in nursing where the pressure of oxygen in contact with the blood is changed. These matters are discussed more fully in Chapter 10, 'Pressure'. The effect of temperature on gas solubility is much less relevant to body function. The temperature of the air which we breathe in may vary greatly, but, by the time it has travelled through the trachea and bronchi to the lungs, it is warmed or cooled to body temperature through its contact with the tissues of those structures.

7.6 Solute Concentration and the Properties of Solutions

7.6.1 *Density and Specific Gravity*

The density of an object is its mass per unit of volume and is obtained by dividing the object's mass by its volume. Thus:

$$\text{density (g/ml)} = \frac{\text{mass (g)}}{\text{volume (ml)}}$$

Density is influenced by temperature because all objects undergo changes in volume as their temperatures change. For this reason, in situations where great accuracy is required, a value for density will be accompanied by the value for the temperature at which it was determined. Thus, the density of water is 1.000 g/ml at 4 °C, but 0.997 g/ml at 25 °C. In most situations this difference is small enough to be ignored.

When a substance is dissolved in a liquid the mass of the solution so formed is exactly equal to the sum of the masses of the liquid and the substance which was dissolved in it. However, the volume of the solution does not change in the same way. The solution does not have a volume which is simply the sum of the

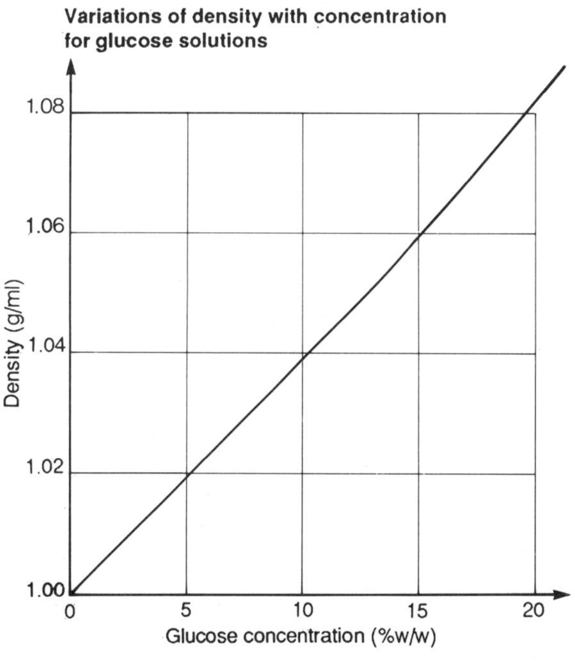

Figure 7.5 *Variation of density with concentration for glucose solutions at 25 °C*

separate volumes. In all cases the change in volume which a liquid undergoes when a substance dissolves in it is less than the corresponding change in mass and so the density of the solution steadily increases as the solution concentration increases. Figure 7.5 displays the relationship between the density of a glucose solution and its concentration.

The relationship between solution concentration and density can be used to determine the concentration of a solution. For example, if we were given a solution of glucose of unknown concentration and asked to determine its concentration we could proceed as follows:

1. Measure out a particular volume of the solution, determine the mass of this volume of solution and calculate the density by dividing the mass by the volume.
2. Use the graph of Figure 7.5 to determine the concentration which corresponds to the measured density.

There are many situations where the concentrations of solutions are regularly checked and quite often the method used depends on the relationship between solution concentration and density. For example:

1. The common car battery contains a solution of sulphuric acid and the concentration of this solution is a good indicator of the state of the battery.
2. Alcoholic beverages have costs which are related to their alcohol concentrations and so all premises licensed to sell alcohol from unsealed containers are visited regularly by inspectors who measure the concentration of alcohol in the drinks being dispensed. In this way proprietors are discouraged from attempting to obtain increased profits by adding water to the drinks which they sell.
3. A healthy person with a normal intake of food and water will produce urine with a density between 1.008 and 1.030 g/ml at 20 °C. If a person's urine is less concentrated than normal its density will be less than 1.008; if it is more concentrated than normal its density will be greater than 1.030. The production of urine with a concentration outside the normal range may be due to disease and warrants further investigation. Thus, urine of low concentration is one symptom of *diabetes insipidus*, while urine of high concentration is a symptom of *diabetes mellitus*.

In order to obtain an accurate measure of a solution's density it is necessary to carry out accurate measures of both volume and mass. This makes density measurement something which is not easy to do outside a laboratory away from carefully calibrated glassware and an accurate balance.

For each of the three situations described above it is not density itself which is determined but another, closely related, quantity called specific gravity. In the case of solutions, this is defined as the ratio of the density of the solution to the density of pure water at the same temperature. Thus:

$$\text{specific gravity} = \frac{\text{density of solution}}{\text{density of pure water}}$$

Being a ratio, specific gravity has no units and it does not matter what units the densities of the solution and pure water are measured in provided that the units are the same in both cases. You may be wondering why anyone would measure a specific gravity instead of a density. After all, it looks as if it is necessary to measure the solution's density in order to calculate a value for specific gravity. This is not so and specific gravity is a useful measure because it can be made very simply using a device called an hydrometer. This device exploits the fact that a floating object will sink to a greater depth in a less dense liquid than in one which is more dense. This is why it is easier to swim

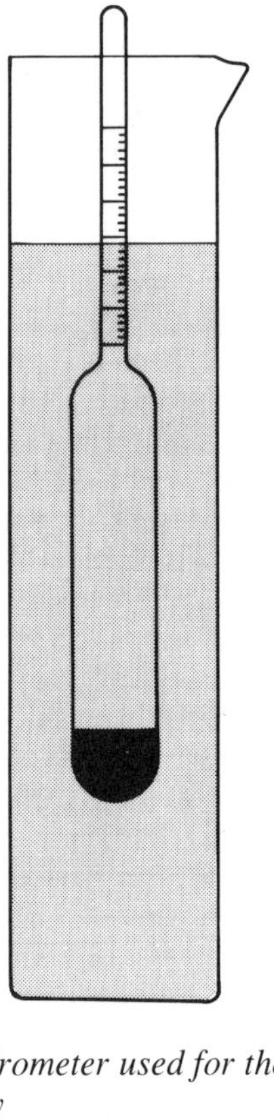

Figure 7.6 *Hydrometer used for the measurement of specific gravity*

in sea water than in fresh water. Sea water is more concentrated and, therefore, more dense than fresh water. Our bodies do not sink as far in sea water as they do in fresh water and so it is easier for us to stay afloat and move about in sea water than in fresh water.

Hydrometers are long, narrow devices heavily weighted at one end so that they will float upright in a liquid (see Figure 7.6). The upper section of the hydrometer has a scale marked on it and the specific gravity is read at the point where the liquid surface intercepts the scale when the hydrometer is floating freely in the liquid. The scale is calibrated at the factory by immersing the hydrometer in solutions of known density and marking it at the appropriate points.

Hydrometers are very convenient devices because they are easy to carry about and can be used anywhere. The specific gravity value which an hydrometer provides so easily is, for most purposes, just as useful an estimate of solution concentration as density itself. If a density value is required it can be obtained from the specific gravity by a simple calculation using a known value for the density of pure water. This is a particularly easy calculation to do when density is measured in g/ml. In these units its value for water may be taken to be one and so we have:

$$\text{specific gravity} = \frac{\text{density of solution in g/ml}}{\text{density of pure water in g/ml}}$$

$$\text{specific gravity} = \frac{\text{density of solution in g/ml}}{1}$$

$$\text{specific gravity} = \text{density of solution in g/ml}$$

This shows that the specific gravity of a solution is numerically equal to its density measured in g/ml.

Hydrometers are usually designed specifically for a particular type of solution. This is the case for the hydrometer which is used to measure the specific gravity of urine. It is given the special name of **urinometer** and a word of caution is needed about the scale which appears on some urinometers. This scale may cover a range of values from 0 to 60 and so when the device is used to determine the specific gravity of a urine sample, a value such as 27 may be obtained. This is not the specific gravity of the urine sample! If it was then the urine would be 27 times as dense as pure water and more dense than gold! To get the specific gravity of urine from the measured value of 27 you must write 1.0 in front of the 27 and so convert it to the value 1.027. The same must be done for all readings which consist of two digits. If the urinometer provides a reading of less than 10 it is converted to a specific gravity by writing 1.00 in front of the single digit of the reading itself. Thus a reading of 4 gives a specific gravity of 1.004.

You are probably thinking that this is all a bit too devious and wondering why the manufacturer of the urinometer did not simply put the correct numbers on the scale of the device. There are two likely reasons for this: the stem of the urinometer is very narrow which would make it relatively difficult to read a four digit number from the scale; and some people using the urinometer might find it difficult to read decimal numbers and so be likely to record an incorrect value.

The specific gravity of urine can also be determined using test strips which are simply dipped into the urine sample. The measurement is made by comparing the colour of the strip with a standard colour key. The strip contains a compound which alters its colour as the concentration of ions in the urine alters. The concentration of the ions affecting the colour of the strip is related to the total concentration of dissolved material present in the urine and therefore to its specific gravity. In this way an estimate of the specific gravity of the urine is obtained. This method is not as accurate as the measurement of specific gravity using a urinometer but it has the following advantages:

1. A few drops of urine are sufficient for the measurement, compared to about 50 ml which are required when a urinometer is used.
2. A fresh test strip is used for each measurement, whereas the urinometer is used repeatedly and must be rinsed and dried between each reading.
3. The urinometer is made of glass and is quite easily broken.

7.6.2 *Melting Point and Boiling Point*

Here we shall restrict our discussion to solutions in which the solute is less volatile than the solvent (meaning that it forms a vapour less readily). This is a reasonable restriction for us to use because, with the exception of materials such as the dissolved gases oxygen and carbon dioxide, most of the solute present in solutions found in the body, or used in intravenous therapy, is less volatile than water.

Solutions containing solutes of low volatility always have lower melting points and higher boiling points than the pure solvent which they contain. In other words, the effect of the solute is to allow the solution to exist as a liquid over a wider range of temperature than the pure solvent. For example, a 10% solution of sodium chloride in water freezes at –3 °C and boils at 101 °C.

The lowering of melting point caused by dissolved substances is the basis of a technique used to determine the concentration of urine and blood plasma. In this technique a small sample of the urine or plasma is placed in contact with a specially designed thermometer. The sample and thermometer are then placed in a chamber held at a low temperature. As the sample cools, the thermometer registers its falling temperature. At the freezing point of the sample the rate of decrease of the temperature slows and in this way the freezing point is determined and compared with that of solutions of known concentration to obtain an estimate of the concentration of the urine or plasma sample.

7.7 Acids and Bases

One of the most useful insights which physical science has provided into the nature of things is that the behaviour of materials may be understood in terms of the properties of the particles of which they are composed. This was illustrated in Chapter 6, 'Water, the Essential Liquid', where the shape of the water molecule was used as the basis for explaining some important features of the behaviour of that substance. Another illustration of the same thing was provided in Section 3.4, 'Types of Chemical Reation', where several different classes of chemical reaction were defined in terms of the type of atom rearrangement which they involved. One of these was the acid–base reaction. This is a very important category of reaction because it occurs frequently in aqueous solutions including those found inside the human body. We shall now consider the topic of acids and bases in more detail.

7.7.1 *Acids*

The term acid is familiar to everyone and most people readily associate acids with corrosive, damaging behaviour. It is certainly true that some acids are capable of rapidly burning their way through almost any substance with which they come in contact. For example, a mixture of nitric acid and hydrochloric acid (called 'aqua regia', a latin term meaning 'royal water') is capable of dissolving gold; hydrofluoric acid is capable of dissolving glass. If acids such as these come in contact with tissue they can cause catastrophic injuries and so they must be handled with great care. Knowing this you may be surprised by the fact that acids are essential to normal body function and that many of the medicines which we take are acids. For example, our stomachs contain hydrochloric acid which is essential for the digestion of food; the common drug aspirin is an acid.

Let us now consider a question which arises quite naturally even at this early stage in our discussion of acids. *What do all acids have in common?* All acids, when mixed with water, react with the water and form the ion $H_3O^+_{aq}$, known as the **hydronium ion**. At the same time, the acid also forms a negative ion in the solution. Two examples are presented below.

$$\underset{\text{sulphuric acid}}{H_2SO_4} + \underset{\text{water}}{H_2O} \xrightarrow{H^+ \text{ transferred}} \underset{\text{hydronium ion}}{H_3O^+_{aq}} + \underset{\text{hydrogensulphate ion}}{HSO^-_{4aq}}$$

$$\underset{\text{acetic acid}}{CH_3CO_2H} + \underset{\text{water}}{H_2O} \xrightarrow{H^+ \text{ transferred}} \underset{\text{hydronium ion}}{H_3O^+_{aq}} + \underset{\text{acetate ion}}{CH_3CO_2^-}$$

In these equations the particle H^+, called the **hydrogen ion**, is shown shifting from the acid molecule to the water molecule thereby changing the water molecule into an hydronium ion. This transfer of H^+ is the essential feature of reactions involving acids. Most hydrogen atoms contain only one proton and one electron and so the particle H^+, which has lost its electron, is usually just a proton. For this reason, reactions involving acids are often called **proton-transfer** reactions.

Many books will simply say that acids produce hydrogen ions in solution, use the formula H^+ in place of H_3O^+ and make no mention of hydronium ions. In most situations this does not matter but there is no evidence for the existence of the hydrogen ion in an aqueous solution while there is considerable evidence for the existence of hydronium ions. For this reason we shall refer to hydronium ions rather than hydrogen ions when discussing the acid–base nature of aqueous solutions.

As well as forming hydronium ions, acids always form another ion when they dissolve in water. This is a negative ion made up of the set of atoms remaining after the acid has lost the particle H^+.

Hydronium Ions, the Essence of Acidity. All the behaviour that is meant when we use the term 'acid' to describe aqueous mixtures is due to the presence of $H_3O^+_{aq}$ ions in the mixture. This particle is the essence of acidity. It will cause the solution to have a characteristic set of properties which include the following:

sour taste
turns blue litmus red
neutralises bases
dissolves metals, causing the production of hydrogen

All these properties, and many others which acids display, are properties of the hydronium ion.

7.7.2 *Strong and Weak Acids*

While it is true that all acids behave similarly in many respects, there are also ways in which they behave quite differently from each other. Most of us have, on numerous occasions, taken some vinegar, sprinkled it on some fish and chips and then eaten the lot thinking that it was a tasty dish. Now, vinegar is a 1–2 mol/l solution of acetic acid in water. If a person did this using a 1–2 mol/l solution of another acid, sulphuric acid, they would not find the meal anywhere near so pleasant in taste and it is quite likely that this acid would cause some damage to the tissues of their mouth and oesophagus.

There are a number of factors responsible for this difference between the effects caused by acetic acid and sulphuric acid when each is consumed as a mixture with water. One of these is that the two acids differ in the extent to which they react with water and produce hydronium ions. Concentrated sulphuric acid reacts completely with water and the only particles present in the solution in significant numbers are $H_3O^+_{aq}$ and HSO^-_{4aq} (hydrogensulphate ion, sometimes called bisulphate). Virtually no unchanged sulphuric acid molecules are present in the solution. Sulphuric acid is referred to as being a **strong acid** because of its complete conversion to hydronium ions. Two other common strong acids are hydrochloric acid (HCl) and nitric acid (HNO_3).

Acetic acid reacts only partially with water and most of the dissolved acid is present in the solution as unchanged acetic acid molecules. Only a small proportion of these molecules react with water to form hydronium ions, and acids which behave this way are called **weak acids**. Some common, weak acids other than acetic acid are carbonic acid, citric acid and lactic acid.

Equations for the reactions of sulphuric acid and acetic acid with water have been rewritten below using the two arrow convention (see Section 3.6) to indicate that each acid reacts to quite a different extent and produces quite a different proportion of hydronium ions.

$$\underset{\text{sulphuric acid}}{H_2SO_4} + H_2O \;\underset{\leftarrow}{\longrightarrow}\; \underset{\text{hydronium ion}}{H_3O^+_{aq}} + \underset{\text{hydrogen-sulphate ion}}{HSO^-_{4aq}}$$

$$\underset{\text{acetic acid}}{CH_3CO_2H} + H_2O \;\underset{\rightarrow}{\longleftarrow}\; \underset{\text{hydronium ion}}{H_3O^+_{aq}} + \underset{\text{acetate ion}}{CH_3CO^-_{2aq}}$$

Whenever the same quantities of strong and weak acid are dissolved in water the solution of the strong acid will always contain a higher concentration of hydronium ions than the weak acid solution. It is the hydronium ion which is the essence of acidity and as its concentration in a solution increases, the typical acid properties of the solution, such as its sour taste and corrosiveness, become more pronounced.

Vinegar gives a meal of fish and chips a pleasant taste when sprinkled on it. The weak acid (acetic acid) present in vinegar forms just enough hydronium ions to produce a pleasant tang when the food is consumed, and nowhere near enough to cause any damage to tissues in the gastrointestinal tract. In a solution containing the same quantity of sulphuric acid the concentration of hydronium ions is much higher, producing a taste which is most unpleasant and a corrosiveness which is damaging to tissue.

This discussion of acids and their strength may be summarised as follows: *an acid is a substance which, when mixed with water, reacts with the water to produce hydronium ions. A strong acid is one which reacts completely with the water and produces a high proportion of hydronium ions. A weak acid is one which reacts only partially with the water and produces a low proportion of hydronium ions.*

7.7.3 *Bases (Alkalis)*

We shall take the two terms 'base' and 'alkali' to mean the same thing but generally use base rather than alkali. A base is a compound which, when added to water, produces **hydroxide ions, OH^-_{aq}**, in solution. The solution also contains some positive ion derived from the base. Two examples of the interaction of a base with water are presented below.

Just as there are strong acids and weak acids there are also strong bases and weak bases, a strong base being one which is completely converted to hydroxide ions when it dissolves in water and a weak base being one which is only partially converted to hydroxide ions. Of the two examples of bases given below sodium hydroxide is strong and ammonia is weak.

$$\underset{\text{sodium hydroxide}}{NaOH} + \text{water} \rightleftarrows \underset{\text{hydroxide ion}}{OH^-_{aq}} + \underset{\text{sodium ion}}{Na^+_{aq}}$$

$$\underset{\text{ammonia}}{NH_3} + \text{water} \leftrightarrows \underset{\text{hydroxide ion}}{OH^-_{aq}} + \underset{\text{ammonium ion}}{NH^+_{4aq}}$$

Just as all acid solutions have a set of properties in common so do all basic solutions and this set of properties includes:

slippery feel
turns red litmus blue
neutralises acids
dissolves fatty (lipid) material

These properties are all due to the presence in basic solutions of the hydroxide ion and so, just as the hydronium ion is regarded as the essence of acidity, so the hydroxide ion is the essence of basicity (alkalinity).

Strong bases are capable of causing severe damage to tissue due to the ability of the hydroxide ion to dissolve fatty material. The membranes of all the body's cells contain a very high proportion of fat and these membranes are quickly destroyed by contact with solutions of strong bases.

The ability of the hydroxide ion to dissolve fat also explains why sodium hydroxide is a common ingredient in the commercial preparations sold as oven cleaners. Ovens are difficult to clean because of the build-up of fat deposits. These are hard to move with just soap or detergent. The sodium hydroxide in the oven cleaning preparation ensures that it contains a high enough concentration of hydroxide ions to dissolve the fat and so facilitate its removal from the oven.

Oven cleaning preparations are hazardous because they are often sold in the form of a spray and it is quite easy for a person accidentally to spray the material in their own, or someone else's, eyes. This is very dangerous because the eyeball is coated with a film of fatty material which, as well as acting as a lubricant, acts as a barrier between the outer tissues of the eyeball and physical agents such as dust. This fatty material also provides some protection against corrosive liquids or gases which make contact with the eye. However, the protection is not effective against strong bases because they quickly strip the layer of fatty material away. This brings the strong base into direct contact with the underlying tissue which may then be extensively damaged.

7.7.4 *Concentrated and Dilute Solutions of Acids and Bases*

It is important to distinguish between the strengths of acids or bases and their concentrations. When we say that sulphuric acid is a strong acid we are referring to an intrinsic property of the pure substance, this property being its ability to react completely with water and form a high proportion of hydronium ions. No matter how much sulphuric acid is added to water nearly all of it is converted from molecules (H_2SO_4) into ions ($H_3O^+_{aq}$ and HSO^-_{4aq}).

When we say that a sulphuric acid solution is concentrated we mean that it contains a large amount of sulphuric acid and, because all this acid will have formed hydronium ions, we can be sure that their concentration in the solution will be high. However, we may choose to make a sulphuric acid solution by adding only a small quantity to water. This solution would be referred to as a dilute solution or a solution of low concentration. All the sulphuric acid molecules added to the water will have changed into the ions $H_3O^+_{aq}$ and HSO^-_{4aq} but, since there were relatively few sulphuric acid molecules to begin with, relatively few $H_3O^+_{aq}$ ions will be present in the solution.

Concentration has a big effect on the behaviour of acid solutions. As the concentration of any strong acid declines its acidic properties become less pronounced and a sufficiently dilute solution of sulphuric acid would be quite mild in its taste and have little effect on tissue. The properties of strong bases also become less pronounced as their solutions are made more dilute.

Solutions of weak acids and weak bases may be highly concentrated and this would mean that a large quantity of the acid or base had been dissolved in water. However, a concentrated solution of a weak acid would not contain a high concentration of $H_3O^+_{aq}$ ions because only a small proportion of the weak acid molecules would have reacted with the water and changed into this form. A dilute solution of a weak acid would, of course, contain even fewer $H_3O^+_{aq}$ ions. In the same way, concentrated solutions of weak bases contain relatively few OH^-_{aq} ions and dilute solutions contain even less.

To summarise, we may say that the terms strong and weak,when used to describe acids or bases, refer to the extent to which the acid or base reacts with water and forms $H_3O^+_{aq}$ and OH^-_{aq} ions respectively. The terms concentrated and dilute refer to the quantity of the acid or base that has been dissolved in water.

7.7.5 *Toxicity of Weak Acids and Weak Bases*

Concentrated solutions of all strong acids and strong bases are hazardous because they contain high concentrations of $H_3O^+_{aq}$ and OH^-_{aq} ions respectively. Weak acids or bases, even when concentrated, do not produce such high concentrations of these ions and so are generally less hazardous on this account. They may, however, be hazardous due to the poisonous nature of the acid or base itself, or of the ions which they form when they dissolve in water. One example of a toxic weak acid is hydrogen cyanide, HCN, which is a gas that dissolves in water to form a solution called hydrocyanic acid. This solution contains the very toxic ion, CN^-_{aq}, called the **cyanide ion**.

$$\underset{\text{hydrogen cyanide}}{HCN} + H_2O \rightleftharpoons H_3O^+_{aq} + \underset{\text{cyanide ion}}{CN^-_{aq}}$$

Cyanides are notorious poisons and hydrogen cyanide is the gas which has been used many times in the United States as the means of executing people in the gas chamber. The fatal dose of cyanide is about 50–60 mg and death occurs very quickly.

In spite of their toxicity cyanides are widely used. Sodium cyanide (NaCN) is used to extract gold and silver from their ores, and in electroplating. Hydrogen cyanide is sometimes used as a fumigant to kill rats, mice and insects in the holds of ships and in grain storage structures such as warehouses and silos.

Another highly toxic weak acid is **fluoroacetic acid** (CH_2FCO_2H). In solution it produces the fluoroacetate ion which, in the form of sodium fluoroacetate (usually called **compound 1080**), has been used to kill animal pests such as foxes and rabbits. To do this the poison must be laid in open country and so it presents a risk to other animals and to humans. This has made its use controversial and unpopular.

An example of a weak base which is toxic is strychnine. It is used to kill rats and has been used many times as an instrument of murder.

7.7.6 *$H_3O^+_{aq}$ and OH^-_{aq}; You Can't Have One Without the Other*

The discussion so far about acids and bases may have created the impression in your mind that solutions of acids contain hydronium ions, but not hydroxide ions while solutions of bases contain hydroxide ions, but not hydronium ions. This is not quite true and all aqueous solutions always contain both types of ion. They form as a result of collisions between water molecules because, in a small proportion of cases, the water molecules collide in just the right orientation, and with sufficient force, to cause a molecule to break apart, forming one hydronium ion and one hydroxide ion. This is known as self-ionisation and the process may be represented as:

$$H_2O + H_2O \rightleftharpoons H_3O^+_{aq} + OH^-_{aq}$$

It is important to emphasise that, in pure water at any instant, there is only a very small proportion of water molecules which have undergone self-ionisation. At a temperature of 25 °C, the proportion is one in about five hundred million and the concentration of each ion is 10^{-7} mol/l. Because of this very low concentration pure water is a poor conductor of electricity even though there are some ions present within it.

Another important point to emphasise is that in pure water the concentrations of hydronium and hydroxide ions are exactly equal. This must be the case because in pure water these ions can only form from water molecules (there are no other particles present) and every time that water molecules undergo self-ionisation one hydronium ion and one hydroxide ion forms.

Although pure water contains hydronium ions, which are the essence of acidity, we cannot say that it is an acidic solution because it also contains an equal concentration of hydroxide ions which are the essence of basicity. Instead we say that pure water is neutral: neither acidic nor basic.

When an acid is added to water it produces hydronium ions in addition to those which have formed by the self-ionisation of water. This ensures that there are more hydronium ions than hydroxide ions present. It is this excess of hydronium ions over hydroxide ions, rather than a complete absence of hydroxide ions, which is responsible for the solution behaving as an acid. Likewise, a basic solution behaves as it does because it contains an excess of hydroxide ions over hydronium ions.

7.7.7 *The Measurement of Acidity, pH*

The concentration of hydronium ions in a solution is often an important factor in determining the effects which the solution produces and this is particularly true of the aqueous solutions found inside the human body. For example, the concentration of hydronium ions in the blood of a healthy person lies in the range 3.6–4.5 × 10^{-8} mol/l. If it should double or halve, and remain at that level for long, then the life of the person affected would be in danger.

For many commonly encountered solutions the concentration of hydronium ions present is very small and awkward to express. For this reason, and others, hydronium ion concentration is usually expressed as a logarithm. The common way of doing this is by means of the term 'pH' which is defined as 'minus the logarithm of the hydronium ion concentration expressed in mol/l'. Thus,

$$pH = -\log[H_3O^+_{aq}]$$

The normal range of hydronium ion concentration in the blood becomes 7.35–7.45 when expressed as pH values and these numbers are much easier to deal with than the unaltered concentration range of 3.6–4.5 × 10^{-8} mol/l. However, there is one point of confusion which can easily arise in the use of this logarithmic method for expressing concentration. As the concentration increases the logarithm term decreases in its value. Thus, low pH values correspond to solutions which contain high concentrations of hydronium ion.

The concentration of hydroxide ions may also be expressed as a logarithmic term and we then have:

$$pOH = -\log[OH^-_{aq}]$$

In the preceding section it was explained that all aqueous solutions contain both hydronium and hydroxide ions. It turns out that there is even a strict numerical relationship between the concentrations of the two ions. In particular, when the temperature is 25 °C and the concentrations are expressed in logarithm form as pH and pOH, the relationship is:

$$pH + pOH = 14$$

When concentrations are expressed simply as moles per litre this relationship becomes:

$$[H_3O^+_{aq}] \times [OH^-_{aq}] = 10^{-14}$$

In Table 7.2 the concentrations of hydronium and hydroxide ions present in solutions having pH values in the range 0–14 are presented together with the corresponding values for pOH. It is possible to have pH values outside the range 0–14 but such solutions are not encountered in human biology and so we shall not be concerned with them.

Table 7.2 *Concentrations of hydronium and hydroxide ion in solutions of different pH*

pH	$[H_3O^+_{aq}]$	pOH	$[OH^-_{aq}]$
0	1	14	10^{-14}
1	10^{-1}	13	10^{-13}
2	10^{-2}	12	10^{-12}
3	10^{-3}	11	10^{-11}
4	10^{-4}	10	10^{-10}
5	10^{-5}	9	10^{-9}
6	10^{-6}	8	10^{-8}
7	10^{-7}	7	10^{-7}
8	19^{-8}	6	10^{-6}
9	10^{-9}	5	10^{-5}
10	10^{-10}	4	10^{-4}
11	10^{-11}	3	10^{-3}
12	10^{-12}	2	10^{-2}
13	10^{-13}	1	10^{-1}
14	10^{-14}	0	1

The data in Table 7.2 show that as the concentration of either one of the ions $H_3O^+_{aq}$ or OH^-_{aq} increases the concentration of the other decreases. The reason for this can be seen by thinking carefully about the self-ionisation of water. Here is the equation for that process written out again.

$$H_2O + H_2O \rightleftarrows H_3O^+_{aq} + OH^-_{aq}$$

If we read this equation from right to left it tells us that the tendency of hydronium ions to react with hydroxide ions and form water is much greater than the tendency of water molecules to break apart and form these ions. The tendency is, in fact, about five hundred million times greater. This is not too surprising because the ions are oppositely charged and so will attract each other. Let us now imagine a situation in which one of the two ions, say, hydronium ions, undergoes an increase in its concentration (an acid must have been added to the solution). The chance now of any particular hydroxide ion colliding with a hydronium ion and forming water must increase. Hydroxide ions will be destroyed at a greater rate and so their concentration must decrease.

7.7.8 *pH of Body Fluids*

The pH of a body fluid is usually one of its most important properties. The normal pH ranges for several body fluids are presented in Table 7.3.

Table 7.3 *Normal pH ranges for body fluids*

Body fluid	Normal pH range
gastric juice	1.6–1.8
saliva	6.2–7.4
urine	5.5–7.0
blood	7.35–7.45
bile	7.8–8.6

Gastric juice is the solution found in the stomach. It is secreted into the stomach from cells of the stomach wall and the rate of secretion is about 2–3 l per day. It contains hydrochloric acid at a concentration of about 0.5% (w/v) which, although low, is sufficient to produce a pH of less than 2 and make gastric juice the most acidic of all body fluids.

Most tissues of the body would suffer severe damage if they were maintained in close contact with gastric juice for an extended period. This does not normally happen to tissues of the stomach wall because it is coated with a layer of mucus and this prevents direct contact between gastric juice and tissue. However, if this layer of mucus is incomplete and gastric juice is able to achieve close and prolonged contact with a section of the oesophagus, stomach or duodenum then tissue damage does occur. This damage is in the form of gastric ulcers which may be described as crater-like holes in the mucus membrane which lines the inner wall of the gastrointestinal tract.

The low pH of gastric juice is essential for the proper digestion of food and it also destroys most bacteria which enter the stomach. Some diseases cause a reduction in the amount of acid which is secreted in gastric juice and a corresponding rise in its pH beyond the upper end of the normal range. This is known as **hypochlorhydria** (less than the normal amount of hydrochloric acid) and it is a condition commonly associated with stomach cancer. In other situations the amount of acid secreted in gastric juice may be increased, causing its pH to fall below the bottom end of the normal range. This condition is called **hyperchlorhydria** and it may be the cause, and indicate the presence, of gastric ulcers or inflammation of the stomach wall. A physician's diagnosis of gastric disease will often involve measurement of the pH of gastric juice which can be obtained by inserting a hollow tube into the stomach and withdrawing the sample by suction.

The normal range for the pH of blood is very narrow in comparison to other body solutions. The consequences of a large rise or fall in the pH of blood are also much more serious and changes larger than about 0.2 are life threatening if they are maintained for an extended period.

The body solution which has a pH subject to the greatest variation is urine. This corresponds to the fact that urine is the means by which the body rids itself of many unwanted substances. Whenever there is an excess of any substance in the body its concentration in urine is likely to increase as the body disposes of it by this route. This applies to excessive amounts of acidic or basic substances and this is why the pH of urine is so variable.

The fact that urine is stored in the bladder where it is out of contact with other body solutions and out of contact with sensitive tissues means that short-term variations in its pH are of much less significance than similar variations in the pH of other body solutions. However, this is not to say that a large variation in urine pH can be ignored. Where such a variation is detected it should be investigated further to rule out the possibility that it is due to some important problem with body function.

The measurement of urine pH is routinely performed by nurses using test strips. These strips are supplied in bottles and the measurement is made by dipping one of the strips into a urine sample and comparing the colour produced on the strip with a colour key which is provided on the bottle. The strip changes colour according to the pH of the urine into which it has been dipped, and this is due to the presence on the strip of chemical compounds which change colour as the pH changes. These compounds are called chemical indicators and two which are frequently used in commercial test strips are methyl red and bromthymol blue. They permit measurements of urine pH in the range 4.5–8.5 which covers most urine specimens.

7.8 Neutralisation and the Formation of Salts

When an acid is mixed with a base a reaction known as **neutralisation** occurs. In this reaction the acid and base destroy each other, forming water and an ionic compound which is usually referred to as a **salt**. The identity of the salt formed depends on which particular acid and base are involved in the neutralisation and sometimes on the relative amounts that are used. However, water is always formed in a neutralisation reaction no matter which acid or base is used.

Neutralisation of a Strong Acid by a Strong Base. With this combination, neutralisation is a reaction between the hydronium ions of the strong acid and the hydroxide ions of the strong base. Thus:

$$H_3O^+_{aq} + OH^-_{aq} \rightleftharpoons 2H_2O$$

The strong acid solution contains a negative ion in addition to the hydronium ion and the strong base solution contains a positive ion in addition to the hydroxide ion. These additional ions remain in the solution after neutralisation has occurred and together they make up the salt which is the other product of neutralisation. If the strong acid used was hydrochloric acid and the strong base was sodium hydroxide then the salt formed would be sodium chloride.

Salts, being ionic compounds, are usually soluble in water. However, any soluble salt can be obtained in pure form by evaporating the water in which it is dissolved until its concentration exceeds its solubility, at which point it will crystallise from the solution.

Neutralisation of a Weak Acid by a Strong Base. In a solution of a weak acid most of the weak acid is in the form of unchanged acid molecules and there are relatively few hydronium ions present. The neutralisation reaction which occurs between a weak acid and a strong base is a reaction between the hydroxide ions of the strong base and unchanged acid molecules. Using acetic acid as an example of a weak acid this neutralisation reaction can be written as:

$$\underset{\text{acetic acid}}{CH_3CO_2H} + OH^-_{aq} \rightleftharpoons \underset{\text{acetate ion}}{CH_3CO^-_{2aq}} + H_2O$$

You can see that water is once again a product of the neutralisation process. The identity of the salt formed depends on which strong base is used for the neutralisation. If it was sodium hydroxide then the salt would be sodium acetate. If it was potassium hydroxide then the salt would be potassium acetate.

Notice also that the arrow pointing from right to left in the equation is longer than it is in the equation for the neutralisation of a strong acid by a strong base. This shows that acetate ions have a significant tendency to react with water, forming hydroxide ions and acetic acid. In other words acetate ions are weakly basic.

Neutralisation of a Weak Base by a Strong Acid. With this combination of acid and base the neutralisation reaction is between hydronium ions of the strong acid and unchanged molecules of the weak base. Using ammonia as an example this neutralisation reaction can be written as:

$$\underset{\text{ammonia}}{NH_3} + H_3O^+_{aq} \rightleftharpoons \underset{\text{ammonium ion}}{NH^+_{4aq}} + H_2O$$

If the strong acid used was hydrochloric acid then the salt formed would be ammonium chloride and if nitric acid was used it would be ammonium nitrate. Notice that the arrow going from right to left in the equation shows that ammonium ions have a significant ability to react with water molecules and form hydronium ions. In other words, the ammonium ion is weakly acidic.

7.9 The Acid–Base Nature of Salts

In Table 7.4 the pH values for solutions containing 0.1 mol/l of several different salts are presented together with some details of the acid and base from which each salt may be obtained by neutralisation.

You can see from the pH values in Table 7.4 that some salts are neutral, some are acidic and some are basic. Now look at the details of the acid and base from which each salt may be obtained by neutralisation. You should notice that the neutral salts in the table are formed from a strong acid and a strong base, the acidic salts from a strong acid and a weak base and the basic salts from a strong base and a weak acid. This pattern is observed with many other salts and it may be accounted for as follows:

1. In the process of neutralisation an acid and a base react with each other in a way which destroys the acid or base nature of each.
2. Neutralisation can be viewed as a contest of strength between the acid and the base and, like all contests of strength, it will have an outcome which can be predicted from a knowledge of the strength of the participants.
3. Neutralisation of a strong acid by a strong base is a contest between equals and so there will be no winner. The salt which is the product of this contest will be neither acidic nor basic. It will be a neutral salt.
4. When a strong acid neutralises a weak base the contest is unequal in favour of the acid which will therefore be the winner. The salt formed will have an acidic nature to reflect this outcome.
5. When a strong base neutralises a weak acid the contest is won by the base and the salt formed is basic.

The acid–base nature of salts may be summarised as follows:

strong acid + strong base ⟶ neutral salt
strong acid + weak base ⟶ acidic salt

Table 7.4 *pH values of 0.1 mol/l solutions of various salts*

Salt	Corresponding acid (strength)	Corresponding base (strength)	pH of 0.1 mol/l solution
potassium acetate	acetic acid (weak)	potassium hydroxide (strong)	8.9
sodium bicarbonate	carbonic acid (weak)	sodium hydroxide (strong)	11.2
ammonium nitrate	nitric acid (strong)	ammonia (weak)	5.2
sodium nitrate	nitric acid (strong)	sodium hydroxide (strong)	7.0
potassium chloride	hydrochloric acid (strong)	potassium hydroxide (strong)	7.0

weak acid + strong base ⟶ basic salt

The fact that weak acids and weak bases form salts which are themselves weakly basic and weakly acidic respectively is very important in the action of chemical systems used to control the pH of aqueous solutions. These chemical systems are known as buffer systems and they are responsible for keeping the pH of blood within the narrow limits 7.35–7.45.

7.10 Buffer Systems and the Control of pH

The pH of a solution is a property which often influences the course of chemical reactions taking place in the solution. This is particularly true of the chemical reactions which take place inside living things. Let us suppose that there is some reaction which we wish to carry out and it requires a solution of pH 4 in order for it to proceed successfully. One way for us to arrange for a solution to have a pH of 4 would be to take some water and add just enough hydrochloric acid to lower the pH to 4.

Another way for us to arrange for the solution to have a pH of 4 would be to add some acetic acid and sodium acetate to water. The acetic acid, being an acid, will tend to make the pH of the solution fall. The sodium acetate, being the salt of a weak acid, is a basic salt and will tend to make the pH of the solution rise. Of course, the solution can only have a single pH value and this value will be determined by the relative amounts of acetic acid and sodium acetate which are present. As the proportion of acetic acid increases the pH will be lower and as the proportion of sodium acetate increases the pH will be higher. It turns out that, for the case of acetic acid and sodium acetate, a pH of 4 is obtained when they are present in the solution in the ratio acetic acid : sodium acetate = 6 : 1. With different ratios different pH values are obtained. This is shown in Table 7.5 and you will notice that as the ratio changes by a factor of 10 the pH of the solution changes by only 1.

Table 7.5 *The effect of changing the ratio of a solution's components on its pH*

Acetic acid : Sodium acetate	Solution pH
100 : 1	2.8
50 : 1	3.1
25 : 1	3.4
10 : 1	3.8
5 : 1	4.1
1 : 1	4.8
1 : 10	5.8
1 : 100	6.8

An important point to make here is that, with this type of solution, it does not matter what the actual concentrations of the solution components are; it is only the ratio of the concentrations that is important in determining the pH. Thus a pH of 4 will be obtained if the two concentrations are acetic acid = 0.06 mol/l and sodium acetate = 0.01 mol/l. If the concentrations are both ten times as great (acetic acid = 0.6 mol/l and sodium acetate = 0.1 mol/l) then the pH will still be 4 because the ratio of the concentrations will still be the same.

If we were dealing with a chemical reaction which required a pH of 9 we could also arrange to obtain this pH in two different ways. Some sodium hydroxide could be added to water, or a mixture of the weak base, ammonia, and its salt, ammonium chloride, could be added in the ratio ammonia : ammonium chloride = 3 : 2 (this is the ratio of these two substances which gives a pH of 9).

If the reactions in which we are interested proceed without producing any additional acid or base, and if no acid or base enters the system in some other way, then it would not matter how we arranged for the pH of the original solution to be at the required value. However, many reactions do produce acids or bases as they proceed and in the human body there are frequent occasions when acidic or basic substances are eaten. These substances are absorbed from the gastrointestinal tract into the blood stream where they may affect the pH of the blood and other solutions in the body. In these situations the way in which the pH of the reaction system has been established makes a great deal of difference. This is shown clearly in Table 7.6, which sets out the changes in pH undergone by several different aqueous solutions when each has a fixed amount of strong base or strong acid solution added to it.

Table 7.6 *The effect of the addition of a fixed quantity of strong acid or strong base on the pH of several different aqueous solutions*

	Substances present in solution[1]			
	HCl	CH_3CO_2H and $NaCH_3CO_2$	NaOH	NH_3 and NH_4Cl
original pH	4	4	10	10
pH after addition of acid[2]	3	3.9	3.1	9.9
pH after addition of base[3]	10.9	4.1	11	10.1

Notes:
1. HCl is the strong acid, hydrochloric acid; NaOH is the strong base, sodium hydroxide; CH_3CO_2H is the weak acid, acetic acid and $NaCH_3CO_2$ is one of its salts, sodium acetate; NH_3 is the weak base, ammonia, and NH_4Cl is one of its salts, ammonium chloride.
2. 10 ml of 0.01 mol/l of the strong acid, nitric acid (HNO_3), is added to 100 ml of solution.
3. 10 ml of 0.01 mol/l of the strong base, potassium hydroxide (KOH) is added to 100 ml of solution.

The acetic acid/sodium acetate and ammonia/ammonium chloride solutions are only slightly affected by the addition of acid or base while both of the other two solutions undergo very large changes when the same amounts of acid or base are added to them. The acetic acid/sodium acetate and ammonia/ammonium chloride solutions are examples of **buffer solutions**. They are given this name because the term 'buffer' means some arrangement for deadening an impact and a buffer solution can be considered to 'deaden the impact' on pH of the addition of acid or base to a solution. There are many buffer systems besides the two which we have considered and any solution which contains significant quantities of a weak acid or base and a corresponding salt will act as a buffer solution.

Whenever a chemical reaction requires the pH of the solution in which it is occurring to remain constant its chances of success will be greatly improved if it occurs in a buffer solution having the appropriate pH. Many of the chemical reactions taking place in solution inside the body require the pH of the solution to remain constant and this is achieved through the presence in those solutions of buffer systems. These buffer systems are discussed in Chapter 9, 'Aqueous Solutions in the Body'.

The main characteristics of a buffer solution may be summarised as follows:

1. It resists a change in pH when either acid or base is added to it.
2. It contains significant concentrations of either a weak acid and one of its salts or a weak base and one of its salts.
3. It has a pH which is determined by the ratio of the concentrations of its two components.
4. In order for the pH of a buffer solution to change by 1 the ratio of the concentrations of its two components must change by a factor of 10.

7.10.1 *Explaining the Action of Buffer Solutions*

Buffer solutions are able to resist a change in pH when either acid or base is added to them because they contain two components and one of these is always capable of destroying hydronium ions while the other is capable of destroying hydroxide ions. Let us consider the addition of strong acid and strong base to the acetic acid/sodium acetate buffer system as an example.

Addition of Strong Acid. This will introduce extra hydronium ions into the solution but these are prevented from causing a large fall in pH because most of them react with the acetate ions present in the buffer and are destroyed.

$$H_3O^+_{aq} + CH_3CO^-_{2aq} \rightleftarrows H_2O + CH_3CO_2H$$

hydronium ion from the added acid	acetate ion present in the buffer	acetic acid

It is very important to realise that the destruction of hydronium ions by this reaction inevitably causes a change in the buffer system: some of its acetate ions are changed into acetic acid molecules and so the ratio of the two buffer components is altered. Since the buffer pH depends on this ratio the ratio must change as well. However, the ratio must change by a factor of 10 in order for the pH to change by 1 and so only a relatively small change occurs.

Addition of Strong Base. This introduces extra hydroxide ions into the solution but they are prevented from causing a significant increase in pH because most of them are destroyed by reaction with the acetic acid component of the buffer.

$$OH^-_{aq} + CH_3CO_2H \rightleftarrows H_2O + CH_3CO^-_{2aq}$$

hydroxide ion from the added base	acetic acid present in the buffer	acetate ion

This destruction of hydroxide ions also causes a change in the ratio of the buffer components but this time the change is in the opposite direction because acetic acid molecules have been changed into acetate ions. Now the pH rises, but by a relatively small amount because a tenfold increase is still required in order to change the pH by 1.

7.10.2 *The Capacity of Buffer Solutions*

It is very easy to form the impression that buffer solutions are completely immune to changes in their pH as acid or base is added to them. This is a false impression and any buffer solution will undergo a large change in its pH if a sufficiently large quantity of acid or base is added to it. If enough is added to change the ratio of buffer components by a factor of 10 then the pH will change by 1; if enough is added to change the ratio by a factor of 100 then the pH will change by 2 and so on.

Just how much acid or base is needed to change the pH of a buffer solution by a given amount depends on the actual concentrations of the components of the buffer system. Let us consider two acetic acid/sodium acetate buffer solutions both of which have a pH of 4 to start with and both of which then have 0.01 mol of strong acid added to them.

Buffer Solution A. This is 1 l of solution which contains 0.12 mol of acetic acid and 0.02 mol of sodium acetate. We added 0.01 mol of strong acid to the buffer and this would produce 0.01 mol of hydronium ion.

If we assume that all of the 0.01 mol of hydronium ion added to the buffer is destroyed by reaction with the sodium acetate component of the buffer then, because the destruction of each hydronium ion uses up one acetate ion and produces one acetic acid molecule, we may say that, after addition of the acid, the buffer contains 0.02 – 0.01 = 0.01 mol of acetate and 0.12 + 0.01 = 0.13 mol of acetic acid. This is a change in the ratio of the buffer components from 6 : 1 to 13 : 1. In Figure 7.7 some of the data in Table 7.5 have been used to draw a graph which displays the relationship between the pH of an acetic acid/sodium acetate buffer solution and the ratio of its components. The graph shows that when the ratio changes from acetic acid : sodium acetate = 6 : 1 to 13 : 1, the pH changes from 4.0 to 3.7.

Buffer Solution B. This is 1 l of solution which contains 1.2 mol of acetic acid and 0.2 mol of sodium acetate. After addition of 0.01 mol of strong acid the amount of acetate present will be 0.19 mol and the amount of acetic acid will be 1.21 mol. The change in ratio that has occurred is much smaller than that which occurred in the other buffer solution. The new ratio is 1.21 : 0.19 which equals 6.4 : 1 and now the graph in Figure 7.7 tells us that the new pH is 3.99.

This shows clearly that the greater the concentrations of the components of a buffer solution the greater will be its resistance to a change in pH.

7.10.3 *The Dilution of Buffer Solutions*

If a hydrochloric acid solution having a pH of 4 is diluted by a factor of 10 its pH would increase to 5.

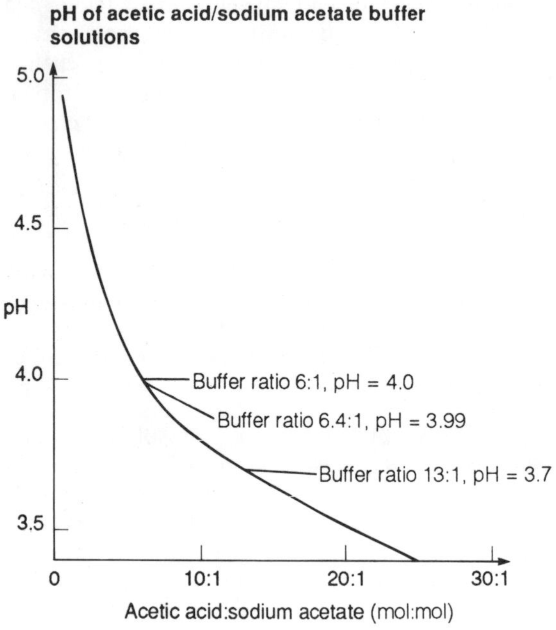

Figure 7.7 *Relationship between the ratio of acetic acid and sodium acetate in a buffer solution and its pH*

The same dilution of a sodium hydroxide solution of pH 10 would see its pH change to 9. However, dilution of any buffer solution will have virtually no effect on its pH. The reason for this is that the pH of the buffer solution is determined by the ratio of the concentrations of its components. When a buffer is diluted the concentration of each component decreases by the same factor, leaving the ratio unchanged and the pH unchanged.

The hydrochloric acid and sodium hydroxide solutions have pH values which depend on the concentration of only one substance in the solution. Dilution reduces the concentration of this one substance and leads to a change in the pH.

7.11 Clinical Uses for Acids, Bases and Salts

7.11.1 *Acids*

Hydrochloric Acid. This acid is administered to people who are suffering from hypochlorhydria. The hydrochloric acid solution used for this purpose is obtained by diluting concentrated hydrochloric acid which has a concentration of about 36% (w/v). The diluted solution has a concentration of about 10% (w/v) and approximately 5 ml is diluted further with water and given as a drink. Thus the concentration of the solution which is drunk is less than 1%. Even so it is sipped through a glass tube to minimise contact with the enamel of the teeth which may otherwise be damaged by the acid.

Sometimes hydrochloric acid solution is introduced directly into the gastrointestinal tract through a tube and in this circumstance it is particularly important that it should be of the correct concentration. A person drinking hydrochloric acid is not likely to drink much of a solution which is so concentrated as to be dangerous because its taste would be intolerable. However, if the solution is being introduced directly into the gastrointestinal tract through a tube then a considerable quantity may enter before the inevitable damage is noticed. A few years ago in South Australia a person died after a solution of hydrochloric acid which had not been sufficiently diluted was administered to him in this way.

Boric Acid (H_3BO_3). This is a weak acid which is a mild germicide. A 1% (w/w) mixture of boric acid with paraffin is used as an ointment. Boric acid is also present in a preparation known as 'Prantal Powder' which is used to control excessive sweating. It is used on the stumps of amputated limbs to control the sweating that can be caused when an artificial limb is fitted.

Boric acid is quite toxic if taken internally and its use is restricted to situations where it is applied to external body surfaces or retained in the mouth for a relatively short period. If it is used as a mouth wash over an extended period symptoms of poisoning may occur if a person regularly swallows significant amounts of the preparation.

Acetylsalicylic Acid (Aspirin). This is a weak acid which is used as a mild analgesic (pain reliever) and anti-pyretic (fever reducer). In recent years some evidence has been obtained which indicates that aspirin, taken regularly in small doses (100 mg/day), reduces the risk of stroke and heart attack. Large doses of aspirin have an anti-inflammatory action and this can be useful in the treatment of arthritic conditions.

7.11.2 *Bases*

Ammonia (NH_3). This substance, which is a gas and a weak base, is responsible for the action of smelling salts. These preparations contain ammonium salts which, on exposure to the air, react with the water vapour contained in it to form ammonia. When inhaled ammonia stimulates respiration.

Magnesium Hydroxide [$Mg(OH)_2$]. This compound is used as an antacid to neutralise excess acid in the stomach. Its solubility in water is low and so there is very little risk of it being absorbed into the circulation where it might upset the body's acid–base balance. Magnesium hydroxide is also used as a laxative. The normal form in which it is administered is as a mechanical suspension in water.

7.11.3 *Salts*

Barium Sulphate ($BaSO_4$). This salt is insoluble in water and opaque to X-rays. It is the main component of the 'barium meal' given prior to X-ray examination of the gastrointestinal tract. After it has been swallowed barium sulphate is not absorbed from the gastro-intestinal tract because of its very low solubility in water. It lines the gastrointestinal tract and when the X-ray is taken its opaqueness ensures that a clear outline of the tract can be seen. A barium sulphate preparation may also be introduced into the body as an enema to obtain clear X-ray images of the lower parts of the gastrointestinal tract.

Morphine Sulphate. Morphine is a weak base which occurs naturally as a component of the juice of the opium poppy. Extracts from this plant have been used for thousands of years to relieve pain and to treat the symptoms of many diseases. In 1803, Friedrich Serturner isolated the pure substance morphine from opium and showed that it had many of the useful therapeutic properties of the crude plant extract. Today morphine is still one of the best agents available for the relief of severe pain such as that experienced by people suffering from terminal cancer.

Morphine is usually administered in the form of a salt such as morphine sulphate. This salt may be formed by neutralising morphine with sulphuric acid. In salt form morphine is more stable and more soluble in water than its base form. The greater solubility in water allows the salt to be easily administered by injection. This is a better route of administration than ingestion because a much smaller dose may be used and the desired therapeutic effects of the drug are achieved more quickly. Another commonly used salt of morphine is morphine hydrochloride. It is often administered as a syrup.

Bibliography

Hoover, J. E. (ed.). *Remington's Pharmaceutical Sciences* (fifth edition). Mack Publishing Company, Pennsylvania, 1975.

Thomas, J. (ed.). *Prescription Products Guide.* Australian Pharmaceutical Publishing Company, Melbourne, 1989.

Questions

1. A pure substance which is a solid at room temperature dissolves in water and produces a solution which conducts electricity. This substance must be
   J. an acid
   K. a base
   L. an electrolyte
   M. an ionic compound
2. Which of the following statements concerning specific gravity is *false*?
   J. It can be measured with a urinometer.
   K. It has no units.
   L. Its value for pure water is 0.000.
   M. It is closely related to density.
3. The body fluid having the lowest pH is
   J. blood
   K. gastric juice
   L. saliva
   M. urine
4. The body fluid which shows the greatest variation in its pH is
   J. blood
   K. gastric juice
   L. saliva
   M. urine
5. Consider the chemical equation

$$C_7H_6O_2 + H_2O \rightleftharpoons C_7H_5O^-_{2aq} + H_3O^+_{aq}$$

   This equation tells us that the substance of formula $C_7H_6O_2$ is a
   J. weak acid
   K. strong acid
   L. weak base
   M. strong base
6. Which of the following statements is true?
   J. Neutral solutions contain neither hydronium nor hydroxide ions.

K. Acidic solutions contain hydronium ions but not hydroxide ions.
L. Basic solutions contain hydroxide ions but not hydronium ions.
M. All aqueous solutions contain both hydronium ions and hydroxide ions.

7. Many drugs are neutralised to form salts and then administered in this form. The main advantage of this is that the salt is usually
J. more pleasant tasting
K. less toxic
L. more soluble in water
M. cheaper to produce

8. A weakly basic solution could have a pH of
J. 1.8
K. 6.8
L. 7.8
M. 13.8

9. A liquid has a pH of exactly 7. This means that the liquid
J. is pure water
K. contains equal numbers of hydronium and hydroxide ions
L. contains no hydronium ions or hydroxide ions
M. contains no ions of any sort

10. A buffer solution has a pH of 4.0 and a small quantity of strong acid is added to it. Which of the following is most likely to be the pH of the buffer solution after this addition?
J. 1.8
K. 3.9
L. 4.1
M. 6.6

11. Identify each of the following aqueous mixtures as being a mechanical suspension, colloidal suspension or solution.
(a) The mixture is unaffected by its passage through paper filters and biological membranes.
(b) The mixture, on standing undisturbed for a few hours, separates into two layers.
(c) The mixture passes through a paper filter unchanged and a light shone through it can be seen from the side.

12. (a) What is the concentration (% w/v) of the following solutions?
(i) 4 g dissolved in 150 ml of solution
(ii) 110 g dissolved in 2 l of solution
(b) What is the mass of solute present in
(i) 250 ml of 6% (w/v) solution
(ii) 5 ml of 15% (w/v) solution
(c) What volume of water must be added to the following solutions to change their concentrations to 5% (w/v)?
(i) 250 ml of 8% (w/v) solution
(ii) 75 ml of 15% (w/v) solution
(d) Normal saline solution is 0.9% (w/v) sodium chloride in water. Calculate the concentration of this solution in moles of sodium chloride per litre.

13. (a) State the relationship between density and specific gravity.
(b) A liquid has a specific gravity of 1.2. What is its density expressed in a metric unit?
(c) Why is specific gravity more commonly measured than density?

14. Write a paragraph which makes clear the meanings of each of the terms:
strong acid
weak acid
concentrated acid
dilute acid

15. List the following substances in increasing order of the pH of the solutions which each would form when added to water.
ammonia, nitric acid, sodium acetate, acetic acid, ammonium chloride

What assumption did you make in formulating your list?

16. A first-aid procedure often recommended for people who have swallowed strong acid or base is for them to drink a large volume of water. If acid is involved they should then drink some milk of magnesia [$Mg(OH)_2$] or limewater [$Ca(OH)_2$]. If base is involved they should drink fruit juice. What is the chemical basis of these procedures?

17. Equal amounts of each of two substances A and B are added to water. In the case of substance A the addition causes a change in the pH of the water from 7 to 1.4. In the case of substance B the addition causes a change in pH from 7 to 4.6. What does this indicate about the nature of the two substances A and B?

18. (a) An ammonia/ammonium chloride buffer solution has its two components present in the ratio ammonia : ammonium chloride = 6 : 1 and its pH is 8.5. Predict the pH the buffer would have if sufficient ammonia was added to change the ratio to ammonia : ammonium chloride = 60 : 1.
(b) If acid was added to this buffer solution what would be the effect on
(i) the pH of the buffer solution
(ii) the value of the ratio ammonia : ammonium chloride

CHAPTER 8

Electricity

Electricity has transformed the way we live. Without it our lifestyle would be so different as to be almost unrecognisable. Despite the way that our use of electricity has pervaded almost every aspect of our lives, probably very few people understand just what it is. This lack of knowledge is not all that surprising because 'electricity' is a term applied loosely to a great many things. This chapter sets out to explain what electricity is by describing how the modern uses of electricity evolved and by explaining the myriad of terms that are used in its description.

Having set the scene, the chapter then explains the effects of electricity on the body and the precautions that are used to ensure human safety. Humans generate their own electricity within the cells of their body, indeed it is essential to our physiology. So we describe the function of this 'bioelectricity' and the usefulness of measuring it. Some of the chapter also deals with the devices used in hospitals that operate on electricity.

Learning Objectives

At the completion of this chapter you should be able to:

1. Define charge, current, potential difference and resistance, and know their units.
2. Know that there are two types of charge and the effect they have on each other.
3. Distinguish between static electricity and current electricity, and between conductors and insulators.
4. Know that electricity is carried by free electrons in wires but by ions in the body.
5. Know the difference between alternating current and direct current.
6. Use Ohm's law.
7. Understand the function of a transformer, a fuse and the earth wire.
8. Distinguish between macroshock and micro-shock.
9. Understand the significance of 'the fatal current' and of ventricular fibrillation.
9. Understand how cells in the body generate a potential across their cell membrane.
10. Describe the conduction of a nerve impulse.
11. Know the bioelectric measurements that are made.

8.1 The Story of Electricity

8.1.1 *The Beginning*

In a Greek-speaking area of what is now called Turkey, at around 500 BC, it was noticed that a type of stone would attract objects if they were made of iron. That is, materials with a large iron content tended to stick to this stone. A man named Thales, from Miletus, called the stone **magnetic** because it was originally found near a city called Magnesia. It was also known as **lodestone**. Thales, in the course of his investigations, noticed that **amber** (a glossy substance with a golden colour) would attract tiny bits of fluff, thread, feathers and other light objects after it was rubbed. These light objects would stick to the amber. In the Greek language amber was called **elektron**.

Amber did not attract iron. Nevertheless the ability of amber and magnetic rock to make other objects stick to them created some confusion between the two phenomena. We now call the attraction of iron to magnetic rock 'magnetism' and the attraction of light objects to amber that has been rubbed 'static electricity'. However, the sciences of electricity and magnetism developed separately. Magnetic rocks could induce magnetism in steel if the steel was stroked with the rock. It was noticed that such a steel magnet would always align itself in the north–south direction if allowed to float on water. By 1400 AD European sailors were using these as 'compasses' to navigate out of the sight of land. However, no use was found for amber's property.

8.1.2 *The Development of the Science of Electricity*

Around 1570 an Englishman called William Gilbert began investigating magnets and amber. He found that materials such as diamonds, opals and other rocky crystals, when rubbed, also attracted light materials. He called all objects with the ability to attract after being rubbed **electrics**. At about 1650 another Englishman named Walter Charleton coined the term **electricity** for the strange power that makes a small scrap of paper cling to rubbed amber. Electric materials could be electrified by rubbing them.

The German Otto von Guericke constructed a simple friction machine in 1663 for producing a large amount of electricity (this was the first of many electricity-generating machines that were constructed in the seventeenth and eighteenth centuries). He used the electric material sulphur, fashioned into a sphere. The sphere of sulphur was electrified by rubbing it as it was made to spin. The ball made loud crackling noises after it was 'filled' or **charged** with electricity and made bright sparks of light when the electricity 'spilled out' or **discharged**. Von Guericke in 1672 also observed repulsion as well as attraction between objects charged with electricity.

Stephen Gray, an Englishman working in 1729, discovered that electricity could travel along a string, away from the material that was rubbed. It could cause another object attached to the string to attract small pieces of feather. He went on to investigate the distinction between materials that allowed electricity to travel through them (**conductors**) and materials that did not allow electricity to flow through them (**non-conductors**). This prompted people to speak of the flow of an 'electric fluid'.

In 1733 Charles-Francois Dufay (a Frenchman) used non-conducting silk threads to hang two tiny pieces of cork (that were covered with gold foil) from the ceiling so that they were very close to each other. He electrified the foil-covered cork by touching each piece with a glass rod that had been rubbed with silk. He found that the two pieces of cork then pushed away from each other, that is, they were **repelled** by each other. Dufay also tried a different experiment. He touched one cork piece with silk-rubbed glass and the other with resin that had been rubbed with wool. This time the two pieces of cork **attracted** each other. Dufay had produced two distinctly different electrical effects. He called the electricity in the glass rod 'glass-electric fluid' and the electricity in the resin 'resin-electric fluid'. Dufay could not find any other kind of electric fluid that was different from these two. Dufay's idea became known as the 'two fluid theory' of electricity.

Benjamin Franklin was a businessman from Philadelphia who had made a considerable amount of money. Consequently he was able to devote some time to scientific investigation. In 1747 he became interested in the electric fluid and its subtle properties. He wondered where it came from. Franklin tried to determine whether the electricity was a product of the action of rubbing or was a material substance that could be taken from silk and transferred to glass.

Franklin obtained two blocks of wax (wax does not conduct electricity) and asked a friend to stand on each one. One of the men rubbed a glass tube with his hand and became electrified. The other, after touching the glass tube, also became electrified. Both men could attract light objects, both men could send a spark to the knuckle of a third man who approached them with an outstretched arm. Furthermore, if the two experimenters on the wax blocks, still electrified, touched each other, a spark jumped between their fingers after which neither was electrified. That is, the spark that jumped between the two men seemed to nullify their electricity. Franklin interpreted the results as follows:

> The electric fire (electricity) is not created by friction but collected, being really an element diffused among matter.

> The electrical matter consists of particles extremely subtle ... Hence have arisen some new terms among us: we say B is electrised positively; A negatively.

To Franklin, all matter contained electricity but was normally neutral. The rubbing disturbed the distribution of 'this subtle fluid' so that it was simply transferred from one body to another during the process of rubbing. He believed that if a body possessed too much electricity, it was charged positive. If it had not enough, it was charged negative but that if it had just enough, it was neutral. Franklin's 'one fluid' electrical theory was not altogether correct because we now know that both positive and negative charges exist in their own right. Nevertheless, his was one of the most fundamental interpretations in the field of electricity.

An Italian obstetrician, Luigi Galvani, showed in 1780 that the leg muscles of a frog would contract when an electrical machine was discharged nearby as long as the frog's spinal cord was electrically connected to the ground. Similar contractions occurred in legs hung by a brass hook from an iron railing, even in the absence of electrical discharge. Galvani attributed the effect to 'animal electricity' in the tissue of the frog. He had shown that electricity played a part in muscular contraction but drew incorrect conclusions as to the origin of the electricity. Nevertheless Galvani is remembered for his contribution by having the **galvanometer**, a device that detects the flow of electricity, named after him.

Allessandro Volta, physics professor at Bologna University, contended that Galvani's electricity came from the contact between two different metals and not from the moist bodies of animals. He proved his point in 1799 when he stacked alternate discs of different metals, for example copper and zinc, in a pile, with each pair of discs separated by moist paper. This 'voltaic pile' caused the copper discs to have a positive charge and the zinc discs to be negative. The positive charges and negative charges respectively added together so that the total charge was greater than that for just one pair of discs. When the discs at each end were connected with a metal wire, the excess negative charge from one end flowed to where there was a shortage of negative charge at the other end. Volta's **battery** of discs produced elec-tricity continuously and it flowed steadily through the wire. He had produced the first continuous 'electric current', and the first electric cell (or battery).

The electric force that we attribute to 'static' electricity (that is, electricity that is not flowing as a current) was measured in 1785 by the Frenchman Charles Coulomb. He devised an extremely sensitive torsion balance to measure the electric force between electrically charged spheres. Using this balance, Coulomb discovered the first quantitative relation in electrical science (that the force between two charges is proportional to the magnitude of each charge and inversely proportional to the square of the distance between them). It is now known as 'Coulomb's Law'. He is also honoured by having the unit of charge named after him (the **coulomb**).

Recall that at one time there was confusion between the electric effect of amber and the magnetic effect of lodestone. Hans Christian Oersted believed that there was a connection between electricity and magnetism. In 1819 in Copenhagen he was able to show that a wire with an **electric current** flowing through it behaved like a **magnet**. The connection was strengthened between 1821 and 1825 by Andre Marie Ampere. He conducted a thorough investigation of the forces between wires that were carrying an electric current, and the force between electric currents and magnets. His research resulted in what came to be known as 'Ampere's Law'. This law relates the magnetic force between two currents to the amount of current flowing. It also provides us with our preferred definition of the **ampere**, the unit of magnitude of electric current (the definition is 'one ampere is that current flowing in each of two long parallel wires, that are separated by a distance of one metre in a vacuum, that produces a force of 2×10^{-7} N on each metre of their length').

At about the same time a German schoolteacher, Georg Ohm, was experimenting with electric current flowing through wires of uniform diameter. He suggested that electricity, in moving through a wire, passed from particle to particle and calculated that the movement must be due to an 'electrical tension' or a difference in potential. In an analogous way, a difference in temperature causes a flow of heat, and a difference in height causes a flow of water. The name given to this electrical 'tension' was **electromotive force** (emf) because a force is required to produce the movement of electricity. The unit of emf is called the **volt** after Alessandro Volta. Ohm is also remembered by the use of his name as a unit. The **ohm** is a measure of the ease (or difficulty) with which electric current moves through a conductor. That is, it is a measure of the **resistance** of a material to the flow of electricity.

8.1.3 *The Development of Electromagnetic Theory*

Michael Faraday, a relatively unschooled Englishman who had a great experimental flair, conducted many experiments to investigate the link between electricity and magnetism. By 1831 he had shown them to be inextricably related so that their combined effects came to be known as electromagnetism. Faraday described the effects of magnets, charged objects and electric currents in terms of lines of force that operated between objects. These force lines existed in a region around the electric or magnetic object which he called a **field**. A strong field had many lines of force and he was able to represent their position and orientation by drawing them on paper. Faraday also coined the term 'ion' for a particle carrying an electric charge. James Clerk Maxwell, between 1855 and 1864, set out to explain mathematically the theories of Faraday. Maxwell sucessfully summarised Faraday's 'electric field', 'magnetic field' and 'lines of force' into mathematical equations. His equations implied that light must be an electromagnetic wave of some kind and indicated that electricity, magnetism and light must all be related phenomena.

Practical applications of electricity and electromagnetic effects seemed to spring forth from inventors with ever-increasing speed and bewildering scope. The electric generator and electric motor were a result of Faraday's work. Samuel Morse built the electric telegraph in 1844, Alexander Bell produced the telephone in 1876. Thomas Edison's laboratory constructed the first viable incandescent light globe in 1879 and DC lightning systems were installed soon after. The first AC lighting system was demonstrated in Paris in 1883. The generator led to a public electricity supply and the use of electric motors in trains, elevators and sewing machines. At about 1890 the New York State legislature passed a law establishing electrocution as a means of applying the death sentence.

The final event in our electrical story, up until the start of the twentieth century, was the discovery of a particle from inside an atom that carried an electric charge. It had been postulated by Helmholtz that a consequence of Faraday's work was that all electrical charges were multiples of some elementary charge. Johnstone Stoney in 1874 suggested the name **electron** for the postulated elementary charge. John Joseph Thomson, in 1897, demonstrated that cathode rays were particles that originated from within atoms and that carried a unit of negative charge. In the same year, John Townsend, a student of Thomson's, obtained an approximate value for the amount of charge on the cathode corpuscles. It was apparent that cathode corpuscles were in fact electrons and are one of the constituents of all atoms.

8.1.4 *Summary of Electrical Terms*

charge (q): That quality (or property) that is responsible for electric effects. Measured in units called coulombs (C).

electron: A 'fundamental' particle that carries the smallest amount of charge (1.6×10^{-19} C).

ion: An atom or molecule that has an electric charge because it has lost one or more electrons (a positive ion) or because it has gained one or more electrons (a negative ion).

positive and negative: The two types of electric charge that exist. Neutral objects have equal numbers of positive and negative charges. An object may be positively charged if it has gained some excess positive charges (a rare occurrence) or if it has lost some of its complement of negative charges (the common occurrence).

current (I): The rate of flow of electric charge, that is, the number of coulombs flowing past a given point in one second. Measured in units called amperes (A).

electric potential (V): The electric potential (or just 'potential') at a point is the amount of energy per coulomb that a charge would possess by being at that point (joules/coulomb). Positive charges, if free to move, will move from a point of high potential to a point of lower potential (negative charges move in the opposite direction). Measured in units called volts (V).

electromotive force (emf): Commonly called 'voltage'. That property that causes charges to move from one place to another in a continuous flow of electric current. A source of emf produces a *difference* in potential between two places so that electric charges tend to move between the places according to their energy. Emf is measured in units called volts (V).

potential difference (V or ΔV): Also commonly called 'voltage', it is the difference in electric potential between two points. Without a difference in potential, no electric current will flow between two points. May be expressed in terms of the work done in shifting one coulomb of charge between the two points (joules/coulomb). Measured in units called volts (V).

resistance (R): Measures the ease of conduction of electric current. The greater the resistance, the smaller the electric current that will flow (all else being equal). Measured in units called ohms (Ω).

electric power (*P*): The rate of flow of energy; or the work done per second in causing electric charge to flow. Measured in units called watts (W).

work (*W*): The kilowatt-hour is the amount of work done (that is, the amount of energy expended) when one thousand watts of power are used for one hour. Measured in units called joules (J). One kilowatt-hour = 3.6 MJ.

electricity: A broad term loosely applied to electrons and ions whether they are stationary (static) or moving (current). Also applied to the interaction that such charges have with each other and the environment. A convenient means by which the energy released by the burning of fuels in a 'power' station is distributed to consumers.

8.2 What is Electricity?

When a plastic object (such as a comb or ruler or biro) is rubbed with some other material (such as hair, wool, silk) the plastic object exhibits a seemingly magical property. It can attract to it, and hold, small pieces of paper (or hair or fluff or dust). This 'magical' behaviour is one of the effects of electricity. A plastic ruler rubbed in this way is said to be electrified. It is also said to be imbued or filled with or charged with electricity (in the same sense as the saying 'charge your glasses' means fill them up).

Electrical charge may be of two types. We know this because two plastic rulers, both rubbed with the same material and suspended so that they are free to swing, will repel each other. But the same two rulers, when rubbed with different materials, will attract each other. Since attraction and repulsion are different manifestations of this 'magical' electrical phenomena, we name two types of electrical charge, viz. positive and negative. It became apparent in 1897 (thanks to J.J. Thomson) that negative electrical charge was carried on a submicroscopic particle, normally found inside an atom, that came to be called an **electron**. By carried on an electron we mean that negative charge can not be separated from the piece of matter that we call an electron, so has no separate existence.

All electrons carry the same amount of charge, and the charge carried by an electron is the smallest possible amount that can be obtained (however, since 1963 the existence of particles called **quarks** has been speculated upon. The theory requires them to carry one third of the charge of an electron, but they have not yet been conclusively detected). All other charges are multiples of the charge on one electron. The SI unit of charge is the coulomb (symbol C) named after Charles Coulomb. It takes 6.25×10^{18} electrons (6.25 million of a million million) to make one coulomb. Clearly the charge on one electron is extremely small when compared to one coulomb. Nevertheless, amounts of charge far smaller than one coulomb produce the many observable effects of electricity. Positive charge is associated with a particle within the nucleus of an atom, called a proton.

Matter in its normal state contains equal amounts of positive and negative electricity and thus is neutral (that is, has no net charge). Neutral matter has electrons and protons present in equal numbers. When glass (for example) is rubbed with silk, electrons will be rubbed off the glass and onto the silk (because the atoms in silk have a greater affinity for electrons than the atoms in glass). Since silk now has more electrons than in its normal state, it is negatively charged. Glass (having lost some of its electrons to the silk) has an excess of positive charge. It is far easier to move electrons around than protons (which carry positive charge) so for our purposes electricity may be thought of as due to an **excess of electrons** (which results in a negative charge), or due to the **loss of electrons** (which results in a positive charge).

8.3 Static Electricity, Insulators and Conductors

Materials that can be charged with electricity by rubbing are called insulators (or poor conductors). These include plastic, rubber, ceramic and wood. Other materials are conductors, for example gold, silver, carbon, copper, aluminium, steel (and other metals or alloys). Still other types of materials are called **semi-conductors** but will not concern us at present. Another way of defining conductors and insulators is: in conductors, electrons are free to move, whereas electrons in insulators cannot move. Even when excess electrons are rubbed onto insulators they do not move along or through the insulator. Thus any charge placed on an insulator (or even placed on a conductor that is separated from other materials by an insulator) remains there. This build up of stationary charge is called **static electricity**, because it is not flowing.

Recall that there are two types of charges, positive and negative. Like charges repel each other (that is, two negatively charged objects would feel a repulsive force from each other) and unlike charges attract each other. In fact the forces between electrical charges are so strong that to keep a charge of 1 C at a distance of 1 m directly above another charge of 1 C of the same sign would require a force equivalent to the weight of 9×10^5 tonnes (equivalent to about 20 000 loaded semi-trailers). Clearly 1 C of charge is an enormous amount of charge. In fact it is not possible to accumulate 1 C of charge at one place because the force of repulsion between the particles would soon dissipate the charge.

Charge (also called static electricity) builds up on door knobs and furniture in rooms with synthetic carpets, on car and aeroplane bodies because air 'rubs' past them and on clothes made from synthetic fibres (to name just a few examples). Static electricity can discharge (momentarily move through air to a nearby object) producing a crackling noise, accompanied by heat and light in the form of a spark. The sound of such discharge may be noticeable when you take your clothes off and if the room is dark you may even see the spark.

Lighting is a dramatic form of electrical discharge from clouds. Positive charge gathers at the top of the cloud (about 40 C) and about the same amount of negative charge at the bottom. Most lightning strokes pass from one cloud to another across potential differences that may be a thousand million volts. Only a few strike the ground, transferring ten or more coulombs of charge to the ground. A stroke of lightning is in fact usually made up of many separate strokes each following the other at intervals of milliseconds, but in opposite directions. As the current passes back and forth between the cloud and the ground, the surrounding air heats up to about 20 000 °C, and it is the rapid expansion of air accompanying this heating which produces the thunderclap. People who survive lightning strikes usually present with burns, fractures and dislocations, neurological damage and eye and ear injuries.

The spark of discharging static electricity is quite hot and can ignite flammable gases, producing explosions and fires. In an effort to reduce the risk of igniting flammable anaesthetic gases in an operating theatre, the floor coverings are made conducting and are grounded (that is, are maintained at zero volts by connecting them electrically to the earth). In addition, the relative humidity of the room is kept above 55% and this prevents the accumulation of large static charges. The patient is connected to a grounded operating table by a conductive rubber mat (the rubber is impregnated with carbon) and a moist bedsheet, and the operating personnel wear conductive clothing. Since precautions against the build up of static electricity are now routine, and ether and other highly flammable gases are no longer used, the dangers of fire and explosion are removed. The nurse may receive a nuisance shock from discharge on making beds, undressing or touching television screens but such shocks do not present any real danger. If anything they add to the interest in life.

8.4 Current Electricity

When electrons move, the charge they carry is said to flow from one place to another. This movement or flow is called a 'current of electricity' or more simply an electric current. The more electrons that move, the greater the charge that is transferred during any specified time interval, and hence the larger in magnitude is the electric current.

electric current = number of coulombs flowing per second

The SI unit of electric current is the 'coulomb per second' and is renamed the **ampere**, or amp (symbol A), in honour of Andre Ampere. One ampere is the amount of current that flows if one coulomb of charge flows past each second. It is the amount of electric current, more than any other measured quantity, that is the most relevant fact when considering the safety or otherwise of an electric shock. Static electricity shocks are generally momentary flows of a few microamps and are not fatal; however, shocks from domestic AC supplies may involve currents of up to 10 A, sometimes more, and are frequently fatal.

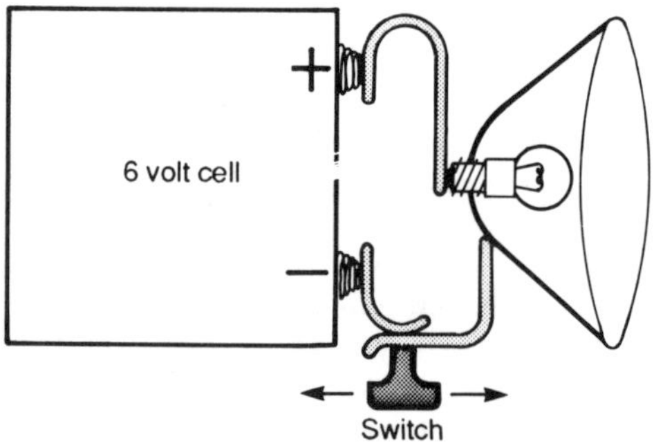

Figure 8.1 *A DC circuit that operates a torch globe. The 6 V cell supplies energy to electrons that circulate from the negative terminal, through the globe to the positive terminal. The circuit is completed or broken by operating the switch*

8.4.1 *Electric Current Needs an Energy Source*

For an electric current to flow, the moving electrons must be supplied with energy (otherwise they can't move). A 'dry' cell, like those that run torches or portable radios, or 'wet' cells, like those in car batteries, can supply this energy from the chemical potential energy stored in them. When their energy is all used up, the cells (or batteries) are 'dead'. In fossil fuel power stations gas, oil or coal is burned; this releases energy as heat to boil water, which creates steam. Steam produced under pressure and directed by nozzles can be made to turn turbines which in turn cause the armatures that are inside 'generators' to spin while subjected to a strong magnetic field. The energy that is harnessed to spin the coiled copper wires of the armature in a strong magnetic field is in part converted into electrical energy for our domestic electrical supply. The **generator** makes electricity circulate through the system.

Devices that supply the energy that makes electrons move are called sources of electromotive force (abbreviated to emf) and are rated according to the amount of energy that they supply to each coulomb of charge (that is, to each 6.25×10^{18} electrons). Australia's domestic AC supply provides 240 J of energy (on average) to each coulomb of charge, that is, is rated at 240 J/C. An automobile battery produces a DC supply. It supplies each coulomb with 12 J of energy. In the SI system of units, the 'joule per coulomb' is renamed the volt (symbol V) after Alessandro Volta. The volt is the unit of the three related quantities of emf, potential and potential difference.

8.4.2 *Electric Current Needs a Continuous Path to Follow*

Electric current will not flow unless there is an energy source (that is, a voltage supply) *and* a complete, unbroken path for electrons to move along. This continuous path is called a **circuit** and is made of conducting materials such as copper wires. Switches are the means by which an electrical circuit is broken (opened/switched off) or made (closed/switched on). Once an energy source (for example, a battery, or cell or a generator) is connected to a complete circuit, electrons will move, and we say that current flows.

8.4.3 *Electric Current Needs a Path of Low Resistance*

If the voltage supply is fixed (at 240 V or some other value), the amount of current that flows is determined by the ease or difficulty that electrons have in moving through the wires and various electrical components in the circuit. The path of the current is usually through materials that allow current to flow, that is, materials that are conductors or semi-conductors. For a fixed voltage, the **resistance** to flow is critical in determining the amount of current that will flow. Electrical components of known resistance are deliberately designed into circuits in order to control the amount of current that flows.

8.4.4 *Ohm's Law*

A high resistance (a hundred thousand ohms) will only allow a small current (a few milliamps) and a low resistance (a few ohms) allows very large currents (60 A or more). The SI unit of resistance is the **ohm** (symbol Ω) named after Georg Ohm. Recall that the current is the primary variable which determines the seriousness of a shock. **Ohm's law** allows us to determine the current that will flow for a given 'voltage' and resistance:

$$\text{current (in amps)} = \frac{\text{potential difference (in volts)}}{\text{resistance (in ohms)}}$$

or in symbolic form

$$I = \frac{V}{R}$$

A 60 W light globe has a resistance of about 960 Ω, so when operated on a 240 V supply would draw a current of 0.25 A. A 1000 W electric radiator would draw 4.2 A.

The electrical resistance of the body varies widely, so the voltage required to produce a dangerous current will also vary widely. Measured from one hand to the other, resistance may be 1 000 000 Ω for very dry skin or as little as 1000 Ω for wet skin. If we choose an intermediate value (say 10 000 Ω), then Ohm's law will show us that a fatal current can flow.

$$I = \frac{V}{R} = \frac{240\ \text{V}}{10\ 000\ \Omega} = 24\ \text{mA}$$

8.5 Alternating Current (AC) and Direct Current (DC)

Electrons in a DC electrical circuit will flow from the negative terminal of a battery, where there is an excess of electrons, to the positive terminal, where there is a lack of electrons. In doing so, they use up all their energy in overcoming the resistance of the conductors that make up the circuit. Their energy is renewed by passing through the battery again. The idea of an electric current was around long before it was discovered that electrons (of negative charge) were the moving objects. Consequently, so-called 'conventional current' was (and still is!) said to flow from the positive terminal (where the 'voltage' is high) to the negative terminal (where the 'voltage' is low). However, electrons actually move in the opposite direction to the so-called conventional current. This apparent anomaly has been allowed to persist because there are situations where positively charged particles (positive ions) are the objects that move under the influence of a potential difference. Positive ions move in the same direction as the 'conventional current'. Note that current will not flow between two points unless there is a difference in voltage between those two points ('purists' would call this difference in voltage a potential difference).

8.5.1 *Direct Current*

Where electrons are flowing in the *one direction* (from negative to positive) through the circuit during *the entire time* that the circuit is operating, we say that the current is **direct current** (DC). The speed of electron movement is very slow — about one tenth of a millimetre per second in an automobile DC system. Nevertheless the number of slow-moving electrons is so vast that a significant current flows. Direct current electricity is quite common and is used in torches, 'walkman' type radios, automobiles and other small-scale or portable electrical devices.

8.5.2 *Alternating Current*

Domestic electricity is called 'alternating' because the electrons move first in one direction through the wire, then in the opposite direction. In fact the direction of motion reverses 100 times each second. Each cycle of motion involves both 'to and fro' motion so 50 cycles occur each second (50 cycles per second is called 50 hertz, or 50 Hz). Thus electrons do not flow from the power lines out of the wall socket along the wires, through the wires of the appliance and then back into the wall. Only *energy* carried by the electric field, at the speed of light, enters the appliance. The electrons in the circuit oscillate about a fixed position without going anywhere. Nevertheless this very rapid to and fro movement by the electrons is a movement of charge and transmits energy. It constitutes an **alternating current** (AC).

8.5.3 *Electric Power*

When we 'use' electricity, the thing that is being used or consumed is energy. Voltage, current or resistance is not consumed, their magnitudes stay the same while the electricity is switched on. Electrical supply companies measure (and charge us for) the amount of energy, in joules, that we use in a given time. How *quickly* we use electrical energy determines the electrical **power** we require. Note that energy is the consumable quantity and that power is the *rate* of consumption of energy.

$$\text{power} = \frac{\text{energy used}}{\text{time taken to use it}}$$

or more usefully,

$$\underset{\text{(in watts)}}{\text{power}} = \underset{\text{(in volts)}}{\text{'voltage'}} \times \underset{\text{(in amps)}}{\text{current}}$$

which stated symbolically is $P = V \times I$. Power is measured in joules per second but this unit is given the name 'watt'. A kilowatt is 1000 W. Suppose that energy is used at the rate of 1 kW for one hour (for example, a 1000 W electric radiator operating for an hour); electric supply companies find it convenient to call this amount of energy consumption a 'kilowatt-hour'. One kilowatt-hour is 3 600 000 J of energy.

8.5.4 *What are the Relative Advantages of AC over DC?*

Direct current is not suited for supplying reticulated domestic electricity, as it cannot be transmitted over long distances economically. AC is easily 'stepped up' to high voltages (200 000 V) for transmission over long distances, and 'stepped down' to 240 V (or any other voltage) for household use. A **transformer** is the device that changes one voltage to another and it does so at the expense of current. That is, the output from the generators of a power station is at *high* voltage but *low* current.

A low current means that relatively few electrons are required to negotiate their way past the atoms of the wires connecting the power station and the substation. Consequently the total energy lost by the few electrons in overcoming resistance while moving through the wires is not much. By the time the wires enter a suburban house, the electricity that they transmit has passed through a 'substation', where the voltage is stepped down, and a local transformer where the electrical supply is again stepped down, to domestic level (240 V in Australia). This relatively *low* voltage allows a *high* current to flow in the house wiring (up to 15 A) so that several appliances can be operated at once. When a large current is flowing, a relatively large number of electrons are negotiating their way through the wires and appliances of the house. As they do so, the energy that they expend is converted into useful forms like light, sound, heat and motion. Consumers pay for the energy that is used inside their house but the power company bears the cost of the energy used by the electrons in delivering the energy to the consumer. It makes good economic and environmental sense to minimise the energy 'lost' in the transmission wires as it merely heats the air surrounding the wires. Thus the transmission of electricity is most efficiently done by using alternating current at very high voltage.

The available power (rate of energy use) is the product of voltage and current, and remains constant. What a transformer does is to increase one of *either* current or voltage while decreasing the other. Thus when the primary voltage (V_p) is transformed to a *higher* secondary voltage (V_s), the current flowing in the secondary coil of the transformer (I_s) is much *lower* than the current flowing in the primary coil (I_p). This is achieved by passing the primary supply into the few coils of the primary winding, but drawing the secondary supply from the many coils of the secondary winding (see Figure 8.2). The four quantities are related by the equation

$$\text{power} = V_s \times I_s = V_p \times I_p$$

The very small secondary current can be transmitted over long distances through copper cables without producing much heat. This means that very little electrical energy is converted to heat energy during the transmission process. So most of it reaches the consumer's meter.

There are several situations where DC is preferred over AC electricity. Where the electrical device is intended to be used in places where there is no reticulated electrical supply, such as at sea, in the air or the desert, then the device needs its own supply of energy. In this case a DC source will do. If the device is intended to be portable (like an automobile, watch, camera, calculator) and needs to operate without the encumberance of power cords trailing after it, it must carry its own source of emf. The source is usually a battery. Thus AC and DC electricity are used as the situation demands. The two methods of supplying electric current are not fundamentally different. In fact, the same electricity generator can produce either AC or DC current by using (respectively) a slip-ring commutator or a split-ring commutator. Furthermore, AC electricity can be converted to DC by a 'full-wave rectifier' and DC electricity can be converted to AC by a device called an 'inverter'.

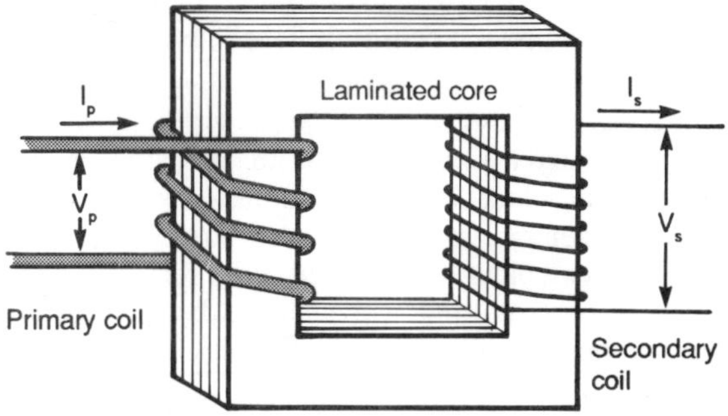

Figure 8.2 *A 'step-up' transformer converts the low-voltage, high-current AC supply into high-voltage, low-current AC. The laminated metal 'core' links the alternating magnetic field of the primary coils to the secondary coils*

8.6 Domestic Electrical Safety

The amount of current that may be drawn by a circuit in a domestic building is limited to about 10 A (sometimes 5 A, sometimes 15 A) by a **fuse** (or an automatic switch called a **circuit breaker**). A fuse is a device that holds a wire (the 'fuse wire') that will get so hot when the predetermined current is exceeded that it melts. This is called 'blowing a fuse' and leaves the circuit 'open' so no more current flows. Since it is cheaper to replace a melted fuse than a melted video recorder, amplifier or X-ray machine, all electrical devices sensitive to large currents have their own fuses (in addition to the fuse or circuit breaker in the house's fuse box) to protect them from large currents.

Domestic electrical devices that plug in to power points have cables that contain three wires, the active, the neutral and the earth. The plastic insulation around the wires is colour coded internationally so that active is brown, neutral is blue and earth is striped green and yellow. The colour coding used to be red, black and green respectively but was changed because of the high proportion of 'colour blind' males.

Domestic power points (sockets) also have three wires connected to them. The **active** or 'live' wire alternates in potential from positive 240 V to negative 240 V. It is connected to the conductors that come from the power station. The switch is also located on the active wire in order to turn the supply on or off. The **neutral** or 'return' wire is at ground potential (zero volts) because it is connected to the earth both at the power station and at the consumer's installation. Thus there is always a potential difference between the active and the neutral wire. When an electrical appliance is plugged in and switched on, the two wires are connected to each other by the circuits in the appliance. Thus the neutral wire 'completes the circuit' by providing electric current with a point of different potential to flow towards. The earth is normally a good conductor of electricity, and therefore provides an alternative return pathway. In other words electric current can 'return' to the generating station via the neutral wire or via the ground. The (bare) neutral wire will not produce a shock if touched, *provided that the wiring is correctly installed*, because it is at the same potential as the person touching it. Since the *difference* in potential is zero, no current should flow.

With the active and neutral wires alone, electrical devices will operate properly. Indeed electric light circuits and so-called 'double insulated appliances' use only these two wires.

The wire connected to the third pin of the power point (the one closest to the floor) is called the **earth** wire. It is also connected via a thick, multi-strand cable, which presents almost no electrical resistance, to a water pipe or an 'earth stem' at the side of a house. The water pipe or earth stem makes good electrical contact with the ground (note that *both* the neutral and earth wires are connected independently to ground). The earth wire in the cord of the electrical appliance is bonded to the inside of the appliance's metal case. Should a malfunction cause the metal case of an electrical device to become 'live', a large current will automatically flow through the earth wire (the path of least resistance) to ground. The large current will exceed the capacity of the fuse in the meter box so the fuse will melt, leaving a gap in the circuit. Since the fuse is on the active wire, the internal wiring will be isolated from the power station and current will immediately cease to flow. Thus a person touching the live metal case will not have a large current flowing through them because:

1. the path through their body has a greater resistance than the path through the earth wire (which has almost zero resistance); and
2. current will cease to flow through the faulty device as soon as the fuse blows so the device will cease to be live.

8.7 The Physiological Effects of Electric Current

The most common type of electric shock that humans receive is called **macroshock**. In this case, electric current has to pass into the body after overcoming the relatively high resistance provided by the skin. The susceptibility of humans to electric shock (macroshock) is not easy to predict because of the variability of individuals and the conditions under which they are exposed. The harmful effects of electricity passing through the body are dependent mainly on the *amount* of electric current, the *duration* of flow through the body and the *path* it follows through the body. In turn, the amount of current flowing is determined by the applied voltage and the resistance of the body between the two points at which the current enters the body and where it leaves the body. It is possible for a fatal shock to occur at 240 V (given a low resistance) but not at 10 000 V (given a high resistance) because current is determined by $I = V/R$ (Ohm's law).

The flow of electric current is usually from a voltage point to ground, so two electrical connections to the body are required for a person to be shocked. A bird sitting on a high-voltage overhead wire is not shocked, even though it may be in contact with 11 000 V, because it has no contact with the ground. Both of the bird's feet are at the same large potential (voltage), thus there is *no difference* in potential between them and current can not flow. However, if one foot was on the wire and the other on the stobie pole, the bird would be electrocuted. For a fatal current to flow, there must be a path, through the victim, connecting the power supply to the ground. This means that there are two contacts to be made, one may be a hand and the other is usually to the other hand or bare feet (there is normally a high resistance between a shod foot and the floor).

Whether contact with the 240 V, 50 Hz domestic power supply will produce a fatal macroshock on a particular occasion is determined by the combination of factors applying at the time. These include whether skin is dry or wet, intact or broken, whether clothing and shoes are worn, whether the floor is wet or dry, whether other parts of the skin are in contact with the ground or walls. In addition the length of time that the current flows and the organs that the current passes through may determine whether the person survives.

Table 8.1 *The effects of 50 Hz current applied externally to the body (macroshock)*

0.5 mA	Approximate limit of perception.
1 mA	Distinct shock perceived.
5 mA	Severe shock, maximum harmless current.
10–100 mA	Severe shock, painful, extreme breathing difficulties, burns, high probability of ventricular fibrillation, muscular paralysis, can not let go, death likely.
100–200 mA	Respiratory paralysis, cardiac arrest, severe burning, death probable.
> 200 mA	Death results.
5–6 A	Sustained myocardial contraction followed by normal heart rhythm if current stops. Temporary respiratory paralysis. Burns. Death occurs if current is not stopped.

The effects of electric current through the body include pain, muscular contraction and burning (see Table 8.1). We do know that *sustained* currents of between 100 and 300 mA are fatal, probably due to **ventricular fibrillation**. Cardiac arrest and cessation of breathing may also be the cause of death. Fibrillation is very high frequency uncoordinated contraction of the walls of the ventricles. Because the heart walls are not contracting simultaneously, no blood is pumped, the ventricles dilate, and after about 90 seconds, are too weak to contract because of the lack of coronary blood supply. Death results. Currents above about 300 mA, while producing severe burns and unconsciousness, do not usually cause death provided that contact with the active wires is severed. Then artificial respiration is applied immediately to restore breathing. Above 300 mA the muscular contraction of the heart is so severe that the heart is forcibly clamped shut during the shock, protecting against ventricular fibrillation.

From a practical viewpoint, it is impossible to tell whether an unconscious person has received a lethal dose of current through the vital organs of the body. Artificial respiration must be applied after removing the victim from the contact. Given appropriate conditions, 75 V may be just as lethal as 75 000 volts, and any electrical device used on a house wiring circuit can, under certain conditions, transmit a fatal current.

8.8 Microshock

When conditions exist such that a patient has an internal electrical path direct to the heart (rather than first having to pass through the skin), the patient may be said to be **microshock sensitive**. Such conditions occur when a pacemaker wire is in place, cardiac catheters are in use, and intracardiac electrocardiograms are being recorded. All these devices bypass the high electrical resistance of the skin by introducing an electrical conductor (a wire or electrolyte solution) which is in direct electrical contact with the heart muscle. Consequently a much smaller current will produce the ventricular fibrillation than is the case for macroshock (Table 8.2).

An additional condition necessary to produce a microshock hazard is the existence of a complete circuit connecting an electrical device to the ground via the patient's internal electrical path. The circuit may be

Table 8.2 *The effects of 50 Hz current applied internally to the body (microshock)*

10 μA	Current limit for design of electrical equipment used for intrathoracic procedures.
20–100 μA	Effects uncertain and will be influenced by cardiac conditions. Likelihood of fibrillation increases with current.
100 μA	Fibrillation likely to occur for currents above this level, followed by death.

completed by someone touching the patient's internal path (if it is not insulated) while touching a grounded object or a second appliance connected to the patient. A wet bed (due to incontinence, spilled liquids, bathing, sweating and so on) may also be the means of allowing a microshock current to flow to ground.

Experiments on several kinds of animals have been used to estimate the fibrillating current levels for humans. Sheep have been found to fibrillate if a current of 1 A is applied for 0.03 s or a current of 100 mA for 3 s. In dogs, a current of 20 μA will induce ventricular fibrillation if applied directly to the heart. In humans, a current of the order of 100 μA may be sufficient to cause ventricular fibrillation if connected to the heart directly. Since such currents are below the threshold of feeling, this current may be transmitted unwittingly through a nurse in electrical contact with the patient, if the nurse is **also** in contact with a faulty device. It may not be obvious that a patient is undergoing micro-electrocution (that is, has 100 μA or so passing through the heart), because no physically visible stimulation or muscle contraction occurs.

8.9 Electrical Safety in the Hospital

To cater for standard modern surgical procedures the operating theatre is packed with electrical equipment. Each of these if used alone presents a negligible risk of electric shock provided that it is in serviceable condition. However, when two or more electrical devices are attached to a patient, an electric shock hazard may be present.

A safe environment is provided if all electrical devices have a fuse as well as a three-wire cord that is securely fastened to a three-pin plug. The patient should have no electrical connection to the ground and should be electrically isolated from the equipment. The ground connections should be periodically examined to ensure their integrity. All exposed conducting wires to the patient should have good insulation. Furthermore the integrity of the power supply can be greatly improved by the measures that are required for 'cardiac protected areas' in hospitals.

8.9.1 *Leakage Current*

The major source of potentially lethal currents in any instrument is leakage current. In a perfect device the current in the neutral wire would be *exactly* the same as the current in the active wire. If not then some of the current that was in the active wire has 'leaked out' into the instrument instead of passing into the neutral wire. Leakage current is an unfortunate name for the phenomena because it implies that something is faulty. This is not so as leakage current exists to some extent in all correctly functioning, AC power-line-operated equipment (except for doubly insulated devices).

Instruments are designed so that this normal leakage current flows to the instrument's metal case and then to ground, through the multi-strand copper earth wire in the three-wire power cord. As long as the instrument is adequately grounded, the leakage current will not flow through a person who touches the case. This is because the electrical resistance of the earth wire between the case and the ground is almost zero, while the resistance of the path to ground through the body

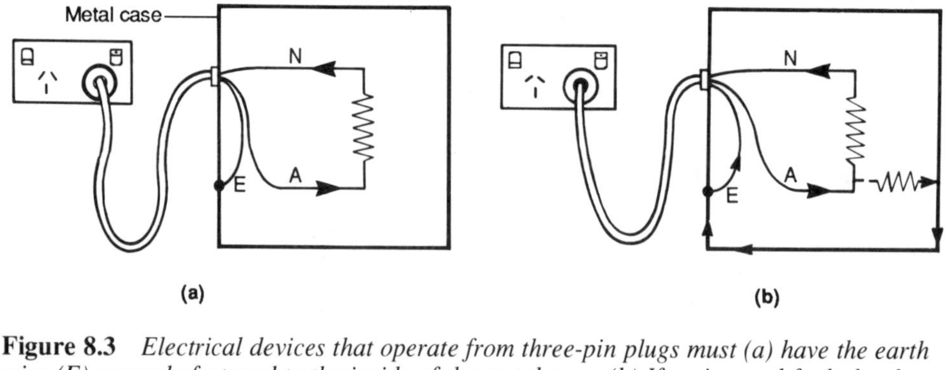

Figure 8.3 *Electrical devices that operate from three-pin plugs must (a) have the earth wire (E) securely fastened to the inside of the metal case. (b) If an internal fault develops, any current transmitted to the case will flow harmlessly to ground via the earth wire*

of someone touching the case is relatively high. By applying Ohm's law it can be seen that the current that flows is inversely proportional to the resistance of the path. Stated another way, current 'takes the path of least resistance'. The integrity of the grounding for a device is the single most important protection system against electrocution.

If an instrument could have perfect insulation (this means that the resistance between the earth wire on the case and the active wire on the internal parts is infinite) then no leakage current will flow (see Figure 8.3). Usually, however, the resistance between the active and the earth wires is not infinite, so some current *will* flow to the case and to ground through the earth wire. This leakage current may be too small (say, 15 mA) when compared to the normal current through the instrument, to cause a fuse to blow. The metal casing of the device will not produce a perceptible shock when touched because the leakage current flows harmlessly through the earth wire to ground. The instrument will not be noticeably faulty, nor would it be regarded as unsafe in a domestic situation, but it will cost a little more to run because of the extra current being drawn.

In a hospital situation 15 mA leakage is not acceptable because it is well above the current that can produce microshock. Note that microshock will not occur unless the grounding of the instrument is inadequate and a patient is sensitive to microshock *and* electrical contact is made between the patient's internal connection and the faulty instrument. Nevertheless the possibility of all these things occurring simultaneously in a hospital is not negligible so the patient deserves to be protected.

8.9.2 *Induced Current*

Some instruments with power transformers inside will 'induce' an electric current in nearby metal parts even when there is no physical contact between the transformer and the metal parts. This induction of electric current is an inescapable feature of AC electricity. The oscillating electric and magnetic fields that constitute the AC electricity supply cause the electrons in nearby conductors to accelerate. This movement of electrons under the influence of the oscillating fields constitutes a current. However, with careful design these instruments can have the level of current that they induce restricted to acceptable levels. In any case this induced electric current will flow harmlessly to ground through the earth wire.

8.10 Electrical Protection Systems

8.10.1 *Adequate Grounding*

For electrical devices to be adequately grounded (or earthed) the following requirements must be met:

1. An earth wire is securely fastened to the inside of the metal case of the instrument and to the earth pin of the three-pin plug that fits into the wall socket. The earth wire in the wall is intact and continuous, making good contact at the power point and eventually with earth at the grounding point. The resistance of the wire and connections between the case and the ground point is very low (less than one ohm).
2. All ground connections should be to the *same* ground potential (zero volts) so that there is no potential difference (at all) between them. Equal ground potential can be achieved by grouping power points together to provide a single grounding point and ensuring that all instruments applying to the one patient are plugged into the same service unit. An 'equipotential earth system' is used to ensure that the metal parts of all equipment are connected to the same good ground. An equipotential earthing system together with either an isolating transformer or an earth leakage circuit breaker will offer protection against microshock.

8.10.2 *Earth Leakage Circuit Breakers (ELCB)*

These devices (also called core balance devices) detect whether the current in the active wire is different from the current in the neutral wire. If the currents differ by 10 mA or more (that is, a leakage current of 10 mA or more exists), within 40 ms a circuit breaker will 'trip' thus cutting off the mains electricity supply. Note that 10 mA is potentially lethal as a microshock; however, the 40 ms delay in cutting the current off is considered to be short enough to prevent the current flowing for long enough to cause fibrillation. Not only is it difficult to design a circuit breaker that will trip at less than 10 mA but where an ELCB is set to trip at lower currents, then 'nuisance tripping' becomes a problem. ELCB systems generally are only suitable in situations where the temporary loss of power (which occurs at each 'trip') can be tolerated.

When a leakage current causes a 'trip', a noticeable 'click' will be heard from a nearby ELCB switch and electric power will be cut off. If this happens, flicking the ELCB switch back up will reset it and restore power. If the ELCB continues to trip then the power plugs at the electrical service outlet should be removed one at a time, and the ELCB reset between each removal. When it does reset then the last item removed may be faulty and should not be used until serviced.

8.10.3 *Isolation Transformers and Line Isolation Monitors*

An isolation transformer provides a 240 V potential difference between the two supply wires of the transformer's secondary coil. Neither wire is earthed, so there is no wire fixed at zero potential. The difference in potential between them is, however, always 240 V. Without a grounded neutral wire, the electrical devices connected to the secondary coil of the transformer are isolated from earth. The effect of such isolation is that a person accidentally touching any one wire while grounded will cause the potential of that wire to be earth potential (zero volts). Thus there is no potential difference between the wire that has been touched and the earth. Without a voltage difference, no current will flow, so no shock can be produced.

The metal casings of devices supplied by an isolation transformer still have an earth wire to ground and a line isolation monitor detects any leakage current flowing in the earth wire. If a predetermined limit is exceeded an alarm sounds indicating a hazard, but power is not automatically cut off. Line isolation transformers are used in supplying power where the loss of supply caused by a circuit breaker cannot be tolerated, for example to life support equipment. Such transformers are more expensive than earth leakage circuit breakers so are less common.

8.11 Classification of Equipment, Procedures and Areas

8.11.1 *Classification of Equipment*

The requirements for all electromedical equipment are specified by Australian Standard 2500 (1986).

Class I: Earthed equipment, having a three-pin plug connected to active, neutral and earth wires.

Class II: Doubly insulated equipment, having a two-pin plug (no earth connection) and a sturdy plastic outer case marked with the symbol ⧈ . Two layers of insulation are used in these devices, the 'functional insulation' around the live parts (the coloured plastic around the wires) and the 'protective insulation' which is the external case made of robust plastic. Failure of either layer alone will not provide a path for current. Failure of both is almost impossible without the complete mechanical fracture of the device, in which circumstance no one (we hope) would attempt to use it.

Class III: Low-voltage equipment (less than 40 V AC or DC) which does not produce a shock so does not require an earth. Equipment in this class has a special plug which can be connected only to its specified power supply.

8.11.2 *Classification of Patient Circuits*

Patient circuits are conductors of electricity that are in contact with patients. These circuits may be electrodes attached to patients for recording signals or delivering current, or parts of equipment which enter the patient or which contact liquid, which in turn enters the patient. Patient circuits within equipment may be classified as **cardiac protected**, **body protected** or **unprotected** (see Figure 8.4 for their symbols). Circuits designated body or cardiac protected meet specified design and construction requirements that cover their degree of insulation, the maximum allowable current in the circuits under normal operating conditions and during fault conditions, and the internal separation of circuits.

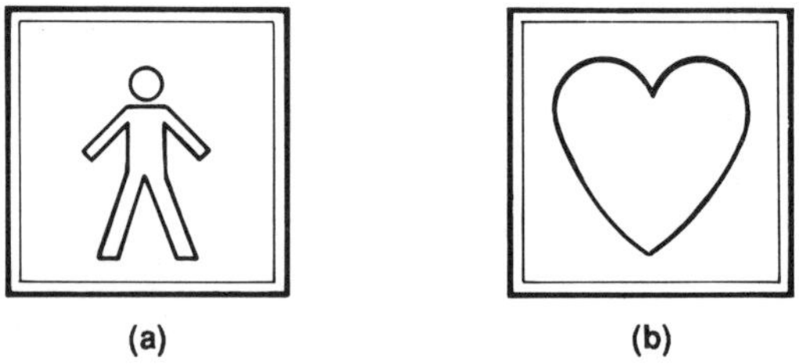

Figure 8.4 *The symbols used to signify (a) body-protected, and (b) cardiac-protected circuits, equipment and treatment areas*

8.11.3 *Classification of Procedures*

Medical procedures involving electricity may be divided into two groups: **cardiac-type procedures** and **body-type procedures**. Cardiac-type procedures are those where the hazard of microshock is present.

That is, they are procedures where a conductor such as a wire or a fluid column is in electrical contact with the heart. It would be possible for an electric current to flow from outside the body along the conductor to the heart without having to overcome the resistance of the skin. Examples are electrocautery, pacemaker leads, thoracic surgery, infusion systems, angiography, cardiology.

Body-type procedures are those where the hazard of macroshock but not microshock is present. Such procedures involve contact between the patient's skin and electrodes or equipment. Thus the skin presents a high resistance barrier to current. Examples are electroencephalogram, electrocardiogram, electromyogram recordings, ultrasound, some physiotherapy procedures and vascular impedance measurements.

8.11.4 *Classification of Areas*

In order to reduce the hazard of shock to patients from electrical equipment, the mains supply of electricity to a room or ward can be designed to meet specific requirements. Areas with electrical services so designed may be classified as **cardiac-protected areas** or **body-protected areas**. Such areas display the symbols in Figure 8.4. In cardiac-protected areas excessive earth leakage currents are guarded against by the use of a line isolation monitor or earth leakage circuit breakers. Furthermore, currents caused by different earth potentials are eliminated by the use of an equipotential earth system. Examples of cardiac-protected areas are operating theatres, intensive care units and coronary care units. The protection in body-protected areas is against macroshock only, so an earth leakage circuit breaker is installed. Examples are electrocardiogram, electroencephalogram, electromyogram clinics and physiotherapy departments.

To ensure the maximum safety during procedures involving mains electrical equipment, procedures of the cardiac type should use equipment having cardiac-protected circuits and a label like those in Figure 8.4. Furthermore the procedure should be carried out in a cardiac-protected area.

8.11.5 *Strategies for the Nurse which Enhance Electrical Safety*

- Ensure that the correct equipment is used for the type of procedure being carried out.
- Ensure that you know how to operate the equipment and that you operate it correctly.
- Do not use damaged equipment
- Do not tamper with equipment.
- Do not touch equipment with wet hands.
- Do not place cups or bottles of liquid, or wet clothes, or small metal objects on top of equipment.
- Remove power cords from the wall socket by pulling on the plug and not on the cord.
- Have frayed cords and damaged plugs repaired.
- Cords and plugs that become hot to touch during use should be removed from service.
- Do not replace fuses without first having the equipment checked.
- Do not use extension cords to plug another item of equipment into a remote power plug.
- Do not touch other pieces of equipment while holding patient circuits in your bare hand.
- Wear dry rubber gloves to handle intracardiac conductors.
- Carry out cardiac-type procedures in cardiac-protected areas.
- Plug patient circuits only into equipment with cardiac-protected circuits.

8.12 Bioelectricity

Many molecules have a net electric charge due to components such as the negative carboxyl group ($R{-}COO^-$) and the positive amino group ($R{-}NH_3^+$). In addition many inorganic substances such as sodium, potassium, chloride, magnesium and calcium are present in solution as ions. These charged particles are found both inside the cell and in the extracellular fluid. Consequently it should not be surprising that electrical phenomena result from the way that these charged particles are distributed and that they play a significant role in cell function.

Bioelectricity refers to any electrical phenomena that are produced within living tissues. The living cell membrane can maintain a difference in charge between the inside of the cell and the outside, the inside being more negative than the outside. This is because there is a slightly greater number of negative charges than positive charges inside the cell, and a slightly greater number of positive charges than negative charges outside the cell. The excess negative ions that are on the inside of the membrane are attracted to the excess positive ions that are outside the membrane. The resultant effect is that the membrane is sandwiched between a thin blanket of negative charge on one side and of positive charge on the other. This maintenance of a charge separation by the cell's membrane constitutes a voltage (its 'real' name is potential difference). Muscle cells and nerve cells generate this voltage or **membrane potential** to a greater extent than other cells so that their interior may be –90 mV with respect to the outside. Bone cells generate a negative potential at areas of active growth and repair. When bone is placed under stress, positive and negative potentials are generated which stimulate the body to remove or to add (respectively) bone at the site of stress (see Section 8.17).

Nerve impulses moving along nerves are just currents of electricity. The largest electric currents are produced in the heart and brain. The electrical impulses generated by the body may be detected by external electrodes as is done by the electrocardiogram (ECG) and electroencephalogram (EEG). Electrical impulses may be generated by instruments such as a pacemaker and applied to the body when it fails to produce its own.

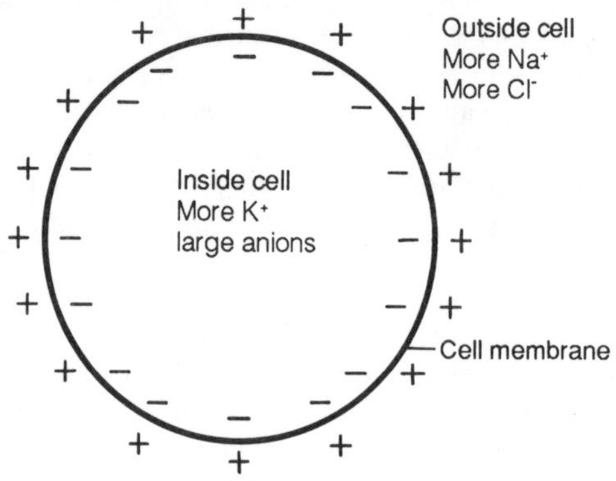

Figure 8.5 *The resting membrane potential is maintained by the differences in the concentrations of large anions, K^+, Na^+, and Cl^- ions on either side of the membrane*

8.13 The Membrane Potential

The membrane potential (also called the 'resting potential'), is not generated by electrons (the negative charge carriers involved in electrical conduction through wires), but by ions. Ions are atoms or molecules that have lost one or more electrons (like sodium (Na^+) and potassium (K^+)), or gained electrons (like chloride (Cl^-) and bicarbonate (HCO_3^-)).

The inside of the cell membrane is more negative than the outside because of the relative abundance of the different ions on each side of the membrane. Large ions such as proteins, phosphate and bicarbonate exist inside the cell and carry a negative charge (hence are called anions). Large ions such as these cannot normally pass through the cell membrane so help maintain the inside of a cell at a negative potential. In addition there are more Na^+ outside than inside (10 times more), less K^+ outside than inside (20 times less) and more Cl^- outside than inside (20 times more). The net result, when all the charges are taken into account, is that inside the cell is more negative than outside, that is, the resting membrane potential (while no nerve impulses are being conducted) is about –90 mV. In this state we say the membrane is **polarised** (see Figure 8.5).

The large differences in the concentration of Na^+ and K^+ ions between the inside and outside of the cell are maintained by the **sodium–potassium pump**. In a normal resting cell, Na^+ is actively transported out while K^+ is pumped into the cell (three Na^+ to every two K^+); that is, energy is expended to maintain the high ion concentrations against the influence of their concentration gradients. On the other hand, Cl^- ions diffuse passively (without the expenditure of energy) into and out of the cell in response to the charge difference between opposite sides of the membrane. The presence of large negative ions (too large to pass through the cell membrane) inside the cell ensures that Cl^- are electrically repelled to the outside.

8.14 Electrical Conduction Along Nerve Fibres

A nerve will transmit an electrical impulse along its length after electrical stimulation of its cell membrane. The electrical stimulation must be sufficient to alter the membrane potential from the resting level (–90 mV) to the threshold level (–75 mV). A stimulus that does not alter the membrane potential by 15 mV does not produce a nerve impulse. However, any stimulus above this value will produce a nerve impulse with a constant magnitude, regardless of the size of the stimulus.

Following a stimulus (which is above the threshold level) to the receptors or postsynaptic terminal of a nerve cell, it 'fires'. That is, the cell membrane lining the axon and dendrites of the nerve cell becomes more permeable to Na^+, so that they flow *into* the cell (along their concentration gradient). The change in permeability is due to the 'opening of the gates to the sodium channels' that exist in the cell membrane. The sudden and rapid inflow of positive charge **depolarises** the cell membrane (that is, changes the potential of the interior of the cell from about –90 mV to about +30 mV). Strictly speaking, the cell, rather than being depolarised, has merely had its polarity reversed. It is still polarised but now the inside is positive rather than negative. Nevertheless, physiologists refer to the effect as a depolarisation.

Following 'depolarisation', the ions that are adjacent to the site of depolarisation migrate along the membrane; that is, the positively charged sodium ions that have just flooded into the cell are attracted to the negative ions next to them on the inside of the cell membrane. This movement of charge alters the membrane potential of the piece of membrane that is next to the original depolarisation site and the potential gradually changes from –90 mV to –75 mV. A 15 mV decrease in membrane polarisation is enough to stimulate the sodium gates across the ion channels in the membrane to open. Thus some sodium ions can move into the cell as a second depolarisation event alongside the first one. This process of sodium ions crossing the membrane and then migrating sideways to trigger another depolarisation causes the depolarisation to propagate, in relay fashion, along the nerve fibre.

Shortly after depolarisation, the membrane becomes more permeable to K^+, so that they flow *out* of the cell (also along their concentration gradient). This sudden and rapid outflow of positive charge **repolarises** the cell membrane (that is, returns the interior of the cell to –90 mV from its depolarised potential of +30 mV).

The sodium–potassium pump continually returns Na^+ to the outside of the cell and K^+ to the inside of the membrane. The variation in the electrical potential across the membrane of the cell that is started by the stimulus, and followed by Na^+ ions moving in and then K^+ ions moving out, is called the **action potential** (see Figure 8.6). The action potential in an axon lasts for about 4 ms. It can recur thousands of times over, even without the sodium–potassium pump returning the Na^+ and K^+ ions to their 'proper' places. This is because there are so many Na^+ and K^+ and only a relatively small number of the sodium ions need to cross the membrane to depolarise it and only a small number of potassium ions need to flow out to repolarise it. Thus the extracellular fluid never runs out of Na^+ ions.

The movement of sodium ions into the nerve axon is the beginning of the action potential (the nerve impulse). At the peak of the action potential, the cell membrane is negative outside and positive inside which

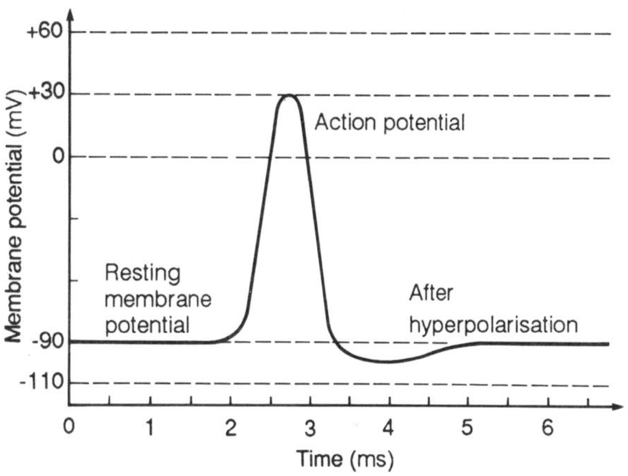

Figure 8.6 *The action potential. The graph displays the changes in potential difference between the inside and outside of an excitable membrane as its permeability to sodium and potassium ions changes*

is the reverse of the resting, polarised state. The reversal (depolarisation) of the cell membrane potential is transmitted along the axon or dendrite from the point of stimulus, as Na^+ move into the axon and then K^+ move out. This shuffling of positive ions across the membrane propagates along the axon and constitutes an electric current.

Myelinated axons are nerve fibres encased in a sheath of myelin (a lipid). The white myelin sheath is segmented, with small gaps called **nodes of Ranvier** between the segments (see Figure 8.7). The nodes of Ranvier are the only sites of depolarisation in a myelinated axon because only at the gaps in the myelin sheath can Na^+ cross the membrane into the cell and the K^- move out. Thus in a myelinated axon, the depolarisation jumps (saltates) from node to node. Axons in myelin sheaths have several advantages over unmyelinated axons:

- The sheath electrically insulates the axon from being depolarised by action potentials from adjacent axons.
- The sheath allows the nerve impulse to propagate at higher speed (by saltatory conduction) because fewer ions leak out of the axon. This leaves more ions moving through the axon towards the site of the next depolarisation so that site reaches its threshold potential sooner.
- Less energy is required to send an impulse along a myelinated axon. This is because fewer ions move across the membrane, so the sodium–potassium

pump has fewer of them to return to their original side of the membrane.

An action potential travels with speeds as low as 0.5 m/s in unmyelinated axons, and up to 130 m/s in myelinated axons. These speeds are far slower than electrical conduction in wires which occurs at almost 300 000 000 m/s. Most nerves have both myelinated and unmyelinated fibres, but myelinated nerves are the more common in humans.

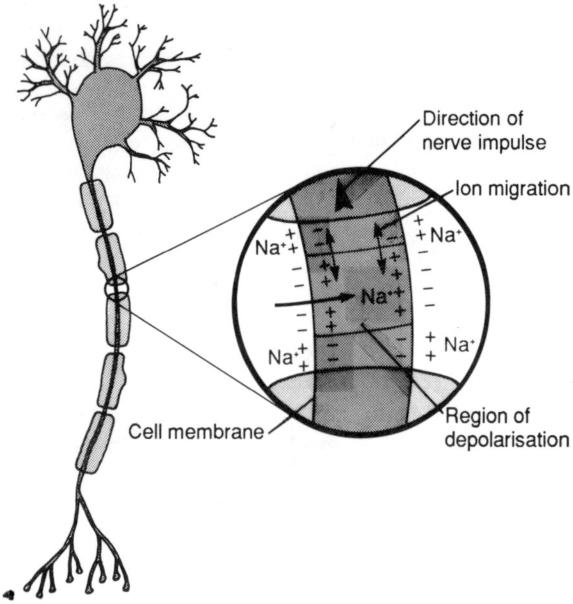

Figure 8.7 *Detail of a multipolar neuron (myelinated) showing that Na^+ ions have moved into the axon across the membrane. This inward movement depolarises the membrane. Ions within the axon then migrate along the axon to stimulate further depolarisation*

8.15 Bioelectrical Measurements

Bioelectricity measurements record the electrical activity by measuring the potentials (voltage) at the surface of the body that result from the electrical activity within the heart, brain and muscles. This is achieved by placing electrodes on the body in various combinations, amplifying the currents produced in them by the bioelectrical activity, and displaying them on a cathode ray tube or on a chart recorder.

8.15.1 *The Electrocardiogram (ECG)*

An electrocardiogram measures the voltage at the body surface that results from the action of the heart. The action potential for cardiac muscle may last from 150 to 300 ms. The electrical activity that starts in one part of a muscle can spread out, like a ripple on a pond, to other parts of the muscle. This causes a large-scale, uniform muscle contraction so that the whole wall of both ventricles contracts at once.

Electrodes are usually placed on the right arm (RA), left arm (LA) and left leg (LL). The measured potentials are 'vector' quantities so must be added via a vector triangle (called the **Einthoven triangle** after Willem Einthoven, a Dutch physiologist who pioneered the technique early this century). Each measurement involves only two of the electrodes at a time. For example, the RA and LA electrodes will produce a vector from right to left, and the LA and LL electrodes will produce a vector directed from shoulder to leg. When these two vectors are added, the result is called the **cardiac vector**. Many other forms of vector ECG are used as well as the one described.

The ECG is not a faithful representation of the action potential produced by the heart but has proved a useful diagnostic tool none the less. A typical voltage produced is 1 mV (see Figure 8.8). Observing the form of ECG traces from many thousands of healthy

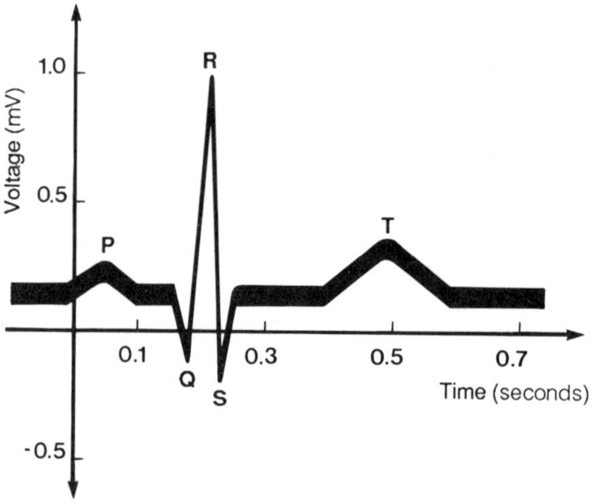

Figure 8.8 *A typical ECG from the right arm and left leg electrodes (lead II). The graph from Q to R to S represents the depolarisation of the ventricular muscle and the graph from S to T represents the change in potential as the ventricles contract*

subjects has resulted in a picture of the 'normal' ECG. Any variation from normal rhythm is known as **arrhythmia** and there are many of these.

8.15.2 *The Electroencephalogram (EEG)*

The electroencephalogram studies the electrical activity of the brain as measured by electrodes placed on the scalp. There are 26 or so sites of electrode placement on the head. Prior to placement, the electrode site is degreased and cleaned with alcohol to provide as good an electrical connection as possible and surface resistance is reduced by the use of a conducting paste. The electrodes are attached to the scalp with a quick-drying adhesive.

The typical EEG produces a relatively smooth oscillation with frequency between 8 and 13 Hz, called the alpha rhythm. The voltage produced is of the order of 50 μV.

8.15.3 *The Electromyogram (EMG)*

The electromyogram records the electrical effects of a muscular contraction by using electrodes placed on the muscle and then amplifying the signal. Alternatively needle electrodes may be inserted directly into the muscle. The signals may be generated by voluntary muscle contraction or by electrically stimulating the muscle to contract. The velocity of electrical conduction, normally between 40 and 60 m/s in healthy nerves in the limbs, may be used to diagnose abnormalities.

8.15.4 *Other Bioelectrical Measurements*

Electrical activity may also be monitored in the eye (electroretinogram), the stomach (electrogastrogram) and on the skin (electrodermal response, EDR). The EDR (also known by several other names) measures the activity of the sweat glands. When the subject is psychologically excited or is in some other elevated state of psychological activity, he perspires. Sweating changes the skin's electrical resistance so a potential may be generated between areas with many sweat glands and areas with few of them.

8.16 Electrical Devices in the Hospital

8.16.1 *The Cathode Ray Tube*

The cathode ray tube (CRT) is used in oscilloscopes, cardiac monitors, computer screens, medical imaging systems, television sets and electronic scoreboards at major sporting venues to provide an electrically controlled picture (Figure 8.9a). The 'cathode rays' are a stream of electrons produced at the cathode (in this case a heated filament with a negative charge) and accelerated by a large voltage to the anode (a positive electrode). After passing through a hole in the anode, the beam of very fast moving electrons hits the display screen of the CRT. On the way, the beam passes between two small, electrically charged, parallel metal sheets called the 'x-plates'. They produce a horizontal deflection of the beam. These plates are connected to

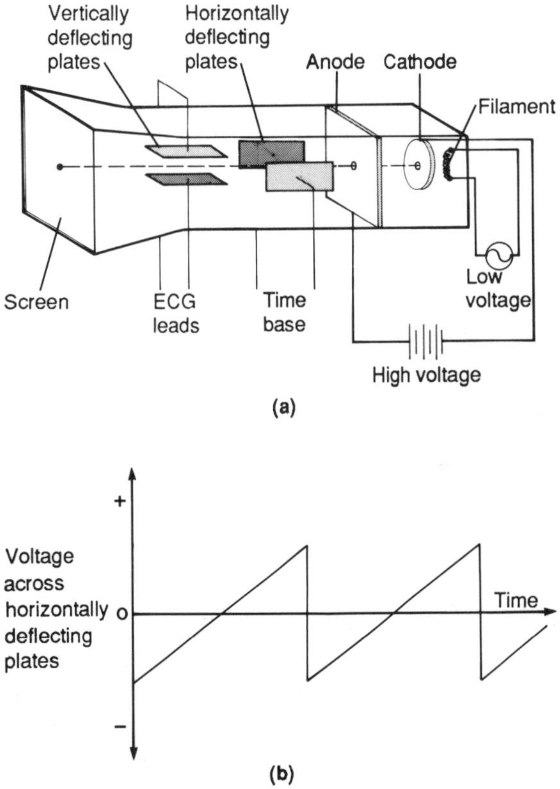

Figure 8.9 *(a) The cathode ray tube. (b) The 'sawtooth' variation in voltage applied to the horizontally deflecting plates with time*

an electrical circuit called the 'time base' which generates a 'sawtooth' voltage. This voltage gradually and steadily increases from a negative value to a positive value and then instantaneously switches back to the negative value to repeat the process (see Figure 8.9b).

The sawtooth voltage may be adjusted to cause the electron beam to sweep from left to right, across the screen, in a time interval that may be varied from microseconds to seconds. The time-base circuit in a cardiac monitor is pre-set so that the beam crosses the screen at the speed of about 25 mm/s. The effect of the time base can be likened to someone standing at the back of a darkened lecture theatre and shining a torch beam at the front wall. The x-plates are the side walls of the theatre, the torch beam represents the electron beam and is swept across the front wall (which represents the screen). A second pair of metal plates called the 'y-plates' are used to deflect the beam of electrons in the vertical direction (these vertically deflecting plates are represented by the floor and ceiling of the lecture theatre). To the y-plates are connected the wires carrying the incoming electrical signal. This may be coming from the electrodes that are attached to the patient undergoing an ECG, for example, or the impulses from a computer.

The screen of the CRT (the front wall of the lecture theatre) is coated internally with a fluorescent material so that a spot of light is produced when the beam of electrons strikes the screen. The fluorescence persists for long enough to show the path taken by the 'spot' of electrons across the screen under the influence of the charged deflecting plates. The screen forms part of a glass case (or 'tube') which surrounds and encloses the cathode, anode and the deflecting plates. The tube is evacuated so that the electrons do not collide with air particles on their way to the screen.

The CRT can be used as a sensitive measuring device as well as a convenient form of visual display. By adjusting the sensitivity control of a cardiac monitor, the ECG voltage (typically 1 mV) can be measured from the screen. When the sensitivity control is set at 2 cm per millivolt, an ECG trace of height 2 cm on the screen represents a normal 1 mV signal from the patient.

8.16.2 *The Defibrillator*

When ventricular fibrillation occurs, a life-threatening situation is present. Defibrillation must be attempted immediately. The process involves placing two electrodes on the bare chest of the patient, one on either side of the heart, and producing a current of several amperes through them. Such a large current momentarily flowing through the heart usually stops the fibrillation, because the cardiac muscle will contract strongly and clamp the heart shut. The pacing centres of the heart will often resume their normal activity when the large current ceases so normal heart beat will be restored.

A defibrillator basically consists of a transformer, a diode, a capacitor, a switch and the electrodes. The transformer converts the 240 V electrical supply to the high voltages required (7000 to 10 000 V). A diode converts the alternating current to a direct current, and a capacitor stores the charge (see Figure 8.10). When the two electrodes are placed on the patient's chest and the switch closed, a current of between 6 and 9 A flows for a few milliseconds (less than five) as the

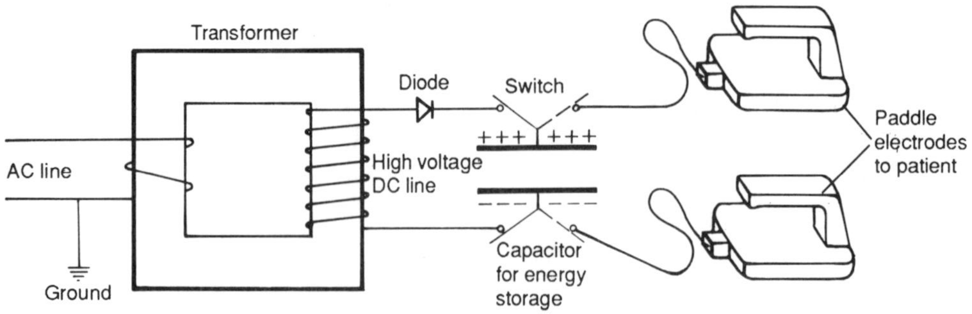

Figure 8.10 *A schematic diagram of a defibrillator. When the switch is thrown, the charge that has accumulated on the capacitor discharges through the paddles to the patient's chest. This produces a momentary, large current*

capacitor discharges through the chest and heart. The adjustable setting of the defibrillator device is calibrated in joules, so that between 200 and 300 J are delivered to the patient's chest, but this amounts to a current of between 6 and 9 A.

The electrodes (or 'paddles') are large (about 8 cm in diameter) and are covered by a conductive medium (pads or paste) to ensure a large area for the current to enter and leave the chest. This prevents an electrical burn to the patient occurring under the paddles. It is also important that the patient not be grounded and that no one touch the patient during discharge. If this is not the case, then some current would flow through the alternative path rather than from paddle to paddle.

8.16.3 *Electrosurgery (Diathermy)*

The body is most sensitive to electrical shock from AC electricity when its frequency is less than 100 Hz (which unfortunately includes the frequency at which domestic electricity is supplied). Nerves and muscles will not react to very high frequencies. High-frequency current will cause burns rather than ventricular fibrillation. It is used to arrest bleeding by closing off blood vessels. The neurosurgeon Harvey Cushing first introduced electrocautery to brain surgery in 1926 after having a device made to his specifications.

Electrosurgical instruments can be used for 'cutting' (electrosurgery) and 'sealing' blood vessels by coagulation of blood and necrotizing tissue (electrocautery and electrodesiccation). The voltages used vary from a few volts to 2000 V depending on the electrosurgical unit and the control settings for various procedures. Typical currents used are about half an ampere for desiccation and about 0.1 A for cutting. The high-frequency AC current (500 to 600 kHz for cutting and 2 to 4 MHz for sealing) is used to heat the probe and so damage tissue in a controlled way.

The electrosurgical probe is narrow (say 0.25 mm diameter) so that the current has a small entry point. This means that the energy is concentrated at a very small area and so produces a burn. The exit point is a large dispersive electrode, attached to the patient's buttock or thigh. It is wide enough to spread the energy over a large area and hence prevent a burn (see Figure 8.11). Good electrical contact on the dispersive electrode is ensured by using an electrically conducting paste, or an adhesive electrode which has been precoated.

Current flows when the probe is immersed in tissue. The instrument settings ensure that a high 'power density' (lots of watts per cubic centimetre) is produced at the probe. The high power densities produce a rapid rise in temperature (to 800 °C) at the probe, but cause an increase of only 0.1 °C at 1.25 cm from the probe. The rapid temperature rise is thought to rupture tissue due to the rapid boiling of the fluids. With proper control, the destruction can be limited to a depth of about 1 mm from the probe. Blood vessels can be closed off by dehydrating the vessel walls, which shrinks the vessel around a clot of congealed blood. This effectively seals off the flow of blood and bleeding is prevented.

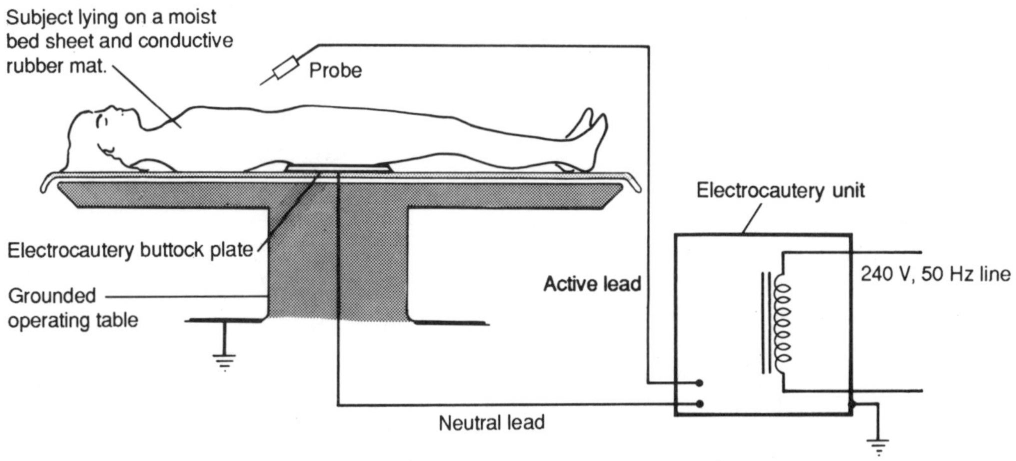

Figure 8.11 *Diagram showing passage of electrical energy during electrosurgery*

8.16.4 *Implanted Pacemakers*

Contractions of the heart are stimulated by an electrical signal that originates at the **sinoatrial** (SA) node of the heart. The depolarisation in the axons travels across the atrial walls causing them to contract. The depolarisation of the atria stimulates the heart's **atrioventricular** (AV) node to begin depolarising the conducting fibres known as **the bundle of His**. These carry the depolarisation to the **Purkinje fibres**. These fibres are muscle fibres which do not contract, but which rapidly conduct the depolarisation to all parts of the ventricle muscle so that all parts contract simultaneously.

If the AV node is damaged, electrical impulses from the atria are not passed onto the ventricles. When this happens, natural pacing centres in the ventricles will produce about 30 beats per minute. Such a low heart beat will produce semi-invalidity in the patient. To improve the quality of life for patients with faulty AV nodes, artificial pacemakers, measuring about 5 cm by 2 cm, are implanted subcutaneously.

In contact with the myocardium are electrodes from the pacemaker and the arrival of an electrical impulse from these causes the heart muscle to contract. The electricity for heart pacemakers can be supplied by lithium batteries, which have a life of up to 10 years, or by nuclear-powered batteries containing plutonium 238. The disintegration of this radioisotope provides the energy to produce the electrical impulses. The life of such batteries is being extended by better design and is currently about 16 years (but may be up to 40 years), after which time they must be replaced surgically.

8.17 Bone Repair by Electrical Stimulation

Bone is a peculiar substance. The collagen in bone gives it a high tensile strength and flexibility. The crystalline bone salt gives it high compressive strength (about 1.7×10^4 N/cm^2 for compact bone). Bone is also elastic. When you stand on one leg, the bone in that leg is shortened (squashed) by about 0.15 mm. Bone is viscoelastic; that is, it can withstand large forces for a short time without breaking, but if the same large force is applied for a longer time the bone will break.

Bone is continually being deposited by **osteoblasts**, and is continually being absorbed where **osteoclasts** are active. The continual deposition and absorption of bone has a number of important functions. First, bone ordinarily adjusts its strength (that is, its thickness) in proportion to the degree of bone stress. Second, even the shape of bone can be rearranged for proper support of mechanical forces by deposition and absorption of bone in accordance with stress patterns. Third, since old bone becomes relatively weak and brittle, a new organic matrix is needed as the old organic matrix degenerates.

When an individual is confined to bed rest, disuse osteoporosis sets in rapidly. With the restitution of weight bearing, the bone soon builds back to normal. This is an example of Wolff's (1892) law (that bone responds to stress by getting stronger). Another example is the straightening of a malunion in the long bone of a child as it grows, even though the bone bears weight. Some signal must arise from the concave side of the malunion 'telling' the osteoblasts there to lay down bone, and a corresponding signal must arise from the convex side of the malunion, 'telling' the osteoclasts there to remove bone.

It is a clinical axiom that bone forms in compression and fails in tension (hence the use of compression plates to promote fracture healing) but biological science could not explain the effect. Nor could it explain Wolff 's law. Since the most important function of bone is physical, namely to bear load, perhaps the 'signal' that directs bone formation and reabsorption is a physical one.

Some materials (called piezoelectric materials) produce an electric charge when a force is applied to

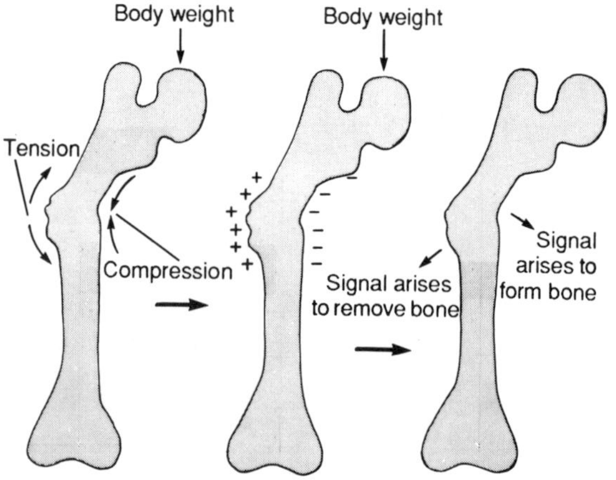

Figure 8.12 *Correction of the malunion in a child's femur, where stress generated by weight bearing produces an electrical potential which is a signal to restructure the bone*

them (see also Section 11.9). Bone is piezoelectric because collagen is a piezoelectric material. An electrical charge is generated on the surface of a bone when it is bent or stressed (see Figure 8.12). It is suggested that this electrical effect is the physical signal for bone growth.

Two types of electrical potentials were found in bones in the 1950s and 60s:

1. Stress-generated (or strain-related) potentials. Bone is a piezoelectric material, areas of compression are negative and areas of tension are positive (these potentials are produced even if the bone is completely decalcified).

2. Bioelectrical or standing potentials. Such potentials are due to living cells. Areas of active growth and repair are negative and less active areas are neutral or positive. Thus the growth plate and metaphyseal regions of a long bone are negative with respect to the diaphyseal and midshaft regions.

Rabbits were used to test whether external electricity applied to bone, given appropriate current and voltage conditions, could induce the formation of new bone. The result was that abundant new bone was formed around the negative electrode (the cathode). The technique was tried on humans in clinical tests from 1970.

Currents of between 10 and 20 μA (depending on the size of the bone) were passed through one or several electrodes inserted near or through the fracture site. The constant direct current was allowed to flow for 12 weeks, and the bone was immobilised for a further 12 weeks. The success rate for the treatment of the non-union of a fracture was between 80 and 85%. In one case union was achieved even after a 12-year non-union! Presently there are a number of methods that use electrical stimulation to heal non-union or congenital pseudoarthrosis or to accelerate fracture healing. They may use continuous direct current, pulsed asymetrical direct current, and pulsed electromagnetic fields. The method may be invasive or non-invasive. The latter uses pulsating electromagnetic fields generated by coils of wire attached to the outside of the cast. In this case the pulsating fields induce an electric current at the fracture site without the need for internal electrodes.

Bibliography

Brighton, C.T., Friedenberg, Z.B., Mitchell, E.I. and Booth, R.E. 'Treatment of non-union with constant direct current', *Clinical Orthopedics and Related Research*, **124**, 106, 1977.

Clare, R. E. and House, M. A. 'Prevention and treatment of lightning injuries', *Nurse Practitioner*, **12**(12), 37–45, 1987.

Standards Association of Australia AS2500. *Electrical Safety in Hospitals*, 1986.

Questions

1. The electrical resistance of the body, measured from hand to hand, will be different on different occasions. This is because the resistance of the skin
   J. increases as the skin gets drier
   K. increases as the skin gets damper
   L. decreases as the skin gets drier
   M. decreases as the hands are brought closer together

2. In order for the 'on–off' switch and the fuse to operate as intended, they should be placed on wires as follows:
   J. switch on active wire, fuse on earth wire
   K. switch on earth wire, fuse on neutral wire
   L. both switch and fuse on active wire
   M. both switch and fuse on earth wire

3. One difference between direct current (DC) and alternating current (AC) is that
   J. DC can produce a fatal shock, whereas AC cannot
   K. AC can supply power to portable devices, but DC cannot
   L. AC can be transmitted over long distances, but DC cannot
   M. DC can be easily transformed to a different voltage, but AC cannot

4. Which of the following statements about the action potential is *false*?
   J. The action potential lasts about 4 ms.
   K. It is triggered by anions crossing the cell membrane.
   L. The sequence: 'Na ions moving in, K ions moving out' constitutes the action potential.
   M. Repolarisation follows depolarisation of the cell membrane.

5. The letters ECG are short for electro-
   J. encephalogram
   K. colonogram
   L. cardiogram
   M. cryogram

6. The deflections seen on an electrocardiogram trace are due to
   J. pressure differences created by ventricular contraction
   K. the closing and opening of heart valves
   L. the transmission of electrical impulses through the conduction system of the heart
   M. variation in the electrical properties of oxygenated blood and deoxygenated blood as it moves through the heart
7. Suppose that while crawling around inside the roof space of your house you touch a bare wire with your bare hand while touching the brick wall with the other bare hand. You are most likely to get a fatal shock if the wire you touched was the
   J. neutral wire
   K. active wire
   L. telephone wire
   M. earth wire
8. Ohm's law relates the three electrical quantities known as
   J. current, resistance and potential difference
   K. potential difference, current and charge
   L. resistance, charge and current
   M. charge, current and potential difference
9. If a person is in contact with the active wire of a domestic 240 V electricity supply, a macroshock will occur if the current that flows is above/below (choose one) 1 mA and there is a second connection between the person and the active/ground wire (choose one).
   J. below........ active wire
   K. below........ ground
   L. above........ active wire
   M. above........ ground
10. In the fluids of the human body the carriers of charge that move through fluids are called
   J. cations
   K. ions
   L. anions
   M. electrons
11. In nerve fibres with myelin sheaths the electrical conduction
   J. is 'saltatory', so propagates at higher speed
   K. requires more energy to send an impulse
   L. between adjacent axons is enhanced ('cross-talk' is increased)
   M. is slower due to the 'nodes of Ranvier'
12. Household three-pin plugs on electrical cords are connected to three wires called
   J. earth, active and fuse
   K. live, return and fuse
   L. active, neutral and earth
   M. active, neutral and live
13. 'Defibrillation' is the process where for a few milliseconds a direct current of about
   J. 6 A is applied directly to the heart through a conducting path that bypasses the skin
   K. 100 mA is applied to the chest wall through two 'paddles'
   L. 6 A is applied the the chest wall through two 'paddles'
   M. a current of about 100 mA is applied directly to the heart through a conducting path that bypasses the skin
14. Choose the statement which correctly completes the following sentence: 'There are two types of electric charge called
   J. protons and electrons and they attract each other.'
   K. positive and negative and they attract each other.'
   L. anions and cations and they repel each other.'
   M. electrons and ions and they repel each other.'
15. A household light globe with a power rating of 60 W operates at a potential difference of 240 V and has a resistance of 960 Ω. Using this information and Ohm's law, the current (I) may be calculated to be:
   J. $I = V \div R = 240 \div 960 = 0.25$ A
   K. $I = R \div V = 960 \div 240 = 4$ A
   L. $I = P \div V = 60 \div 240 = 0.25$ A
   M. $I = V \div P = 240 \div 60 = 4$ A
16. A correct definition of macroelectrocution could be: 'that phenomenon which results from a prolonged macroshock produced by
   J. an electric current flowing directly to the heart without having to cross the skin.'
   K. the contact of bare skin to alternating voltages of over 100 000 V.'
   L. a fatal current in direct contact with unprotected skin.'
   M. switching on a faulty device that was earthed and had a fuse on the active wire.'
17. Some cells in the body can maintain an electric potential across their cell membrane. They do this by
   J. using the sodium–potassium pump to continually eject positive sodium and potassium ions from the cell
   K. allowing negative chloride ions to enter the cell along their concentration gradient
   L. trapping large cations inside the cell membrane
   M. keeping unequal concentrations of various ions on each side of the cell membrane
18. When making an electrocardiogram, to what part of the cathode ray tube in the cardiac monitor are the patient leads connected?

J. The vertically deflecting plates.
K. The horizontally deflecting plates.
L. The time base.
M. The anode and cathode.

19. An action potential is initiated when
J. the resting membrane potential changes from –90 mV to +30 mV
K. a nerve impulse has caused some muscle action to be produced
L. the potassium 'gates' in the cell membrane open and potassium ions flood into the cell
M. a stimulus, which is above the threshold level, is applied to a receptor

CHAPTER 9

Aqueous Solutions in the Body

The body of an adult human being contains about 42 l of aqueous solutions. This includes the blood plasma which plays a central role in the maintenance of good health although it makes up only a small proportion of the body's aqueous solutions. The importance of blood has been appreciated, in a general way, since ancient times, but it is only over the last century or so that we have been able to obtain particular knowledge of the changes it undergoes when health is impaired. These changes may be the result of health impairment or they may be its cause. In either case, when they can be measured they are of great value in diagnosis and therapy.

Another aqueous solution of the body is urine. Until about a century ago this was regarded, even by many physicians, with a mixture of disgust and disinterest. Now we know that urine is derived from the blood and that it also is a valuable source of information concerning a person's state of health.

The principles of physical science, although formulated mainly on the basis of observations made through the study of non-living systems, are applicable to living things. In this chapter we make an attempt to show how a knowledge of the chemistry of simple aqueous solutions has been combined with a knowledge of the anatomy and physiology of the human body to provide effective strategies for the diagnosis and treatment of disease.

Learning Objectives

At the completion of this chapter you should be able to:

1. Name the different fluid compartments of the body and describe some important differences in composition between the aqueous solutions found in different compartments.
2. Describe the processes of filtration, diffusion, facilitated diffusion, active transport, osmosis, dialysis and give examples of the operation of these processes in the human body.
3. Use a knowledge of the nature and concentration of solutes in a solution to determine its tonicity and predict the effect that it would have on the movement of water across a biological membrane.
4. State the relationship between the concentration units mol/l, osmol/l and equiv/l.
5. Explain what is meant by the phrase 'fluid and electrolyte balance' and describe, in general terms, the way in which the kidneys contribute to the maintenance of this balance.
6. Explain what is meant by the phrase 'acid–base balance' and describe the ways in which this balance is maintained.
7. Describe the common purposes for which intravenous therapy is used.

8. Describe some common causes and remedies for fluid and electrolyte disturbances including dehydration, hypo- and hyperkalemia, hypo- and hypernatremia, acidosis and alkalosis.
9. Describe the important features of the techniques of haemodialysis and peritoneal dialysis.

9.1 Fluid Compartments of the Body

The 42 or so litres of aqueous solution in the body are distributed into compartments and these are referred to as the body's **fluid compartments**. The walls of the fluid compartments are capillary and cell membranes. The **intracellular compartment** consists of the contents of all cells and it has a volume of about 27 l. The **extracellular compartment** consists of all the aqueous solutions found outside the body's cells. It has the following subdivisions.

1. **Plasma compartment:** This is the aqueous solution existing outside cells and confined within the blood vessels. It has a volume of about 3 l.
2. **Interstitial compartment:** This is the aqueous solution which fills the spaces between cells. Its volume is about 11 l.

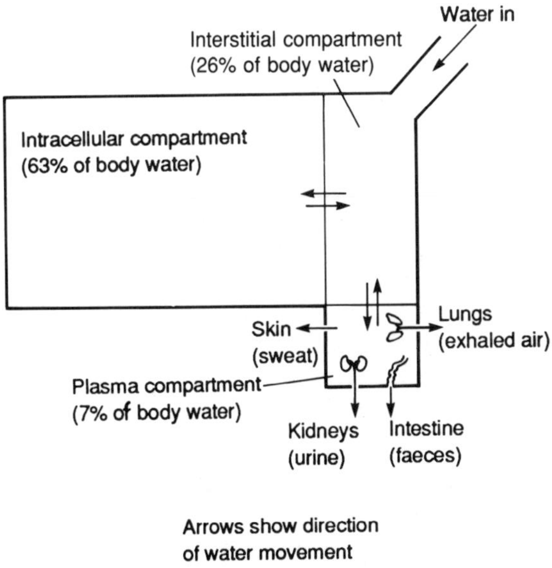

Figure 9.1 *Diagrammatic representation of the relationship between the body's fluid compartments*

3. **Transcellular compartment:** This consists of aqueous solutions located in quite different and specific parts of the body. These solutions are secretions of epithelial tissues. They differ from other extracellular solutions in that they do not bathe cells. Solutions in the transcellular compartment include **gastrointestinal fluid**, **intraocular fluid**, **cerebrospinal fluid**, **sweat** and **urine**. This is the smallest fluid compartment, having a total volume of between 1 and 2 l.

Figure 9.1 shows the relationship between these different fluid compartments. You will notice that the plasma and intracellular compartments do not share a boundary line and this emphasises the fact that within the body they are always separated by fluid of the interstitial compartment.

The compartmentalisation of the body's aqueous solutions does not mean that the contents of each compartment are entirely separate. There is constant movement between compartments across the membranes which separate them. However, in a healthy person the volume and composition of the solutions in each compartment remain the same.

9.1.1 *Movement of Water and Solutes Between Fluid Compartments*

This occurs via two quite different processes, **filtration** and **diffusion**.

Filtration. This is the process whereby a gas or a liquid is made to pass across a porous barrier by a pressure difference. The direction of movement is always from the side of higher pressure to the side of lower pressure. In the body aqueous solutions are filtered in the capillary bed of the circulatory system and in the glomerulus of the kidney. Filtration in capillaries causes movement of water and solutes other than protein (which consists of molecules too large to pass through the pores of capillary membranes) between the plasma and interstitial compartments. At the arterial ends of capillaries the pressure inside a capillary is greater than that outside and so movement is *from* the plasma *to* the interstitial compartment. At the venous end of a capillary the pressure difference is reversed and so is the direction of movement of water and solutes. In the glomerulus of the kidney, water and solutes other than protein move by filtration from the plasma to the transcellular compartment (urine).

Diffusion. This is the process whereby a gas or a dissolved substance moves *from* a region where its concentration is high *to* a region where it is lower. This direction of movement is often described as being movement **down a concentration gradient**. Diffusion occurs simply as a result of the random motion of the particles of the substance involved. It requires no pressure difference and continues until the concentration of the substance is uniform throughout the system.

A familiar situation involving the diffusion of a gas is when a bottle of perfume is opened in a room. It is not long before the perfume is detectable all through the room. Diffusion within a liquid may be demonstrated by dropping a crystal of some coloured, soluble substance, such as copper sulphate, into water. First of all, the blue colour of the copper sulphate is only seen in the immediate vicinity of the crystal. Then it begins to spread uniformly throughout the water showing that the copper sulphate is diffusing from the immediate vicinity of the crystal to all parts of the system.

The time taken for copper sulphate to diffuse through water, even when the volume of water is only a litre or so, is much greater than the time it takes for perfume to spread throughout a room even though the room may have a volume of many thousands of litres. Diffusion always occurs much less rapidly in liquids than it does in gases and if we wish to have a substance dissolve and spread throughout even quite a small volume of liquid we normally speed up the process by stirring. We do this when we have added sugar to a cup of coffee or tea. If we waited until the sugar had spread throughout the cup by diffusion we would have a cold cup of coffee or tea to drink by the time this had happened! Likewise, most cells of the human body would have a very long wait if they had to rely on diffusion to bring them nutrients from the gastro-intestinal tract or carry their toxic wastes to the kidneys for excretion. For movement over these long distances within the body something analogous to the stirring of a cup of coffee must occur. This is why we have a circulatory system which, through its capillaries, makes close contact with all cells of the body. This ensures that water and solutes only need to move tiny distances by diffusion in order to shift between the largely still intracellular and interstitial compartments and the constantly moving (stirred) plasma compartment.

While diffusion is not sufficiently rapid to move water and solute over large distances it is the first, indispensible step in this movement and we shall now look more closely at diffusion in the human body.

9.1.2 *Diffusion in the Human Body: Osmosis and Dialysis*

We begin here by pointing out that every solution must have at least two components: the solvent and one or more solutes. When we specify the concentration of a solution we normally focus our attention on the solute, but if you think carefully about concentration you will realise that it also says something about the solvent component of the system. A 0.9% (w/v) solution of sodium chloride is one in which we have 0.9 g of sodium chloride (the solute) dissolved in enough water (the solvent) to produce a total volume of 100 ml. Clearly, a solution which is 9% (w/v) sodium chloride contains a higher proportion of sodium chloride than the 0.9% (w/v) solution and a lower proportion of water. Thus, we may say that *the concentration of solvent in a solution decreases as the concentration of solute increases.*

Another important, general point to be made is that the essential difference between diffusion in a simple system such as a cup of tea and diffusion in the body is that the body contains semi-permeable membranes which are a barrier to movement of some components of the body's aqueous solutions. As a matter of fact, membranes hinder the movement of all components of a solution but they hinder some components more than others. Biological membranes are usually most permeable to water.

There are some rather striking observations which are made when whole blood is mixed with various solutions. For example, mixture with sodium chloride solutions having concentrations greater than 0.9% (w/v) causes the cells in the blood to shrink and change shape. This process is called **plasmolysis** or **crenation**. It also occurs when glucose solutions more concentrated than 5% (w/v) are used. If blood is mixed with sodium chloride or glucose solutions having concentrations substantially less than 0.9% (w/v) and 5% (w/v) respectively, the cells are observed to swell up and burst. This process is called **haemolysis**. Mixture of blood with either 0.9% (w/v) sodium chloride or 5% (w/v) glucose has no effect on its cells. These observations can be explained in terms of diffusion as follows.

From the fact that there is normally no net movement of water into or out of blood cells we conclude that the concentration of water inside and outside the cells is normally the same. When the highly concentrated solutions which cause plasmolysis are mixed with blood they raise the concentration of solute and, therefore, lower the concentration of water in the solution surrounding the cells. This creates a situation in which the concentration of water inside the cell has become higher than that outside. The cell membrane is permeable to water and so water diffuses from inside the cell to outside. This reduces the volume of the cell contents, causing it to shrink and change shape (plasmolysis).

When blood is mixed with solutions of low concentration this causes the solute concentration outside the blood cells to fall and the water concentration there to rise. Water diffuses from the outside of the cell to the inside. This increases the volume of the cell contents causing them to swell and eventually burst (haemolysis).

This diffusion of water across a cell membrane from the side where solute concentration is lower to the side where it is higher is called **osmosis**. You should always remember that it is simply a case of water diffusing from where its concentration is high to where its concentration is lower (that is, down its own concentration gradient). Water is not soluble in the material of which membranes are composed and it is usually assumed that it passes across them by moving through small channels which they contain.

Osmotic Pressure. Osmosis can be prevented by applying pressure to the solution on the side of the membrane towards which the water is moving. If a solution is placed on one side of a membrane and pure solvent on the other there will be a tendency for the pure solvent to move across the membrane into the solution. If a hydrostatic pressure is then applied to the solution it will oppose this movement and the applied pressure which is just sufficient to stop all net movement of water is called the **osmotic pressure** of the solution. Osmotic pressures for several aqueous solutions are presented in Table 9.1.

Table 9.1 *Osmotic pressures for different solutions*

Solution	Osmotic pressure (kPa)
1% sodium chloride	844
1% glucose	138
1% sucrose	72

A higher osmotic pressure for an aqueous solution means that more pressure must be applied on the solution side of the membrane in order to prevent movement of water into the solution. Thus, *the osmotic pressure of an aqueous solution may be taken as a measure of the tendency of water to move into the solution.*

When a membrane separates two solutions having different osmotic pressures water will always move *from* the solution having the lower osmotic pressure (and, therefore, the lower tendency for movement of water in) *into* the solution having the higher osmotic pressure (and, therefore, the higher tendency for movement of water in). Later in this chapter we will see that it is also possible to predict the direction of osmosis using a knowledge of solution concentration expressed in units known as osmoles. However, there are situations in the body where the movement of water occurs by a combination of filtration and osmosis. The tendency of water to move by filtration can only be measured in terms of a pressure difference between the two sides of the membrane through which the solution is filtering. This makes it essential to express the tendency for water to move by osmosis in pressure units also. Otherwise there is no way of knowing which effect, filtration or osmosis, is more important. In particular, if the situation is one in which filtration and osmosis are working against each other it will not be possible to predict the net effect.

Movement of Solutes Across Membranes. Water is not the only substance which is capable of passing across biological membranes and many solutes can do so. This is easily demonstrated by taking a bag made out of a membrane, filling it with plasma, and placing it in distilled water. It is not long before many components of the plasma are detected in the water outside the bag. The bag also swells because water moves into it by osmosis. We explain the presence of plasma components outside the bag by saying that the membrane is permeable to those components and they have diffused from inside the bag where their concentrations are high to the outside where they are lower.

There are two means by which water-soluble substances move across membranes. Simple ions and some small molecules pass through channels in the membrane. Other substances, which consist of particles too large to pass through these channels manage to get across by attaching to **carrier compounds** in the membrane. These are usually proteins (see Section 13.8.4) and movement by this method is called **facilitated diffusion**.

Dialysis. This is the name given to any process in which solute travels across a membrane from the side where its concentration is high to where it is lower.

Dialysis is exploited in techniques used to treat impaired kidney function (see Section 9.6). It is also used to separate proteins from the other components of biological fluids. The fluid is enclosed in a membrane bag which is then placed in a stream of running water. Protein molecules inside the bag are too large to pass across the membrane and so they are retained inside. Those components of the biological fluid which consist of smaller particles are able to pass across the membrane and so they move out of the bag by dialysis.

The processes of osmosis and dialysis are summarised in Figure 9.2.

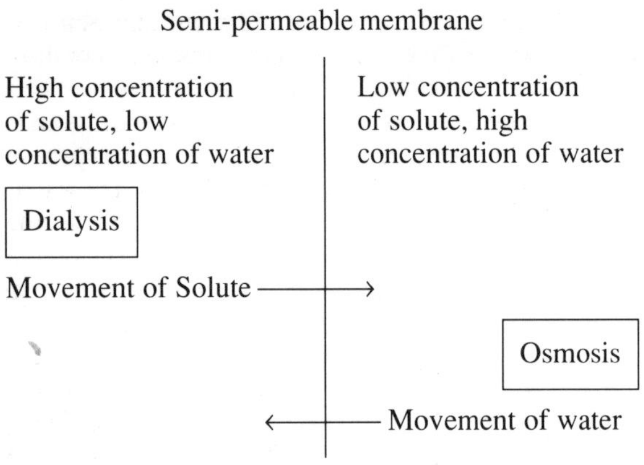

Figure 9.2 *Osmosis and dialysis*

9.1.3 *Tonicity: Isotonic, Hypotonic and Hypertonic Solutions*

Tonicity is a term used to describe the effect which a solution has on the movement of water into or out of cells with which it is in contact. A solution may be **isotonic**, **hypotonic** or **hypertonic**.

Isotonic Solutions. These cause no net movement of water into or out of cells. The two most commonly encountered examples are 0.9% (w/v) sodium chloride and 5% (w/v) glucose. An isotonic sucrose solution has a concentration of 9.5%.

Hypotonic Solutions. These cause a net movement of water into cells. A hypotonic solution always has a lower concentration than an isotonic solution of the same substance. Thus hypotonic solutions of sodium chloride, glucose and sucrose always have concentrations less than 0.9, 5 and 9.5% (w/v) respectively.

Hypertonic Solutions. These cause a net movement of water out of cells. A hypertonic solution always has a higher concentration than an isotonic solution of the same substance. Thus hypertonic solutions of sodium chloride, glucose and sucrose always have concentrations greater than 0.9, 5.0 and 9.5% (w/v) respectively.

It is clear that tonicity is controlled by concentration and a question which now arises is: 'Why do isotonic solutions of different substances have different concentrations?' They all have the same effect on water movement and so one might expect that they would all have the same concentration. The answer to the question is that they *do* all have the same concentration. To show that this is so we must make use of the *mole* to express concentration. (If you are not clear about what a mole is you should go back and read Section 3.5.)

The percentage (w/v) concentrations of isotonic glucose and sucrose can be converted to concentrations expressed in moles per litre by proceeding as follows.

For isotonic glucose:

1. 5.0% (w/v) means 5.0 g of glucose dissolved in every 100 ml of solution which, in turn, means 50 g of glucose dissolved in every litre (1000 ml) of solution.
2. The formula of glucose is $C_6H_{12}O_6$, while C, H and O have relative atomic mass values of 12, 1 and 16 respectively. Therefore, glucose has a formula weight of $6 \times 12 + 12 \times 1 + 6 \times 16 = 180$.
3. A mole of any substance is a sample having a mass, in grams, equal to its formula weight and so a mole of glucose is 180 g of glucose. Put another way we may say that glucose has a molar mass of 180 g/mol.
4. The number of moles in 50 g of glucose is $50/180 = 0.28$.
5. The concentration of a 5% (w/v) solution of glucose when expressed as moles per litre is, therefore, 0.28 mol/l.

For isotonic sucrose:

1. 9.5% (w/v) means 9.5 g of sucrose dissolved in every 100 ml of solution which, in turn, means 95 g of sucrose dissolved in every litre (1000 ml) of solution.
2. The formula of sucrose is $C_{12}H_{22}O_{11}$, while C, H and O have relative atomic mass values of 12, 1 and 16 respectively.Therefore sucrose has a formula weight of $12 \times 12 + 22 \times 1 + 11 \times 16 = 342$.
3. A mole of any substance is a sample having a mass, in grams, equal to its formula weight and so a mole of sucrose is 342 g of sucrose. Put another way we may say that sucrose has a molar mass of 342 g/mol.

4. The number of moles in 95 g of sucrose is 95/342 = 0.28.

5. The concentration of a 9.5% (w/v) solution of sucrose when expressed as moles per litre is, therefore, 0.28 mol/l.

So, we see that isotonic glucose and sucrose solutions have the same concentrations when concentration is expressed in moles per litre. Perhaps now you will want to ask: 'Why should we take any more notice of a solution concentration expressed in moles per litre than one which is expressed as percentage (w/v)?' The answer to this question is that a mole of any substance always contains the same number of particles (the Avogadro number which equals about 6×10^{23}). Isotonic glucose and sucrose therefore contain the same number of particles. In the glucose solution the particles are $C_6H_{12}O_6$ molecules while in the sucrose solution they are $C_{12}H_{22}O_{11}$ molecules. We need 9.5 g of sucrose dissolved in every 100 ml portion of solution but only 5 g of glucose because each sucrose molecule has nearly twice the mass of each glucose molecule.

For isotonic sodium chloride:

1. 0.9% (w/v) means 0.9 g of sodium chloride dissolved in every 100 ml of solution which, in turn, means 9 g of sodium chloride dissolved in every litre (1000 ml) of solution.

2. The formula of sodium chloride is NaCl, while Na and Cl have relative atomic mass values of 23 and 35.5 respectively. Therefore, sodium chloride has a formula weight of 23 + 35.5 = 58.5.

3. A mole of any substance is a sample having a mass, in grams, equal to its formula weight and so a mole of sodium chloride is 58.5 g of sodium chloride. Put another way we may say that sodium chloride has a molar mass of 58.5 g/mol.

4. The number of moles in 9.0 g of sodium chloride is 9.0/58.5 = 0.15.

5. The concentration of a 0.90% (w/v) sodium chloride solution when expressed as moles per litre is, therefore, 0.15 mol/l.

Now it looks as though we have run into a problem with this attempt to show that all isotonic solutions have the same concentration. The concentration of isotonic sodium chloride, expressed in moles per litre, is about half that of isotonic glucose and isotonic sucrose! However, there is a very important difference between the behaviour of sodium chloride and these other two compounds when each is dissolved in water. Sodium chloride forms separate sodium and chloride ions whereas the glucose and sucrose go into solution as intact molecules. The situation is summarised in Table 9.2.

So we see that every mole of sodium chloride which dissolves in water produces twice as many dissolved particles as a mole of either glucose or sucrose. Thus, while an isotonic sodium chloride solution has a concentration in moles per litre which is only about

Table 9.2 *Summary of the number and nature of particles which form as sodium chloride, glucose and sucrose dissolve in water*

		Number and nature of dissolved particles		Total number of particles
1 mole of sodium chloride	⟶	Na^+ ions + Cl^- ions		
6×10^{23} NaCl units	⟶	$6 \times 10^{23} + 6 \times 10^{23}$	⟶	12×10^{23}
1 mole of glucose	⟶	$C_6H_{12}O_6$ molecules		
6×10^{23} $C_6H_{12}O_6$ units	⟶	6×10^{23}	⟶	6×10^{23}
1 mole of sucrose	⟶	$C_{12}H_{22}O_{11}$ molecules		
6×10^{23} $C_{12}H_{22}O_{11}$ units	⟶	6×10^{23}	⟶	6×10^{23}

half that of isotonic glucose and sucrose solutions, the number of dissolved particles which it contains is about the same. It turns out that this is the feature which all isotonic solutions have in common: they contain the same concentration of dissolved particles.

Osmosis, then, is a phenomenon controlled by the concentration of solute particles. Water moves from regions where the concentration of solute particles is low (and the concentration of water particles is high) to regions where solute particle concentration is high (and water particle concentration is low). The nature and identity of the solute particles does not matter. Any property of a solution which depends on the concentration of solute particles and is independent of their nature is called a **colligative property**. Other examples of colligative properties are the depression of freezing point and elevation of boiling point of a liquid which occur when solutes are dissolved in it (see Section 7.6.2).

Osmoles, Units for Particle Concentration. Because the concentration of particles in a solution is so important in determining the effect it has on cells there is considerable value in having a way of expressing concentration which makes this explicit. This is achieved through the use of a unit called the **osmole** which may be defined as 'an amount of substance which must be dissolved in order to produce 6×10^{23} separate solute particles'.

For substances such as glucose and sucrose, which have molecules that remain intact when they dissolve, an osmole is the same as a mole. For ionic substances which form separate ions when they dissolve the relationship between moles and osmoles is:

$$\text{number of osmoles} = \text{number of moles} \times \text{number of ions in the formula}$$

or

$$\text{concentration in osmoles per litre} = \text{concentration in moles per litre} \times \text{number of ions in the formula}$$

All the different ways in which we have now expressed the concentrations of isotonic sodium chloride, glucose and sucrose solutions are set out in Table 9.3.

You may be wondering why isotonic sodium chloride does not have a concentration, in osmoles per litre, which is *exactly* equal to that of isotonic glucose and sucrose solutions. The reason is that the oppositely charged ions in the sodium chloride solution have an attraction for each other and this makes them associate to some degree. At any one moment there is always a small number of the ions which are organised as Na^+, Cl^- pairs. This reduces the number of completely separate particles present in the solution and accounts for the isotonic sodium chloride concentration being slightly higher than that of glucose and sucrose. These two substances exist in solution as neutral molecules and have a much smaller tendency to associate with each other.

Table 9.3 *Isotonic concentrations expressed in different units*

	Concentration		
Dissolved substance	% (w/v)	mol/l	osmol/l
sodium chloride	0.9	0.15	0.30
glucose	5.0	0.28	0.28
sucrose	9.5	0.28	0.28

Isotonic Solutions and Blood Plasma. Having established what all isotonic solutions have in common with each other, we are now in a position to go on and establish what they all have in common with blood plasma. First of all though, let us make perfectly clear what they do *not* have in common with blood plasma.

Plasma does not contain sodium chloride at a concentration of 0.9% (w/v) or glucose at a concentration of 5% (w/v) or sucrose at a concentration of 9.5% (w/v). There is no sucrose at all in blood plasma and the concentration of glucose present is about 0.0006-–0.001% (w/v). The concentration of sodium chloride in plasma is quite high but still significantly less than 0.9% (w/v).

The thing that plasma has in common with any isotonic solution is that it contains the same *total number* of separate solute particles. The majority of these particles are sodium and chloride ions but there are smaller numbers of each of many other particles also present. The composition of plasma is very similar to that of interstitial fluid, the main difference being that plasma contains an appreciable amount of protein whereas interstitial fluid contains very little. Plasma and interstitial fluid are both very different in composition from intracellular fluid and this is shown in Table 9.4.

Equivalent, Another Concentration Unit. In many American textbooks you will encounter electrolyte concentrations expressed in terms of **milliequivalents per litre** rather than millimoles or milliosmoles per

Table 9.4 *Electrolyte composition of the body's aqueous solutions*

Solute	Concentration in mmol/l	
	Extracellular fluid	Intracellular fluid
sodium	142	10
potassium	4	160
magnesium	1	30
calcium	2	0.5
chloride	100	4
bicarbonate	24	10
monohydrogenphosphate	2	32
dihydrogenphosphate	0.5	8
protein	0.5 (plasma) 0 (interstitial fluid)	1.5

litre. The equivalent is a unit which is used to specify the amounts of single ions and it emphasises the fact that ions vary in the amount of electric charge which they have associated with them. For example, the potassium ion has a single positive charge while the magnesium ion has a double positive charge and so a given number of magnesium ions will carry twice as much electric charge as the same number of potassium ions. One equivalent of any ion is an amount which carries the Avogadro Number (6×10^{23}) of electric charges and equivalents are related to moles as follows:

$$\text{number of equivalents of an ion} = \text{number of moles of the ion} \times \text{number of charges on the ion}$$

In Table 9.4, the concentrations of potassium (K^+) and magnesium (Mg^{2+}) in intracellular fluid are reported as 160 and 30 mmol/l respectively. In milliequivalents per litre (mEq/l) they have the values 160 and 60 respectively. The proteins in biological fluids usually exist as negative ions and there are many charges on each ion. Consequently, when protein concentrations are reported in milliequivalents per litre the values are much higher than when reported in millimoles per litre. The equivalent is not a particularly useful unit and its use is discouraged in Australia. It will not be used again in this book.

The most obvious differences in the compositions of the body's aqueous solutions are:

1. the much greater concentration of sodium ions outside cells (in the plasma and interstitial fluid) than inside and vice versa for potassium ions;
2. the much greater concentration of chloride ions outside cells than inside and vice versa for phosphate ions;
3. the lower concentration of protein in interstitial fluid compared to plasma and intracellular fluid.

The membranes of cells and capillaries are usually impermeable to many proteins and this explains why there is so little protein in interstitial fluid. Its high concentration in intracellular fluid simply corresponds to the fact that protein production occurs inside cells. The protein in plasma is produced in the liver by cells which are able to transport it across their cell membranes into the blood. Once there it is prevented from entering the interstitial fluid by the low permeability of capillary membranes.

It is rather more difficult to account for the striking differences between the concentrations of simple ions in different fluid compartments. Let us take, as examples, sodium and potassium ions. These enter the body in food and so they soon enter the plasma. A small proportion of the sodium in plasma finds its way into cells but most stays in the plasma and interstitial fluid. On the other hand, nearly all the potassium which enters the plasma finds its way into cells, leaving only a small proportion in the plasma and interstitial fluid. The cell membranes are certainly permeable to sodium and potassium otherwise both these ions would only be seen in plasma and interstitial fluid. But this raises the question of why each ion does not diffuse across cell membranes in the direction which would see its concentration become equal on both sides? The answer is that each ion does diffuse in this direction but the equalisation of concentration is not achieved due to the fact that cells are equipped with a means of constantly returning each type of ion to the side of the membrane where its concentration is greater. This is movement of material in the 'unnatural direction' and it is called **active transport**.

If we liken diffusion to the flow of water downhill then active transport is analogous to the flow of water uphill. Furthermore, we all know that water needs energy in order to flow uphill (it needs to be pumped) and the maintenance of concentration differences by active transport also requires energy. As a matter of fact, the amount of energy which the body uses for this purpose represents a significant percentage of its minimum requirement.

9.2 Fluid and Electrolyte Balance

In a healthy person the volume of all aqueous solutions and the concentrations of all the components of those solutions in every fluid compartment of the body stay within fairly narrow ranges. This is called **fluid and electrolyte balance**. It is largely (but not entirely) maintained by the **urinary system** which consists of the **kidneys**, **ureters**, **urinary bladder** and **urethra** (see Figure 9.3). The most important parts of the urinary system are the kidneys, which determine the composition of urine. The ureters, bladder and urethra simply provide for the storage of urine and its flow from the kidneys to the outside. The general structure of a kidney is shown in Figure 9.3.

It is the task of the urinary system to remove from the body all those substances which are toxic to it, while minimising the loss of all those other substances which the body requires in order to function properly. Each day a healthy person, eating a normal diet, eliminates 1000–2000 ml of urine. This consists of 96% water and 4% solutes. The identities and the amounts of the main solutes present in urine are given in Table 9.5 and compared with the total amounts which are initially removed from the blood as it flows through the kidneys. The comparison highlights the remarkable ability the kidneys have for recovering solutes from urine.

The functional unit of the kidney is the **nephron** which consists of a **capsule** and **tubule**. The capsule, known as **Bowman's capsule** surrounds a tiny network of capillaries called the **glomerulus**. The capsules of all nephrons are located in the cortex of the kidney. Those located well away from the medulla are called **cortical nephrons** and those that are located within the cortex, but close to the medulla, are called **juxtamedullary nephrons** (juxta means 'near to'). The tubule, usually called the **renal tubule**, leads from the capsule to a **collecting duct** which, in turn, leads towards the pelvis of the kidney and the ureters. Between Bowman's capsule and the collecting duct

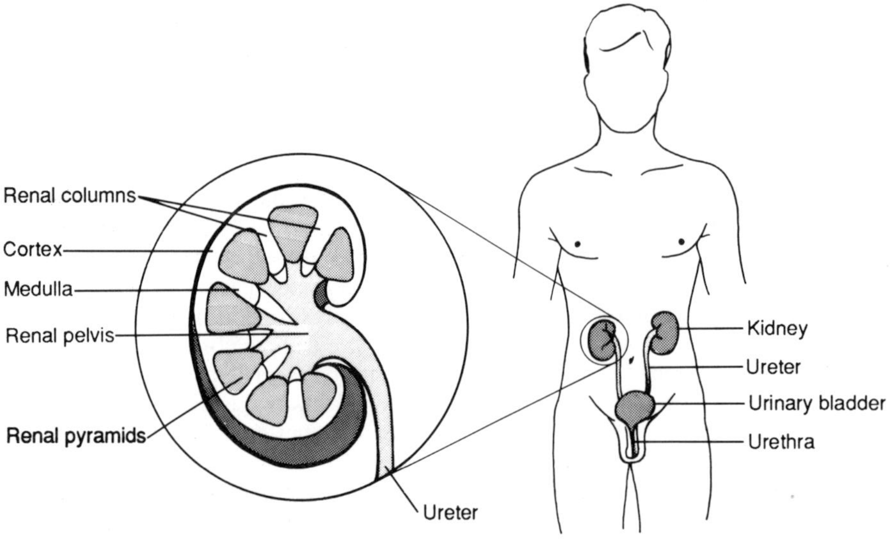

Figure 9.3 *The urinary system and kidney structure*

Table 9.5 *Solute components of urine*

Plasma component	Amount entering the kidneys (g/day)	Amount excreted in urine (g/day)
water	180 000	1000
Cations		
sodium, Na^+	540	4
potassium, K^+	28	1.5–2
calcium, Ca^{2+}	9	0.15
magnesium, Mg^{2+}	4	0.1–0.2
Anions		
chloride, Cl^-	630	7–10
bicarbonate, HCO_3^-	300	0.3
Organic compounds		
urea	53	30
uric acid	8.5	0.6

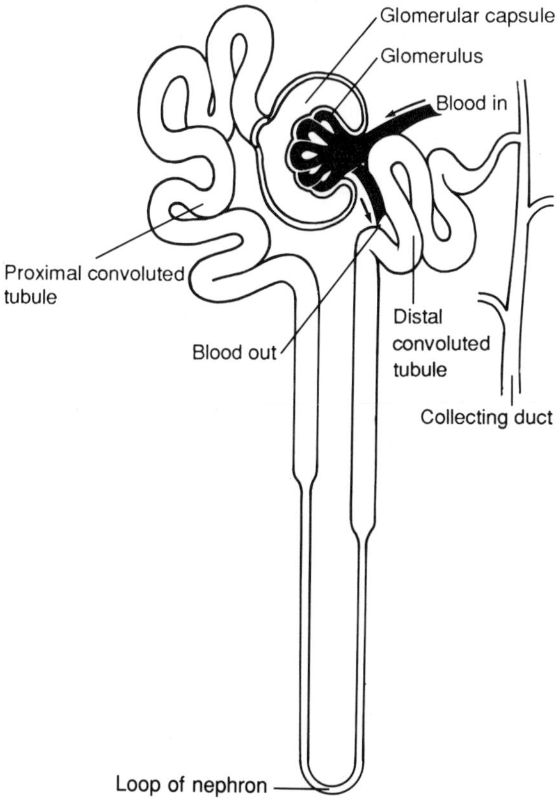

Figure 9.4 *Nephron structure*

(which is a part of the tubule) the renal tubules adopt the very characteristic shapes shown in Figure 9.4. Along the entire length of the tubule there exists a network of capillaries which ensures intimate contact between the tubules, blood supply and interstitial fluid.

The nephron is a remarkably versatile and efficient regulatory device. Every day about 180 l of aqueous solution move from the blood into the capsules of the kidneys' two million nephrons. All but about one litre of this is reabsorbed as it passes along the tubule. This one litre is the normal daily output of urine. Its formation involves all the processes which have been described above for the movement of material across membranes.

Filtration in the Nephron. In the capsule of the nephron the hydrostatic pressure of the blood inside the glomerular capillaries tends to push water and solutes across the capillary membranes into the fluid which surrounds them. However, the protein component of blood, being composed of very large particles, cannot cross the membranes and so the fluid inside Bowman's capsule, but outside the glomerular capillaries, has a lower concentration of solutes than the blood. This creates an osmotic pressure difference between the fluid and the blood. This pressure difference is often called the **blood colloid osmotic pressure** because it is due to protein which is present in the blood as a colloidal suspension.

Because the osmotic pressure of the blood is higher than that of the capsular fluid it tends to cause a movement of water *from* the capsular fluid *into* the blood. The capsular fluid has an hydrostatic pressure which also tends to send water and solutes back into the blood. However, the sum of these two pressures tending to send water and solutes back into the blood is less, by about 1.3 kPa, than the hydrostatic pressure of the blood which is tending to push water and solutes into the capsular fluid and so there is a net movement of water and solutes *from* the blood *into* the capsular fluid. This is shown diagrammatically in Figure 9.5. The proportion of the plasma which is filtered into the capsular fluid and then begins to move through the renal tubules is called the **glomerular filtrate**. It represents about 20% of the volume of the plasma flowing through the glomeruli each day.

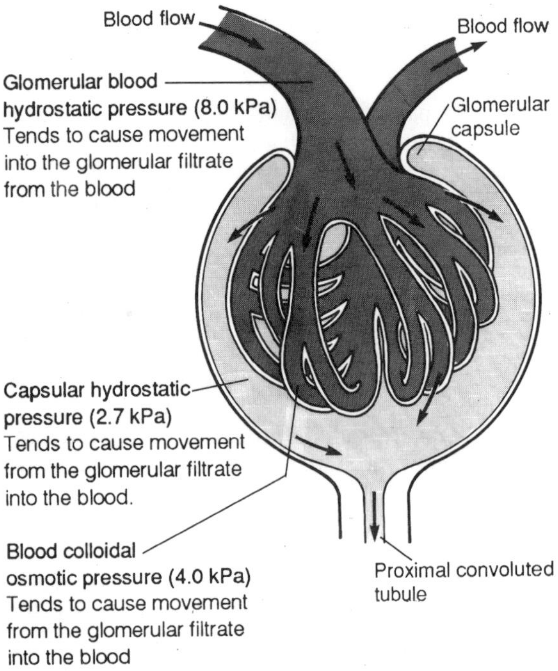
Blood flow
Blood flow
Glomerular blood hydrostatic pressure (8.0 kPa)
Tends to cause movement into the glomerular filtrate from the blood
Glomerular capsule
Capsular hydrostatic pressure (2.7 kPa)
Tends to cause movement from the glomerular filtrate into the blood.
Blood colloidal osmotic pressure (4.0 kPa)
Tends to cause movement from the glomerular filtrate into the blood
Proximal convoluted tubule

Figure 9.5 *Glomerular filtration*

Active Transport in the Nephron. In the glomerular filtrate which enters the proximal convoluted tubule (see Figure 9.4) the concentrations of most electrolytes and simple organic compounds such as amino acids, urea and glucose are about the same as they are in the plasma. With the exception of urea, most of these electrolytes and organic compounds are moved back into the plasma as the glomerular filtrate flows along the tubule. Active transport is very important in this process. It shifts a high proportion of sodium and chloride ions, which are the most abundant ions in plasma, back into the plasma. It also shifts virtually all glucose back into the plasma provided that the concentration of glucose in plasma is less than 10 mmol/l. At this concentration the ability of the tubule to recover all the glucose in urine is exceeded and some escapes. The plasma concentration of 10 mmol/l is called the **renal threshold** for glucose. It is exceeded in *diabetes mellitus* and may be exceeded in a healthy person who rapidly consumes a large quantity of glucose. In pregnant women the renal threshold may be lowered with the result that glucose appears in urine even when the intake of glucose is normal. In elderly people the renal threshold may be elevated and glucose may not appear in urine even when its concentration in blood is above normal. Most active transport occurs in the proximal convoluted tubule but it also occurs to varying degrees in other parts of the tubule. For example, active transport of chloride ions occurs in the ascending limb of the loop of the tubule and, in the presence of the hormone aldosterone, active transport of sodium occurs in the distal convoluted tubule and collecting duct.

Osmosis in the Nephron. Most of this occurs in the wake of the active transport of sodium and chloride ions. As these ions are transported out of the tubule into the surrounding fluid the concentration of that fluid increases and this leads to an osmotic shift of water out of the tubules.

Passive Diffusion of Solute in the Nephron. This also occurs in the wake of active transport. Where sodium ions are actively transported out of the tubule they produce a slight electrical charge difference between the solutions on the inside and outside of the tubule (sodium ions are positively charged and so the solution on the outside becomes positive compared to the solution on the inside). This causes ions which are negatively charged to follow sodium ions. In sections of the tubule where active transport of chloride ions occurs it is accompanied by diffusion of positively charged ions in the same direction.

This shift of water and solutes out of the glomerular filtrate back into the blood is usually called **tubular reabsorption**.

Not all the activity of the nephron is directed towards removal of water and solutes from the glomerular filtrate. Some solutes are added to the filtrate as it moves through the nephron and this is called **tubular**

secretion. The potassium content of urine is largely due to tubular secretion because most of the potassium originally present in the glomerular filtrate is reabsorbed in the proximal convoluted tubule. Tubular secretion of hydronium ions is important in the maintenance of a constant blood pH.

Urea Concentration in the Nephron. Wherever water is able to move across a biological membrane so can urea. However, the data in Table 9.5 show that while about 99% of the water in the glomerular filtrate returns to the blood less than 40% of urea does. The concentration of urea in blood is about 0.3 g/l and in urine it is about 25 g/l. All this raises the question: 'How does the nephron manage to produce such a high concentration of urea in urine?' Part of the answer is that water moves more rapidly than urea across biological membranes.

All along the nephron there is active transport of solutes (other than urea) out of the filtrate. In some regions where this occurs the walls of the nephron are permeable to water and urea. In these regions, water leaves the filtrate by osmosis and urea also diffuses in the same direction because its concentration is higher in the filtrate than outside the nephron. However, the movement of urea is slower than the movement of water and so more water than urea leaves the filtrate. This assists in the concentration of urea but it is only a small part of the explanation for the nephron's ability to concentrate urea. The anatomical relationship between the nephron and its blood supply is a major factor and there is also the fact that very high urea concentrations are found in interstitial fluid in some parts of the kidney. This high concentration reduces movement of urea out of the filtrate.

Water Balance in the Body. Although the kidneys have an impressive ability to excrete urine that is much more concentrated than plasma, thereby conserving water, this ability is limited. Every day a human being must produce at least 500 ml of urine otherwise there will be undue retention of urea and an increase in its plasma concentration. This is called **uremia** which means 'urine in the blood'. Water is also lost from the body by exhalation in air, by sweating and in the faeces. A human being cannot survive long without replacing these inevitable losses of water and a 'balance sheet' for the body's loss and gain of water is presented in Table 9.6.

The most variable components of water intake and output are, respectively, the quantity of water drunk and the amount of urine produced. The component of intake labelled 'metabolism' is water which forms as a result of the body's metabolic activity. Glucose, for example, is combined with oxygen to form carbon dioxide and water. In the body this takes place in many separate steps but the overall process is:

$$\underset{\text{glucose}}{C_6H_{12}O_6} + \underset{\text{oxygen}}{6O_2} \longrightarrow \underset{\text{carbon dioxide}}{6CO_2} + \underset{\text{water}}{6H_2O}$$

For every 100 g of glucose metabolised 55 ml of water are produced. Metabolism of the same quantities of fat and protein produce 107 and 41 ml of water respectively. On the output side of the water balance sheet the losses from the skin and from the lungs are often referred to as **insensible water losses** because they occur without a person being aware of the loss. If the rate of loss of water through the skin is greater than the rate at which it evaporates from the surface of the body then liquid water (perspiration) is evident on the body's surface and this is no longer an insensible loss.

In a healthy person water balance is achieved through the sensation of thirst and the secretion of anti-diuretic hormone (ADH). Both of these occur as soon as the concentration of plasma has increased by about 1–2%. This change stimulates the so-called 'thirst

Table 9.6 *Gain and loss of water in the body*

Water input	Amount (ml)	Water output	Amount (ml)
drink	1500	kidneys	1500
food	700	lungs	350
metabolism	300	skin	450
		intestine	200
total	2500		2500

centre' which is located in the hypothalamus, the person feels thirsty and drinks. It also stimulates the pituitary gland to release ADH which, in turn, stimulates the kidneys to retain more water.

Electrolyte Balance. Hormonal control is also important in the maintenance of electrolyte balance. The best example is the influence exerted over sodium and potassium concentrations by the hormone **aldosterone** which is produced in the adrenal gland. The effect of aldosterone is to stimulate the kidneys to retain sodium ions and eliminate potassium ions. In a healthy person aldosterone is secreted in response to a decrease in plasma sodium concentration. It stimulates the kidneys to retain more sodium and so shifts the plasma concentration of sodium back towards its normal value. As this happens, though, potassium is lost at a greater rate than normal and so it is often said that the kidneys tend to 'spill' potassium. If you look back at Table 9.5 you will see that the amount of potassium excreted in urine each day is a much bigger proportion of the amount which enters the kidneys than is the case with most other plasma components.

9.3 Acid–Base Balance

One of the most important electrolytes present in aqueous solutions of the body is the hydronium ion, $H_3O^+_{aq}$. This particle is the essence of acidity and it always co-exists in aqueous solution with another electrolyte, the hydroxide ion, OH^-_{aq}, which is the essence of basic (alkaline) nature. As the concentration of hydronium ions in a solution increases the concentration of hydroxide ions decreases and vice versa. Solutions which contain more hydronium ions than hydroxide ions are said to be acidic solutions, those which contain more hydroxide than hydronium ions are said to be basic or alkaline and those which contain exactly equal concentrations of the two ions are said to be neutral. In Chapter 7 we saw that it is usual to indicate the acid–base nature of a solution using the term pH, which is a logarithmic measure of the hydronium ion concentration. A pH value below 7 indicates an acidic solution, a pH value above 7, an alkaline or basic solution and a pH of exactly 7, a neutral solution.

In a healthy person the aqueous solutions in the three main compartments of the body all have a pH of 7.4 and so are very slightly basic. The concentrations of hydronium ions and hydroxide ions corresponding to this pH are:

hydronium ion concentration = 4.0×10^{-8} mol/l
hydroxide ion concentration = 2.5×10^{-7} mol/l

An obvious thing about these concentrations is that they are both very small in comparison to the concentrations of other electrolytes. For example, the magnesium ion, Mg^{2+}, is one of the less abundant electrolytes found in blood plasma but its concentration is 1×10^{-3} mol/l, which is about 25 000 times larger than the concentration of the hydronium ion.

However, the importance of the hydronium ion is out of all proportion to its concentration in the body's aqueous solutions. If the concentration doubles or halves, and stays that way for long, the person affected is likely to die. Because it is so small to start with, the doubling of the hydronium ion concentration in all the body's 42 l of aqueous solution only requires the addition of about 1.7×10^{-6} moles of the ion. This is much less than the amount which is present in a 500 ml carton of fruit juice, or which is produced when two aspirin tablets are dissolved in water. Since we often do such things as drink 500 ml of fruit juice or take two aspirin tablets, without suffering any ill effects at all, it is clear that these materials do not produce much of a change in the hydronium ion concentration of the body's aqueous solutions. The reason is that these aqueous solutions are all buffer solutions. The ability of the body to maintain the pH of the aqueous solutions which it contains close to the normal value of 7.4 is referred to as **acid–base balance**. In the next section we look closely at the buffer systems present in the body and the way in which they are used to maintain acid–base balance. If you are not clear about the action of buffer solutions you should go back and read Section 7.10.

9.3.1 *Buffer Systems of the Body*

The three main buffer systems of the body are: carbonic acid/bicarbonate buffer, phosphate buffer and protein buffer.

Carbonic Acid/Bicarbonate Buffer. This consists of the weak acid, carbonic acid (H_2CO_3), and its bicarbonate salts, sodium bicarbonate ($NaHCO_3$) and potassium bicarbonate ($KHCO_3$). At the pH of 7.4 the mole ratio of carbonic acid to bicarbonate salts is 1 : 20 and so body fluids contain about 20 times as much bicarbonate salt as carbonic acid.

The carbonic acid/bicarbonate buffer system is the major buffer system of the extracellular compartment. The concentrations of its components are about three times as great in this compartment as they are in the intracellular compartment (remember, that it is the *ratio* of buffer component concentrations that determines pH, not their magnitudes).

We saw in Section 7.10 that one component of a buffer system is capable of destroying hydronium ions and the other is capable of destroying hydroxide ions. In the case of the carbonic/bicarbonate buffer it is the bicarbonate component which destroys hydronium ions and the carbonic acid which destroys hydroxide ions.

$$\underset{\text{bicarbonate ion}}{HCO_3^-} + H_3O^+ \longrightarrow \underset{\text{carbonic acid}}{H_2CO_3} + H_2O$$

$$\underset{\text{carbonic acid}}{H_2CO_3} + OH^- \longrightarrow \underset{\text{bicarbonate ion}}{HCO_3^-} + H_2O$$

Since the buffer contains 20 times as much bicarbonate as carbonic acid it has a much greater capacity to protect the body against hydronium ions than against hydroxide ions. This is very appropriate because a normal diet supplies the body with more acidic material than basic material and normal metabolism produces more acid than base.

Phosphate Buffer. This buffer is a mixture of two different types of phosphate salts, dihydrogenphosphate ($H_2PO_4^-$) and monohydrogenphosphate (HPO_4^{2-}). Both types of salt are present predominantly as sodium salts in the extracellular compartment and potassium salts in the intracellular compartment. The buffer component capable of destroying hydronium ions is monohydrogenphosphate and the component capable of destroying hydroxide ions is the dihydrogenphosphate. At a pH of 7.4 the ratio of the two is monohydrogenphosphate : dihydrogenphosphate = 1 : 4. Once again, the component that is capable of destroying hydronium ions is present in larger amount. The phosphate buffer system is located largely within the intracellular compartment.

$$\underset{\text{monohydrogen-phosphate}}{HPO_4^{2-}} + H_3O^+ \longrightarrow \underset{\text{dihydrogen-phosphate}}{H_2PO_4^-} + H_2O$$

$$\underset{\text{dihydrogen-phosphate}}{H_2PO_4^-} + OH^- \longrightarrow \underset{\text{monohydrogen-phosphate}}{HPO_4^{2-}} + H_2O$$

Protein Buffer. Proteins have the capacity to act as buffers because they consist of very large particles within which are located acidic and basic groups of atoms. The acidic groups are usually carboxylic acid groups ($-\overset{O}{\overset{\|}{C}}-OH$) and the basic groups are usually amine groups ($-\underset{|}{N}-H$). These groups give each protein molecule the capacity to destroy both hydronium and hydroxide ions. The buffer action of a protein molecule is illustrated in Figure 9.6.

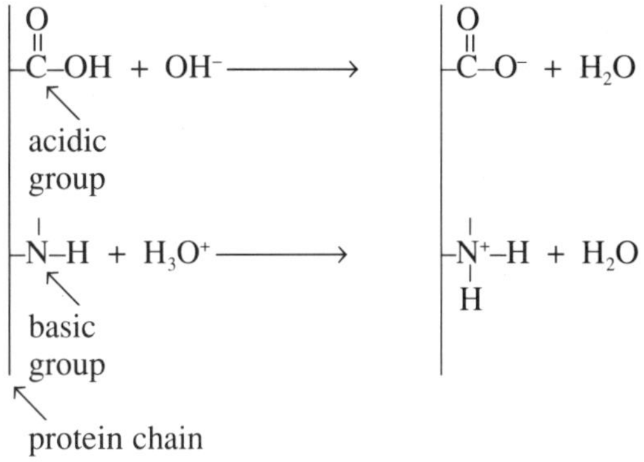

Figure 9.6 *Buffer action of a protein molecule*

The protein buffer system is located mainly in the plasma and the intracellular compartment.

9.3.2 *Long-term Maintenance of Acid–Base Balance*

We saw in Section 7.10 that the capacity of buffer solutions to resist a change in pH is limited. As acid or base is added to any buffer it will destroy most of the additional hydronium or hydroxide ions which enter the system, but as it does so one component of the buffer is changed into the other. This changes the ratio of the buffer components and so the pH changes. The ratio must change by a factor of 10 in order for the pH to change by 1 and this is why buffer solutions are resistant to a change in pH. However, the amount of acid which enters the body every day in food, or which is produced as a result of the body's metabolic activity, is more than sufficient to bring about such a change in the ratio of the components of the body's buffer systems. And yet in a healthy person there is no significant change observed in the pH of the body's aqueous solutions. This can be explained by taking account of the actions of the lungs and the kidneys.

The problem of maintaining acid–base balance is the problem of ensuring that the components of the body's buffer systems are maintained in their correct ratios (the ratios which correspond to a pH of 7.4). As more acid enters the body it reacts with the bicarbonate component of the carbonic acid/bicarbonate buffer, changing it into carbonic acid. This increases the value of the ratio carbonic acid : bicarbonate and leads to a fall in pH. Likewise, the monohydrogenphosphate component of the phosphate buffer is changed into dihydrogenphosphate, the ratio dihydrogenphosphate : monohydrogenphosphate increases and the pH decreases. In a healthy person the change in the ratios of the buffer components is never very substantial because the lungs and the kidneys work to restore them to their normal values.

The Lungs and Acid–Base Balance. The lungs contribute to the maintenance of acid–base balance because they control the rate at which carbon dioxide (CO_2) is removed from the body. This substance is formed constantly in all cells as a product of respiration and a proportion of it reacts with water to form carbonic acid.

$$\underset{\text{carbon dioxide}}{CO_2} + \underset{\text{water}}{H_2O} \rightleftharpoons \underset{\text{carbonic acid}}{H_2CO_3}$$

As acidic substances enter the body and cause a build-up of the carbonic acid component of the carbonic acid/bicarbonate buffer the rate and depth of breathing increases slightly. This results in an increase in the rate at which carbon dioxide is eliminated in exhaled air and leads to a drop in the concentration of carbon dioxide dissolved in the blood. This, in turn, produces a reduction in the concentration of carbonic acid, restoring the carbonic acid/bicarbonate ratio and the pH back to their normal values.

When a base enters the body its hydroxide ions are destroyed by reaction with carbonic acid. The carbonic acid is converted into bicarbonate, the ratio carbonic acid : bicarbonate decreases and the pH rises. Now the lungs respond with a reduced rate and depth of breathing. The rate of carbon dioxide elimination decreases, the concentration of dissolved carbon dioxide increases, leading to an increase in the concentration of carbonic acid. This restores the carbonic acid/bicarbonate ratio and the pH to their normal values. For a person in good health, eating a normal diet, the lungs are able to adjust the concentrations of buffer components quickly enough to ensure that they stay very close to the normal values.

The Kidneys and Acid–Base Balance. The kidneys also contribute to the maintenance of acid–base balance but the mechanisms involved are more complicated than those involved in pH control by the lungs. We need only say that the kidneys assist in the maintenance of acid–base balance due to the ability of the nephron tubule to control the movement of hydronium, bicarbonate, dihydrogenphosphate and monohydrogenphosphate ions between the glomerular filtrate and blood plasma. This control is exerted after glomerular filtration has occurred and so involves tubular reabsorption and secretion. The response of the kidneys to a change in acid–base balance is much slower than that of the lungs.

The direction in which different ions move under conditions of increasing acid or base load are shown in Table 9.7.

Table 9.7 *The kidneys and acid–base balance. Direction of movement of hydronium ions and buffer components*

	Increasing acid load		Increasing base load	
Ion	Urine	Plasma	Urine	Plasma
hydronium	⟵		⟶	
bicarbonate	⟶		⟵	
dihydrogenphosphate	⟵		⟶	
monohydrogenphosphate	⟶		⟵	

The Protein Buffer and Acid–Base Balance. In a healthy person there is very little excretion of protein and so the protein buffer is not influenced by the body's excretory processes. Nevertheless, the protein buffer plays an important part in the maintenance of acid–base balance. It does so because of the large number of acidic and basic groups attached to the protein molecules which are present in plasma and intracellular fluid. This adds significantly to the capacity of the body's buffer systems so that a given increase in acid or base load produces an immediate change in pH which is smaller than it would be in the absence of protein. It also means that the amount of adjustment which the lungs and kidneys need to make to the concentrations of the components of the carbonic acid/bicarbonate and phosphate buffers is smaller than it otherwise would be. In some situations the protein content of the blood may decrease and when this happens the person affected is rendered more vulnerable to disturbances of acid–base balance.

9.4 Solutions Used in Intravenous Therapy

Intravenous therapy is used to restore water to the body, to restore or maintain electrolyte balance and to provide nutrients. The first priority is always the restoration of water (rehydration). This will allow an assessment of kidney function to be made and this is essential before there is any significant addition of electrolytes to the blood.

The solutions used for water replacement and for the restoration or maintenance of electrolyte imbalances are usually isotonic or moderately hypertonic. Their rate of entry to the body is controlled to ensure that hypertonic solutions do not produce any significant increase in plasma concentration (which might cause crenation) and to ensure that the total volume of the plasma compartment does not become too great.

Rehydrating solutions usually contain glucose at a concentration of about 5% (w/v) and in addition they may contain a low concentration of sodium chloride. A commonly used mixture contains 4% (w/v) glucose and 0.18% (w/v) sodium chloride. Once it is circulating in the blood, glucose is subject to removal by metabolism and so the net effect of administration of the glucose solution is to increase the amount of water in the circulation by a larger margin than the amount of solutes. Pure water cannot be introduced directly into the bloodstream because it is so hypotonic that it would cause haemolysis.

Intravenous solutions administered to maintain electrolyte balance are referred to as 'balanced solutions'. They usually contain sodium, potassium, calcium and chloride ions. One example is **Ringer's Solution**, in which these ions have the concentrations 147, 4, 2.25 and 155.5 mmol/l respectively. Glucose is also often present in a balanced solution.

Where a person is unable to take food and drink by mouth for an extended period their nutritional needs can be met using intravenous solutions. This is called **parenteral nutrition**. However, the energy value of a solution which contains 5% (w/v) glucose is only 714 kJ per litre and the maximum amount of intravenous solution which can be administered each day is 3 l. The minimum daily nutritional requirement for a male having a mass of 75 kg is about 7200 kJ. It is perfectly clear from these figures that strongly hypertonic solutions must be used if a person's energy requirements are to be met by use of intravenously administered solutions. Of course, for a person receiving nourishment this way over an extended period the solutions used would need to contain other nutrients besides glucose.

The solutions used in parenteral nutrition usually contain high concentrations of glucose and lower, but still significant, concentrations of amino acids. Significant concentrations of electrolytes are also usually present. The total concentration of solutes in one of these solutions may be greater than 1000 mosmol/l which is more than three times as great as the concentration of solutes in plasma (280–300 mosmol/l). If such a solution was to be administered through a small peripheral vein (as most isotonic solutions are) it would significantly increase the concentration of plasma in the relatively small volume of blood with which it first mixed. This would cause crenation of blood cells and, to prevent this, solutions for parenteral nutrition are usually administered through the subclavian vein via a tube which empties into the superior vena cava, a very large vein. Furthermore, administration is usually controlled by an automated pump which ensures that the rate of entry of the parenteral nutrition solution is appropriate. These things guarantee that the highly concentrated, parenteral nutrition solution is always mixing with a large volume of blood and so its effect on the concentration of plasma is kept at a minimum.

9.5 Common Disturbances of Fluid and Electrolyte Balance

9.5.1 *The Role of Laboratory Measurements*

An observant clinician will often be able to detect cases of fluid and electrolyte disturbance by taking account of the procedures which a person has undergone and clinical signs such as body temperature, blood pressure, heart rate, skin turgor (the ability of the skin to resume its normal shape after pinching) and so on. For example, a person who has lost a large amount of fluid from their gastrointestinal tract as a result of vomiting, or diarrhoea, or gastric suctioning is prone to dehydration, changes in blood pH and reduced levels of sodium and potassium in plasma. A decrease in skin turgor often accompanies dehydration.

However, changes in skin turgor and in other traditional clinical signs are only ever indicative of fluid and electrolyte imbalance. Confirmation must be obtained through laboratory measurements. These unambiguously reveal the concentrations of the different components of the body's aqueous solutions and provide clinicians with objective data on which they may base their decisions about a person's condition and the treatment it requires. In a large, modern hospital there are always laboratory services available to provide rapid measurement of the concentrations, in blood and urine, of all the solutes we have been discussing and many others besides. This is a far cry from the days when the physician could do little more than use the colour of blood to judge its level of oxygenation and the sweet taste of glucose in urine to diagnose *diabetes mellitus*.

Sampling of Body Fluids for Laboratory Measurements. The body fluid most commonly examined is blood. Measurements are also commonly performed on urine. Other less accessible body fluids such as gastric juice or cerebrospinal fluid are only collected and examined in special circumstances.

Most solutes have the same concentration in both venous and arterial blood. However, it is usually venous blood which is used to determine these concentrations because the high pressure inside arterial vessels makes the sampling of arterial blood a more difficult and more risky procedure. Arterial blood samples are taken when the concentrations of blood gases (oxygen and carbon dioxide) are required. These concentrations are quite different in venous and arterial blood and the values for arterial blood provide more information about lung and heart function.

If a person is receiving intravenous therapy then any blood sample should be taken well away from the point at which the intravenous solution is entering the circulation. Otherwise there is the possibility that the blood sample obtained will be significantly diluted with the intravenous solution. If so, the concentrations obtained may be quite misleading. Another possible source of contamination is the anti-coagulant which is present in some syringes and sample tubes used to obtain and store blood. For example, the anti-coagulant heparin, which is a complex organic acid, is obtained in the form of sodium and potassium salts. In either of these forms it is unsuitable as an anti-coagulant for blood which is to be used in the determination of sodium or potassium concentrations. Care must also be taken to minimise the haemolysis of cells in a blood sample. This releases large quantities of potassium ion into the plasma (remember, the concentration of potassium inside cells is about 160 mmol/l and only about 4 mmol/l outside).

When laboratory measurements are performed on urine it is usual to collect all urine excreted over a 24 hour period. This minimises the chance of obtaining misleading values for the concentrations of components which are subject to variation in the rates at which they are excreted during the day (diurnal variation).

9.5.2 *Dehydration, an Example of Water Imbalance*

Dehydration occurs when the intake of water is reduced below the output. A person's intake of water may fall due to an impaired thirst sensation, reduced availability of water or due to severe weakness which prevents drinking. Output of water may be increased by an increase in urine production or abnormal loss of other body fluids through vomiting, diarrhoea and sweating.

Two laboratory measurements which indicate dehydration are the **haematocrit** and **osmolarity** of plasma. The haematocrit is the measure of the proportion of the volume of whole blood which is occupied by cells. It is obtained by placing a small sample of whole blood in a capillary tube and subjecting it to high-speed centrifugation. This packs all cells in a block at one end of the tube. Calibration lines on the tube are then used to estimate the proportion of the blood sample's volume which is due to the cells. In dehydration this proportion increases. Osmolarity is a measure of the total concentration of all solutes. It is usually determined by measuring the freezing point of the solution. Dissolved material always reduces the freezing point of a solution compared to that of the pure solvent (see Section 7.6.2) and this reduction in freezing point is proportional to the osmolarity of the solution. In dehydration, osmolarity of plasma is increased beyond the normal range of 280–300 mosmol/l.

Dehydration is corrected by an increase in water intake. This may simply involve an increase in the quantity of water which is drunk or it may be achieved by intravenous administration of a glucose solution.

9.5.3 *Sodium Imbalance, Hyponatremia and Hypernatremia*

Hyponatremia is said to exist when the concentration of sodium in plasma falls below 130 mmol/l. This may be due to an excessive intake of water in which case it is called **dilutional hyponatremia** because the amount of sodium in the plasma has not declined, it has simply been diluted by the extra water which is present. Sometimes a dilutional hyponatremia is caused by undue secretion of anti-diuretic hormone (ADH) which promotes excessive reabsorption of water from urine. This is known as **syndrome of inappropriate secretion of ADH** (SIADH) and it is caused by certain tumours and brain disorders. Another example of hyponatremia which does not involve a reduction in the amount of sodium present in plasma occurs in uncontrolled *diabetes mellitus* where blood glucose concentration increases greatly. This produces an increase in the osmolarity of the plasma and causes an osmotic shift of water from the other fluid compartments of the body into the plasma compartment. Hyponatremia may result from excessive losses of sodium such as those which occur with burn injuries and with prolonged vomiting and diarrhoea. In such cases the hyponatremia corresponds to a reduction in the amount of sodium which is present in the blood.

Correction of dilutional hyponatremias is best achieved by restricting water intake and, in these cases, the administration of additional sodium is usually avoided. However, in cases of SIADH, sodium intake may be increased by the addition of salt to the diet. If the hyponatremia is caused by uncontrolled diabetes then the level of glucose in the blood must be reduced by administration of insulin. Where hyponatremia is due to excessive losses of sodium, replacement by intravenous therapy is used.

Hypernatremia is said to exist when the concentration of sodium in plasma rises above 145 mmol/l. Its most common cause is excessive loss of water (dehydration) rather than an increase in the total amount of sodium. However, hypernatremia occasionally occurs as a result of the administration of intravenous solutions containing sodium. Hypernatremia is corrected by reducing the sodium intake and increasing the intake of sodium-free water.

9.5.4 *Potassium Imbalance, Hypokalemia and Hyperkalemia*

Hypokalemia exists when potassium plasma levels fall below 3.5 mmol/l. There are several common causes of hypokalemia. Administration of diuretic drugs promote excretion of relatively large amounts of urine and since the kidneys tend to spill potassium this is often accompanied by excessive potassium loss. In congestive heart failure there is increased excretion of the hormone aldosterone by the adrenal glands. This hormone promotes the reabsorption of sodium and the loss of potassium. Gastrointestinal fluid usually contains a higher concentration of potassium than plasma and so hypokalemia may be seen when there is excessive loss of gastrointestinal fluid.

Hypokalemia is usually corrected by increasing the intake of potassium. This may be achieved orally by consumption of potassium-rich foods such as fruits and vegetables, or by consumption of commercial potassium supplements. If the hypokalemia is severe then replacement by intravenous administration of solutions which contain potassium may be warranted. However, this must be done carefully. The rate of addition of potassium should not exceed 20 mmol/h and a check should be made to ensure that urine is being produced at a substantial rate. These precautions will help ensure that the hypokalemia is not converted into hyperkalemia.

Hyperkalemia exists when the potassium plasma level rises above 5 mmol/l. It is seen in a condition known as **Addison's Disease** in which aldosterone secretion is reduced causing excessive loss of sodium and retention of potassium. It is also seen in situations where a person has suffered a severe crushing injury. Here the hyperkalemia is due to the destruction of cells and the release of the potassium which they contain. This is also the cause of hyperkalemia seen in a condition known as **tumour lysis syndrome**. In this condition, large numbers of cancer cells die, break up and release their contents into the plasma.

Correction of hyperkalemia may be achieved by restricting the potassium intake and increasing the intake of water. The increased water intake stimulates urine production and increases the rate of excretion of potassium.

An interesting method sometimes used to correct hyperkalemia is the oral administration of **ion-exchange resin**. This is a type of material often used in water softeners. The resin consists of very large molecules which contain many negative groups of atoms bound by covalent bonds to the rest of the molecule. Each negative group is neutralised by one or more positive ions which sit within the material but are not bound to the resin molecules by covalent bonds. If the resin is placed in contact with a solution which contains positive ions different to those present on the resin an exchange occurs. In a home water softener the aim is to reduce the concentration of calcium ions in the water since these are responsible for water 'hardness'. The water softener is loaded with a resin in which sodium ions are present and as the water runs through the softener the calcium ions which it contains are exchanged for sodium ions. These do not cause hardness and so the water is 'softened'. The ion-exchange resin administered in the correction of hyperkalemia contains sodium ions and as it passes through the gastrointestinal tract it exchanges these for potassium ions which are present in the gastrointestinal fluid. This potassium is carried out of the body, allowing more potassium to move from the plasma into the gastrointestinal fluid thereby lowering the plasma level. This ion-exchange process is illustrated in Figure 9.7.

Hyperkalemia may be associated with impaired kidney function and it is often seen in dialysis patients,

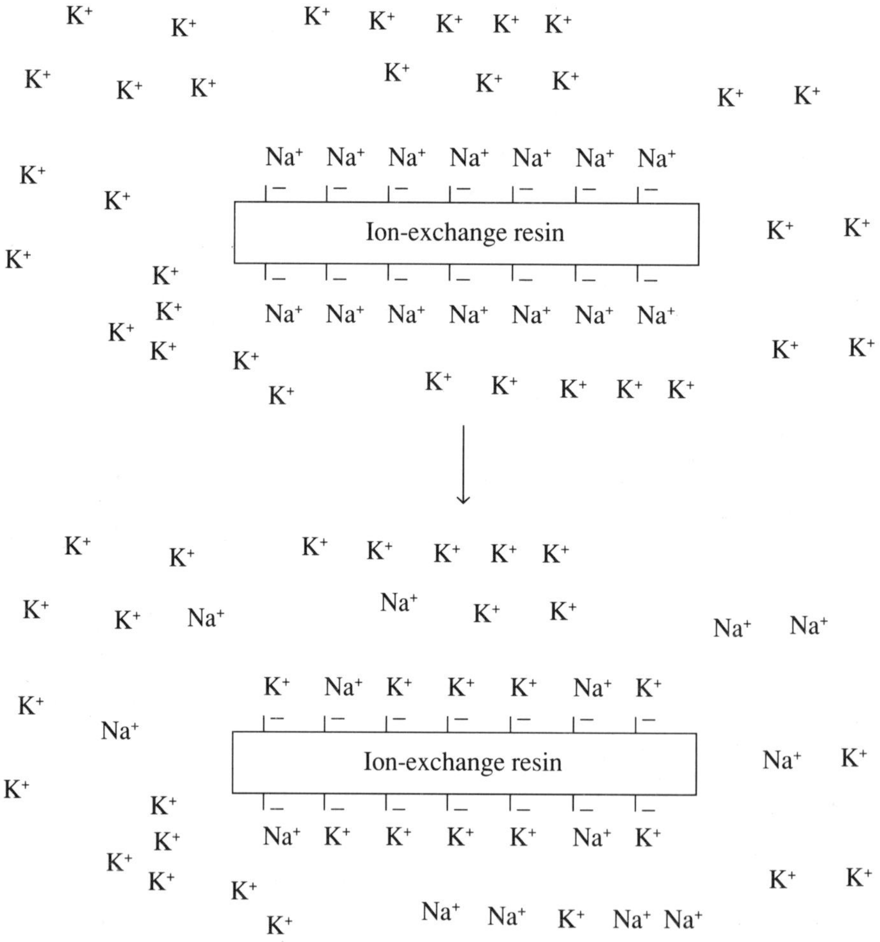

Figure 9.7 *Replacement of potassium ions by sodium ions using ion-exchange resin*

particularly if they miss a dialysis session or fail to maintain a low-potassium diet. In such cases the hyperkalemia is corrected by dialysis.

Although its concentration in plasma is much lower than that of sodium, potassium is often considered to be the plasma electrolyte of greatest importance. This is due to the fact that it affects the action of the heart and when a person is already in poor health quite small changes in the plasma concentration of potassium may have catastrophic consequences. Developing potassium imbalances are most readily detected by examination of the electrocardiogram (ECG) trace and a close watch is kept on this whenever there is reason to believe that a potassium imbalance may develop in a seriously ill person. The drawings in Figure 9.8 show the differences between a normal ECG trace and those seen as hypo- and hyperkalemias develop.

The effect which changes in plasma potassium concentrations have on heart action explains why it is a dangerous practice to use diuretic drugs as a means of weight control. This practice is adopted (often unwisely) as an alternative to diet and exercise. It may be adopted for very practical reasons by people such as boxers and jockeys who need to meet strict weight limits in order to earn a living. For these people the practice is particularly dangerous as they may suffer an episode of hypokalemia at the same time as their hearts are required to work very hard. This combination of circumstances occasionally proves to be fatal.

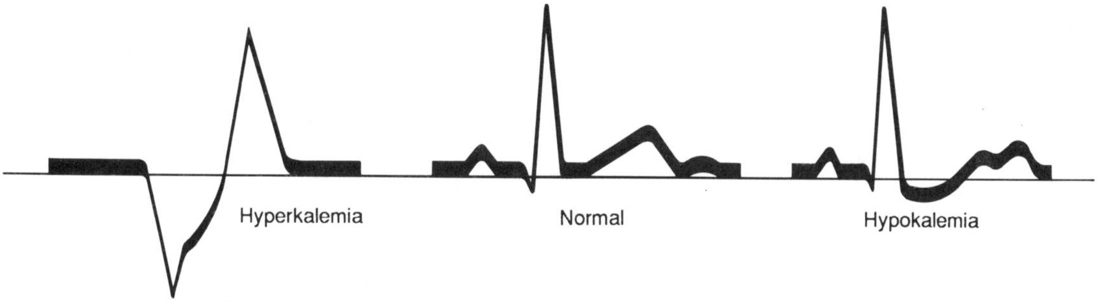

Figure 9.8 *Changes in ECG trace which occur in hypokalemia and hyperkalemia*

9.5.5 *Acid–Base Imbalance, Acidosis and Alkalosis*

Acidosis and alkalosis are usually defined as the conditions in which the pH values for arterial blood are below 7.3 and above 7.5 respectively. In strict chemical terms a solution is not acidic unless it has a pH below 7.0 and it is very rare for the pH of blood to be this low. Thus, acidosis does not mean that the blood is acidic in chemical terms. It means that it is less alkaline than normal. This is due to there being a larger proportion of acidic material in the body than normal and the term acidosis is used to signify this.

The acid–base status of the body is assessed on the basis of measurements performed on arterial blood, in particular pH, dissolved carbon dioxide concentration and bicarbonate concentration. You may be wondering why assessment of the body's acid–base status involves measurements other than pH. The reasons are that the blood is a buffer solution and many of its buffer components are subject to adjustment by action of the lungs and kidneys. This allows the possibility of blood pH being in the normal range even when there are processes occurring that have added or removed abnormal amounts of acid or base to or from the blood. In such situations there is the potential for acidosis or alkalosis but the conditions are not apparent from pH measurement alone because of compensatory activity by the lungs and kidneys. In these situations we say that **compensated acidosis** or **compensated alkalosis** exists. If the condition has been fully compensated for then the *ratio of the concentrations* of the components of the blood's buffer systems will be normal but the *actual concentrations* will not. This is discussed in more detail below.

Disturbances of acid–base balance are usually categorised according to their origin. If the disturbance arises due to some change in lung function it is a **respiratory acidosis** or **respiratory alkalosis**. If it arises from any other cause it is known as a **metabolic acidosis** or **metabolic alkalosis**.

Respiratory Acidosis. The cause of this is always **hypoventilation**, a reduced rate of excretion of carbon dioxide by the lungs. This may occur in people with respiratory impairment if their bronchodilator therapy is inadequate. In respiratory acidosis carbon dioxide concentration in the blood increases, causing an increase in the concentration of carbonic acid. Without compensation the ratio carbonic acid : bicarbonate increases above its normal value of 1 : 20 and pH falls. Compensation is made through action of the kidneys and this involves excretion of hydronium ions and retention of bicarbonate ions. The excretion of hydronium ions reduces the concentration of carbonic acid by causing it to undergo ionisation in an attempt to replace the hydronium ions that have been excreted. The retention of bicarbonate ions causes an increase in plasma bicarbonate concentration. Both these effects operate to move the ratio carbonic acid : bicarbonate and the pH back towards their normal values.

Respiratory acidosis is often accompanied by hyperkalemia and this is usually explained by saying that in acidosis hydronium ions diffuse into cells and displace potassium into the plasma in order to maintain the balance of electric charge inside and outside cells. The hyperkalemia is significant because it may have serious effects on heart action. To avoid this, a severe respiratory acidosis may be corrected by intravenous administration of sodium bicarbonate. In less severe cases, though, correction is attempted simply by taking steps to improve the rate of ventilation.

Respiratory Alkalosis. This is caused by **hyperventilation**, an increased rate of excretion of carbon dioxide by the lungs. This is much less common than hypoventilation but it may occur during episodes of severe anxiety, strenuous exercise or in the initial stages of asthma.

When hyperventilation is occurring the carbon dioxide concentration in the blood falls and this, in turn, causes a fall in carbonic acid concentration. If there is inadequate compensation by the kidneys then the ratio carbonic acid : bicarbonate decreases and the pH rises. Compensation by kidney function involves increased retention of hydronium ions and increased excretion of bicarbonate ions. The retention of hydronium ions leads to an increase in the carbonic acid concentration as the retained hydronium ions combine with bicarbonate ions to form carbonic acid. The increased excretion of bicarbonate leads to a decrease in the plasma bicarbonate concentration. The overall effect is to restore the carbonic acid/bicarbonate ratio and the pH to their normal values.

Most examples of respiratory alkalosis are self-limiting in the sense that if the episode of anxiety or strenuous exercise continues long enough the person will lose consciousness and so the cause of the hyperventilation will have been removed. Where hyperventilation has been caused by generalised anxiety it can be corrected by rebreathing from a paper bag. This raises the concentration of carbon dioxide in the blood, increases the concentration of carbonic acid and so corrects the alkalosis.

In Table 9.8 the values for pH, carbonic acid concentration and bicarbonate concentration in situations of uncompensated and partially compensated respiratory acidosis and alkalosis are presented. The table also contains a value for the concentration of carbon dioxide in the blood which is expressed as a **partial pressure** (see Section 10.8). This value is the one actually measured and the carbonic acid concentration is calculated from it. In many books you will see partial pressure represented using the symbol pCO_2. In this book we use the symbol $ppCO_2$ so that partial pressure is not taken to be a term of the same type as pH.

Table 9.8 *Carbonic acid, bicarbonate concentrations and pH values in respiratory acidosis and alkalosis*

	$ppCO_2$ (mm of Hg)	H_2CO_3 (mmol/1)	HCO_3^- (mmol/1)	$H_2CO_3 : HCO_3^-$	pH
normal values	40	1.2	24.0	1 : 20	7.4
uncompensated acidosis	90	2.7	24.0	1 : 9	7.2
compensated acidosis (partial)	80	2.5	38	1 : 15	7.3
uncompensated alkalosis	20	0.6	24.0	1 : 40	7.6
compensated alkalosis (partial)	25	0.8	20.0	1 : 25	7.5

Metabolic Acidosis. There are three common causes for metabolic acidosis. It may be caused by accumulation of acids in the blood such as occurs in *diabetes mellitus*. In this condition glucose is prevented from moving into cells where it is normally metabolised and so fat is metabolised instead. The end products of fat metabolism are mainly acidic substances and these enter the plasma. Once there, they react with the bicarbonate component of the carbonic acid/bicarbonate buffer system, converting some of it into carbonic acid. Metabolic acidosis may also arise from excessive loss of bicarbonate which can occur with severe diarrhoea. Gastrointestinal fluid (but not gastric juice) contains a higher concentration of bicarbonate than blood plasma and so loss of this fluid depletes the plasma of bicarbonate. The third common cause of metabolic acidosis is the ingestion or intravenous administration of acidic substances. These react with bicarbonate ion, converting it into carbonic acid.

No matter what the cause of metabolic acidosis there is a decrease in the plasma concentration of bicarbonate. If compensation by the lungs and kidneys is inadequate then the ratio carbonic acid : bicarbonate will increase and the pH will fall. The lungs compensate for a metabolic acidosis by increasing the rate of excretion of carbon dioxide. This lowers the concentration of carbonic acid in the blood. Compensation by the kidneys involves increased retention of bicarbonate and enhanced excretion of hydronium ions. All this moves the ratio of buffer components and the pH back towards their normal values.

Metabolic Alkalosis. This occurs when relatively large amounts of basic substances enter the body, for example when a person consumes a large amount of sodium bicarbonate in an attempt to relieve the symptoms of indigestion. Prolonged episodes of vomiting may also produce a metabolic alkalosis because the gastric juice which is lost contains a high concentration of hydronium ions which ultimately comes from the plasma.

Compensation for metabolic alkalosis involves the same mechanisms which are used to correct a metabolic acidosis. The rate of excretion of carbon dioxide via the lungs is reduced causing an increase in the carbonic acid concentration. The kidneys excrete bicarbonate at an enhanced rate and hydronium ions at a reduced rate. The combined effect of these compensating activities is an increase in the carbonic acid/bicarbonate ratio and a fall in pH.

Table 9.9 contains values for pH, carbonic acid concentration and bicarbonate concentration of plasma in metabolic acidosis and alkalosis.

Depending on the efficiency of compensating mechanisms, the pH of blood plasma may be very close to normal even when there is a substantial underlying tendency to alkalosis or acidosis. In such cases, however, the underlying conditions always leave their marks in the form of abnormal values for carbonic acid and bicarbonate concentrations (see Tables 9.8 and 9.9) and this is why these concentrations are determined in addition to pH.

Table 9.9 *Carbonic acid, bicarbonate concentrations and pH values in metabolic acidosis and alkalosis*

	$ppCO_2$ (mm of Hg)	H_2CO_3 (mmol/1)	HCO_3^- (mmol/1)	$H_2CO_3 : HCO_3^-$	pH
normal values	40	1.2	24.0	1 : 20	7.4
uncompensated acidosis	40	1.2	15.0	1 : 13	7.2
compensated acidosis (partial)	30	0.9	17.2	1 : 19	7.4
uncompensated alkalosis	40	1.2	38.0	1 : 32	7.6
compensated alkalosis (partial)	45	1.3	35.0	1 : 27	7.5

9.6 Dialysis and Impaired Kidney Function

The kidney is the only organ whose function can be replaced for an indefinite period by artificial means. The two techniques most commonly used for this purpose are **haemodialysis** and **peritoneal dialysis**. In both of these techniques poisonous materials are removed from the blood by their diffusion across a semi-permeable membrane from the side where their concentrations are higher to the side where they are lower.

9.6.1 *Haemodialysis*

This technique is **extracorporeal** which means that dialysis occurs outside the body. It makes use of a **dialyser** and this part of haemodialysis equipment is often referred to as an **artificial kidney**. The essential component of a dialyser is a semi-permeable membrane, usually cellulose. This membrane may be in the form of sheets or hollow tubes and the dialyser is constructed so that blood flows on one side of the membrane while a **dialysing** solution, often called the **dialysate**, flows on the other.

In haemodialysis access to the patient's bloodstream is usually obtained through an artery in the lower leg or arm. Blood flows from the artery through the dialyser and back into the body through a vein. The dialysate flows from a reservoir into the dialyser and then to a drain (see Figure 9.9).

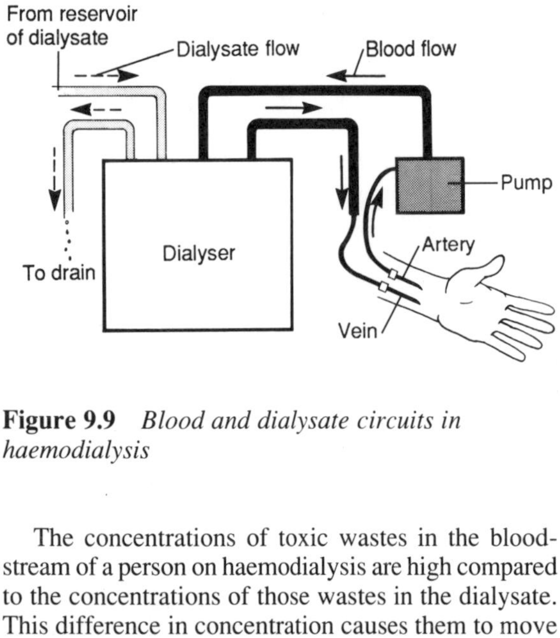

Figure 9.9 *Blood and dialysate circuits in haemodialysis*

The concentrations of toxic wastes in the bloodstream of a person on haemodialysis are high compared to the concentrations of those wastes in the dialysate. This difference in concentration causes them to move out of the blood into the dialysate which is drained away. After a while, usually 2–4 hours, the concentrations of waste materials in the blood are reduced to normal. The concentrations of electrolytes in the dialysate are close to normal and there is relatively little net movement of these between the blood and the dialysate.

When there is impaired kidney function water accumulates in the body and it must be removed during the haemodialysis session. This removal is achieved as a result of the pressure difference which exists across the dialyser membrane. On the blood side of the membrane the pressure is always higher and so there is a movement of water (and small solutes) out of the blood into the dialysate. The pressure difference across the membrane of a dialyser is called the **transmembrane pressure** (TMP) and it can be adjusted to control the rate at which water is removed during haemodialysis.

Although the dialyser is the working unit in haemodialysis its use requires a great deal of other equipment. A blood pump is used to move the blood through the dialyser at the appropriate rate (usually 200–300 ml/min). Mixing equipment is required to produce the dialysate from its component solutions. The dialysing solution must be warmed to body temperature before it comes in contact with the blood in the dialyser. Monitoring devices are required to detect air bubbles in the stream of blood returning to the body, to provide information concerning the pressure at various points in the blood circuit, to detect blood leaks within the dialyser and so on. This complexity of the equipment used in haemodialysis makes it a technique which is usually carried out in hospitals under the control of specially trained medical and nursing staff. However, many health services do offer home dialysis programs and the number of people using these is increasing.

9.6.2 *Peritoneal Dialysis*

With this technique the semi-permeable membrane used is the **peritoneum**. This is the membrane which lines the abdominal (often called the peritoneal) cavity and covers the organs within it (stomach, intestines, liver and so on). Entry is gained to the peritoneal cavity by making a small incision in the skin on the anterior surface of the body about 3 cm below the umbilicus. A catheter is then inserted through the abdominal wall using a sharp metal tool called an **obdurator**. The dialysate is instilled into, and withdrawn from, the peritoneal cavity by gravity flow. Prior to instillation it must be warmed to body temperature because infusion of cold dialysate causes distress. The time the dialysate remains in the peritoneal cavity is usually about 30–40 min. During this time, waste materials move out of the blood and into the dialysate. As was the case with haemodialysis the concentrations of the electrolytes in the dialysate are similar to those normally found in the blood. Consequently there is minimal movement of these electrolytes between the blood and the dialysate. Peritoneal dialysis, because of its lower dependence on complicated equipment, lends itself more readily to management at home and there are many people who are able to see to their own peritoneal dialysis while going about the ordinary activities of daily life.

An important difference between haemodialysis and peritoneal dialysis is that the pressure difference across the peritoneal membrane is too small to cause filtration of water into the dialysate. In peritoneal dialysis this movement of water is achieved osmotically by including a relatively high concentration of glucose in the dialysate. This may range from about 80–250 mosmol/l. The compositions of typical dialysates used in haemodialysis and peritoneal dialysis are given in Table 9.10. The exact composition used for a particular dialysis treatment will depend on the circumstances which apply.

Table 9.10 *Compositions for typical dialysates*

	Concentration (mosmol/l)	
Component	Haemodialysis	Peritoneal dialysis
sodium ion	135–145	132
potassium ion	0–4	—
calcium ion	1.25–1.75	1.25–1.75
magnesium ion	0.25–0.5	0.25–0.5
chloride ion	100–124	98
bicarbonate ion	30–38	—
acetic acid	2–4	—
glucose	11	80–250
lactic acid	—	40

Bibliography

Daurgidas, J. T. and Ing, T. S. *Handbook of Dialysis*. Little, Brown and Company, Toronto, 1988.

Delaney, C. W. and Lauer, M. L. *Intravenous Therapy. A Guide to Quality Care*. J. B. Lippincott, Philadelphia, 1988.

Hamilton, Helen (ed.). *Monitoring Fluids and Electrolytes Precisely*. Intermed Communications, Pennsylvania, 1981.

Lamb, Jane. *Laboratory Tests for Clinical Nursing*. Brady Communications Company, Maryland, 1984.

Porth, Carol M. *Pathophysiology. Concepts of Altered Health States* (second edition). J. B. Lippincott, Philadelphia, 1986.

Sherman, A. and Sherman, Sharon. *The Elements of Life. An Approach to Chemistry for the Health Sciences*. Prentice-Hall, New Jersey, 1980.

Tortora, G. J. and Anagnostakos, N. P. *Principles of Anatomy and Physiology* (fifth edition). Harper and Row, New York, 1987.

Questions

1. The largest fluid compartment of the body is the
   J. intracellular compartment
   K. plasma compartment
   L. interstitial compartment
   M. transcellular compartment
2. The main process occurring in the glomerulus of the kidney is
   J. concentration
   K. diffusion
   L. filtration
   M. secretion
3. Which of the following components of urine is reabsorbed to the greatest extent in the kidneys?
   J. bicarbonate
   K. chloride
   L. sodium
   M. water
4. Which of the following components of urine is concentrated to the greatest extent in the kidneys?
   J. phosphate
   K. potassium
   L. protein
   M. urea
5. The hormone aldosterone acts on the kidneys to increase reabsorption of
   J. chloride
   K. sodium
   L. potassium
   M. phosphate

6. Which of the following combinations of blood plasma concentrations is most indicative of compensated respiratory acidosis?
   J. pH below normal, bicarbonate concentration above normal, carbon dioxide concentration above normal
   K. pH below normal, bicarbonate concentration normal, carbon dioxide concentration above normal
   L. pH normal, bicarbonate concentration below normal, carbon dioxide concentration below normal
   M. pH below normal, bicarbonate concentration below normal, carbon dioxide concentration normal

7. Which of the following combinations of blood plasma concentrations is most indicative of an uncompensated metabolic alkalosis?
   J. pH above normal, bicarbonate concentration above normal, carbon dioxide concentration below normal
   K. pH above normal, bicarbonate concentration normal, carbon dioxide concentration below normal
   L. pH above normal, bicarbonate concentration above normal, carbon dioxide concentration normal
   M. pH above normal, bicarbonate concentration below normal, carbon dioxide concentration below normal

8. In blood plasma which of the following ions has the lowest concentration?
   J. chloride
   K. hydronium
   L. potassium
   M. sodium

9. Write a paragraph which distinguishes clearly between the processes of diffusion, osmosis and dialysis.

10. Both of the observations described below are related to the phenomenon of osmosis. Suggest an explanation for each.
   (a) Many plants die when salt is sprinkled on them.
   (b) Dilute solutions of carbohydrate, if left exposed to the air, soon have substantial numbers of microorganisms growing in them but honey, which is a very concentrated solution of carbohydrate, may be exposed to the air for a long period without this happening.

11. Indicate whether each of the solutions listed below is isotonic, hypotonic or hypertonic.
   (a) 3% (w/v) sodium chloride (NaCl)
   (b) 3% (w/v) glucose ($C_6H_{12}O_6$)
   (c) 7% (w/v) fructose ($C_6H_{12}O_6$)
   (d) 0.9% (w/v) potassium chloride (KCl)

12. The two solutions, 5% (w/v) glucose and 9.5% (w/v) sucrose, are each isotonic with the blood. Therefore, blood contains 5% (w/v) glucose and 9.5% (w/v) sucrose. Is this correct? Explain your answer.

13. A solution is prepared by dissolving 55.5 g of calcium chloride ($CaCl_2$) in 400 ml of water. Calculate the concentration of this solution in
   (a) moles/l
   (b) osmoles/l
   (c) equivalents/l

14. Why are the intravenous solutions used in total parenteral therapy run directly into the superior vena cava rather than into a peripheral vein?

15. The total concentration of the dialysate used in peritoneal dialysis is usually much higher than that used in haemodialysis. What is the purpose of this?

16. (a) Explain the meaning of the terms acid–base balance, acidosis, alkalosis.
   (b) Describe some ways in which the body is able to respond to (i) respiratory acidosis; (ii) metabolic alkalosis.

CHAPTER 10

Pressure

Pressure is a word of very extensive application in our language. It may be associated with the use of force, but it is also means to attempt to influence and it may convey a sense of urgency or stress. In science, the word is restricted in meaning to convey a sense of 'weightiness'. Pressure is defined as the ratio of force to area. The *force* being exerted is most commonly (but not only) the force of gravity acting on a solid, liquid or gas. The *area* is the extent of the surface in contact with the force.

Quantities in science are by definition able to be measured and expressed in appropriate units. The original unit of pressure (mm Hg) was derived from the first means by which air pressure was measured. We now have several ways to measure pressure and this has allowed the units assigned to pressure to be standardised. We will spend some time describing the various pressure units.

Pressure can be exerted by solids, liquids or gases so we will discuss the effect that the state of matter has on the pressure being exerted. Solids are rigid, but fluids can flow. A consequence of the freedom of movement within fluids is that pressure considerations are different in fluids that are static when compared to fluids that are flowing. The study of the latter is called fluid dynamics and will occupy us later in this chapter.

Learning Objectives

At the completion of this chapter you should be able to:

1. Define pressure and its unit the pascal in terms of newtons per square metre.
2. Understand fluid pressure in terms of the force exerted by a column of liquid.
3. Be aware of the meanings of the terms standard atmospheric pressure, gauge pressure, positive pressure and negative pressure.
4. Know the special considerations that apply to pressure in liquids.
5. Apply the laws of Boyle and of Charles and Gay-Lussac.
6. Define 'partial pressure' and apply Dalton's law of partial pressures.
7. Know the significance of Henry's law to the concentration of respiratory gases in solution.
8. Use pressure considerations to describe the act of breathing and gas exchange in the lungs.
9. Apply Pascal's principle.
10. Realise the significance of the dependence of flow rate on the fourth power of radius (Poiseuille's law).
11. Understand capillary exchange in term of pressure gradients.
12. Know the Bernoulli effect and its use to explain entrainment and the action of a Venturi mask.

10.1 Definition of Pressure and Pressure Units

Pressure is a derived quantity relating a force to the area on which it is acting. Consequently it is defined mathematically by the formula

pressure = force/area $P = F/A$

and defined in words as 'the force acting per unit area'.

The dependence of pressure on area means that in different situations, the amount of pressure that a given force can exert can be different, even though the force producing the pressure is constant. This is possible because pressure depends inversely on area. In the case of the pressure that a nail exerts while being driven into a block of wood, 'area' is the area of the nail point. The block of wood, in turn, exerts a pressure on the workbench on which it rests. In this case, the 'area' is the size of the surface of the block of wood that is in contact with the bench. Since the area of the nail point is far less than the area of the block of wood in contact with the workbench, the nail is able to exert much more pressure than the block. This is so, even though the force that the nail exerts on the wood block is the same as the force that the block exerts on the workbench. Consequently the nail can be hammered into the block of wood but the block can not be hammered into the workbench.

Note that pressure and force are not the same thing and so are measured by different units. The SI unit for force is the newton (N) and for area is the square metre (m^2). So the SI unit for pressure is the **newton per square metre** (written in symbols as N/m^2 or Nm^{-2}). This unit is renamed **pascal** (Pa) in honour of the seventeenth-century French scientist Blaise Pascal; thus 1 N/m^2 = 1 Pa. The pascal is a very small unit so you will usually see gauges calibrated in units of kilopascals (kPa); 1 kPa = 1000 Pa.

Unfortunately there are, for historical reasons, many other units of pressure in common usage, and these will probably continue to be used until the equipment carrying the gauges is replaced. The other units are:

- millimetres of mercury (mm Hg) (sometimes renamed as 'torr' after Torricelli)
- centimetres of water (cm H_2O)
- standard atmospheres (atm)
- bars (1 bar = 10^5 Pa)
- pounds per square inch (1 psi = 6.89 kPa)

You will come across kPa, mm Hg and cm H_2O in clinic. Often a gauge will carry a scale calibrated with two sets of units to enable easy conversion between them. Some conversion factors are:

1 kPa = 7.50 mm Hg = 10.2 cm H_2O = 10^3 N/m^2
1 mm Hg = 0.133 kPa = 1.36 cm H_2O = 1 torr
1 cm H_2O = 0.098 kPa = 0.735 mm Hg
1 psi = 6.89 kPa = 51.7 mm Hg

An arterial blood pressure reading may be 120 over 80 (in units of mm Hg); the same reading would be close to 16 over 10.6 (in units of kPa).

10.2 Atmospheric Pressure and 'Gauge Pressure'

10.2.1 *Atmospheric Pressure*

The air around us is a gas and so exerts a pressure equally on every part of us and from every direction. This pressure is called 'atmospheric pressure' and arises because of the weight of air in an imaginary vertical column from sea level to the 'top' of the atmosphere. The exact height of the atmosphere has no real meaning, because even though the density of the atmosphere decreases rapidly with distance above sea level, there are some molecules present at any height. Even in interplanetary space there is about one molecule of hydrogen per cubic centimetre. We do know that 50% of the atmosphere lies within 5.6 km of sea level, and 99% is below a height of 30 km. A 'column' of air of one square metre cross-section would weigh approximately 101 000 N (and have a mass of about 10 000 kg). Thus the 'standard' atmospheric pressure is 101 000 N/m^2. Daily atmospheric pressure varies from this standard because the atmosphere tends to 'pile up' at some places, producing a higher pressure, and to be shallower at others, producing a lower pressure. The 'standard atmosphere' converted into all the common units that we have discussed is:

1 atm = 101 000 N/m^2 = 1.01×10^5 Pa
= 101 kPa = 1.01 bar
1 atm = 760 mm Hg = 1030 cm H_2O
= 14.7 psi = 760 torr

The weather report would state this atmospheric pressure as 1010 **hectopascals** (hPa), where 1 hPa is equal to 100 Pa. Weather reports in the days before the conversion to metric units called the same pressure 1010 'millibars', which is the same as 1.01 bar.

Evangelista Torricelli (1608–1647) first devised a method for measuring atmospheric pressure by using a glass tube, about 80 cm long, filled with mercury (symbol Hg), which was then inverted into a container of mercury. He used mercury because it was the densest liquid readily available in the seventeenth century (1 ml has a mass of 13.6 g). Despite the subsequent usefulness of Torricelli's device in predicting changes in the weather, it was the *space* above the column of mercury that was more significant at the time than the ability to measure atmospheric pressure. The space developed at the closed-off upper end of the tube as the mercury fell down the tube. The space 'contained' a near-perfect vacuum (apart from the mercury vapour present). The production of a vacuum created a sensation in the seventeenth century because it ended the 2000-year-old notion of Aristotle that a vacuum could not exist.

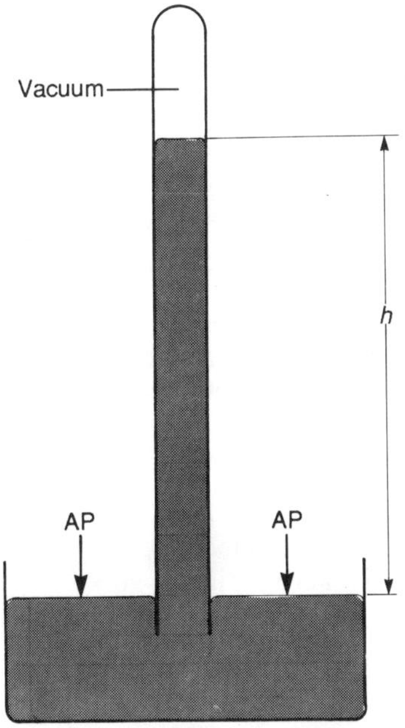

Figure 10.1 *A Torricelli barometer. The weight of the atmosphere produces atmospheric pressure (AP) which is able to prevent the mercury from flowing down the tube. The height, h, of mercury in the tube is a measure of atmospheric pressure*

Torricelli reasoned that the mercury that remained in the inverted tube, was prevented from draining out by the gases of the atmosphere pressing on the mercury in the container. Hence the column of mercury in the tube was held up by the atmosphere. The pressure of the atmosphere was exactly equal to the weight of mercury being supported in the tube, divided by the cross-sectional area of the tube. Dividing weight by area is mathematically the same thing as multiplying the density of mercury, d, by the strength of gravity, g, and by the height of the column of mercury in the glass tube, h (see Fig.10.1). Thus

$$\text{atmospheric pressure} = d \times g \times h$$

Since d and g are constants (at 0 °C and at sea level) ($g = 9.8$ and $d = 13.6$) only the height of the mercury column changes as atmospheric pressure changes.

Blaise Pascal realised that atmospheric pressure should change as the depth of the layer of atmosphere above the ground changes. He demonstrated that it did, by measuring h on an apparatus in Paris and again when the apparatus was assembled on a high mountain. As the column height is measured in millimetres, the measure of atmospheric pressure was stated as 'millimetres of mercury'. In fact millimetres of mercury was renamed as the unit **torr** in view of Torricelli's contribution to pressure measurement. Even though millimetres of mercury sounds like a length, pressure is not a length, it is the *ratio* of force to area. Water could be used to replace mercury in Torricelli's inverted tube, but since water is 13.6 times less dense than mercury, a tube 13.6 times longer than the one used by Torricelli would be required. Such a 10 m long tube would be cumbersome to say the least. Nevertheless, Pascal constructed a device similar to Torricelli's, but used red wine instead of mercury and a glass tube 14 m long.

We are used to living in an atmosphere of about 101 000 N/m^2 of pressure, produced because of the 10 100 kg of atmosphere above each square metre of area. Atmospheric pressure is equivalent to a mass of one kilogram pressing on each square centimetre of body surface. This causes us no discomfort, because the pressure inside the body is approximately equal to that outside. In fact considerable discomfort is felt if the body is not subjected to the pressure of the atmosphere. Under normal conditions the walls of the capillaries in the nose, ears and lungs are subjected to the approximately equal pressures of the blood supply within and the air pressure without. At high altitudes, the external pressure due to the atmosphere is so much reduced that the internal pressure of the blood causes the blood vessels to expand. Thus a sudden decrease in pressure, as may happen when the body of an aircraft flying at high altitude is pierced, may cause bleeding.

The body has a mechanism in the ear that is very sensitive to small but rapid changes in air pressure. The middle ear is a small, air-filled chamber, behind the ear drum, that can be vented through the eustachian tube. Normally the air pressure in the chamber is the same as the atmospheric pressure. However, if you rise a few hundred metres above ground level, by taking off in an aeroplane (or driving in a car up a range of hills), there will be an uncomfortable difference in pressure between each side of the ear drum. It will bend outwards (painfully) under the greater internal pressure until the middle ear space is vented by opening the eustachian tube. We can usually achieve this by swallowing or yawning.

10.2.2 *Pressure Gauges*

A **manometer** is a device that measures pressure by means of a vertical column of liquid. 'Sphygmos' is a Greek word for 'the pulse', thus the word **sphygmomanometer** was coined to describe a device used to count arterial pulsations. If the liquid in the manometer is relatively dense, as mercury is, the height of the vertical column is minimised. A stethoscope, together with a mercury sphygmomanometer, is used to determine arterial blood pressure by the auscultatory method. If water was used in a sphygmomanometer to measure arterial blood pressure, a reading of 140/80, in millimetres of mercury, would become about 1900/1100 in millimetres of water, and would require a glass tube 2 m long for a reading.

A **barometer** is a device for measuring atmospheric pressure. It takes its name from the old unit of pressure, the bar (perhaps the device should be renamed a 'pascalometer' now that the bar is no longer the unit of pressure!). Torricelli invented the mercury barometer in 1643. It measures atmospheric pressure by the height of a column of mercury. More recent barometers dispense with the mercury and measure atmospheric pressure from its effect on a sealed evacuated box (an aneroid barometer). The pressure of the atmosphere causes the surface of the box to bend. The extent of the bending is amplified and transmitted to a pointer. The pressure value is then displayed on the dial of the gauge.

Most pressure gauges use atmospheric pressure as a reference level and measure the *difference* between the actual pressure and atmospheric pressure. Manometers, the Bourdon gauge and the hand-held gauges used to check the pressure in automobile tyres all measure the difference between pressure and atmospheric pressure. The difference is called the **gauge pressure**, but usually the word 'gauge' is dropped and we just say 'pressure'. Thus the systolic pressure may be 120 mm Hg, but is actually 120 mm Hg *more* than atmospheric pressure (that is, 120 + 760 = 880 mm Hg). Such a pressure is also called a 'positive pressure', because it is greater than atmospheric pressure. Negative pressures are pressures that are less than atmospheric pressure. They are also referred to as 'suction'.

The process of filling a hypodermic syringe by withdrawing the plunger creates a negative pressure in the syringe. The negative pressure is produced because the volume inside the syringe has been increased without allowing any more air inside. Since the liquid into which the needle is dipped is pressed upon by atmospheric pressure, it will be forced, by this greater pressure, into the region of lower pressure thus filling the syringe.

10.3 Pressure Exerted by Solid Objects

For a solid object resting on a bench, the pressure it exerts on the bench depends on:

1. the object's weight (as weight increases so does pressure); and
2. the area of the object in contact with the bench (as area increases, pressure decreases).

Note that it is possible for a large force to exert only a small pressure. For example, a building worker may walk across wet concrete (without sinking in) by stepping on wide, flat boards. Some calculation will emphasise the point:

$$\begin{aligned}\text{if the worker's mass} &= 90 \text{ kg}\\ \text{then the worker's weight} &= 90 \times 9.8\\ &= 882 \text{ N (a large force)}\\ \text{area of board} &= 30 \text{ cm} \times 50 \text{ cm}\\ &= 1500 \text{ cm}^2 = 0.15 \text{ m}^2\end{aligned}$$

$$\begin{aligned}\text{pressure} = \frac{\text{force}}{\text{area}} &= \frac{882 \text{ N}}{0.15 \text{ m}^2}\\ &= 5880 \text{ N/m}^2\\ &= 5.88 \text{ kPa}\end{aligned}$$

Thus a large force (882 N) exerts only a small pressure (5.88 kPa) so that the stepping boards will not sink (very far) into the wet concrete. A large elephant (of mass seven tonnes) would exert about 240 kPa on the ground when standing on all its feet. Since the mass of the elephant is large, the area supporting its weight must also be large to prevent it from sinking into the ground. Conversely, if the area is very small, then even small forces will result in very high pressures, for example inserting a hypodermic needle through a patient's skin. The area of the point of the needle is very small (the needle is sharp) and may be as small as one thousandth of a square millimetre.

$$\begin{aligned}\text{area of needle point} &= 0.001\ \text{mm}^2\\ &= 0.000\ 000\ 001\ \text{m}^2\\ &= 10^{-9}\ \text{m}^2\end{aligned}$$

force with which needle is pushed = 100 N

$$\begin{aligned}\text{pressure} = \frac{\text{force}}{\text{area}} &= \frac{100\ \text{N}}{10^{-9}\ \text{m}^2}\\ &= 10^{11}\ \text{Nm}^{-2}\\ &= 10^{11}\ \text{Pa}\\ &= 10^{8}\ \text{kPa}\end{aligned}$$

One hundred million (10^8) kilopascals is a large pressure for such a small force (100 N) to exert, hence the hypodermic needle easily pierces the skin. A 50 kg woman who rocks her weight back onto her heels while wearing stilettos can exert a pressure of 2500 kPa on the ground because of the very small area of her stiletto heels.

One object may exert several different pressures depending on the way it stands. In Figure 10.2, the greatest pressure is exerted when the smallest area is in contact with the supporting surface. Any sharp object such as a scalpel, pin, scissors or knife cuts or pierces because its 'sharp point' ensures that a very small surface area is in contact with the object to be cut. Consequently any force applied over such a tiny area produces very large pressures, large enough to 'push through' the material being cut.

The highest pressures in the body are found in the weight-bearing bone joints. As you walk, there are times when all your weight is on one leg. At these times, the pressure in the knee joint may be greater than 1000 kPa (more than 10 atm). Since pressure is force per unit area, the pressure would be even higher were it not for the large area of the knee joint. When necessary, the pressure in the weight-bearing joints may be decreased by leaning on crutches or a walking stick. This decreases pressure by decreasing the weight acting on the area of the joints.

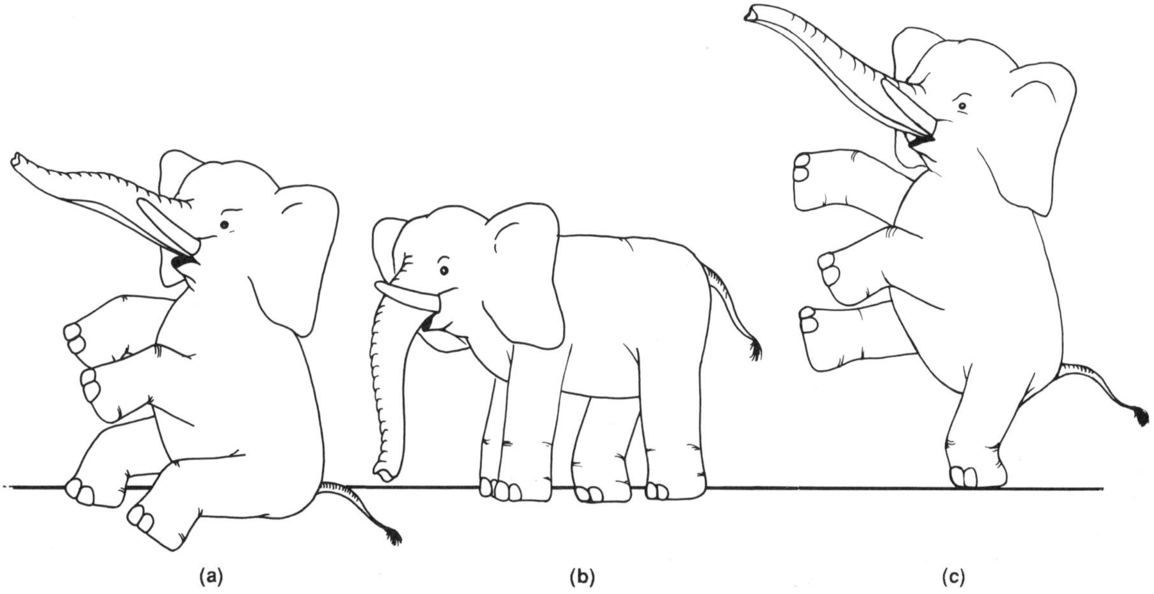

Figure 10.2 *One object can exert several different pressures depending on the way that it stands. The elephant exerts a constant force on the ground. However, the pressure it exerts is greater in (b) than in (a) and greatest in (c)*

10.4 Pressure Exerted by Liquids

10.4.1 *Special Considerations for Liquid Pressure*

Pressure in liquids increases with depth. This is due to the weight of liquid above that particular depth. The pressure increase with depth is often illustrated (and often incorrectly illustrated!) in textbooks by the familiar diagram of the can with three holes (Figure 10.3). The can contains water at a depth of h, which is kept constant by an incoming stream of water and an overflow. The three holes are at distances of $h/4$, $2h/4$, and $3h/4$ below the surface, that is, if $h = 40$ cm, the holes would be 10 cm, 20 cm and 30 cm respectively below the water surface. The increased pressure with depth is indicated by the greater *speed* with which water spurts from the lower holes (Figure 10.3a). In fact the actual speed of exit (v) is given by Torricelli's law ($g = 9.8$):

$$v = \sqrt{2gh}$$

Note also that the streams of water follow parabolic paths and that it is the stream from the middle hole (not the lowest hole) that has the greatest range (Figure 10.3b). This somewhat unexpected result arises because the lowest hole is so close to the ground. Water flowing through it will curve parabolically and strike the ground before it has travelled far.

The increase of pressure with depth can also be illustrated by attaching manometers to each of the three holes (Figure 10.3c). In this case the pressure at levels 1, 2 and 3 is indicated by the 'head of water' in each manometer: 30 cm H_2O at level 3, 20 cm H_2O at level 2 and 10 cm H_2O at level 1.

The deeper you go underwater, the greater is the weight of water above you. Since the weight of liquid also depends on its density the complete relationship between pressure and depth is:

$$\text{pressure (Pa)} = 9.8 \times \text{density (kg/m}^3) \times \text{depth (m)}$$

The densities of some liquids are:

pure H_2O (at 37 °C)	= 0.993 g/ml
cerebrospinal fluid	= 1.007 g/ml
pleural fluid	= 1.015 g/ml
urine, about	= 1.020 g/ml
blood, about	= 1.060 g/ml
mercury (at 37 °C)	= 13.51 g/ml

Consider the pressure at the bottom of a tub containing water 20 cm deep. Using the conversion factors given earlier, the pressure of 20 cm H_2O = 14.7 mm Hg = 1.96 kPa more than the water at the top of the tub. The enclosed fluids in the human body are of relatively small capacity so the variation in their pressure due to depth is negligible. However, the pressure readings in blood vessels and cerebrospinal fluid are subject to increase due to the head of liquid. To eliminate this

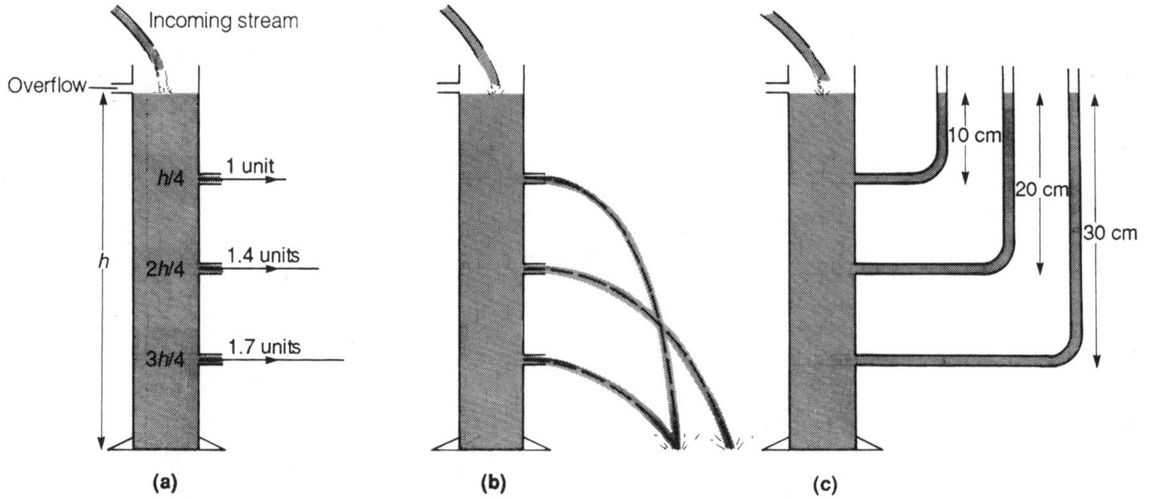

Figure 10.3 *(a) The speed of flow is greater the further the exit hole is below the water surface. (b) The streams of water have a parabolic shape and the middle stream has the greatest range. (c) It can be seen that the pressure at the lowest hole is greatest*

effect, blood pressures in the legs and the pressure of cerebrospinal fluid are measured when the patient is supine.

Three special considerations need to be borne in mind when dealing with pressures exerted by liquids:

1. The pressure at any point in a liquid at rest acts equally in all directions (otherwise the liquid would not be at rest!).

2. At different points in the same horizontal plane, pressures are equal.

3. Pressure increases with depth. Vertical pressure differences do not depend on the shape of the containing vessel, nor on the volume of liquid. They depend only on the vertical depth below the surface of the liquid.

For example, in Figure 10.4 the vessels contain water to depths of 15, 10, 5, 3 and 2 cm. The greatest pressure occurs at the bottom of the container with 15 cm of water; at the bottom of the other vessels the pressure is less, with the least pressure being at the bottom of the vessel containing water to a depth of 2 cm. The volume of liquid and the shape it forms in the container do not affect the pressure. Furthermore, the pressure in all containers at a depth of 2 cm below the surface has the same value, and that is 2 cm H_2O (196 Pa).

10.4.2 *Pascal's Principle*

In addition to these three considerations, Pascal's principle is useful in understanding static fluid pressures. Pascal's principle (*c.* 1650) is:

> 'When pressure is applied to any point of an enclosed fluid at rest, it is transmitted undiminished to every portion of the fluid and to the walls of the containing vessel' (that is, every part of the fluid experiences the increase in pressure).

Consider the pressure exerted on those parts of the body that bear the weight when you lie down, the buttocks, heels and shoulders. Decubitis ulcers (bed sores) may form on these and the other bony projections of bed-ridden patients, because the weight of the patient is being supported on relatively small areas. The pressure produced is given by weight divided by area. The abnormally high pressure on these bony areas, which are not adapted for weight bearing, reduces the blood flow to the area, which then blisters and ulcerates. To some extent the likelihood of bed sores can be reduced by the use of an air or water mattress. Such a mattress consists of a 'bag' that is filled with air or water, so it contains an 'enclosed fluid'. By Pascal's principle, the pressure in the fluid-filled mattress is uniform (apart from the increase in pressure with depth). The patient's weight displaces the fluid in the mattress and exerts a pressure on the fluid. The pressure is equal to the patient's weight divided by the area of the patient that contacts the mattress. This pressure is transmitted throughout the fluid and to the

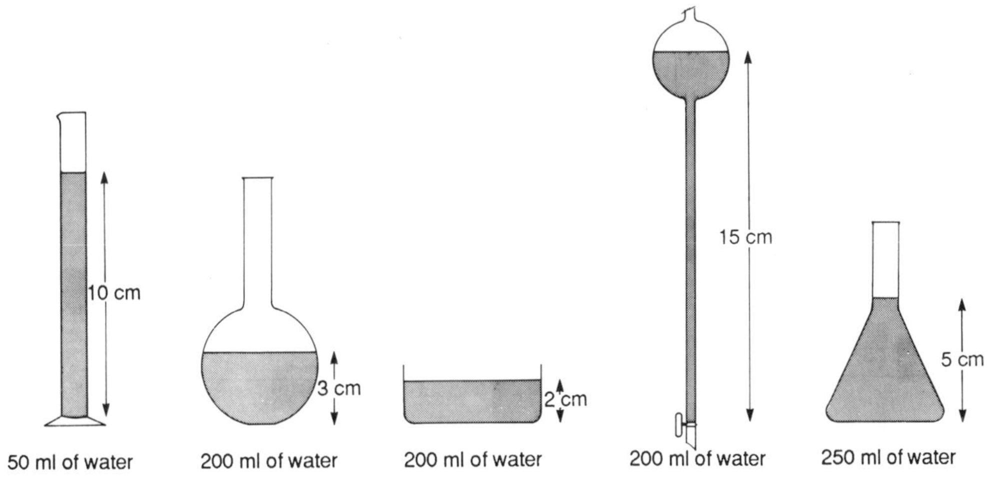

Figure 10.4 *The pressure at a point in a liquid is determined solely by the depth of that point below the surface. The volume of water or shape of the container has no effect*

walls of the mattress. Thus the mattress exerts this same pressure back onto all parts of the body that are in contact with it. Provided that the material of the mattress 'bag' is flexible enough to follow the contours of the body, the patient would experience a uniform pressure over most of their lower body surface. This surface has a much larger area than just the bony projections. The increase in contact area has the effect of decreasing the pressure to below that which would have been experienced by the bony projections on an ordinary mattress. The lower pressure may allow sufficient blood flow to prevent bed sores.

The body's 'enclosed' fluids include cerebrospinal fluid, urine in the bladder, fluid in the eyeball, amniotic fluid around the foetus and synovial fluid in joint cavities. Blood is not included as it is a circulating fluid and involves some additional considerations that do not apply to 'static' fluids. Pressure considerations are also useful in understanding the 'potential spaces' of the pleural, peritoneal and pericardial cavities. Note that none of the body's fluids are *strictly* static or enclosed, as they are continually being replaced in a normally functioning body.

Cerebrospinal fluid (CSF) is normally at a pressure of about 13 cm H_2O (plus or minus 5 cm H_2O) for a person lying *horizontally* (that is important!). In metric units the normal range is between 0.8 and 1.8 kPa. Brain tumours, inflamed meninges, haemorrhage or infection can increase the pressure of the CSF to between 3.9 and 5.9 kPa (40 and 60 cm H_2O). Measurement of CSF pressure may be made by inserting a spinal needle into the spinal cavity (between the third and fourth lumbar vertebrae) and allowing the CSF pressure to cause saline to rise in a glass tube. For each centimetre that the saline rises above the level of the needle, the pressure is approximately 100 Pa (1 cm H_2O). Such measurement can be a useful diagnostic tool.

Queckenstedt's test involves compressing the jugular veins. This causes the venous sinuses in the cranium to swell, which in turn will press against the CSF. According to Pascal, this increased pressure should be transmitted throughout the enclosed fluid, thus CSF pressure should immediately rise to two or three times normal. If it doesn't, then a blockage of fluid flow in the spinal canal is indicated.

Glaucoma is a condition caused by increased pressure in the eye. The space between the cornea and the lens of the eye is filled with a liquid-like substance called **aqueous humour** at a pressure of about 2 kPa (15 mm Hg) with a range of from 1.3 to 4.0 kPa (about 10 to 30 mm Hg). This substance is continually being produced and the surplus escapes through a drainage tube called the **canal of Schlemm**. Blockage of this tube can produce pressure in the eye of up to 9.3 kPa (70 mm Hg). Such very high pressure is transmitted (by Pascal's principle) to the **vitreous humour** in the rear chamber of the eye. This decreases the blood supply to the retina and can cause permanent blindness within a few days. Eye pressure is measured with a **tonometer** and if excessive, may be relieved by drugs.

Pascal's principle tells us that liquids are virtually incompressible, so a sharp blow to the eye or head will cause the pressure to be transmitted to the opposite side. Thus the optic nerve may be damaged by a sharp blow to the *front* of the eye, or by an eye irrigation at too high a pressure. Boxers suffer brain damage to the occipital regions rather than the frontal lobes (where they get hit). On the other hand, amniotic fluid provides protection for the foetus against a sharp blow to the mother's abdomen. The force of such a blow would produce a pressure in the amniotic fluid that is transmitted to all the surface area of the foetus and the surrounding uterus. Thus the force is dissipated into the mother's abdomen while the whole foetus, rather than that part that was adjacent to the blow, experiences a reduced force.

One of the more noticeable internal pressures is the pressure that builds up in the bladder due to the accumulation of urine. The micturation reflex becomes more insistent when bladder pressure rises above 30 cm H_2O (3 kPa). The resulting muscular contraction in the bladder wall can be made large enough to provide a momentary pressure of up to 150 cm H_2O (14.7 kPa). This is about how high up a wall boys can urinate when they experimentally determine their bladder pressure.

10.5 Osmotic Pressure

In 1748 Abbe Nollet found that if a membrane separated a dilute solution from a more concentrated one, the solvent would pass from the dilute solution through the membrane and into the more concentrated one. For example, if a tube is closed at one end with a membrane, partly filled with a sugar solution and then placed in a vessel of pure water so that the level of sugar solution in the tube is the same as the level of water in the vessel, there is a net flow of water molecules through the membrane (Figure 10.5). Although water molecules pass through the membrane the sugar molecules cannot. Membranes that allow the passage of some molecules but not others are called semi-permeable membranes.

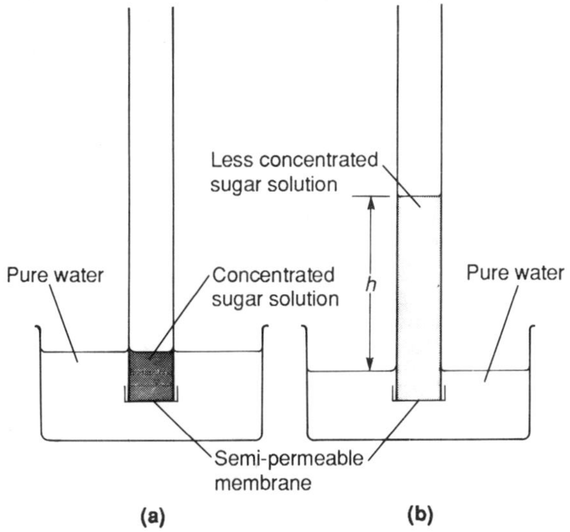

Figure 10.5 *(a) A concentrated sugar solution separated from pure water by a semi-permeable membrane. (b) More water molecules will enter the sugar solution than will leave it. The height h is a measure of the osmotic pressure of the original sugar solution*

There are more water molecules per millilitre in pure water than there are in a sugar solution. Therefore the number of water molecules passing into the sugar solution exceeds the number passing out so that the level of liquid in the tube rises. The difference in height between the level of pure water and the level of liquid in the tube means that the liquid in the tube exerts a hydrostatic pressure. The hydrostatic pressure is equal to the head of liquid. This pressure is called **osmotic pressure**. The osmotic pressure of blood is about 4.0 kPa (30 mm Hg or 41 cm H_2O) so that if normal blood is used instead of sugar solution in the example above, the level in the tube would rise to 41 cm above the level of pure water in the vessel. For further discussion on osmosis, see Chapter 9.

10.6 Factors Affecting the Pressure in Gases

10.6.1 *The Atmosphere*

The considerations that apply to the pressure in static liquids also apply to enclosed gases, since both liquids and gases are fluids. These considerations are restated below.

1. The pressure at any point in a gas 'at rest' acts equally in all directions. Thus atmospheric pressure acts equally on the floor and the ceiling of a room, and on the walls too.
2. The pressure in a gas increases with depth. This is a negligible consideration for air enclosed in the body because the depths of any enclosed gases are so small, but is critical when considering the atmospheric pressure at a particular location. On the earth's surface we are at the bottom of an 'ocean of air', so the local atmospheric pressure decreases as we climb above sea level.

For example, at sea level the daily atmospheric pressure varies around an average value of about 101 kPa. However, on the top of Mt Everest the atmospheric pressure varies around an average value of about 33 kPa. A lowered atmospheric pressure has significant effects on gaseous exchange in the lungs. In fact if the atmospheric pressure drops to below about 70 kPa, as it does in mountain ranges above 3000 m, then 'mountain sickness' becomes a problem for un-acclimatised people.

3. Pascal's principle applies to enclosed gases. That is, any pressure applied to an enclosed gas at rest is transmitted undiminished to every portion of the gas and to the walls of the container.

In addition to the three properties above, *gases are compressible* and so behave differently from liquids in a number of respects.

4. If the amount of gas in an enclosed space is increased, by pumping more air into a tyre, for example, then the pressure in the space will increase as the original gas molecules move closer together to allow more molecules in.

10.6.2 *The Gas Laws*

Boyle's Law (c. 1660). This can be stated as follows:

> Provided that the temperature of the gas does not change, then the pressure, P, of a fixed amount of gas will increase as the volume, V, decreases (and vice versa).

Boyle's law may be stated symbolically as

$$P \propto 1/V$$

An example of this law is the increase in pressure in the bulb of a sphygmomanometer as the bulb is squeezed (which causes its volume to decrease).

Another example is in the filling of a syringe. As the plunger of the syringe is withdrawn, the volume of the syringe increases, therefore the pressure must decrease, allowing atmospheric pressure to force liquid into the syringe.

The Law of Pressures. This can be stated as follows:

> Provided that the volume of gas does not change, then the pressure of the enclosed gas will increase when the absolute temperature, T, of the gas increases (and vice versa).

In symbols, the law of pressures may be stated (T in kelvin)

$$P \propto T$$

It can now be understood that gas cylinders (which confine an enclosed gas to a fixed volume) should be stored away from heat sources otherwise the pressure inside full cylinders may rise to unsafe levels. Furthermore the pressure gauges on a heated cylinder would read a higher value, giving the impression that the cylinder contains more compressed gas than is the case.

The Law of Charles and Gay-Lussac. This law states:

> Provided that the pressure in a gas does not change, the volume of a fixed amount of gas will increase as the (absolute) temperature of the gas increases.

Charles and Gay-Lussac discovered this relationship independently of each other in about 1802. When stated in symbols it is (T in kelvin)

$$T \propto V$$

An elastic gas container, such as a balloon or an air mattress, will expand if its temperature rises (for example, if it is exposed to strong sunshine), and may pop. Conversely it will contract as its temperature drops (as an air mattress does after a cold night when camping). If you inhale deeply and quickly on a cold morning, the air that enters your lungs is much colder than the temperature of your alveoli. At the end of your inhalation, the air in your lungs is at the same pressure as the atmosphere. The inhaled air will increase in temperature as it is warmed by your alveoli and by Charles' law, will also increase in volume.

The three laws stated above may be combined into the 'ideal gas equation' which may be stated as

$$\frac{PV}{T} = \text{constant} \qquad \text{or} \quad \frac{P_1V_1}{T_1} = \frac{P_2V_2}{T_2}$$

where P_1 and P_2 are initial and final pressures respectively, V_1 and V_2 are initial and final volumes respectively and T_1 and T_2 are initial and final kelvin temperatures respectively.

10.6.3 *Work Done by an Expanding Gas*

The work done by a gas on its surroundings as it expands may be used to understand the production of solid carbon dioxide ('dry ice'). Solidified carbon dioxide is at such a low temperature that it is used to kill warts by freezing them. The liquid in the cells of the wart expands when it freezes, rupturing the cell walls so that on thawing, the ruptured cells die and eventually drop off the skin. Strangely this process is known as 'burning off' the wart. Carbon dioxide is a gas at normal temperatures, but solidifies (without passing through a liquid phase at atmospheric pressure) at –78.5 °C. This temperature is easily obtained by allowing compressed carbon dioxide, held at high pressure (18 000 kPa) in a gas cylinder, to rapidly expand into a 'sock' attached to the outlet. Since the pressure of the gas in the cylinder is large (about 180 atmospheres) when compared with atmospheric pressure (101 kPa), the carbon dioxide rushes out of the cylinder, 'pushing back' the atmosphere. In doing so, the expanding gas 'does work' on the atmosphere. This means that the carbon dioxide must expend some of its energy in pushing the atmosphere back. From kinetic theory, we know that the energy in a gas is kinetic energy and that temperature is a measure of the average kinetic energy of a gas. If the gas loses some of its energy in pushing against the atmosphere, the result is a decrease in the temperature of the carbon dioxide, to below the point of solidification. 'Dry ice' is then collected from the sock at the nozzle of the cylinder.

10.7 Kinetic Molecular Theory

The kinetic molecular theory of gases culminated from the work of Boyle, Dalton, Gay-Lussac, Charles, Regnault, Bernoulli, Joule and probably many others. However, R. Clausius in 1857 set out the theory that has been shown by experiment to describe the behaviour of gases extremely well. It may be summarised as follows:

> Gases are composed of a great many particles — called molecules — (of the order of 10^{20} per cubic

centimetre), that are continually moving with a range of speeds (average speed of hundreds of metres per second at 20 °C), in straight lines, in random directions. There are no appreciable intermolecular forces, and the particles neither gain nor lose energy during collisions. The particles occupy a negligible volume compared to the volume of their container.

By comparing the behaviour of a real gas (as described by the gas laws in Section 10.6.2) with the theoretical behaviour of an 'ideal' gas (one that conforms to the kinetic molecular theory for gases), two important results emerge:

1. The pressure that a gas exerts is explained in terms of the collisions of its molecules with the container walls.
2. The temperature of a material is determined by the average kinetic energy (which is proportional to absolute temperature) of the molecules of the material. That is, absolute temperature (°C plus 273) is proportional to the average kinetic energy of the particles.

Gases differ from liquids because their particles are much further apart and they exert negligible forces of attraction on each other. Consequently gases may be compressed or expanded (but liquids can't). Gas particles will collide with their container's walls (and bounce off!) and so exert a force on the wall. The act of bouncing off a wall constitutes an acceleration and by Newton's second law, all accelerations are caused by an unbalanced force. In this case it is the wall that is exerting a force. By Newton's third law, each particle will exert an equal but oppositely directed force on the container wall. When the force of all collisions with the walls, in a one second time interval, are added together and then divided by the area of the container's walls, a value for the pressure exerted by the gas particles may be calculated (pressure = force/area). According to the kinetic molecular theory, gases at higher temperature have particles travelling at higher average speeds, hence they undergo greater accelerations on collision with the walls. Consequently they exert more force per collision and so exert more pressure.

10.8 Partial Pressure

Air is a mixture of gases. Each gas contributes to the total atmospheric pressure in proportion to its concentration. Approximately 21% of the volume of dry air is oxygen, so 21% of the average atmospheric pressure (101.3 kPa) is due to the pressure being exerted by oxygen: 21% of 101.3 kPa = 21.2 kPa (158 mm Hg). Since 21.2 kPa is that part of the total pressure that may be attributed to oxygen, we call 21.2 kPa the **partial pressure** of oxygen (ppO_2). The major constituents of dry air and their approximate partial pressures are displayed in Table 10.1.

Atmospheric pressure is the sum of all the partial pressures exerted by the individual gases. Thus

$$\text{total } P = pp_A + pp_B + pp_C + pp_D + \ldots$$

Thus standard atmospheric pressure = 101.3 kPa, and 79.1 + 21.2 + 1.0 + 0.03 kPa adds approximately to 101.3 kPa. The addition is only approximate because the concentration of carbon dioxide varies, and the partial pressure of water vapour changes according to the humidity. Furthermore, the gases that occur in the atmosphere in very small quantities (krypton, xenon, neon and helium) have not been taken into account.

Table 10.1 *Partial pressures of the major constituents of dry air*

Gas	Proportion of atmosphere (% of vol.)	Partial pressure (kPa)
oxygen	21	21.2
nitrogen	78	79.1
argon	0.95	1.0
carbon dioxide	0.3–0.03	0.3–0.03

The idea that total gas pressure is the sum of the parts is formalised as **Dalton's law of partial pressure**:

> In a mixture of gases, the total pressure is the sum of the pressures exerted by each of the gases alone.

Or, stated in another way:

In a mixture of gases, the partial pressure of gas A is that pressure that would be exerted by A alone, if all other gases were removed from the container.

Thus, if all the gases except for oxygen could be removed from a room full of normal air, then the pressure in the room would be about 21 kPa. If we consider only the two most abundant atmospheric gases, a cubic metre of air at 101 kPa may be thought of as a mixture of one cubic metre of oxygen at 21 kPa and one cubic metre of nitrogen at 80 kPa.

All gases enclosed in the body (in the lungs, stomach and bowel) are in direct contact with water and will, therefore, be saturated with water vapour. This gas exerts a pressure of 6.2 kPa at body temperature (37 °C) and will cause the partial pressures of other gases to be less than their dry air values stated above. That is, the partial pressures of the other gases will total 95.1 kPa rather than 101.3 kPa.

Consider the air contained in a relaxed lung. It will be saturated with water vapour, and contain more carbon dioxide (about 5% of the total) than atmospheric air. Nevertheless the pressure of the air in the lungs is the same as atmospheric pressure and by Dalton's law, each of the constituent gases contributes its partial pressure to the total. Thus the contributions of water vapour and carbon dioxide to air pressure in the lungs are at the expense of oxygen and nitrogen. The concentrations of these last two gases is lower in the lungs than in atmospheric air. Of course, another factor contributing to the reduced concentration of oxygen in the lungs is its absorption into the capillaries lining the alveoli.

10.9 Respiratory Gas Exchange

10.9.1 *Henry's Law*

Of great interest in respiratory physiology are the quantities of oxygen and carbon dioxide that will dissolve in the blood. **Henry's law** relates the amount of gas that will dissolve in a liquid to its partial pressure.

The mass, C, of a gas that will dissolve in a millilitre of water at a given temperature is proportional to the partial pressure, pp, of the gas and to its 'solubility coefficient', k. (More gas will dissolve at lower temperatures.)

$$C = k \times pp$$

In order for oxygen to diffuse into the capillaries of the alveoli, it must first dissolve in the liquid that lines the alveoli. From Henry's law, the mass of oxygen that is able to dissolve depends only on its partial pressure in the alveoli (since the temperature of the lungs is constant and the solubility coefficient of oxygen is fixed).

10.9.2 *Alveolar Air is Different from Atmospheric Air*

It is important to note that the concentration of oxygen in the air of the alveoli is different from its concentration in atmospheric air. The difference arises from three sources.

Firstly, atmospheric air becomes humidified before it enters the alveoli. Inhaled air passes over wet membranes to get to the lungs so becomes saturated with water vapour. In fact, all gas in the human body contains water vapour at its saturation partial pressure of 6.2 kPa (47 mm Hg). According to Dalton's law, the partial pressure of oxygen must be less in humidified air than in dry air. For humidified air, $ppO_2 + ppN_2 + ppH_2O = 101.3$ kPa, but for dry air, $ppO_2 + ppN_2 = 101.3$ kPa. The presence of water vapour in air means that the total contribution of the partial pressures of oxygen and nitrogen to air pressure is 6.2 kPa less than it is in dry air. This means that water vapour is present at the expense of the other gases and that there is less oxygen in humidified air.

Table 10.2 *A comparison of the partial pressures of gases in atmospheric air, humidified atmospheric air and alveolar air. Pressures are stated in kPa, with mm Hg in parentheses*

	N_2	O_2	CO_2	H_2O
atmospheric air	79.1 (597)	21.0 (159)	0.04 (0.3)	0.5 (3.7)
humidified air	74.1 (563)	19.7 (149)	0.04 (0.3)	6.2 (47)
alveolar air	75 (569)	14.0 (104)	5.3 (40)	6.2 (47)

Secondly, oxygen is continually being absorbed from the alveoli into the blood capillaries, and carbon dioxide is continually diffusing into the alveoli from the blood. Thus 14% of alveolar air is oxygen, which is significantly less than the amount of oxygen (21%) in the atmosphere.

Thirdly, alveolar air is different to atmospheric air, also because it is only partially replaced by humidified atmospheric air with each breath. In the absence of vigorous exercise (which promotes deeper breathing), about one seventh of the volume of air in the lungs is expired with each breath. This is called the tidal volume and is approximately 500 ml.

10.9.3 *Gases Dissolved in the Blood*

The partial pressure of oxygen in the oxygenated blood that leaves the lungs will be slightly less than that of the alveolar air (14 kPa). However, more oxygen may be made to dissolve in the arterial blood by administering air containing oxygen at a higher concentration than in atmospheric air (that is, more than 21%), but at normal pressure (101 kPa). Alternatively, air may be administered at pressures greater than atmospheric pressure, that is, at hyperbaric pressure. If the air is enriched with oxygen and at greater than atmospheric pressure, the procedure is called hyperbaric oxygen therapy. In each case the partial pressure of oxygen will be more than 21 kPa, which is what it is in atmospheric air, so by Henry's law, more oxygen will dissolve in the blood.

An air mixture with oxygen at greater than atmospheric concentration may be used to treat the hypoxia and anoxia which can arise in high-altitude flying, mountain climbing, firefighting and from shock. In an hyperbaric chamber, oxygen at greater than atmospheric pressure and at high concentration is used to treat anaerobic infection (gas gangrene), carbon monoxide poisoning and decompression sickness.

The amount of oxygen that normally dissolves in the blood is much less than that required by the body. In fact haemoglobin in the red blood cells can carry 97% of our oxygen requirements. Of course, before oxygen can bind to haemoglobin it must dissolve in the liquid lining the alveoli and then diffuse into the blood across the walls of the capillaries. One of the reasons that haemoglobin is required to supply adequately our body with oxygen is that oxygen is not very soluble in water (or blood). On the other hand, carbon dioxide is sufficiently soluble to be carried away from the cells in solution without the need for a special binding protein. Thus there is more carbon dioxide than oxygen dissolved in arterial blood.

We can estimate how much more carbon dioxide than oxygen is carried in solution in the blood from the solubility of those gases in water at 40 °C and using the partial pressures of oxygen and carbon dioxide in the alveoli. From Henry's law:

$$\text{concentration} = \text{partial pressure} \times \text{solubility coefficient of gas}$$

For oxygen,

$$C = 14\ \text{kPa} \times \frac{3.08 \times 10^{-5}}{93.6\ \text{kPa}}$$
$$= 0.46 \times 10^{-5}\ \text{g of } O_2 \text{ per gram of } H_2O$$

For carbon dioxide,

$$C = 5.3\ \text{kPa} \times \frac{97.3 \times 10^{-5}}{93.6\ \text{kPa}}$$
$$= 5.5 \times 10^{-5}\ \text{g of } CO_2 \text{ per gram of } H_2O$$

Thus about 12 times more carbon dioxide will be in solution than oxygen. [The figure of 93.6 arises by subtracting the partial pressure of water vapour at 40 °C (7.4 kPa) from atmospheric pressure (101 kPa). This figure (93.6) is then divided into the solubility coefficient of oxygen in water at 40 °C (3.08×10^{-5}) because the coefficient was calculated for an atmosphere of pure oxygen (apart from the water vapour) at a pressure of 101 kPa over the water surface.]

The number of molecules of gas that are dissolved in a liquid is a dynamic equilibrium between the number of gas molecules that collide with the surface of the liquid (and subsequently dissolve) and the number of already dissolved gas molecules that escape from the liquid's surface. The amount of gas that has dissolved in a liquid is stated as a 'partial pressure' in respiratory physiology. So the amount of oxygen dissolved in blood can be stated as an oxygen partial pressure of 5.3 kPa (40 mm Hg). This means that the blood contains as much oxygen as if it was in contact with a gas mixture in which oxygen exerted a partial pressure of 5.3 kPa (and equilibrium had been reached). If this blood is now brought into contact with air containing oxygen at a higher partial pressure, then more oxygen would dissolve. On the other hand, if blood with an amount of dissolved carbon dioxide stated as 6.1 kPa (46 mm Hg) comes into contact with carbon dioxide gas at a lower partial pressure (as is the case in the alveoli), then some carbon dioxide would come out of solution.

Our bodies are used to working at an atmospheric pressure of about 101 kPa (760 mm Hg) of which about 21 kPa is due to oxygen. If we experience air at a markedly different pressure (for example, while mountaineering, flying, diving underwater or inside hyperbaric chambers), or if the relative concentrations of the gases that we breathe are different from normal, then significant deleterious or beneficial effects occur.

Decompression sickness (caisson disease or 'the bends') is a risk faced by underwater divers who breathe air at high pressure. Their air must be at high pressure in order to balance the hydrostatic pressure exerted on their chest by the surrounding water. Hydrostatic pressure is proportional to depth, thus an extra atmosphere of pressure is exerted by each 10 m depth in water. So at 30 m depth, a diver would experience a pressure of approximately 4 atm (405 kPa). It is difficult to expand the chest against the hydrostatic pressure of the water in order to breathe in unless the air breathed in is at the same pressure as the surrounding water.

Since the bottled air breathed by the underwater diver is at high pressure, the partial pressures of the constituent gases is also high. Normally very little nitrogen dissolves in blood at atmospheric pressure. However, the concentration of dissolved gas increases as the partial pressure of gas increases (Henry's law), hence significant amounts of nitrogen do dissolve in the blood of divers while they are submerged. On slowly ascending to the surface, dissolved nitrogen comes out of solution as the pressure falls, and is breathed out. If the ascent is too rapid, nitrogen comes out of solution in the tissues and forms bubbles in the blood vessels. These cause great pain and can block blood vessels.

The effect of rapid decompression on dissolved gases can easily be demonstrated by removing the top from a bottle of carbonated soft drink. Carbon dioxide was dissolved in the drink at high pressure, so by Henry's law a large amount was forced into solution. Consequently a much smaller amount of carbon dioxide will remain in solution if the pressure is suddenly relieved by opening the bottle. The gas comes out of solution so rapidly that gas bubbles are evolved. Much the same thing occurs in the bloodstream of divers who come to the surface too rapidly.

Breathing in a chamber with a pressure of 3–4 atm (a hyperbaric chamber) is an effective treatment of decompression sickness. The increased pressure causes the bubbles of nitrogen to dissolve in the blood and, by slowly reducing the pressure, the excess nitrogen can gradually diffuse from the tissues into the blood and move with it to the lungs. There it can come out of solution at a rate which allows it to be expired through the lungs.

Henry's law tells us that the amount of oxygen that dissolves in the blood can be increased without increasing air pressure or the use of hyperbaric chambers, if the concentration of oxygen in the air is increased. Thus in an atmosphere at standard pressure but containing 30% oxygen, rather than the standard 21%, the partial pressure of oxygen is increased by about 50% (to about 30 kPa from 20 kPa). Consequently, 50% more oxygen will dissolve in the blood than does at normal concentration.

10.10 Breathing

Breathing may be thought of as a repetitive change in the balance between opposing forces. Muscular force expands the chest against the elasticity of the lungs and ribs. Air moves in the direction of the pressure gradient, into the lungs. In the absence of the muscular expanding force, the elasticity of the chest causes it to contract and this reverses the pressure gradient, so forcing air out.

During inhalation, the volume of the thoracic cavity is increased, thus decreasing the pressure inside the lungs (Boyle's law) to below atmospheric pressure. Hence air is forced into the lungs by the greater pressure outside (see Figure 10.6). The pressure difference is only 400 or 500 Pa (a few mm Hg below atmospheric), but may reach –5.6 kPa (–80 mm Hg) at maximum effort. During exhalation, the volume of the thoracic cavity decreases as muscles relax and the lungs 'recoil' elastically. This causes the pressure in the lungs to increase above atmospheric pressure and air is forced out of the lungs. Again, the pressure gradient required is only a few hundred pascals but may reach +13 kPa (+100 mm Hg) during maximum effort.

In a resting man or woman, about 500 ml of air is inhaled and exhaled with each breath via the nostrils or mouth. This is called the **tidal volume**. Of the 500 ml that is expired, 350 ml comes from the alveoli and 150 ml comes from the conducting passages that are outside the lungs. This latter volume is called the **anatomical dead space**. The 150 ml is fresh air, as it has not entered the alveoli. On inhalation, 500 ml of air is taken in, consisting of 150 ml of previously expelled alveolar air that remained in the conducting passages, and 350 ml of fresh air. The end result is that 150 ml of the fresh air in each inhalation never reaches the alveoli, but simply moves in and out of the airways. Hence a deep breath (say 1000 ml) provides a greater proportion of fresh air than a shallow breath (500 ml) because the anatomical dead space remains constant.

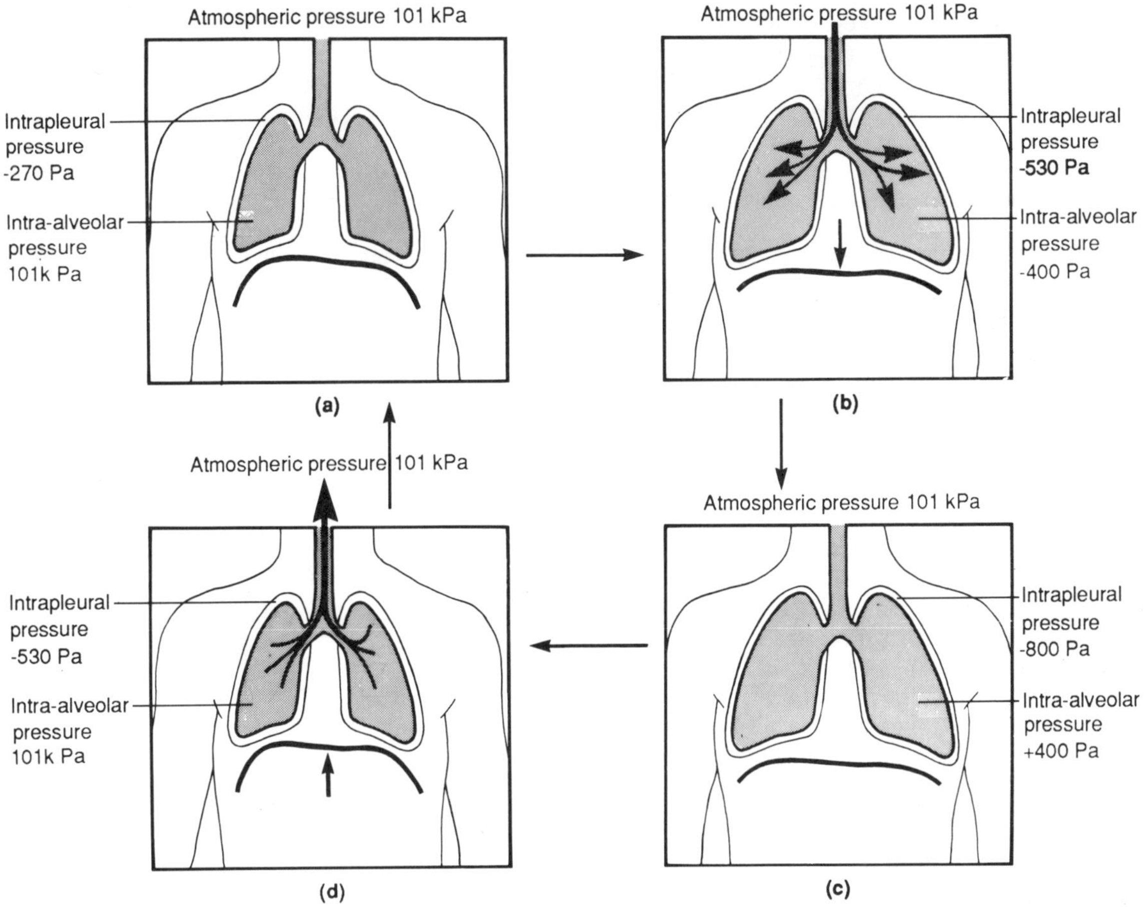

Figure 10.6 *(a) As the volume of the spaces in the alveoli increases, by Boyle's law, the air pressure in the alveoli will decrease. (b) The pressure gradient produced is sufficient to force atmospheric air into the alveoli*

In order for the lungs to expand and contract along with the chest, they must be 'stuck' to the chest. This is achieved by a negative pressure (a suction) between the lungs and the chest wall. The normal pressure in the intrapleural 'space' (that is, the *potential* space between the outer, parietal pleura and the inner, visceral pleura) while the lungs are resting is about –400 Pa (–4 mm Hg). It falls to about –800 Pa during inhalation because the pressure in the lungs also falls during inhalation. This negative intrapleural pressure acts as a suction to hold the visceral pleura of the lungs tightly against the parietal pleura of the chest wall. The 'gluing' together of the chest wall, parietal pleura, visceral pleura and lung walls is necessary in order to expand the lungs when the chest expands, and to keep the lungs expanded to normal size. They collapse in the absence of the negative pressure. Lung collapse can occur when the chest is opened during surgery or by a stab wound.

A **surfactant** (also called a detergent) is a substance that reduces the surface tension of a liquid. In the lungs, a phospolipid (dipalmitoyl lecithin) is the surfactant which decreases the surface tension of the liquid lining the alveoli. A low surface tension prevents the alveoli from contracting too far during exhalation and thus prevents them from sticking together. The alveoli may be pictured as air-filled bubbles lined with water. At the air–water interface of bubbles, the attractive forces between water molecules (which are relatively strong) cause them to squeeze in on the air within the 'bubbles', thus tending to decrease their volume (and increase the pressure within them). This 'squeezing force' is due to surface tension. Inhalation requires considerable energy to expand the alveoli against surface tension. The presence of the surfactant reduces the cohesive forces between water molecules, thereby lowering the surface tension and increasing the compliance of the lungs (that is makes them easier to expand).

If the alveoli did collapse (a condition called atelectasis) a large effort during inhalation would be required to reinflate them. The lungs of premature babies (with gestation periods of less than about 30 weeks) may lack sufficient surfactant to allow their lungs to expand; such a condition is called respiratory distress syndrome. The infant's lungs collapse with each breath and the effort required to expand them leads to difficult and laboured breathing. Positive pressure ventilation is used to keep the infant alive until surfactant production reaches normal levels. Surfactant from the amniotic fluid of full-term infants can be administered as an aerosol by the ventilator.

If a patient is unable to breathe normally, or the effort required to expand the chest is beyond the patient's capability, positive pressure ventilation (intermittant positive pressure breathing) may be used. Air is applied to the patient at a pressure greater than atmospheric to force it into the lungs, without the patient having to produce the effort to actively expand the chest. The air is turned off as the patient exhales. That is, the air is applied intermittently and the chest allowed to contract elastically by itself. It is essentially the same technique as 'mouth to mouth' resuscitation.

10.11 Ideas About Air Pressure Applied to Nursing Equipment

10.11.1 *Intravenous Infusion Bags*

When infusion containers were made of glass, the containers required two separate tubes for proper operation (see Figure 10.7). This was because the glass provided a rigid container that maintained a constant volume inside its walls. One tube allowed the infusion to flow out of the bottle (under the influence of gravity), and the other allowed air into the bottle to take up the volume vacated by the liquid of the infusion. That is, the second tube was an air vent through which air could enter the bottle to ensure that the air space above the infusion liquid remained at atmospheric pressure. If the air space was not vented, then the pressure of the air enclosed in the bottle would fall as its volume expanded (Boyle's law). Eventually it would become low enough to prevent any more liquid from flowing from the bottle. In this steady-state situation, the outside atmospheric pressure is able to prevent the liquid from flowing through the tube despite the force of gravity. This is because the negative pressure in the air of the container when added to the pressure due to the head of infusion liquid, is equal to atmospheric pressure. Without a pressure difference at the end of the infusion tube, there can be no flow.

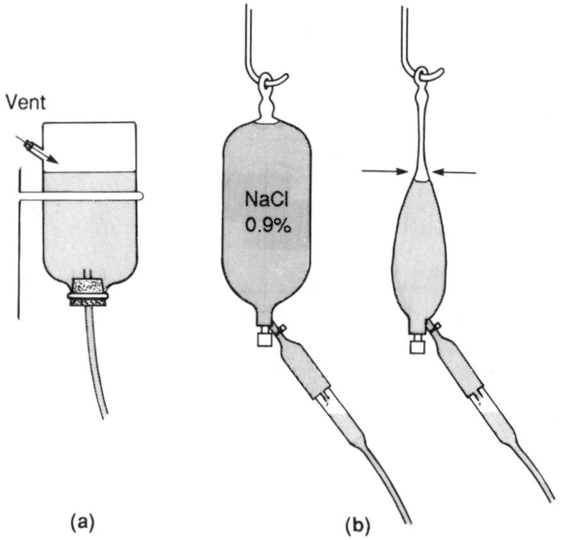

Figure 10.7 *(a) A rigid glass infusion bottle requires a vent to the atmosphere. (b) A flexible infusion bag collapses as the infusion flows out, thus remains at atmospheric pressure without the need for a vent*

Modern infusion containers are disposable soft plastic bags. The soft plastic of the bag allows it to collapse as the volume of liquid in the bag decreases. This means that the interior of the bag is maintained at a constant pressure. These bags require only one tube for proper operation. As gravity causes the infusion to flow out of the bag via the tube, the volume vacated by the liquid is eliminated because the soft walls collapse inwards under the influence of the external atmospheric pressure. The pressure of the small amount of air in the bag always remains at atmospheric pressure.

10.11.2 *Wagenstein's Gravity Suction Apparatus*

The apparatus for Wagenstein's gravity suction technique for draining the stomach consists of three interconnected bottles (see Figure 10.8). Bottles A and B are both fitted with airtight stoppers through which a short tube and a long tube are inserted. The short tubes of each bottle are connected by a tube which can be clamped shut. These two bottles produce the negative pressure necessary for 'suction'. Bottle C also has an airtight stopper but with two short tubes through it. One tube is connected to the long tube of bottle A while the other is connected to a tube that passes into the stomach. Bottle C receives the contents drained from the stomach. Suction commences when the clamp on the tube connecting bottles A and B is removed.

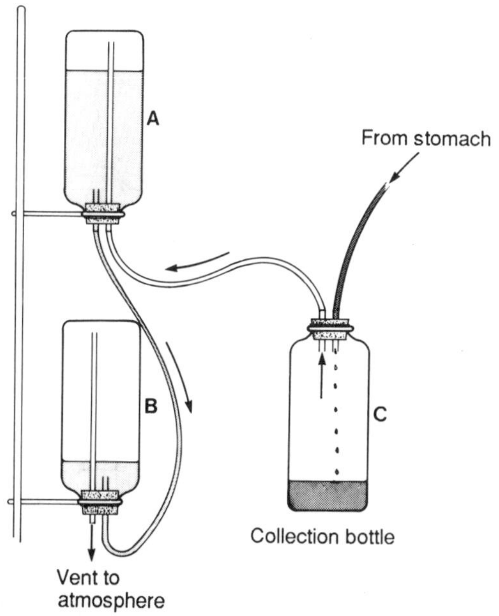

Figure 10.8 *Wagenstein's gravity suction apparatus*

Water from bottle A drains into bottle B under the force of gravity. That is, the volume of liquid in bottle A decreases while the volume of the air space increases. Negative pressure is produced in the air space of bottle A as the air expands into the volume created by the draining water (Boyle's law). Bottle B is vented to the atmosphere so that as it fills with water, the air in bottle B can escape from the bottle. This ensures that the air in bottle B is always at atmospheric pressure. Without a vent, the water flowing into bottle B causes the volume of air to decrease. The increase in pressure that would result, will halt the flow of water, and prevent a sufficiently large negative pressure being produced in bottle A.

The air space in bottle A is a continuation of the air space in bottle C (the collection bottle) because the two are connected by a tube. Since they are the one air space, the pressure in bottle A and bottle C (and in the tube connecting them!) is always the same. As a negative pressure is produced in bottle A, the same negative pressure is produced in bottle C. Bottle C is connected to a tube that enters the patient's stomach so that the pressure on the stomach contents (which is slightly above atmospheric pressure) forces the contents into bottle C. Suction will continue until the stomach is drained or until the water from bottle A has all run into bottle B. In the latter case, suction can be restored by interchanging bottle A and bottle B.

Note that the collection bottle C need not be lower than the stomach. However, it should not be so much higher that gravity acting on the liquid flowing from the stomach to the collection bottle can overcome the force on the liquid produced by the suction of the collection bottle. If the collection bottle is lower than the stomach, then once drainage has commenced it will continue by 'siphon action' until the stomach is drained, whether suction is continued or not.

10.11.3 *Siphon Flow in Liquids*

The siphon is a bent tube through which a liquid will flow under the influence of gravity (see Figure 10.9). The tube (labelled ABC in the diagram) is open at both ends, with the vertical height from B to C being greater

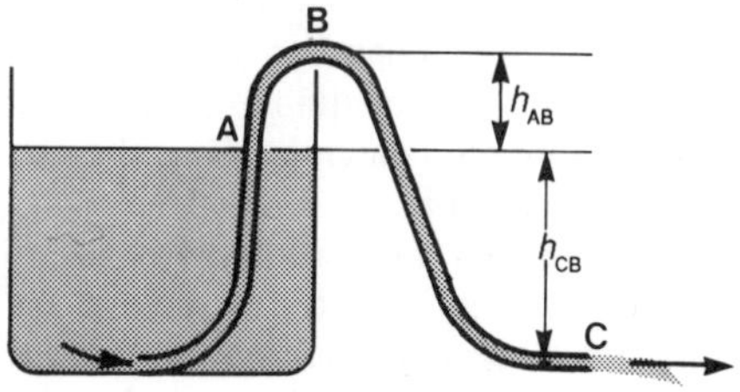

Figure 10.9 *Siphon flow. A liquid can be drawn from a container through a tube as long as the outflow of the tube, C, is below the level of liquid, A, in the container*

than the height from A to B. If the tube is filled with liquid (either by pouring some in or by drawing liquid into the tube by suction), and the opening of one end is dipped under the liquid, then liquid will flow 'uphill' from A to B and then 'downhill' from B to C. This apparently gravity-defying flow of liquid 'uphill' before it flows downwards, is called siphon flow.

The pressure at A tending to force liquid into the tube is equal to atmospheric pressure minus the weight of the head (h_{AB}) of liquid in the tube AB. The pressure at C tending to force liquid up the tube is equal to atmospheric pressure minus the weight of the head (h_{CB}) of liquid in the tube CB. Since h_{CB} is greater than h_{AB}, the pressure forcing the liquid in at A is greater than at C, so the liquid will flow from A to C (in the direction from higher pressure to lower pressure).

Siphon flow can be used for gastric lavage. The washing liquid is poured into the stomach through a flexible tube inserted into the stomach. When filling is complete, the end of the tube is placed in a collecting vessel located at a level below the patient's stomach, and the stomach contents will siphon into the container. The process may be repeated if necessary.

10.11.4 *The Hydraulic Lift*

This device can be used to shift heavy patients who are not able to walk or to lift themselves out of bed. The hydraulic lift (or press) multiplies the force that we exert by an amount equal to the ratio of the cross-sectional areas of its two fluid-filled chambers.

An incompressible fluid fills the two connected chambers. One of the chambers has a small cross-sectional area while the other has a large cross-sectional area (see Figure 10.10). A lever acting on a piston can be used to exert a force on the liquid in the small chamber, thereby increasing the pressure in it. Since the two chambers are connected by a small passage, then, according to Pascal's principle, the pressure exerted in the small chamber will be transmitted undiminished through the liquid to the larger chamber and to the walls of the container. Thus the pressure is the same in both chambers.

One of the walls of the large chamber is a movable piston of larger area than the piston in the small chamber. The amount of pressure in the liquid is determined by the force that is exerted by the lever on the area of the small piston. The same pressure will act on the large piston of the other chamber. The weight that can be lifted by the large piston depends on its cross-sectional area. We know that pressure = force/area, thus

$$\text{constant pressure} = \frac{\text{force}}{\text{small area}} = \frac{\text{weight to be lifted}}{\text{area of larger chamber}}$$

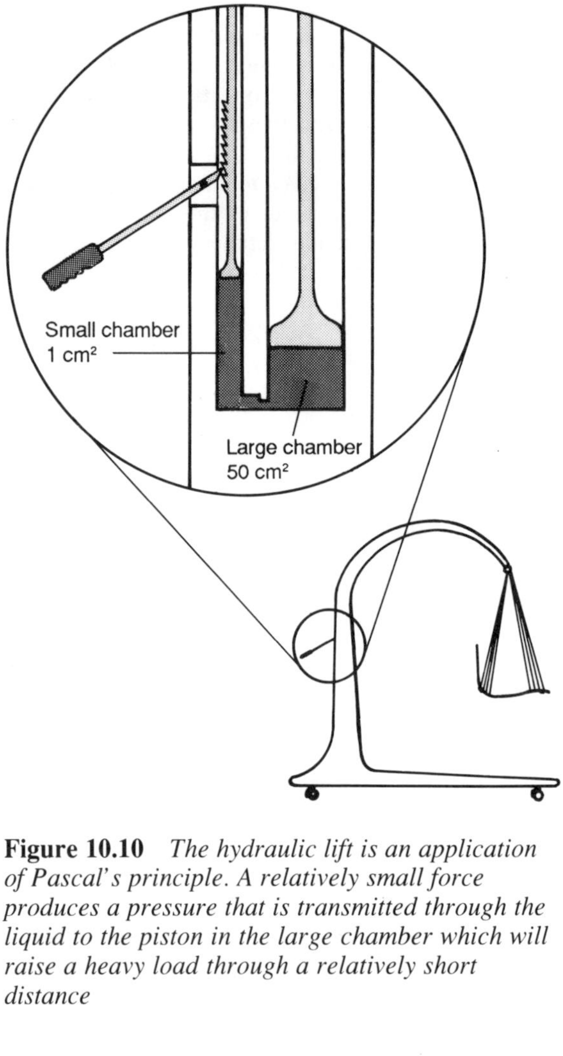

Figure 10.10 *The hydraulic lift is an application of Pascal's principle. A relatively small force produces a pressure that is transmitted through the liquid to the piston in the large chamber which will raise a heavy load through a relatively short distance*

If the cross-sectional areas of the two chambers are 1 cm^2 and 50 cm^2, then a force of 30 N acting on the 1 cm^2 chamber can be used to lift a person weighing up to 1500 N who is supported on the 50 cm^2 chamber (a mass of about 150 kg). This is more than enough to cope with anyone a nurse is likely to need to lift. The exertion of 30 N on the small piston is quite simple provided that a lever (of the first or second class) is used to gain mechanical advantage.

Note that even though our 30 N force is multiplied by 50 to give a resultant force of 1500 N, energy has been conserved. The 30 N force must move the small piston 50 times as far as the large piston moves the 1500 N force. So

energy used = work done
= small force × large distance
= large force × small distance

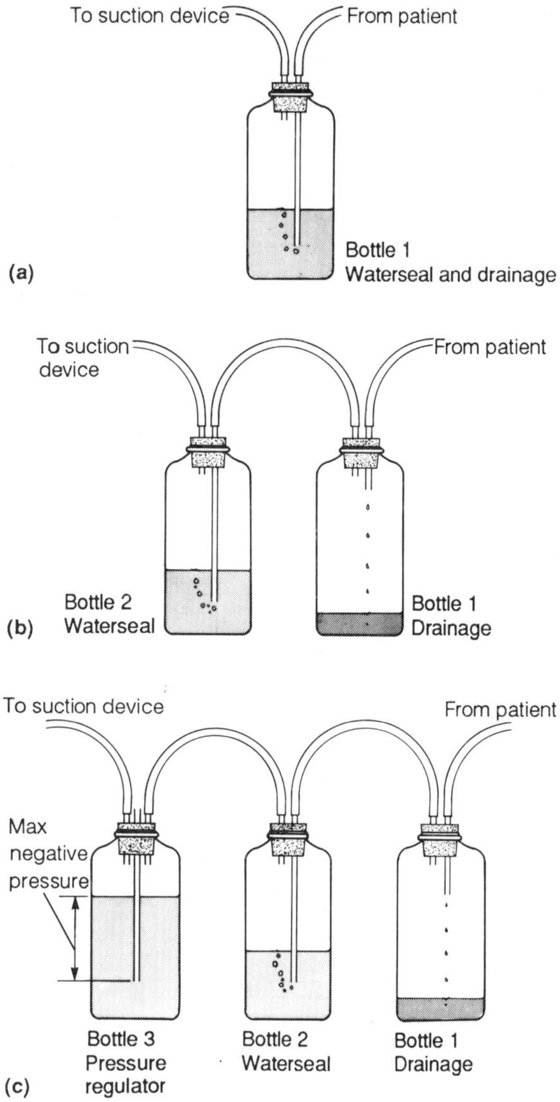

Figure 10.11 *(a) The waterseal prevents air re-entering the chest cavity in the event of suction ceasing. (b) Separate bottles produce the waterseal and collect the drained fluid. (c) A third bottle with an underwater vent to the atmosphere will limit the amount of negative pressure produced*

10.11.5 *Watersealed Chest Drainage*

Breathing is only possible because of the negative pressure that exists between the visceral pleura and the parietal pleura that surround the lungs. The negative intrapleural pressure ensures that the visceral pleura moves outwards with the parietal pleura as the chest expands during inhalation. The negative pressure also means that the lungs will not collapse during exhalations instead they are held against the parietal pleura. Closed waterseal drainage is a method of restoring negative pressure after some intrathoracic procedures (see Figure 10.11). The drainage is called 'closed' because the end of the drainage tube is kept under water so that air cannot be drawn up the catheter into the intrapleural space. That is, the drainage bottle is closed to the atmosphere.

The **one-bottle system** combines the drainage bottle and the waterseal bottle into one. The drainage tube from the patient extends below the water level in the bottle, so that air bubbles out as it escapes from the chest. The water level in the tube rises as the patient breathes in and falls as the patient breathes out. A short tube through the stopper of the bottle acts as a vent for the air drawn from the chest.

In the **two-bottle system** the drainage bottle and the waterseal bottle are separate. The separation of bottles allows the drained fluid to be measured accurately and its colour and character observed effectively. The tube from the patient passes through an air-tight stopper into the drainage bottle but *does not extend to the level of liquid.* Another short tube connects the drainage bottle to the waterseal bottle and this tube does extend to below the water level to provide a seal. Again the level of water in the sealed tube rises and falls with the patient's breathing cycle and again the waterseal bottle is vented to the atmosphere.

The **three-bottle system** entails a third bottle being added to the two-bottle system if a suction device is used to empty the pleural cavity. The third bottle is a pressure-regulating bottle and ensures that a constant negative pressure is maintained in the system and applied to the pleural space. Three tubes pass through the air-tight stopper of the pressure-regulator bottle: a short tube from the waterseal bottle, another short tube from the bottle to the suction device, and a long tube that acts as a pressure regulator. The regulating tube extends to below the water level of the bottle and is vented to the atmosphere.

The depth to which this regulating tube is immersed below the water determines the pressure in the system. Each centimetre below the surface is equivalent to a negative pressure of 1 cm H_2O (98 Pa). If the suction device is applying more than the predetermined amount of suction, the pressure of the atmosphere will bubble air into the pressure-regulator bottle through the long tube, which ensures that the pressure drops no further. If the suction is turned off, then the pressure-regulator bottle should be disconnected from the waterseal bottle. Otherwise the return of atmospheric pressure to the pressure-regulator bottle may force water to overflow from the immersed tubes.

10.12 Introduction to Fluid Dynamics

We have already discussed the pressure that arises in static liquids and gases. Now we need to consider the factors which affect fluids when they are in motion. Fluid dynamics, the study of flowing fluids, is mathematically and physically very complex and at its heart lies Bernoulli's law. This law deals with *ideal* fluids (homogeneous, incompressible and non-viscous) and so serves as a first approximation when applied to a real fluid. In the study of the fluid dynamics of the circulatory system, in which the pressure that produces blood flow is limited to that achievable by the heart, the law of Poiseuille is of particular interest. It relates the volume of flow to the size of the 'pipes' through which the liquid moves. Our discussion will make particular reference to the human circulatory system and its non-ideal fluid (blood). In addition, some devices make use of the consequences of fluid flow in their operation and we will look at these.

10.13 Poiseuille's Law

Jean Poiseuille studied the flow of water through rigid tubes of different sizes, and in 1844 formulated an equation that now bears his name. Before discussing his equation, we need to define some new terms.

10.13.1 *Pressure Gradient*

Recall Pascal's principle: 'any change in pressure in an enclosed fluid is transmitted equally and undiminished to every part of the fluid and to the walls of the container'. Furthermore, the pressure at any point in a *non-flowing* liquid is dependent on the height, h, of the 'column' of liquid above that point, and the density, d, of the liquid ($P = h \times d \times 9.8$). However, once a fluid starts to flow (for example, when the intravenous infusion starts to flow into the patient), there is a drop in the pressure difference between the start of the tube (the liquid level in the drip chamber) and where the fluid leaves the tube (at the canula). Thus the pressure in the liquid of the infusion as it enters the vein is less than it was ($h \times d \times 9.8$) prior to flow commencing. Evidence of this pressure drop at the onset of flow is the decrease in bladder pressure that occurs at the onset of urination.

The decrease in pressure occurs because the molecules in the fluid are no longer just pushing against the container wall and against the molecules above. Instead of bouncing back from the wall to support the molecules in the column of fluid above them, some of their energy is used to move into the opening. Without molecules rebounding from the container wall, the pressure at the opening is lessened. The decrease in the pressure in liquids once they start flowing may also be understood from the Bernoulli effect, that is, pressure is least where the speed of flow is greatest (see later). The onset of flow means that the speed of flow is increased from its previous value of zero, so the pressure (according to Bernoulli) must decrease.

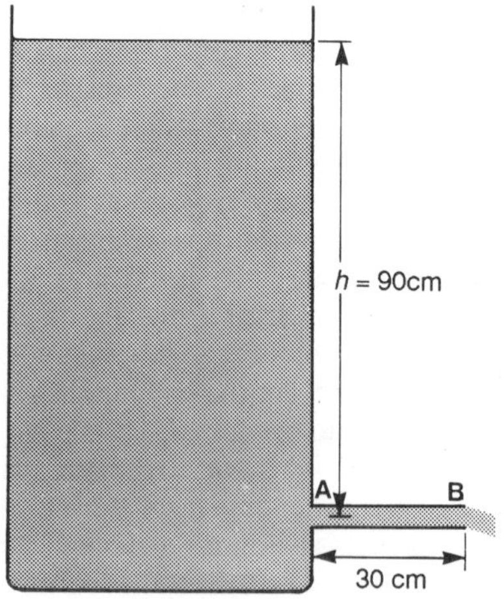

Figure 10.12 *The pressure at B is atmospheric pressure. The pressure at A is atmospheric pressure plus 90 cm H_2O. Thus the pressure gradient between A and B is 90 cm H_2O/30 cm, or 3 cm H_2O per centimetre (in SI units 30 Pa/m)*

The change in pressure along a tube divided by the length of the tube is called a **pressure gradient** and causes the fluid to flow (see Figure 10.12).

$$\text{pressure gradient} = \frac{\text{pressure difference between ends of tube}}{\text{length of tube}}$$

10.13.2 *Volume Flow Rate*

We need to distinguish between the *speed* of flow of liquid and the *volume* of liquid that is flowing. It is possible for the speed of flow to be high while the volume of flow is low, and vice versa. Water coming from the nozzle of a garden hose may be squirting out with a speed of 10 m/s and take one minute to fill a 15 l bucket. In this case the speed of flow is 10 m/s and the volume of flow is 15 l/min. A river meandering towards the sea may have the relatively slow speed of flow of 0.2 m/s but the volume of flow may be tens of thousands of megalitres per minute.

volume flow rate = no. of litres per minute

10.13.3 *Resistance to Flow*

Poiseuille's law relates the pressure gradient (P/L) to the volume flow rate, V.

The volume flow rate (V), will be equal to the pressure drop (P), divided by the resistance to flow ($2.54 \times n \times L/R^4$).

Intuitively we would expect that if pressure increases, then more fluid will flow and also that 'thicker' fluids flow more slowly than 'thinner' fluids. That is, water flows more freely than paint, which in turn flows more easily than honey. If paint gets too stiff, we add a thinner to make it easier to brush. The stiffness in a liquid is referred to as its viscosity. We can also understand that a tube of larger radius should allow a greater flow of liquid, all else being equal. Perhaps not so obvious is that a longer tube should produce more friction between the tube and the flowing fluid. The increased resistance to flow should cause the rate of flow to decrease. All these considerations are combined to form Poiseuille's law. In symbolic form, it may be represented as

$$V = \frac{R^4P}{2.54nL}$$

where R = radius of tube, L = length of tube and n = viscosity of fluid.

Blood is the flowing liquid holding greatest interest for us. Blood is a complex liquid, that is, one composed of many different molecules, some of which are very large. Furthermore, it contains a variety of cells in suspension. A consequence of this lack of homogeneity is that the viscosity of blood changes with pressure (pressure changes do not affect the viscosity of water). In addition, the vessels that blood flows through are not rigid tubes, so their radius may change. Yet another complicating factor is that the flow of blood is pulsatile in nature rather than smoothly continuous. Because of these considerations Poiseuille's law does not apply strictly to blood flow. Nevertheless the law does have some general application, and we will use it to discuss the factors which affect blood flow.

10.14 Factors Which Affect Fluid Flow

10.14.1 *Pressure Gradient*

If a person is lying horizontally we may ignore the slight differences in blood pressure due to the 'head of liquid' between the patient's lowermost surface and their uppermost surface. In the horizontal position the pressure gradient in the circulatory system is due to the pumping action of the heart. Typical pressures in the arteries may be about 16 kPa (120 mm Hg) in the aorta, and about 4 kPa (30 mm Hg) at the start of the capillaries. Venous blood pressure is about 2 kPa (15 mm Hg) at the end of the capillaries and drops to about 0.5 kPa (4 mm Hg) or less at the right atrium.

According to Poiseuille's law, if the pressure drop doubles so does the volume flow rate. That is, V is proportional to P, other things being equal. However, in the circulatory system, other factors *do* change with pressure. Doubling the pressure difference between the ends of a blood vessel does not double the flow, it may triple it or even quadruple it. The viscosity of blood decreases (as does that of synovial fluid) as the shearing force (caused by pressure) on it increases. The decrease in viscosity arises because the long rod-like molecules of plasma proteins in suspension will tend to align themselves, due to the shear force, parallel to the direction of flow. This presents less resistance to flow hence decreasing viscosity. A decrease in viscosity leads to an increase in the volume flow rate (see Poiseuille's law) which is in addition to the increase in flow rate caused by the pressure gradient. Thus a doubling of the pressure gradient will more than double the flow rate.

Raising the container of an intravenous infusion will increase the pressure gradient (because the column or head of liquid increases), and also the rate of flow into the patient. The relationship between head of fluid and flow rate for an intravenous infusion is not a simple one. However, if the head of fluid is between about 20 cm and 120 cm, the relationship between them is almost linear. If the head of fluid is doubled, the flow rate increases to about 1.4 (square root of 2) times its former value; if the head of fluid is tripled then flow increases by a factor of about 1.8 (square root of 3). That is, the velocity of flow (and hence the flow rate) increases as the square root of the head of fluid. The relationship is known as Torricelli's law.

Note that the increased pressure that accompanies the increase in flow rate, when the infusion bag is raised, may be avoided by using a catheter of larger internal diameter. Larger-bore tubes allow for much greater volume flow rates for the same pressure gradient, so are used in preference to larger pressure gradients, when the situation calls for it.

10.14.2 *Friction Between the Fluid and the Walls of the Tubing*

The *material* from which the tubing is made affects the amount of friction. For example, rubber tubing produces more friction than plastic tubing. The *length* of tube affects friction. A longer tube results in more friction; in fact if tube length is doubled, then Poiseuille's law tells us that flow rate is halved ($V \propto 1/L$). In practice the decrease is actually less than half. The *radius* of the tube has a large influence on flow rate, a wider tube producing less friction.

According to Poiseuille's law, flow rate varies as the fourth power of radius. Consequently the effect of a change in radius easily outweighs the effects of changes in the other variables which affect flow rate. Such a strong dependence on one variable is unusual in physical laws. In this case it means that flow rate will double if the radius increases by only 19%. If the radius is doubled, flow rate increases by 16 times! ($V \propto R^4$). Thus a wider-bore catheter will allow an increased flow rate without an increase in pressure (or suction). In intravenous drip equipment, the rate of flow is regulated by constricting the plastic tube (that is, by decreasing its radius) in the line above the catheter, rather than raising the container or using a catheter of different gauge. Since the rate of flow is so sensitive to the radius of the tube, needle or catheter, the most efficient way to increase flow rate is to increase the internal diameter of the tube.

The fourth power dependence of flow rate on tube radius has some dire consequences for blood flow. If a condition exists that results in the internal radius of an artery decreasing, or in the artery walls becoming less flexible, then the amount of blood that can pass through the artery is drastically reduced. For example, if the radius of the aorta decreases from 10 mm to 9 mm (Figure 10.13), the flow rate will decrease from about 90 ml/s to about 60 ml/s, only two thirds of the original value. Coronary artery disease is commonly caused by the build-up of plaque in the wall of the coronary artery. The narrowing of the passage results in a decreased flow rate of blood and will result in angina pectoris when the heart is stressed. Atherosclerosis (the build-up of plaque) is the major cause of strokes and myocardial infarcts.

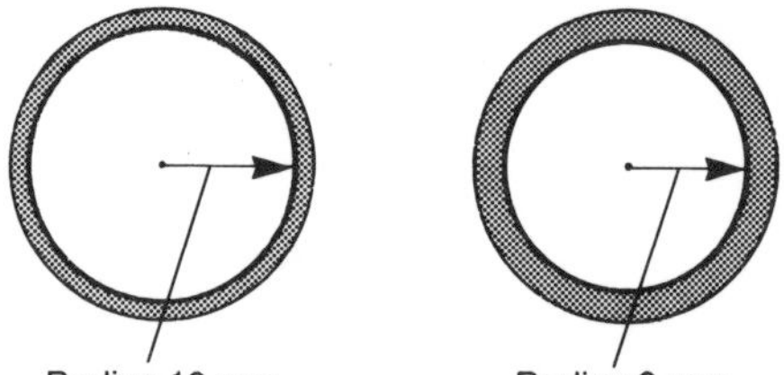

Figure 10.13 *The dependence of volume flow rate on radius is so strong that a decrease of 10% in radius will produce a decrease of 33% in flow rate*

10.14.3 *Fluid Viscosity*

The ease or difficulty with which a fluid can flow affects its flow rate. A fluid's ability to flow is called its **viscosity** and is determined by the internal friction in a fluid. For example, water flows quite freely but honey flows slowly, so honey is more viscous than water. Viscosity arises from the mutual cohesive forces between molecules of liquid; the stronger these forces are, then the more viscous the liquid is. From Poiseuille's law, the higher the viscosity, n, of a liquid, then the lower its flow rate ($V \propto 1/n$).

Apart from at the start of the aorta, where the velocity of flow is high (30 cm/s), blood flow may be considered to be *streamlined*, that is, the flow of blood is smooth and without turbulence. Concentric 'cylinders' of blood in the vessel may be imagined to be sliding one inside the other with the cylinder with greatest speed in the centre of the artery and the slowest cylinder closest to the walls. Blood viscosity is determined by the friction between adjacent 'cylinders' of blood as they flow through the arteries. This friction increases with the percentage of cells in the blood (99% of which are red blood cells). So whole blood is more viscous than plasma, which in turn is more viscous than water (the ratio is approximately 3.5:1.7:1). Typical values for blood and plasma viscosity are 0.004 Pascal seconds (Pas) and 0.0015 Pas respectively (viscosity is sometimes stated in centipoise (cP) where 1 cP = 0.001 Pas). A 'normal' man or woman has about 42% of his or her blood volume taken up by cells (that is, has a haematocrit of 42). A haematocrit may vary from 15 (in anaemia) to 70 (in polycythemia). With a high haematocrit, blood viscosity is so high that its flow through blood vessels is retarded. Dehydration increases blood viscosity, because as the amount of water in the blood decreases, so the proportion of cells increases.

Saline solutions have a lower viscosity than blood or plasma thus tend to flow more readily. This means that blood or plasma require a wider-bore tube to produce the same flow as for saline. The viscosity of blood may be increased by giving a transfusion of packed red blood cells rather than whole blood. Some athletes have tried to enhance their performances by 'blood doping', that is, their own packed red blood cells are retransfused into their system prior to a contest. In theory, the extra red blood cells enable a larger amount of oxygen to be circulated without much increase in blood volume; presumably the increased viscosity does not bother them. An infusion of stable plasma proteins solution will also affect blood viscosity.

Temperature affects blood viscosity. As blood gets warmer, its viscosity decreases. Muscular activity will raise the local muscle temperature and also the temperature of the blood flowing through the muscle. Hence blood viscosity will decrease there. Exposure or shock will lower body temperature and so increase the viscosity of blood, so shock victims need to be kept warm. The increase in blood viscosity in the extremities is a significant factor in the reduction of the circulation in cases of frostbite. The viscosity of blood apparently decreases as it flows through the capillaries which means that less work is required from the heart to drive blood through the narrow blood vessels.

10.14.4 *Laminar or Turbulent Flow*

Laminar (smooth or streamline) flow is usual in long smooth blood vessels. With laminar flow, blood flows in concentric cylindrical layers within the vessel, with each layer remaining the same distance from the wall. The path followed by liquid particles is a smooth line called a streamline, and these paths never cross or intermingle. The liquid molecules touching the wall hardly move because of adherence to the vessel wall. The next layer slips over this almost stationary layer, the third layer slips over the second and so on until at the middle of the blood vessel, blood velocity is greatest (see Figure 10.14).

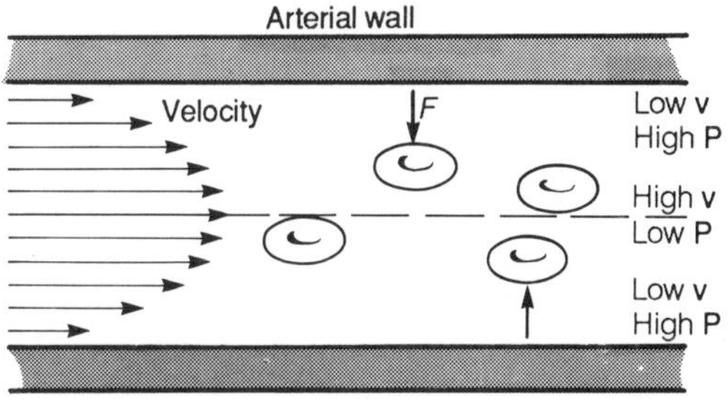

Figure 10.14 *A fluid flowing through a smooth pipe has a parabolic spread of speeds in its streamlines. This gradation in speed within an artery produces a difference in pressure. Consequently, red blood cells are forced into the middle of the artery*

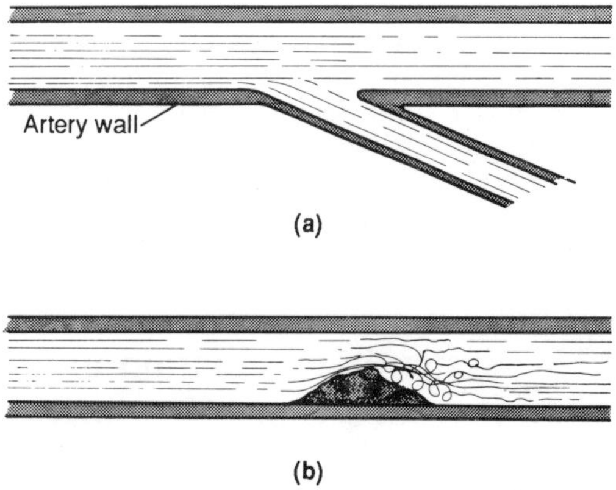

Figure 10.15 *(a) Streamline flow. (b) Turbulent flow caused by a plaque deposit in an artery*

Turbulent flow is when fluid moves in all directions within the vessel and continually mixes in swirls and eddies (Figure 10.15). Turbulence increases the resistance to blood flow by increasing friction. Thus if flow is turbulent the volume of flow is less than for laminar flow at the same velocity. Turbulent flow will occur if blood velocity is high (for example, 30 cm/s in aorta), when blood passes through a narrowing or constriction in a vessel (a stenosis), over a rough surface or makes a sharp turn. Plaque or cholesterol deposits and atherosclerosis can produce turbulent flow and hence a decrease in flow rate (as well as decreasing the radius of the vessel and decreasing the flow rate still further!). Turbulent flow may even release sufficient energy to rupture platelets and cause a blood clot in a vessel.

Another difference between laminar and turbulent flow is that the former is silent while the latter is 'noisy'. By listening with a stethoscope, the sound produced by turbulent flow may be heard. The opening and closing of the heart valves produces turbulent flow, hence noise, so the healthy sound that should be produced may be listened for.

During auscultatory blood pressure measurements the constriction produced in the brachial artery by the pressure cuff causes turbulent flow. The air pressure in the cuff is increased until it is sufficient to collapse the artery and stop all flow. As pressure in the cuff is allowed to decrease, it eventually falls to below the maximum pressure exerted on the blood by the heart muscle. When this occurs, blood is forced through the constricted artery and blood flow is restored. This flow is turbulent, hence relatively noisy and can be heard with a stethoscope. The sounds produced are called the **Korotkoff sounds**. The pressure in the cuff at the restoration of flow is called the **systolic pressure**. As the cuff pressure decreases further, the flow of blood remains turbulent until the pressure in the cuff is too low to produce a significant constriction in the artery. The pressure in the cuff when the sound of turbulent flow ceases is recorded as the **diastolic pressure**.

10.15 Systemic Circulation and Pressure Considerations

Arterial blood pressure arises from the action of the heart pumping blood into the branching system of arteries, which are already filled with blood. It is maintained because this blood is prevented from draining away rapidly by the high resistance to blood flow that is offered by the arterioles. Thus arterial blood pressure is determined by how quickly blood is pumped into the aorta by the heart and by how rapidly it is allowed to leave.

The volume flow rate of blood is called the cardiac output (and is measured in litres per minute). It is calculated by multiplying the heart rate by the stroke volume. Flow rate may be 5 l/min while resting and up to 35 l/min in a well-trained, vigorously exercising athlete.

10.15.1 *The Control of Blood Pressure*

Blood pressure is monitored by **baroreceptors** located in the major arteries in the aortic arch and in the carotid sinus. The baroreceptors are sensitive to the distention of the arterial walls that is caused by pressure and generate action potentials in sensory nerves, which are conducted to the control centre in the medulla of the brain.

The regulation of blood pressure is a complicated topic, but briefly, cardiac output may be decreased and blood vessels dilated to decrease pressure. During exercise, vasodilation causes a decreased resistance to blood flow so more blood can flow back into the heart. The ventricles thus fill to a greater extent before each contraction, and a greater volume of blood is pumped at each stroke. The observation that stroke volume increases as the ventricles receive a greater volume of blood is sometimes called **Starling's law of the heart**. Vasodilation can occur by autoregulation, in which the local release of vasodilator substances can increase blood flow to particular tissues. In addition both arteries and veins may alter their radius by constricting, and pre-capillary sphincters may open or close to regulate blood flow. Since flow varies so strongly with radius (Poiseuille's law), vasodilation and vasoconstriction is a powerful method of blood flow control.

The arterioles play an important role in controlling blood flow. They are lined with muscle that can alter the diameter of the blood vessels. By increasing the radius of the arterioles, the resistance to blood flow is markedly decreased. Thus the volume flow rate of blood increases without the heart having to work harder. The heart maintains an average resting pressure of about 13.3 kPa (100 mm Hg) in the blood of the arteries; this pressure drops as blood passes through the arterioles (due to the resistance that they present to flow) to about 3.3 kPa (25 mm Hg) at the start of the capillaries. Thus, it is in the arterioles that most (about 70%) of the blood pressure is lost.

10.15.2 *The Pressure Gradient and Capillary Exchange*

The transfer of molecules between blood and the tissues, across the capillary walls, occurs along the pressure gradient. That is, the molecules are forced from regions of high pressure, across the capillary wall, to regions of low pressure (Figure 10.16). The net pressure inside the capillary at the arteriole end is *greater* than the pressure outside the capillary, so fluid moves into the tissues at the arteriole end of the capillary. However, at the venule end, the net pressure in the capillary is *less* than the outside pressure, so fluid moves out of the tissues and back into the capillary. The pressure drop between the ends of the capillary (from about 3.3 kPa at one end to about 2.0 kPa at the other) is due to the resistance to flow presented by the capillary. The osmotic pressure difference between the inside and the outside of the capillary remains constant at about −2.9 kPa (the negative sign indicates that osmotic pressure is greater outside the capillary than inside). By adding blood pressure to osmotic pressure difference, the net pressure difference between the capillary and the surrounding tissues can be found. Thus, using the numbers in Figure 10.16, the net pressure difference at the arteriole end is 3.3 − 2.9 = 0.4 kPa (from capillary to tissues) and at the venule end 2.0 − 2.9 = −0.9 kPa (from tissues to capillary).

The average blood velocity in a capillary is 1 mm/s and this low velocity allows time for the diffusion of molecules across the capillary walls to occur. The fluid lost from the capillary at the arteriole end is almost exactly the same (apart from a small amount of fluid and protein that returns to the heart via the lymph) as the amount of fluid that is returned to the capillary at the venule end. This statement is also known as **Starling's law of capillaries**, and means that the volume of blood is maintained at a normal level.

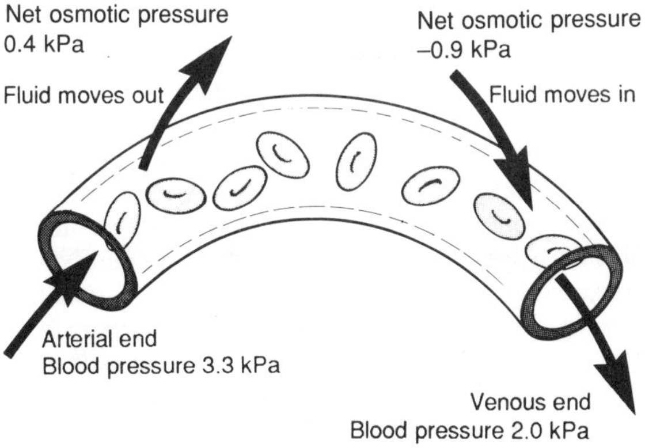

Figure 10.16 *Liquid flows out of the arterial end of a capillary along the pressure gradient and in at the venous end, also along the pressure gradient. The pressure gradient changes from being outwardly directed to inwardly directed because blood pressure falls along the capillary* (see Errata)

10.15.3 *Venous Return*

Blood is forced through the arteries by the pressure gradient produced by the heart. Venous return also occurs along a pressure gradient. For veins, the gradient is produced by the action of the surrounding skeletal muscles. At various points along the veins there are one-way flaps (valves) that prevent blood from flowing away from the heart. The contraction of skeletal muscles causes the muscles to squash on the blood held by the valves in veins and results in an intravenous pressure of about 2.7 kPa (20 mm Hg) during exercise. Thus the 'skeletal muscle pump' produces the pressure gradient between valves that causes the return of venous blood. Since the skeletal muscle pump only operates while the muscles are contracting, standing strictly to attention for an extended period can cause blood to pool in the legs rather than return to the heart. The reduced supply of blood to the rest of the body, the brain in particular, may produce fainting. Once a person has fainted, the horizontal position adopted allows the blood that has pooled in the legs to flow, more or less horizontally, back to the heart and normal circulation is restored.

A varicose vein is one in which the valves are not functioning correctly. They allow blood to flow the wrong way, back through them (away from the heart), causing blood to 'pool' in the legs. The added pressure causes the veins to stretch and to lose their elasticity. In veins close to the surface, a varicose vein may be dilated and discoloured. Pregnant women who sleep on their back will find that the additional abdominal weight of the foetus will press on the veins near the spinal cord and restrict venous return. Consequently on awakening, they may find that their legs are 'asleep'.

When lying down, pressure in the circulatory system is mainly the result of the pumping action of the heart. The resistance to flow in the large blood vessels is low. As a result only small pressure drops result from the flow of blood through the large arteries and veins. Therefore if the body is lying in a horizontal position the average arterial pressures at the upper and lower extremities are the same. However, when standing, hydrostatic pressure, due to the 'head' of blood, is an additional significant factor. The arterial pressure in the brain is reduced while that in the feet is increased, simply because of blood draining under the influence of gravity. In the standing position, the pressure in the right atrium is approximately 0 kPa, because the heart pumps into the arteries any excess blood that accumulates there. However, in an adult who is standing absolutely still the pressure in the veins of the feet is approximately 12 kPa (90 mm Hg). This is simply because of the vertical distance from the heart to the feet and the weight of the blood in the veins. The 'hydrostatic factor' also affects the peripheral pressures in the arteries and capillaries. For example, a standing person who has an average arterial pressure of 13.3 kPa (100 mm Hg) in the aorta would have an arterial pressure of 13.3 + 12 = 25.5 kPa (190 mm Hg) at the feet (the sum of pressure due to the heart and pressure due to the hydrostatic factor). The pressure in an artery that is 40 cm above the heart would be about 4.2 kPa less than that in the aorta. Therefore arterial pressures are stated by reference to the hydrostatic level of the heart, that is, as if the subject was lying horizontally.

If the circulatory system is viewed as a closed system of tubes through which a liquid flows, it can be understood that any increase in volume of fluid without an increase in the size of the vessels must result in a build-up of pressure. Thus if blood volume was to increase, as it does when the diet has an excessive amount of salt (sodium chloride), then blood pressure would increase. Conversely, a decrease of more than 15% in blood volume, due to a haemorrhage for example, would cause blood pressure to drop. For smaller blood losses, a drop in arterial blood pressure is prevented by the constriction of arteries and veins. However, heart rate will increase and cardiac output will fall.

The resistance to blood flow in the systemic circulation is much greater (about six times) than in the pulmonary circulation because of the much greater total length of blood vessels (resistance to flow increases with length of tube). Consequently the left heart pump must raise the pressure of blood in the systemic circulation to a higher level (average 13.3 kPa) than the right heart pump. Blood that leaves the heart to enter the pulmonary circulation is at a pressure of only 3.4 kPa (25 mm Hg). The pulmonary vascular bed can accommodate large changes in blood volume with only small changes in pressure. This is because the pulmonary arterioles have relatively little smooth muscle and are highly elastic, while the capillaries and veins are relatively short and easily distended.

10.16 The Bernoulli Effect

Daniel Bernoulli published his treatise *Hydrodynamica* in 1738, in which he reported his law:

> At any two points along the same streamline in a non-viscous, incompressible fluid in steady flow, the sum of the pressure, the kinetic energy per unit volume, and the potential energy per unit volume, has the same value.
>
> $P + KE + PE = \text{constant}$

Bernoulli's law applies to ideal fluids and so provides only a first approximation to the flow of real fluids. Corrections for the effects that occur in real fluids must be made after experimental investigations.

10.16.1 *Consequences of Bernoulli's law*

An experimental observation of Bernoulli's was that the pressure in fluids that are flowing is least where the speed of flow is greatest. This phenomenon is now known as the **Bernoulli effect**. Bernoulli was able to show that this effect was consistent with his law.

Consider a fluid that is flowing steadily through a horizontal pipe (so that the gravitational potential energy of the fluid does not change). Steady flow means that the same volume per unit time flows past every point of the tube (no fluid leaks out and fluid cannot be compressed). The speed of flow can be increased in a section of the pipe by replacing that section with a pipe of smaller diameter. In order for the volume flow rate to be maintained, the fluid must speed up while passing through the narrower pipe (see Figure 10.17). However, the kinetic energy of the fluid depends on the mass that is moving and its speed ($KE = 0.5 \times m \times v^2$). Thus an increase in speed will mean that kinetic energy per unit volume must also increase, since the mass that is moving (the volume flow rate) does not change. Recall that Bernoulli's law states that the sum of pressure and energy remains constant, thus if one of them (kinetic energy) increases, then the other (pressure) must decrease in order for their sum to be unchanged. Hence pressure must decrease as fluid velocity increases (the Bernoulli effect).

An alternative explanation of the Bernoulli effect can be made using pressure gradients. Consider Figure 10.18. The pressure in the fluid at point A (the start of the tube) is atmospheric pressure plus the hydrostatic pressure due to the head (h) of fluid. The pressure in the fluid at C (the end of the tube) is atmospheric

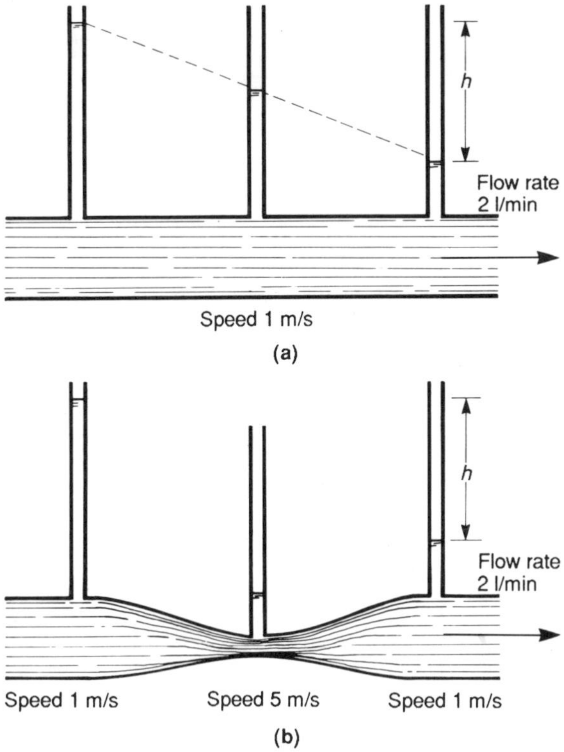

Figure 10.17 *(a) Initially a pressure difference maintains a flow rate and fluid speed. (b) A constricted pipe causes fluid speed (and kinetic energy) to increase at the expense of pressure while flow rate is unchanged*

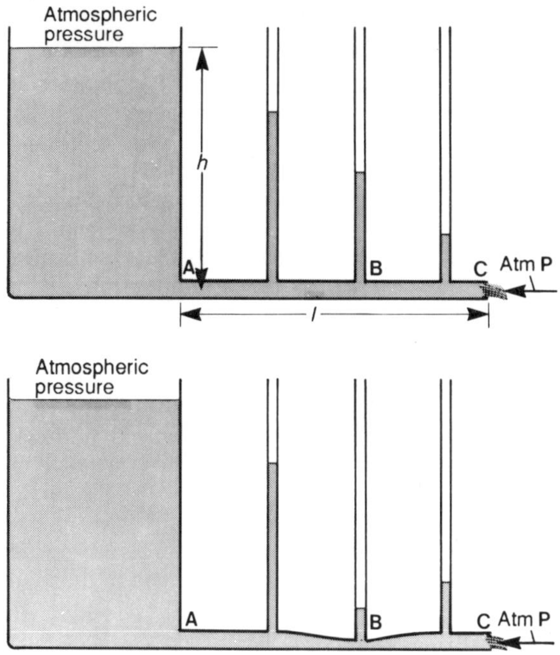

Figure 10.18 *The increase in speed at B is accompanied by an increase in pressure gradient between A and B*

pressure because the fluid is open to the atmosphere. Hence the pressure gradient is h divided by l (the length of the tube from A to C).

$$\text{pressure gradient} = \frac{\text{pressure at A} - \text{pressure at C}}{l}$$
$$= \frac{\text{atm. pressure} + h - \text{atm. pressure}}{l}$$
$$= \frac{h}{l}\ \text{Pa/m}$$

The pressure gradient is in the direction from A to C because the pressure at A is greater than at C. Hence fluid will flow steadily from point A through point B to point C. In other words, fluid flows in the direction of the pressure gradient (from high pressure to low pressure). If the pressure gradient is increased, then the speed of flow must also increase. The pressure gradient can be made greater by increasing the pressure at A, by decreasing the pressure at C, or by shortening the tube.

If the tube at B is replaced by a narrower piece of tube, we notice that the speed of flow of fluid increases. Bearing in mind the above discussion about pressure gradient, the increase in speed must have been in response to an increased pressure gradient. Remember also that fluid flows towards the point of low pressure, so if the fluid now flows faster through B, then the pressure at B must be even lower than before (since the pressure at A has not changed). That is, the region of tube with a faster speed of flow through it must be a point of lower pressure. If, after passing through B, the tube increases in diameter then the speed of flow will decrease and the pressure in the fluid must be greater than at B (but not greater than at A).

It may help your understanding if you think of a weather map (a synoptic chart) showing pressure isobars. High-pressure systems are associated with calm weather. You know that low-pressure systems are associated with strong winds, storms and tropical cyclones. Thus where the atmospheric pressure is low, the speed of fluid flow (the wind) is greatest.

A common example of the Bernoulli effect is the displacement of a shower curtain inwards when the shower is turned on. The downward rush of water draws a stream of air with it. This fast-moving stream of air creates a low pressure, consequently the air outside the shower enclosure (which is at normal atmospheric pressure) pushes the curtain in.

Recall from Section 10.14.4 that blood flows with the greatest speed in the centre of arteries and that speed decreases as we move towards the artery walls. This difference in speed produces a difference in pressure (by the Bernoulli effect) between the blood flowing near the artery walls and the blood flowing through the middle. Pressure is lowest in the mid-line of arteries. Consequently red blood cells experience a net force towards the middle of the artery which causes them to congregate there and leaves a deficit of cells near artery walls (Figure 10.14). This 'axial accumulation' of red blood cells results in a smaller number of red blood cells occurring in the blood flowing through the side branches of arteries than in the total circulation.

10.16.2 *Entrainment*

Consider a fluid flowing steadily at a certain speed due to a pressure gradient through a tube that has a constriction in it (but is otherwise uniform). The speed of fluid movement through the constriction must be greater than in the rest of the tube in order for the constricted tube to pass the same volume of fluid in a given time as the rest of the tube (Figure 10.19a). The pressure in the fluid when it is moving at higher speeds is less than at lower speeds (the Bernoulli effect). As the fluid leaves the constriction it will slow down and its pressure will rise. If the constriction in the tube narrows gradually and expands gradually, the tube is called a venturi tube, after Giovanni Venturi, and flow will remain laminar despite the increase in speed. If the narrowing of the tube is sufficient (that is, the fluid speed is made high enough), the fluid pressure may be decreased to below atmospheric pressure. In this case, a second fluid will be pushed into the fluid by the pressure of the atmosphere if an entry point is made in the constriction. In this way, a liquid or gas can be mixed in with a fast-flowing fluid stream. The introduction of one fluid (whether it be liquid or gas) into another by utilising the Bernoulli effect is called **entrainment**. Nebulisers are devices that entrain water or a medicated solution, in the form of small droplets, into the stream of oxygen or gas flowing into a patient (Figure 10.20).

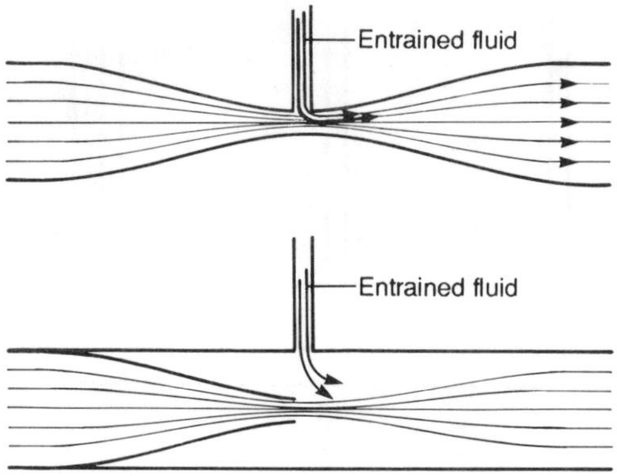

Figure 10.19 *The entrained fluid is forced into the region of low pressure, which was created by increasing the speed of the majority fluid. (a) Entrainment by venturi tube; (b) entrainment by using a nozzle*

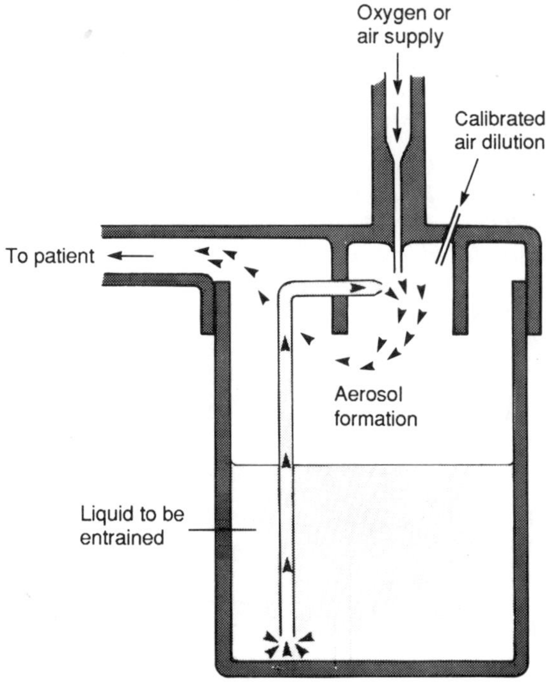

Figure 10.20 *A nebuliser. The high speed of flow through the nozzle produces a sufficient pressure drop for the liquid to be forced upwards against gravity and into the air stream*

When oxygen is administered to a patient at greater concentration than occurs in the atmosphere, it comes from the cylinders as a dry gas. Consequently there is less humidity in the inspired gas mixture than in normal atmospheric air. The dry air would be humidified as it passes over the membranes of the air passages. In order to avoid the resultant excessive drying of nasal membranes, a nebuliser is used to introduce water droplets into the air stream and thus humidify the gas mixture before it enters the patient.

Asthma or chronic obstructive airways disease are treated with medications that work faster if administered to the respiratory tract as an 'aerosol', via a nebuliser. Nebulisers can be used with intermittent positive pressure respirators to push water and medication deeper into the respiratory system. This is very useful where the patient is weak because the therapy is not dependent on the patient's ability to inhale deeply.

More sophisticated entrainment devices are calibrated so that the amount of entrained fluid can be varied. Sometimes they are called **injectors** and are used to mix gases in the administration of anaesthetics.

A venturi mask, used in oxygen therapy, utilises a nozzle (a constriction in the tube) with the shape of a venturi tube (to prevent turbulent flow) to increase the speed of oxygen flow. The increased speed of flow creates a low-pressure region in front of the nozzle (the Bernoulli effect). This allows air to be entrained with the oxygen as it blows onto the face. By selecting another venturi mask with a nozzle of smaller diameter, the speed of the oxygen molecules through the venturi tube can be increased and more air will be entrained. Note that the selection of a different venturi mask does not alter the volume flow rate of oxygen, it alters the speed of the oxygen molecules through the nozzle. The increase in speed of oxygen produces a larger drop in pressure at the nozzle opening, which in turn entrains more air into the mask, so decreasing the concentration of oxygen that is delivered to the patient.

Questions

1. When an 80 kg person is seated on a stool so that the area of contact is 400 cm^2, the pressure on the stool due to the person's weight is very nearly
   J. 2 kPa
   L. 20 kPa
   L. 200 kPa
   M. 2000 kPa
2. If the pressure between the visceral pleura of the lungs and the parietal pleura of the thoracic cage is –8 mm Hg, then
   J. the lung will collapse
   K. exhalation is occurring
   L. the pressure is above atmospheric pressure
   M. the lungs will fill with air
3. Which of the following statements about pressure is true?
   J. As boxes are stacked on top of each other, the pressure being exerted on the floor decreases.
   K. Very small forces will exert small pressures.
   L. By standing on flat boards, the pressure being exerted on the floor decreases.
   M. Objects of large mass produce large pressures.
4. Which of these statements about pressure in static liquids is *not* true ? Pressure at a point in a liquid
   J. depends on the height of liquid above it
   K. acts equally in all directions
   L. depends on the depth it is below the surface
   M. depends on the volume of liquid above it
5. Given that 20% of the air at the normal pressure of 100 kPa is oxygen, then the partial pressure of oxygen is
   J. 0.2 kPa
   K. 2.0 kPa
   L. 20 kPa
   M. 80 kPa
6. Boyle's law states 'when the volume of a fixed amount of gas decreases, its pressure will increase, and vice versa (provided that the temperature doesn't change)'. In symbols, this law is
   J. $P \propto V$
   K. $P \propto T$
   L. $P \propto 1/V$
   M. $P \propto VT$
7. Henry's law may be stated as
   J. The partial pressure of a gas, in a mixture of gases, is the contribution it makes to the total pressure of the mixture.
   K. In a mixture of gases, the total pressure is the sum of the pressures exerted by each of the gases alone.
   L. Pressure applied to any point in a gas is transmitted equally and undiminished to all parts of the gas and to the walls of the container.
   M. The quantity of gas that will dissolve in a liquid at a given temperature is proportional to the partial pressure of the gas and to its solubility coefficient.
8. A statement of Boyle's law is 'the volume of a fixed amount of gas is inversely proportional to the pressure of the gas, as long as temperature does not change'. This means that
   J. a balloon would expand to a larger volume in a hyperbaric chamber

K. the air pressure in the lungs would decrease if the diaphragm is contracted
L. the pressure inside a gas cylinder remains constant while some gas is let out, because the volume of the cylinder has not changed
M. if the lungs could expand to twice their volume, they would contain air at twice the pressure

9. A bed-ridden patient is less likely to develop bed sores while lying on a water bed. This is because
J. the force applied to their bony projections is acting over a tiny area
K. the flexibility of the bed assists the blood circulation
L. the weight of the patient is being supported by parts of the body that are adapted for weight bearing
M. the patient experiences a uniform pressure over most of the lower surface of their body

10. The measurement of cerebrospinal fluid (CSF) pressure is made while the patient is lying down rather than sitting up. The horizontal posture prevents a false high reading due to
J. the weight of the 'head' of CSF in the spinal cord
K. possible movement of the patient while sitting up
L. pressure on the lumbar vertebrae when the back is vertical
M. the greater muscle tone needed to maintain a sitting position

11. The quantity called 'pressure' is defined as the
J. mass per unit area
K. force per unit area
L. height of mercury supported by the atmosphere
M. newton per square metre

12. If the partial pressure of oxygen in the atmosphere was halved, the amount of oxygen that would now dissolve in the alveolar fluid of the lungs would
J. decrease to one quarter of its former value
K. decrease to one half of its former value
L. be about the same as before
M. increase to one and a half times its former value

13. Boyle's law may be stated 'provided that the temperature does not change, the volume of a fixed amount of gas decreases as its pressure increases (and vice versa)'. Which statement concerning the pressure of the air in the lungs is consistent with Boyle's law?
J. It will decrease as the chest expands.
K. It decreases as we breathe out.
L. It increases when we contract our diaphragm.
M. It decreases as our intercostal muscles relax.

14. The consideration of pressure in gases differs from pressure in liquids because
J. pressure at any point in a gas acts differently in different directions
K. in gases, the pressure exerted by each different gas must be considered
L. the pressure in a liquid increases with depth
M. liquids are virtually incompressible

15. Consider an arteriole that is 50 cm distant from the aorta. If blood pressure is 130 mm Hg in the aorta and 30 mm Hg in the arteriole, what is the *pressure gradient* between the two?
J. 2 mm Hg/cm
K. 30 mm Hg/cm
L. 100 mm Hg/cm
M. 130 mm Hg/cm

16. If a stenosis reduces the size of a blood vessel to half of the original diameter, the volume flow rate through the vessel will be reduced. The extent of the decrease in flow can be determined by
J. Poiseuille's law
K. Bernoulli's theorem
L. Dalton's law
M. Pascal's principle

17. During an auscultatory blood pressure determination, the Korotkoff sounds that are listened for are produced because
J. the partial pressure of the blood has been increased
K. the blood flow is turbulent
L. of the viscosity of the blood
M. the volume flow rate has decreased

CHAPTER 11

Waves and Hearing

One of the most sensitive and sophisticated means by which we gather information about our environment is via our sense of hearing. Consequently the loss of this sense constitutes a considerable disability and requires major adjustments to lifestyle. This chapter will deal with how our ear hears, why it fails to hear and how we describe the sounds that we hear. In addition we will explain how the stethoscope allows us to hear the sounds produced by the functioning of our bodies.

There are limits to our sense of hearing. The basis for these limits will be explored. Beyond the range of frequencies that humans can hear is the sound energy carried as ultrasound. This chapter will also focus on the medical uses that have been made of ultrasound.

However, before we investigate sound and hearing, we must establish some basic knowledge about waves in general and about the waves that carry sound energy in particular. To that end we will discuss waves first.

Learning Objectives

At the completion of this chapter you should be able to:

1. Define a wave, a medium, oscillation, direction of propagation.
2. Distinguish between longitudinal waves and transverse waves (and between sound and light).
3. Understand the meaning of wavelength, frequency, period, speed, amplitude and intensity (you should be able to identify them on a diagram).
4. Be familiar with the inverse relationship between period and frequency and with the wave equation.
5. Know that sound intensity is an objective measure of the energy carried by a sound wave (specifically the power per unit area in W/m^2).
6. Know that sound level is a subjective measure, in decibels, that approximates the sensation of loudness.
7. Describe, with the aid of diagrams, the passage of sound energy from the air through the ear to the vestibulocochlear nerve.
8. Be familiar with the common forms of hearing loss and how they may be treated.
9. Appreciate how the stethoscope works.
10. Know the distinction between sound and ultrasound and to be aware of the use of ultrasound in diagnosis.

11.1 Definition of a Wave

We are all familiar with water waves, which travel along the surface of an expanse of water, and with sound waves, which travel through air. Both of these types of waves are **mechanical waves** because they require a material **medium** to travel through. That is, they require some solid, liquid or gas to act as the medium through which they move. For waves on the sea, the medium is sea water. For sound waves, the medium is air, or if you press your ear to the bench, the medium is the material of the bench. On the other hand, light waves are not mechanical, they are one type of **electromagnetic wave** (see Section 12.6). Such waves do not require a medium, since they can travel through a vacuum (empty space) as well as space filled with a medium.

11.1.1 *Waves are a Periodic Phenomenon*

When referring to waves we say a wave travels through the medium, or the empty space. That is, we refer to something that moves (the energy in the wave) and to something that is being passed through and hence does *not* move (the medium). For mechanical waves, the medium does not move in the macroscopic sense of travelling from one place towards another; however, its particles do vibrate. The particles of the medium **oscillate** about an average position. They move in one direction then slow down and stop before retracing their path in the opposite direction. They again slow down and stop before moving once again in their original direction. This to and fro motion continually takes them through the spot where they would be resting if no wave were present. That is, they oscillate about their rest position, taking a certain amount of time to do so.

The continual and repeated disturbance to the position of the particles of the medium constitutes a periodic disturbance, and the time between repeats of the disturbance is called the **period** of the wave (see Section 11.3.3).

11.1.2 *Waves Transmit Energy*

Moving objects such as bullets, stones, tennis balls and the wind all transfer energy to the objects that they hit. In doing so, matter (that is, the moving object) has also been transferred from one place to another. On the other hand, *all waves transfer energy without transferring matter*. Water rushing out from a firehose may knock over someone standing in its path. In this case the water is transferring energy by transferring matter (the water is actually changing its location from inside the water main to the place in front of the hose). Energy transfer without matter transfer occurs when a cargo ship is continually heaved up and down by the swells on the ocean. In this case the water wave is transferring energy to the ship while the medium (the sea water), despite heaving, remains more or less where it is.

Mechanical waves originate when a part of the medium is displaced from its normal position, causing it to oscillate about the 'normal' or 'rest' position. For example, the surface of a swimming pool is at its resting position (if there are no ripples) until someone jumps in (which displaces the particles of the medium), causing waves to radiate out. Since the medium is elastic the disturbance is transferred to adjacent particles of water. Note that the medium as a whole doesn't move (so the swimming pool doesn't move to another part of the backyard) but some of its particles move up and down or to and fro and backwards and forwards. That is, the medium remains relatively at rest while energy is transported through the medium due to the oscillation of the particles of the medium.

Electromagnetic waves also transport energy but without the requirement of oscillating particles of a medium. The magnitudes of the electric 'field' and magnetic 'field' are the things that oscillate. Note that electromagnetic waves can travel through a medium as long as the medium is transparent for the appropriate wavelengths, but that they are not prevented from travelling by the absence of a material medium.

When a wave encounters a surface between two different media, not all of the energy of the wave will pass into the new medium. Some will be reflected. Reflected light is seen as glare or as an image of the surroundings. An echo is reflected sound. The extent of the reflection depends on the characteristics of the two media. For sound, a quantity called impedance (the product of the density of the medium and speed of sound in the medium) determines the amount of reflection that occurs (see Section 11.5.3). If two media have greatly differing impedance, then most of the sound energy will be reflected. If the impedances are similar, the two media are said to be 'impedance matched', and most of the sound energy will pass through their interface. Impedance matching is discussed further in Section 11.5.3.

11.1.3 *The Definition of a Wave*

Now that we have some understanding of what a wave is, we can summarise what we mean by wave motion. A wave may be defined simply as *a mechanism for the transfer of energy without the transfer of matter*, or with greater precision as *the propagation of a periodic disturbance, in some property of a medium, or through space. The medium is unchanged by the passage of the wave motion through it.* Sound travels through air but the air remains still. The energy carried by water waves can propel a surfer, erode a coastline and buffet a massive ship. The energy carried by sound waves can damage ears, rattle windows and stun fish underwater. The energy carried by electromagnetic waves can stimulate vision, warm our bodies, cook our food, transmit our communication, heat our water or burn our skin.

11.2 Longitudinal Waves and Transverse Waves

Sound waves (as well as being mechanical) are termed **longitudinal waves** while light waves are termed **transverse waves**. The direction in which the wave is transferring its energy is called the **direction of propagation**. Longitudinal and transverse are terms used to describe the orientation of the direction of oscillation of the particles in the medium, with respect to the wave's direction of propagation (see Figure 11.1). Longitudinal waves cause a displacement of the particles in the medium that is in a direction parallel to (or along) the direction of propagation. This causes the medium to 'squash up' (forming a **compression**) and to 'stretch out' (forming a **rarefaction**) as the particles move backwards and forwards along the line that the wave travels. Transverse waves in a medium (waves on water, for example) cause a displacement that is in a direction perpendicular to (or across) the direction of propagation. The displacements form **crests** and **troughs** and these displacements move through the medium in the direction of the wave.

Electromagnetic waves (of which light is but one example) are also called transverse even though they don't require a medium. They are difficult to visualise because they are not mechanical waves, so exactly what is oscillating is difficult to understand. In the case of electromagnetic waves, the properties that undergo oscillation are the direction and magnitude of the electric field and the direction and magnitude of the magnetic field. The direction of these two fields are at 90° to the direction of propagation of the wave (and to each other) and their magnitudes continually oscillate from a positive value through zero to a negative value and back again (see Figure 11.2).

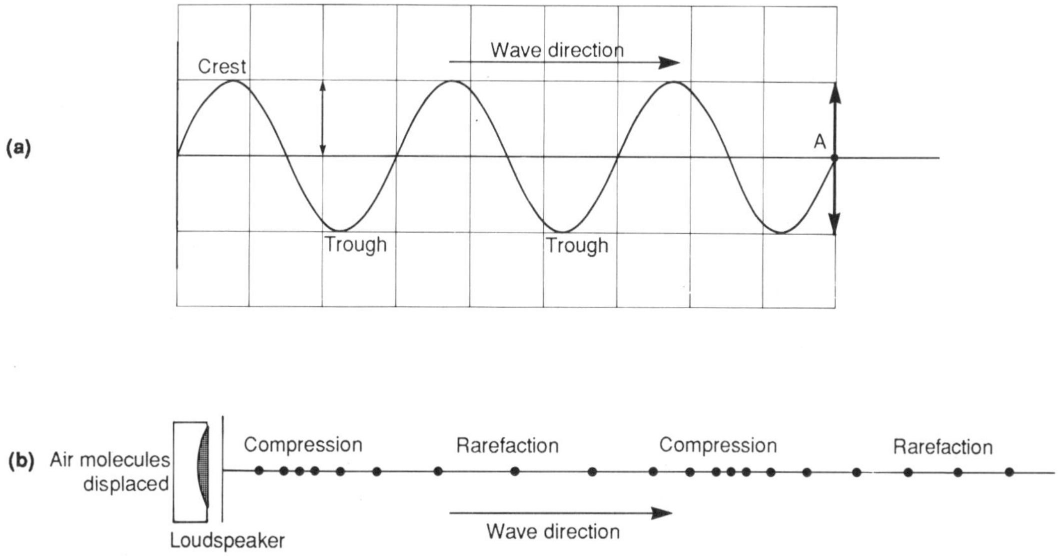

Figure 11.1 *(a) A transverse wave consisting of crests and troughs that are moving from left to right. The particle at A would move down and up as first a trough and then a crest passes by. (b) A longitudinal wave consisting of compressions and rarefactions. A particle of the medium will move left then right as first a compression and then a rarefaction passes by*

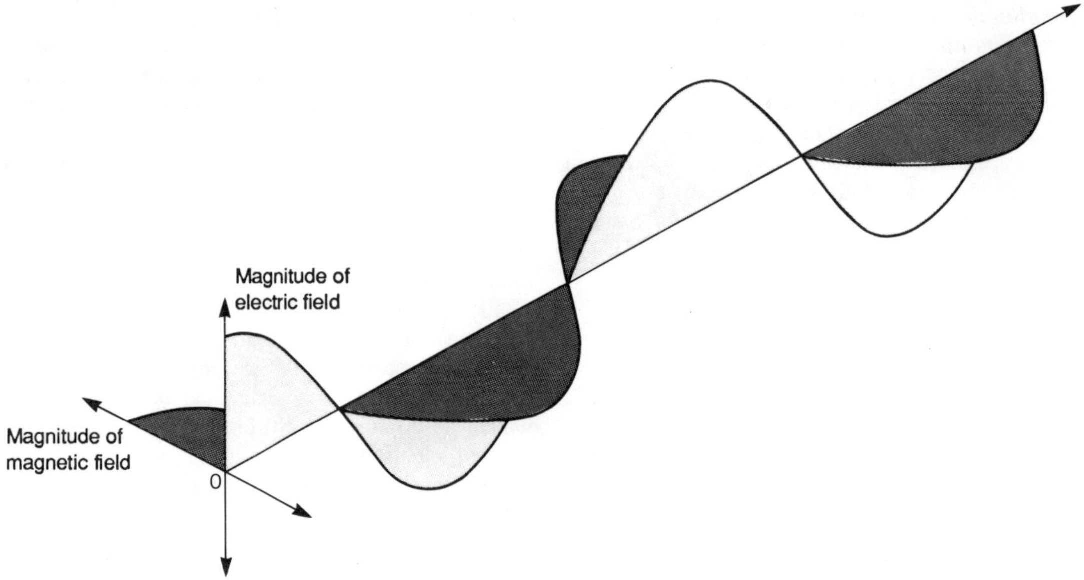

Figure 11.2 *An electomagnetic wave consists of an oscillating electric field whose direction is at right angles to an oscillating magnetic field*

11.3 Properties of Waves

There are several technical terms that are used to refer to those properties of waves that can be measured. Some of these properties are represented on the pictorial representation of a wave in Figure 11.3.

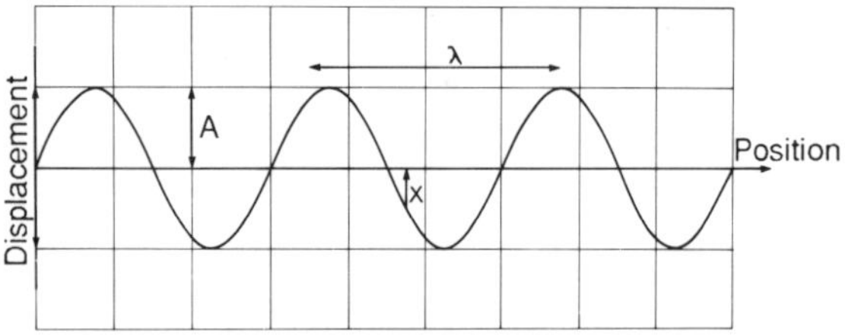

Figure 11.3 *Wavelength (λ) is the distance between adjacent crests. Amplitude (A) is the maximum displacement of the medium as the crest (or trough) passes by. The displacement of a point X is the distance that it is from the middle position*

11.3.1 *Wavelength*

The length of a wave is the distance between two successive crests (or troughs), or any other two successive points in phase (see Section 11.3.8). It is symbolically represented by the Greek letter lambda, λ (an upside down y). In longitudinal waves, wavelength is the distance between successive compressions or rarefactions. Being a distance, wavelength is measured in metres, m. Wavelength will change when a wave moves into a medium in which its speed of travel is different. It decreases as the speed of the wave decreases (and vice versa). Typical values for the wavelength of light and sound are 0.000 000 5 m (500 nm) and 0.4 m respectively.

11.3.2 *Frequency*

Frequency, symbol *f*, is how many wavelengths pass by in one second. Alternatively, it may be thought of as how many crests move by in one second (or how many compressions). Frequency used to be expressed as 'cycles per second' but this unit has been renamed the **hertz** (Hz), after Heinrich Hertz. Thus if 400 crests per second pass by, 400 wavelengths have passed by in one second and the frequency is 400 Hz. The 'pitch' of a pure musical note is equivalent to its frequency. Frequency does not change if the wave moves into a different medium. A typical value for the frequency of light is 10^{14} hertz (100 000 000 000 000 Hz) and for sound is 1000 Hz.

11.3.3 *Period*

The period (T) of a wave is the time, in seconds, it takes for one complete wavelength to pass by. Period is the inverse of frequency. Thus

$$T = \frac{1}{f} \text{ and } f = \frac{1}{T}$$

For example, if a wave has a frequency of 400 Hz, then its period is 1/400 = 0.0025 s. One wavelength of sound (of frequency 1000 Hz) takes 0.001 s to pass by while light is much faster; in one second, 10^{14} wavelengths can pass by.

11.3.4 *Speed*

The speed of a wave (v) is how fast the wave (or a crest on the wave) is moving in the direction of propagation, in other words, the distance it moves in a certain time. Speed is related to frequency and wavelength by a formula which is often called the 'wave equation'.

$$v = \frac{\text{distance moved}}{\text{time taken}} = \frac{\lambda}{T} = f\lambda$$

so speed = frequency × wavelength.

The speed of a wave is not necessarily a constant quantity. It changes if the wave moves into a different medium. Light travels at 3×10^8 m/s through air (as does all electromagnetic radiation), but is slower in more dense media. For example, in glass the speed is 2×10^8 m/s. The speed of sound in air increases as the temperature of the air increases: at 0 °C, v = 331 m/s, at 20 °C, v = 343 m/s. The speed of sound increases also as the density of the medium increases: in sea water (at 20 °C) v = 1540 m/s, in human tissue v = 1550 m/s, in steel v = 5200 m/s.

11.3.5 *Displacement*

We have said that particles in the medium vibrate or oscillate about their rest position (their undisplaced position). The displacement of a particle (or the medium) is the distance that a particle has moved from its rest position. Strictly speaking it is the *distance* and the *direction* in which it has moved, so a positive displacement occurs when a particle moves to one side of the rest position, and a negative displacement occurs when the particle is displaced to the other side.

11.3.6 *Amplitude*

The amplitude (A) of a wave is the **maximum displacement** of a particle of the medium from its rest position. In the case of a water wave, the amplitude is half the vertical distance moved by a boat floating on the water as a crest 'turns into a trough'. Amplitude is a distance so is measured in metres. Amplitude is related to intensity (in fact, intensity is proportional to the square of amplitude). Thus, the louder a sound or brighter the light, the greater is the intensity (and amplitude) of the wave. The amplitude is also related to the amount of energy being transported by the wave. The amplitude of the loudest sound the ear can bear is about 0.01 mm while for the softest sound, amplitude is as small as 10^{-10} m (the diameter of an atom).

11.3.7 *Intensity*

The intensity of a wave refers to the amount of energy being carried by the wave. The intensity is expressed in terms of the amount of energy passing through an area (one square metre) at right angles to the direction of propagation in one second. Thus the sound wave produced by someone talking may have an intensity of 0.000 001 J/s/m², or more concisely, 10^{-6} W/m² (one watt = one joule per second). If you look at a 60 W light globe from a distance of 2 m, the intensity of the light entering your eye is about 1.2 W/m². Of course since your pupil is much less than one square metre in area, the actual amount of energy that enters your eye in one second is a very small fraction of 1.2 J.

11.3.8 *Phase*

The term **phase** refers to the particular stage of the cycle of oscillation that a particle or field may be in. A complete cycle, starting from a crest, moving through the rest position into a trough and then back through the rest position to a crest again, can be related to the 360° of a circle. If a particular particle is at its rest position, then a particle halfway up the following crest is said to be 45° behind the phase of the particle at the rest position. If two parts of a medium are moving up and down 'in step' with each other, they are said to be in phase. Two particles that are completely 'out of step' are said to be 180° out of phase. Differences in the phase of sound waves allow us to determine from which direction a sound is coming. Phase considerations are also important when we discuss lasers in Section 12.10.

Of the eight listed wave properties, which is the one most characteristic of the wave? The frequency (and hence the period) of a wave remains constant no matter how many different media the wave may pass into (but read about the Doppler effect in Section 11.11). However, all the others change when a different medium is entered. For this reason the frequency of a wave is the characteristic quantity that is most often referred to. However, for light waves, wavelength is more easily measured than frequency, so the wavelength in air is often quoted.

11.4 Range and Sensitivity of Human Hearing

11.4.1 *The Relationship Between Sensitivity and Range*

The range of human hearing lies within the frequencies of 20 to 20 000 Hz but the exact end points vary with different individuals and contract with age. Low-frequency sounds are 'deep' or of low pitch while high-frequency sounds are 'shrill' or of high pitch. Sound waves with a frequency that is less than audible sound are called **infrasonic** while those with frequencies above 20 000 Hz are **ultrasonic**.

The sensitivity of human hearing lies between the sound intensities of about 10^{-12} W/m^2 and 1 W/m^2, but the lower limit increases with age or noise damage to the ear. Above an intensity of 1 W/m^2 sound becomes painful. Hearing sensitivity is not uniform across the range of audibility (see Figure 11.4). That is, we can hear sounds of intensities as low as 10^{-12} W/m^2, as long as the frequency is in the range of 1000 to 6000 Hz. However, in order to hear sounds of lower or higher frequency, their intensity must be raised. Thus the intensity threshold of hearing for sounds of frequency 16 000 Hz and 180 Hz is 100 times higher (10^{-10} W/m^2) than for a 2000 Hz sound. Moreover, the difference in sensitivity between frequencies *decreases* as the intensity level of the sound is increased. In other words, if the intensity is high (say 10^{-2} W/m^2), sounds of all frequencies will be heard as approximately of equal loudness.

The complex relationship between human hearing range and our sensitivity to different frequencies within the range is complicated further by the human *perception* of sound. The greatest intensity of sound

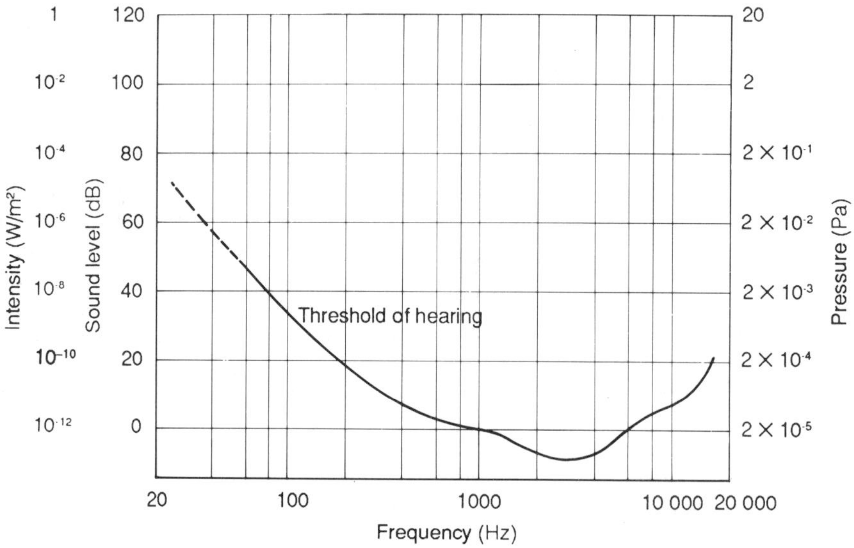

Figure 11.4 *The sensitivity of the ear is not the same at every frequency. The '0 dB phon' shows how the threshold of hearing varies. That is, different frequencies must have different intensities in order to be heard*

that we can bear is a million million times more energetic than the faintest sound (a factor of 10^{12}), yet the loudest sound we can bear seems nowhere near this many times as 'loud' as the faintest. The relationship between intensity and loudness involves physiological and psychological processes in the ear and brain.

11.4.2 *Sound Intensity and Sound Level*

Sound intensity is defined as the acoustic power per unit area, hence is measured in watts per square metre, W/m^2. It is the amount of energy crossing one square metre in one second. As such it is an objectively measurable quantity. On the other hand, *perceived loudness* is a subjective judgement that depends the brain's interpretation of aural stimulation (as well as on the state of health of the hearing mechanism). Hence to decide whether a particular sound is twice as loud as another is not straightforward and the relative loudness of the two sounds will be adjudged differently by different individuals.

The human hearing mechanism does not respond very well at very low frequency, so in order to detect a sound of 20 to 50 Hz it has to be relatively intense. As sound frequency increases so does the sensitivity of our ear, so that we can hear sound waves which carry progressively less energy. Our sensitivity increases for frequencies up to about 4000 Hz after which it decreases (see Figure 11.4). How loud a sound seems to be depends on its frequency *and* its intensity. Thus a 4000 Hz note 'sounds louder' at an intensity of 10^{-8} W/m² than it does at 10^{-11} W/m² *because it carries more energy*. However, a note of 100 Hz will 'sound fainter' than a note of 4000 Hz even if they are both at an intensity of 10^{-6} W/m² because our ears don't hear as well at 100 Hz.

Since the human ear is not equally sensitive to all of the frequencies that are audible, we use a quantity called **sound level**, instead of sound intensity, to try to represent the 'loudness' response of the ear. Sound level is thus a measure of our sensation of loudness, albeit an approximate one. Sound levels are expressed as **decibels**, dB, rather than watts per square metre (which is the unit of sound intensity). A decibel is one tenth of a **bel**, a unit that is named after the American, Alexander Bell. For example, if a 100 Hz sound carries energy amounting to 10^{-9} W/m² we can barely hear it (it has a sound level of about zero decibels), but a 1000 Hz sound of the same energy would be perceived to be much louder (about 30 dB).

Because our sensation of loudness is *subjective* (is produced in the mind of the hearer), it does not correspond to the *objectively* measurable quantity of sound intensity. For a sound to be heard as 0.1 dB louder than another (of the same frequency) when the intensity is 0.05×10^{-3} W/m², the first sound must carry 0.001×10^{-3} W/m² more energy. At higher intensities, sound perception changes. For a sound to be heard as 0.1 dB louder than another when the intensity is 50×10^{-3} W/m², the first sound must carry 1.165×10^{-3} W/m² more energy. At the higher intensity, the intensity difference is 1165 times the difference at the lower intensity. We can summarise the result as follows: the difference in intensity, between two sounds that we can barely perceive as being of different loudness, increases as intensity increases. The increase is approximately logarithmic. So we define the difference in sound level between two sounds in terms of their intensities in the following way. The number of decibels by which a sound of intensity I exceeds I_0 is

$$\text{dB} = 10 \times \log_{10}\left(\frac{I}{I_0}\right)$$

If I_0 is set at 10^{-12} W/m² (the accepted threshold of hearing), and I is the intensity (in W/m²) of the sound being compared to I_0, the formula defines sound level in dB.

Since the response of our ear is roughly logarithmic, equal ratios of intensity are interpreted by the ear as equal increments of loudness. For example, each time that sound intensity increases by a factor of 10, sound level increases by one bel. Thus if a sound is 10 times more intense than another, it sounds one bel (10 dB) louder. If it is 100 times more intense, it sounds two bels (20 dB) louder, if it is 1000 times more intense it sounds three bels (30 dB) louder and so on. The size of one bel is slightly large for reporting changes in loudness so the decibel equal to 0.1 bel is used. Note that the bel rating of sound level is not true psychological loudness, but it is close enough to justify calling it the loudness. Hence it is common to specify sounds by their sound level (in decibels) rather than their intensity (in watts per square metre) as in Table 11.1.

11.4.3 *Equal-Loudness Curves*

We have said that sound level only approximates to our sensation of loudness. The exact nature of the difference between them is determined by testing an individual. An experiment may be performed where

Table 11.1 *Sound levels and sound intensities of various sounds*

Intensity (W/m^2)	Level (dB)	Source of sound
10^{-12}	0	Threshold of hearing or complete silence
10^{-11}	10	Rustling paper or leaves
10^{-10}	20	Whispering (at 1 m)
10^{-9}	30	Ticking watch 1 m from ear, city street no traffic
10^{-8}	40	Quiet home, church or garden, very soft music
10^{-7}	50	Quiet conversation, office, classroom
10^{-6}	60	Normal conversation at 1 m
10^{-5}	70	Loud conversation, city street with traffic
10^{-4}	80	Heavy traffic noise at 5 m, class lecture, loud radio
10^{-3}	90	Engineering workshop. Pneumatic drill at 3 m. Hearing damage occurs
0.01	100	Boilermakers workshop and riveting, loudest passages of orchestra for close observer
0.1	110	Pneumatic drill at 1 m. Loud indoor rock concert
1	120	Threshold of pain and discomfort, jet engine at 50 m
10	130	Jet engine noise at 5 m
100	140	Shotgun blast causing pain and which perforates the ear drum
10^8	200	Saturn rocket at 50 m

the subject compares a standard sound (1000 Hz at 60 dB) to a test sound of frequency *f*. The intensity of the test sound is varied until the subject judges it to have the same loudness as the standard sound. The process is repeated for other test sounds of frequency above and below 1000 Hz and covering the audible range until an 'equal-loudness curve' can be drawn. Such a curve is called the 60 dB phon because the standard

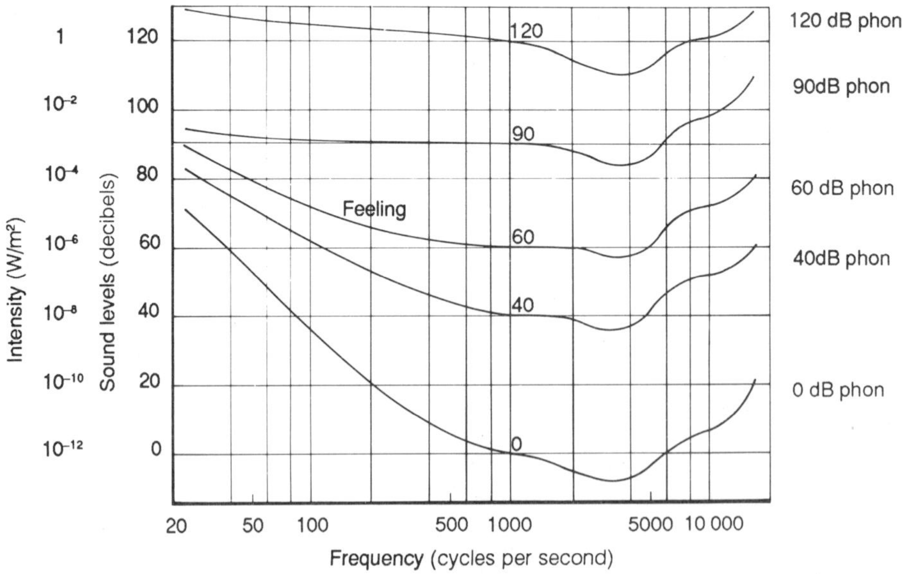

Figure 11.5 *Equal-loudness curves (phons) for five loudness levels. The line of the 60 dB phon indicates the intensity that a particular frequency must have in order for that frequency to sound as loud as 1000 Hz at 60 dB*

sound was at the 60 dB level (see Figure 11.5). If the standard sound used is 1000 Hz at 40 dB, the equal-loudness curve would be called the 40 dB phon.

By following the 60 dB phon curve from low frequencies to high frequencies, we can determine that even though we may adjudge loudness to be constant (at 60 dB phon), the sound level varies from 77 dB when frequency is 60 Hz, down to 57 dB at 4000 Hz and back up to 72 dB at 10 000 Hz. The intensity of sound (and hence the energy) impinging on our ear drums varies over a much larger range. The 60 dB phon ranges in sound level over 20 dB but ranges in intensity over 100 W/m^2.

It is easy to be confused by sound measurements, but try to remember that frequency (in Hz) and sound intensity (in W/m^2) are objective physical measurements of the disturbance in the medium caused by the sound wave. Sound level (in dB) attempts to scale sound intensity into a more human-sized range, and is an *approximation* to the sensation of loudness. Since our ear responds to different frequencies by producing different sensations of loudness, the loudness phon curves are used as a relative measure of loudness over the range of frequencies. Note also from the previous paragraph that a sound level of 60 dB does not necessarily produce the loudness of the 60 dB phon.

We have discussed the response to sound of an ear with a healthy, young hearing mechanism. The ability of a particular individual's ear to respond to sound depends on many things. These include:

- the frequency of the sound (the human ear is most sensitive in the range between 800 Hz and 6000 Hz);
- the intensity of the sound (the apparent difference in loudness between frequencies decreases as sound intensity increases);
- the age of the ear (old age decreases the ability to hear low-intensity sounds and high-frequency sounds);
- noise-induced ear damage (decreases the loudness of frequencies near 4000 Hz the most);
- congenital differences.

11.5 The Physics of Hearing

11.5.1 *The Mechanism of Hearing*

Recall that sound waves are a series of compressions and rarefactions travelling through air (or some other medium). A compression causes air molecules to come closer together and so the air will momentarily be at an increased pressure. A rarefaction causes molecules to move further apart to produce a momentary, local, low pressure. The pressure variations produced by sound waves on the eardrum vary from 2.0×10^{-5} Pa for the faintest to about 28 Pa for the loudest tolerable sound.

The eardrum (**tympanic membrane**) separates the air in the ear canal from the air in the middle ear cavity. The air in the middle ear cavity is maintained at atmospheric pressure because it is vented to the

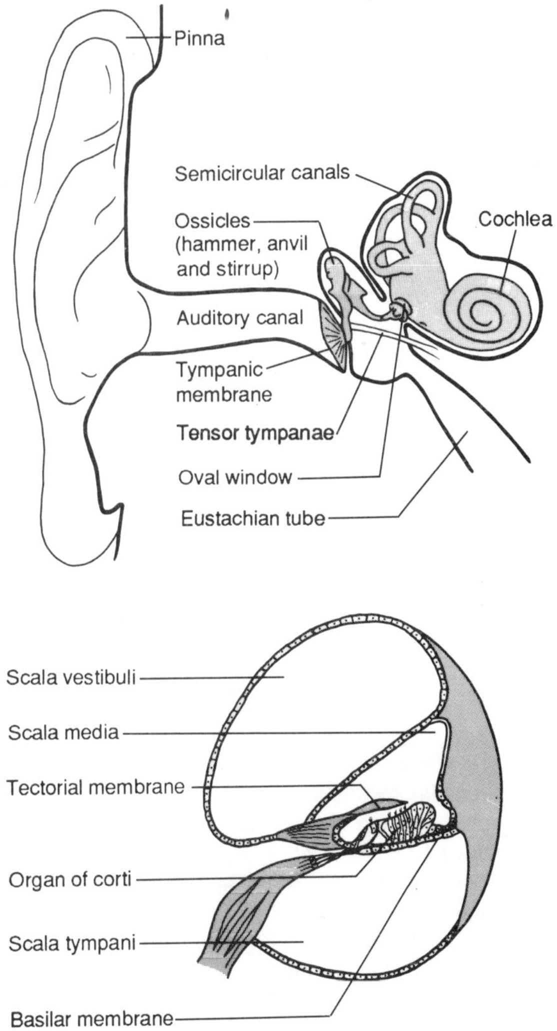

Figure 11.6 *Top: schematic diagram of the ear. Bottom: a cross-section through the scalae of the cochlea*

atmosphere by the eustachian tube. The local increase in air pressure that is associated with the compression of a sound wave will cause the eardrum to bulge inwards. The eardrum will then bulge outwards as the lower pressure that is associated with the rarefaction arrives. The rapid and continuous displacement of the tympanic membrane inwards and outwards, in time with the arrival of the compressions and rarefactions of the sound wave, constitutes a vibration. This vibration of the tympanic membrane, in turn, causes the three **ossicles** of the middle ear (the malleus, incus and stapes) to move. The movement of the ossicles passes the vibration of the eardrum, through the air-filled cavity of the middle ear, to the **oval window**. This 'window' is a small, membrane-covered 'opening' to the organ called the **cochlea**, in the inner ear (refer to Figure 11.6). The cochlea consists of three parallel tubes (the scala vestibuli, the scala tympani and the scala media) that are coiled upon themselves in the way a snail shell coils. The tubes are filled with fluid, perilymph in the scalae vestibuli and tympani, and endolymph in the scala media. The passage of sound energy through the perilymph of the scala vestibuli is due to the propagation of the compressions and rarefactions that make up the longitudinal wave. These compressions and rarefactions are in fact pressure variations and are transmitted throughout the perilymph (recall Pascal's principle, Section 10.4.2). The walls of the scala vestibuli will press against the endolymph in the scala media.

The scala media is separated from the scala tympani by the basilar membrane. In the scala media, mounted on the basilar membrane is the **organ of Corti**. The basilar membrane is set in motion by the pressure variations in the perilymph. The organ of Corti has some cells with hair-like projections which are rubbed by the moving basilar membrane. The hair cells are connected to nerve endings so that the movements of the 'hairs' somehow trigger the nerve cells to send an impulse to the brain.

The basilar membrane is thin and tight near the oval window and thickens and slackens as the coil of the cochlea tightens. The thin part responds best to high frequencies while the thicker part responds to the low frequencies. Consequently a sound wave will produce a response in the basilar membrane at a place where the thickness is optimal for the frequency of the sound. In this way different hair cells are stimulated to send impulses to the brain and the brain is able to distinguish different sounds.

The benefit of having two ears is that we can tell where sound is coming from. Sound coming from one side will not affect both ears the same way because the ears will differ in their sensation of loudness. The waves will arrive at the ears at different times and the *phase* of the waves will differ. That is, as a compression is entering one ear, a different compression or a rarefaction or something in between, is entering the other ear. From this information we are able to localise the source of sound in space.

11.5.2 *Pressure Amplification*

Sound waves approach our eardrum through the ear canal, a 2.7 cm long pipe, closed at one end by the eardrum. Such a tube will resonate (see Section 11.7.2) for a sound of wavelength 10.8 cm (four times the length of the tube). This wavelength corresponds to a frequency of 3000 Hz as calculated below:

$$f = \frac{v}{\lambda} = \frac{340 \text{ m/s}}{0.108 \text{ m}} = 3000 \text{ Hz (approximately)}$$

When resonance occurs in the air in the ear canal, a larger vibration than results from a non-resonant frequency is passed on to the eardrum. This in part accounts for the ear's greater sensitivity for frequencies near 3000 Hz.

The passage of sound from the outside air to the cochlear fluid is accompanied by considerable amplification of the amplitude of vibration. Resonance in the ear canal produces a times two multiplication of amplitude. The area of the oval window (about 3 mm^2) is 20 times smaller than the area of the tympanic membrane (about 60 mm^2) thus the pressure on the oval window is about 20 times that at the eardrum. However, we have so far ignored the leverage system of the ossicles. They produce a mechanical advantage of about two. Thus the total pressure amplification for a 3000 Hz sound is about $2 \times 20 \times 2 = 80$ times. This amplification of pressure is required for impedance matching (see below). Sound intensity varies as the pressure squared, so a 40 times amplification can be shown to result in a sound level increase of about 30 dB. So were it not for the leverage of the ossicles and the small area of the oval window, sounds would seem 30 dB softer than they do.

11.5.3 *Impedance Matching*

Whenever a sound wave meets an interface between two media (such as air and water) some of the energy will be reflected and so will not enter the new medium.

The amount of energy that is reflected depends on the density and the elasticity of the two media. **Impedance**, Z (the product of density and speed of sound in the medium), is a measure of these properties. The greater the *difference* in impedance between two media is, the greater the amount of energy reflected from the interface will be. The impedance of air at 20 °C and atmospheric pressure = density × speed = 1.205 × 340 = 410 kg/m^2/s, while the impedance of water is about 1 400 000 kg/m^2/s. The difference in impedance between air and water is enormous and means that almost all of the sound energy falling on water would be reflected. Consider now the problem of transferring the energy of the sound wave in *air* to a sound wave in the *liquid* of the cochlea in the inner ear. Sound would be reflected right back out of the ear were it not for the mechanism of three ossicles in the middle ear. These small bones provide the link between the tympanic membrane and the oval window that enables the transfer of sound energy from air to the perilymph. In other words, the hearing mechanism is an impedance-matching device. Without it we would be insensitive to sound energy.

11.6 Noise and Hearing Loss

Occasional loud sounds won't harm our hearing much, as the muscles in the middle ear (the tensor tympanae and the stapedius) pull sideways on the ossicles to restrict their movement. This muscle action reduces the sound levels reaching the inner ear by about 15 dB but it may take 15 ms for this reaction to occur, which is sufficient time for some damage to occur. Long-term exposure to steady 90 dB noise will cause hearing loss. However, since pain isn't felt until about 120 dB, and the day to day deterioration in hearing is not noticed, it is difficult to convince those at risk that their hearing is in danger. Nevertheless it is very common nowadays to see workers wearing earmuffs when operating noisy equipment.

When considering the effects of industrial noise it is important to know the type of noise, the level of noise and its duration. For reasons that are not known, noise damage has the effect of reducing our ability to hear frequencies near 4000 Hz. That is, sounds at this frequency have to be increased in intensity to be audible. On an audiogram, the damage appears as a peak at 4000 Hz. The 4000 Hz 'notch' in the hearing chart of the subject who has suffered noise trauma is characteristic of all forms of noise-induced hearing impairment.

Most of the sound energy used in conversational speech falls between the frequencies of 300 and 3000 Hz and the sound levels of 50 and 60 dB. A person insensitive to frequencies above 4000 Hz or sound levels below 40 dB would not be called 'deaf' or even hard-of-hearing since they could understand normal conversations. Hearing impairment due to ageing (presbycusis) is the progressive deterioration of the ability to hear high frequencies. A normal 70 year old, without hearing damage, would have lost about 10 to 15 dB of hearing, while a hard-of-hearing person would have a 60 dB hearing loss. A 60 dB hearing loss means that in order for the sound to be heard, the sound level must be increased by 60 dB above the level that an average young person (15–25 years old), of normal hearing can just detect. A person with such a hearing loss can still hear if they are spoken to in a loud voice and can be assisted in hearing by a 'hearing aid'.

Conductive 'deafness' results when sound, although undistorted, is not transmitted well to the inner ear. You can experience conductive deafness by putting your fingers, or ear plugs, in your ears. Indeed an obstruction in the ear canal produced by the build-up of wax is a common form of temporary conductive hearing loss. Middle ear inflammation was once a principal cause of conductive deafness but with modern antibiotic drugs this is no longer the case. Otosclerosis is an important cause of conductive deafness. It is a progressive disease in which a spongy growth near the foot of the stapes gradually hardens into bone, immobilising it, thereby impairing the ability of the ossicles to pass vibration to the inner ear. Otosclerosis can be treated surgically by the procedures of:

- Stapes mobilisation. The stapes is jarred loose from its horny growth, removed and replaced with a plastic substitute.
- Fenestration. If stapes mobilisation fails, the malleus and incus are removed and a direct connection made between the outer ear and one of the semi-circular canals, thus bypassing the inoperative stapes. Normal hearing, however, can never be restored.

Sensorineural loss (nerve deafness or perceptive deafness) results from congenital factors and from disorders of the cochlea or the auditory nerve. If the auditory nerve is intact it can be stimulated electrically by a cochlear implant to give a sensation of hearing. A cochlear implant consists of electrodes placed in the cochlea (22 electrodes in the Australian device) at various locations, which are stimulated by electrical signals from the receiver buried under the skin behind the ear. An external microphone, sound processor and transmitter sit behind the ear to detect sound, process it and transmit it as electromagnetic waves to the receiver underneath the skin. The receiver picks up electromagnetic waves from the microphone and sends signals to the 22 electrodes implanted in the cochlea. The cochlear implant does not restore normal hearing, but with practice and training some recognisable hearing sensation is enjoyed by people with this implant.

Hearing aids consist of a microphone (to pick up sound) connected to an amplifier which feeds an earphone (to play the amplified sound) at the eardrum. They simply amplify all sounds or some range of frequencies by a set level (say 30 dB). These aids are useful to ameliorate conductive hearing loss and for some forms of sensorineural hearing loss. However, the amplification is dependent on frequency, so considerable distortion to the quality of the sound received can occur.

11.7 The Stethoscope

We have seen that vibrations of the particles in material media produce sound waves. Within the body there are several sources of sound, usually associated with the turbulent movement of fluids. Thus blood rushing through the heart valves, air moving through the bronchi and food moving through the digestive tract all produce audible sounds. These sounds are not normally heard outside of the body as the very different impedance of the body compared with the impedance of air means that almost all of the energy is reflected from the skin, back into the body. However, the use of the stethoscope permits the sounds made in the body to be listened to easily.

The stethoscope was invented and named by R. Laennec in about 1818 ('stethos' is Greek for chest). Prior to this time, the methods for examining the chest were by feeling with the hand, percussion and immediate auscultation by placing the ear directly on the patient's chest. Laennec found these methods inconvenient, and 'in the case of females indelicate and often impracticable'. Furthermore the standards of cleanliness of the early nineteenth century often made close contact with '. . . that class of persons found in the hospitals, disgusting'. Laennec developed a hollow wooden tube about 30 cm long that allowed him to listen to the sounds of heart, lungs and voice. The interpretation of these sounds requires considerable experience with normal and pathological sounds and will not be discussed here. We will consider how the stethoscope works and how to optimise the sound produced at the listener's ear drum.

Almost all the sounds of interest in auscultation lie below 1000 Hz in frequency. The sensitivity of the human ear decreases rapidly as frequency falls below 1000 Hz, so listening conditions must be optimised if sounds are to be clearly distinguished. Different sound sources within the body produce different frequencies. Heart murmurs are mainly low frequency sounds while lung sounds have a higher pitch. The sounds may travel by different paths to reach the skin surface and must pass through bones, fluid and tissues, and some paths result in clearer sounds than others. Fatty tissues cause the amplitude of the sound waves to decrease rapidly.

Modern stethoscopes consist of ear pieces, flexible rubber tubes and open or closed bells (see Figure 11.7). The ear pieces should fit snugly into the ear canal so that there are no sound leaks. It may be necessary to obtain alternative ear pieces that fit your ear canals properly. Poorly fitting ear pieces allow noise from the room to enter the ear and mask the sounds being listened to and also allow some of the body sounds to escape. The ear canal slopes forwards, downwards and inwards so it is possible to insert the ear pieces incorrectly (backwards).

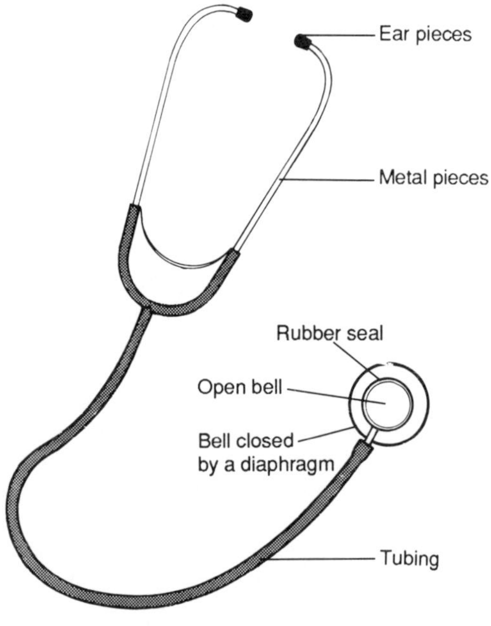

Figure 11.7 *The stethoscope. The open bell is smaller in diameter than the closed bell*

11.7.1 *The Stethoscope Tubes*

The rubber tubes conduct the sound waves from the bell to the ear pieces. These sound waves, if not confined within the tubes, would spread out spherically from the bell into the open air. Instead the energy is reflected from the internal surfaces of the tube. Consequently sound travels along the tube with little reduction in amplitude. The sound waves in the air of the tubes are almost completely reflected by the boundary between air and rubber (because the speed of sound is so different in air and in rubber) and so proceed down the tube with little loss of energy. In other words the sound heard in the ear pieces is as loud as if the ear pieces were attached directly to the bell.

Tubes of small diameter cause significant energy losses through friction, while larger-diameter tubes hold too large a volume of air. A compromise may be reached by using two tubes with an internal diameter of about 4 mm. The efficiency of sound transmission decreases as the length of the tubes increases, so a length of about 25 cm is a good compromise between efficiency of energy transmission and enough manoeuvrability to reach all body sites.

11.7.2 *The Stethoscope Bell*

Most of the sound energy that originates from within the body is reflected back into the body at the skin because of the great difference between the speed of sound in tissue (1540 m/s) and the speed of sound in air (340 m/s). As mentioned earlier, it is the difference in speed that determines the amount of sound energy that is reflected and transmitted at a boundary. In order to produce audible sounds at the ear, the difference in sound speeds at the boundary must be reduced. The bell of the stethoscope performs this function. The bell matches the impedence of the skin to that of the air. Impedance matching is achieved by having a diaphragm over the bell that **resonates** with sounds from the body. Resonance occurs when the diaphragm has a natural frequency of vibration that is the same as the frequency of the sounds coming from the body. At resonance, the vibration of the diaphragm is amplified, and causes the air behind it, in the stethoscope tube, to vibrate as well.

There are often two bells on a stethoscope. The larger-diameter bell is closed with a stretched diaphragm of plastic or metal, which resonates with a frequency near 1000 Hz. This is the end of the body sounds' spectrum to which the ear is most sensitive and is used for listening to the faint higher-frequency sounds produced from the lungs and heart. The open bell uses the skin as its diaphragm and the flesh under the skin acts as a damper to the vibration. The rubber ring ensures a good seal between the bell and skin. The open bell is mainly used for the lower frequencies produced by heart murmurs.

Note that the resonant frequency of the 'skin diaphragm' is governed by several factors:

- the diameter of the bell (the larger the diameter the lower the resonant frequency);
- the taughtness of the skin (the more tension the higher the resonant frequency);
- the reciprocal of the mass per unit area of skin.

Thus it is possible to enhance the sound range being listened for by pressing the bell more firmly, thus stretching the underlying skin more taughtly, or by changing to a bell of different diameter.

11.8 Ultrasound Waves

Mechanical vibrations such as those in a vibrating guitar string, piano wire, tuning fork or a whistle produce audible sound. That is, the frequency of vibration is between 20 Hz and 20 000 Hz and so stimulates the human hearing mechanism. Longitudinal, mechanical vibrations of higher frequency than 20 kHz are inaudible to humans and are called ultrasound. Some ultrasonic frequencies are clinically useful. The ultrasound scans used for medical diagnostic purposes utilise frequencies in the range 1 000 000 Hz to 15 000 000 Hz (1–15 MHz).

Ultrasound can provide an image of internal body structures in a non-invasive manner and without the use of introduced substances such as a barium meal. Furthermore the associated hazard that the ionizing radiation used in radiography presents is absent with ultrasound. Internal soft tissues of different types can be visualised provided that they differ either in elasticity or density.

Most of the diagnostic uses of ultrasound employ echo techniques similar to the SONAR (SOund Navigation And Ranging) echo-location of underwater objects by submarines and fishing vessels. An 'echo' is the sound that returns to the source after being reflected by some object or different medium. For example, sound will reflect from a cliff or large structure and return as an echo. By measuring the time elapsed between sending an ultrasound 'pulse' and receiving its echo, and knowing the speed of sound in tissue, the distance to the object causing the echo can be calculated. For example, in soft tissue the speed of ultrasound is approximately 1540 m/s, so if the echo returned after 100 μs, then the distance travelled by the ultrasonic wave is calculated as follows:

$$\begin{aligned} \text{distance} &= \text{speed} \times \text{time} \\ &= 1540 \times 0.0001 \\ &= 0.154 \text{ m} \\ &= 15.4 \text{ cm} \end{aligned}$$

Half of this distance is travelled by the original ultrasound pulse and half by the returning echo. Thus the ultrasound has reflected from a structure that lies 7.7 cm below the body surface.

When ultrasonic waves are directed into the body, reflections occur at interfaces between different tissues and fluids. Some of the energy is transmitted through the interface to be reflected by other interfaces deeper in the body. A reflection will occur at any interface when the speed of sound changes. The speed of sound is dependent on density of the tissue to a large extent, but also on the elastic properties of the tissue. Echo-producing interfaces consist of organ boundaries, blood vessels and small groups of cells. Diseases within an organ will be detected if the lesion or tumour has a density different from the rest of the organ. In this case, the tumour will reflect ultrasound and so show up amongst the healthy tissue.

The amplitude of the reflection depends on the difference in the speed of sound in the tissues on either side of the interface (see Table 11.2 for the speed of sound in various media in the body). Since the difference in speed of sound between air and tissue is so great, air causes almost total reflection. Consequently ultrasound examination can not take place through the lungs or a gas-filled bowel.

Table 11.2 *Speed of sound in various body structures*

Structure	Speed (m/s)
air	340
fat	1450
liver	1549
kidney	1561
blood	1570
muscle	1585

Within the body, most reflections are relatively weak, so sensitive equipment is required to detect the echos from internal boundaries. The greater the reflected amplitude, the lighter will be the image. To ensure that ultrasound enters the body rather than being reflected by air between the skin and the ultrasound probe, an acoustic gel is spread on skin. Sometimes a water bath is used to exclude air from between the sound source and the body surface and to avoid the distortion of the body surface that results through contact with the probe.

11.9 Production of Ultrasound

The very rapid mechanical vibrations that produce ultrasound are produced in a crystal mounted in the ultrasound 'transducer' (also called a scanner or a probe). Transducer is the name given to any device that converts energy from one form to another. An ultrasound transducer (see Figure 11.8) converts electrical energy into the kinetic energy of vibrating particles. Another transducer, often on the same probe, converts the reflected ultrasound energy back into electrical energy.

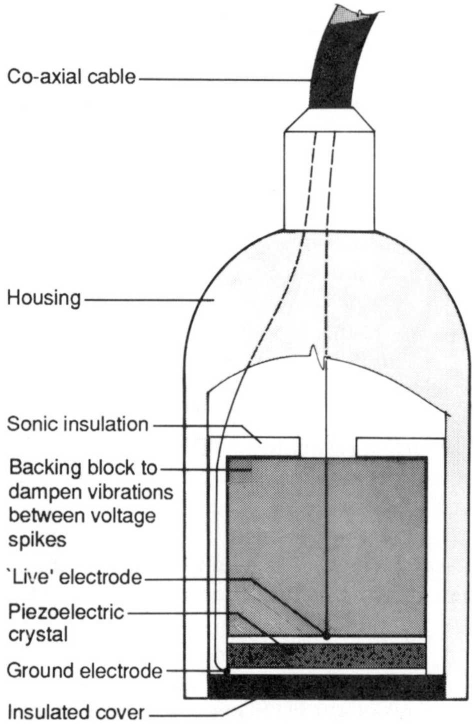

Figure 11.8 *An ultrasound transducer*

Pierre and Paul-Jacques Curie (in 1880) discovered that when a deforming force was applied to certain crystals (such as Rochelle salt, quartz or tourmaline) a small voltage was generated between the ends of the crystal. These crystals are termed **piezoelectric** and the effect is called the **piezoelectric effect**. Note that human bone is a piezoelectric material. The compression in bones that arises because they support the body generates a negative charge at the areas of compression and stimulates the production of more bone. The reverse piezoelectric effect also happens (see Figure 11.9). When a voltage is applied to the crystal, it expands or contracts depending on the polarity. If the applied voltage is an alternating one (for example, 2 MHz AC voltage) then the crystal will not just deform, it will *vibrate*. Because the frequency of vibration is high (2 MHz), ultrasound is produced.

During World War I, P. Langevin first used the piezoelectric effect to generate ultrasound for the detection of submarines (SONAR). Following improvements in technique after World War II, ultrasound was successfully used for the detection of internal body structures. Manufactured ceramics are now used as the piezoelectric material.

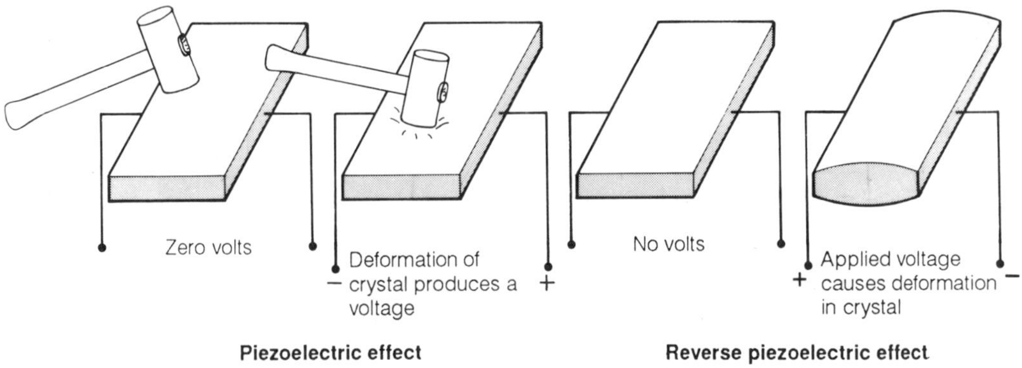

Figure 11.9 *Ultrasound is generated by the reverse piezoelectric effect*

11.10 Clinical Applications of Ultrasound

Obstetrics. The most widespread use of ultrasound occurs on pregnant women where it is used to form an image of the developing foetus (Figure 11.10). The scan is performed after the patient has drunk a considerable amount of water. This ensures that the urinary bladder is full so that it displaces the bowel (which may contain air). The urine-filled bladder also acts as a 'window' that lets ultrasound through and allows the uterus to be examined. Ultrasound can be used on pregnant women to:

1. detect pregnancy;
2. detect multiple foetuses;
3. determine the age of the foetus (by measuring the biparietal diameter of the skull and the length of the femur);

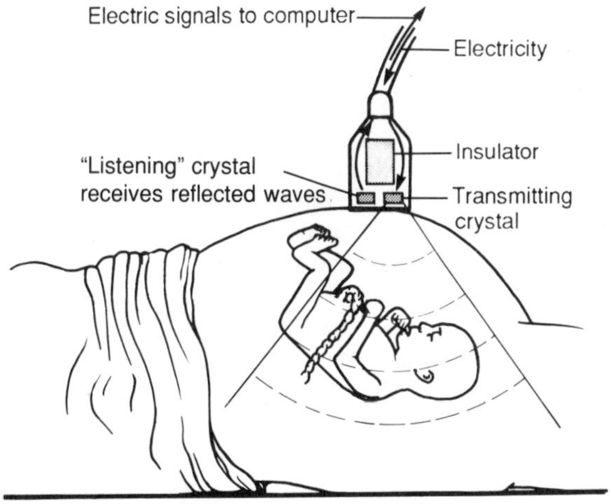

Figure 11.10 *Imaging the foetus is a major application of ultrasound*

4. detect foetal abnormalities (anencephaly, hydrocephaly, spina bifida, growth retardation);
5. sometimes identify a male foetus;
6. determine the position of the placenta (placenta praevia).

Organ and Tissue Pathologies. Various structures in the abdomen can be visualised, and examined for abnormality. These include the kidney, liver (detection of cysts, primary and secondary malignant tumours, cirrhosis), gall-bladder (gall stones, chronic inflammation and tumours), spleen (enlargement), pancreas (cysts, abscesses, tumours, inflammatory disorders), thyroid. Breasts when allowed to hang freely in a water bath may show carcinomas, haematomas, enlarged ducts, fatty deposits, fibrocystic disease.

Surgical. At sufficiently high levels of intensity, using continuous wave ultrasound, enough energy can be concentrated into a small volume to damage tissue. In this way ultrasound can be used as a precision surgical tool. Menière's syndrome (a disease of the labyrinth of the inner ear) may be treated this way. Ultrasound at about 40 000 Hz is used to shatter a cataract in the lens of the eye, whereupon the fragments are drawn out using a thin tube and a plastic lens is inserted.

Kidney Stones. Kidney stones can be shattered by ultrasonic 'shock waves' of high intensity but very short duration. The process is known as lithotripsy. The ultrasonic waves are accurately focused on the kidney stones with the aid of X-ray cameras.

11.11 Doppler Ultrasound

Christian Doppler, in 1842, proposed that the frequency of a wave was dependent on the velocity of the source of the wave. Thus a train's bell or whistle sounds at a *higher* frequency if travelling *towards* you, but at a *lower* frequency when travelling *away*. Someone on the train will hear the natural frequency (which is between the two) because the source of the wave and the observer are moving together. We call the *change in frequency* of a sound or electromagnetic wave, when the source of the wave is moving relative to the observer, the **Doppler effect**. This 'Doppler shift' in frequency (to a higher or lower value) is also observed in the sound that is *reflected* from a moving object.

When two waves of similar frequencies overlap, they 'interfere' with each other. In much the same way that the waves in the wakes of two speed boats will produce a double-sized wave where the wakes meet, overlapping sound waves add on to each other. For example, if the original ultrasound pulse has a frequency of 8 000 000 Hz and the reflected pulse has a frequency of 8 000 200 Hz (a Doppler shift of 200 Hz), the two signals will interfere with each other in a regular way. Sometimes the disturbances in the medium will reinforce each other to produce an even larger disturbance, and sometimes they annul each other so that there is no disturbance. The resultant effect of the annulling and reinforcing is to produce evenly timed 'beats' (200 per second in the example above). Beats are the high intensities of sound (the reinforcements) that follow the low intensities of sound (the annulments). The number of beats per second is the 'beat frequency'.

beat frequency = difference between the original frequency and the Doppler-shifted frequency

Note that the beat frequency would be 200 Hz whether the reflected wave had a frequency of 8 000 200 Hz or 7 999 800 Hz. Since the beat frequency is in the audible range it can be heard even though the two interfering ultrasound frequencies cannot! The resulting beat frequency depends on the size of the Doppler shift in the reflected wave. The Doppler shift depends in turn on the speed of the object that produced the echo. In 1959 S. Satomura (of Japan) first successfully measured the velocity of blood in a particular vessel, non-invasively from the surface of the body, using a 'Doppler shift flow-velocity meter'. In operation the device produces pulses of ultrasound of about 10 MHz. When directed at an angle to the blood vessel, the ultrasound pulses 'scatter' from the moving red blood cells. That is, they are reflected in all directions from the cells (see Figure 11.11). The frequency of the reflected pulse is measured within the device and the Doppler shift in frequency calculated. Assuming that ultrasound has a frequency of 10 MHz, and travels at 1540 m/s through the body at an angle of 30° to the blood vessel, then the approximate blood velocity can be calculated as below:

$v = 0.002 \times \text{Doppler shift}$

A vascularscope using the Doppler ultrasound technique to detect blood flow can be used to search for abnormalities in venous blood flow (caused, for example, by a thrombosis) or arterial disease (a stenosis or occlusion). If a blood vessel is constricted at some point the blood velocity must increase at that point otherwise less blood will be flowing in the vessel after

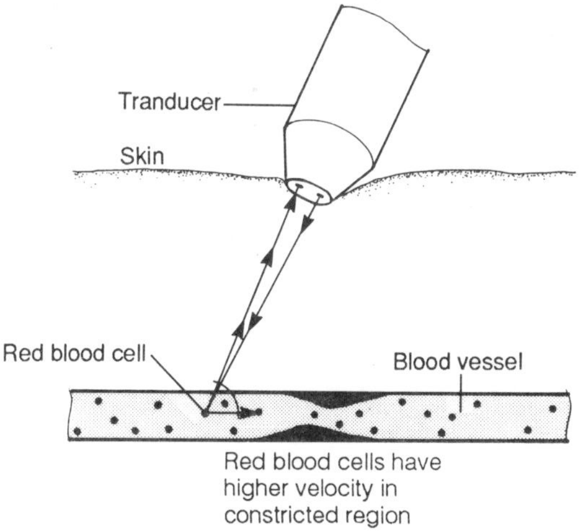

Figure 11.11 *Doppler ultrasound techniques can detect vascular constrictions by measuring the speed of blood flow. The transducer has two piezoelectric crystals, one for producing the ultrasound and another for receiving the echo*

the constriction. This increase in velocity can be detected from the increased Doppler shift in the reflected ultrasound. That is, the echo from faster-moving red blood cells will be at a different frequency than the echo from red blood cells of 'normal' speed. In both cases, the echo has been Doppler-shifted in frequency, but one echo more so than the other. The reflected frequency produces beats as it interferes with the incident frequency. The beat frequency is audible, even though the two ultrasound waves are not, and will be higher for places of high blood speed. With practice, an abnormal sound, indicating a sudden constriction in a blood vessel, can be distinguished from the normal sound of blood flowing through a healthy vessel.

Doppler techniques can also be used to monitor foetal heart rate and respiration and in cardiology to investigate the motion of the heart valves.

Bibliography

Devey, G. B. and Wells, P. N. T. 'Ultrasound in medical diagnosis', *Scientific American*, **243**(5) 98–112, 1978.

Questions

1. A wave may be defined as
   J. the oscillation of a particle of the medium
   K. a series of crests and compressions that propagate through space
   L. a mechanism for the transfer of energy without transferring matter
   M. the transport of the medium due to the oscillation of its particles
2. The quantity that most closely describes the amount of energy that is transported by a sound wave is
   J. frequency
   K. amplitude
   L. wavelength
   M. velocity
3. Noise-induced hearing loss
   J. affects sound frequencies near 4000 Hz most
   K. is also called presbycusis
   L. is likely to be caused by sounds above 65 dB
   M. is due to otosclerosis
4. Hearing aids are most successful when used by people with
   J. conductive hearing loss
   K. perceptive deafness
   L. nerve deafness
   M. sensorineural hearing loss
5. The unit called the decibel (dB) is used in the measurement of
   J. sound frequency (pitch)
   K. sound intensity (energy)
   L. sound pressure
   M. sound level (loudness)
6. Which of the following is not a small bone involved in hearing?
   J. meatus
   K. malleus
   L. stapes
   M. incus
7. If the frequency of a sound is 1000 Hz, its period will be
   J. 1 second
   K. 0.1 second
   L. 0.001 second
   M. 0.0001 second
8. A sound of frequency 250 000 Hz will be
   J. audible
   K. painful to listen to
   L. ultrasonic
   M. close to the threshold of hearing

9. As the frequency of a sound in air is made to decrease, which of the following will happen?

   J. The period will decrease.
   K. The wavelength will decrease.
   L. The amplitude will decrease.
   M. The velocity will decrease.

CHAPTER 12

Waves and Sight

Sight is of such immense importance and interest to us that it would be hard to imagine life without it. There can be few interrelationships as complex as that between light and people. The sun of course is the dominant source of light. It pours out radiations that have defined our environment and to which we have responded by developing our sense of vision.

Our earliest recorded ideas about vision are attributed to Pythagoras (560–500 BC). His belief was that vision was caused solely by something emitted from the eye. Empedocles of Acragas (492–432 BC) held the view that luminous objects emit something that meets with rays that come from the eyes. He also reasoned that light takes time to travel through space. The Islamic physicist al-Haytham (965–1020?) rejected as absurd the idea that vision emanated from the eye. He realised that light was emitted from every self-luminous object. He also gave us the concept of 'a ray of light'. Our modern understanding of light is based on the ideas of Christian Huygens (1629–1695) and Isaac Newton (1642–1727). According to Huygens, light was a series of shock waves that moved through an invisible substance, the aether. Newton's idea was that light was a stream of corpuscles.

In this chapter we will discuss whether either of these models of light are of use to us today. Wc will also discuss the physical principles in the optical system of our eye. In doing so, considerable space will be devoted to describing electromagnetic radiation and the uses to which it is put in medicine.

Learning Objectives

At the completion of this chapter you should be able to:

1. Define what electromagnetic radiation is.
2. Be aware of the place of visible light in the electromagnetic spectrum.
3. Define reflection and refraction by referring to the interface between two media, angles of incidence, reflection and refraction and to velocity.
4. Understand the relevance of oscillations and of material media to the propagation of light.
5. Understand what is meant by a lens and the terms concave, convex, focal length and dioptres.
6. Label a diagram of the eye and describe how lenses can correct some vision defects of myopia, hyperopia and astigmatism.
7. Be aware of the theory of colour vision and of defective colour perception.
8. Gain a working knowledge of the common vision defects of presbyopia, cataracts, glaucoma.
9. Be familiar with the principles of laser action.
10. Distinguish between ionising radiation and non-ionising radiation.
11. Know that the energy of electromagnetic radiation increases as its frequency does.

12.1 Properties of Light

Light may be thought of as energy that is being transferred by a wave motion. For some phenomena, however, it is necessary to think of it as an energy transfer brought about by the movement of 'particles' called **photons**. The notion of light being photons will be discussed in greater detail in Section 12.7. For the present we will treat light as if it is a wave motion of the type also referred to as 'electromagnetic radiation'. Radiation refers to emissions that travel away from their source in all directions so that the energy is spread over a sphere whose radius is ever increasing. Consequently the intensity of the radiation decreases with distance from the source. The word 'electromagnetic' is a combination of the words electricity and magnetism. In fact electricity and magnetism do not have an existence separate from each other (although this is not immediately apparent). So combining the two words into one is a good way of reminding ourselves that two seemingly very different phenomena are very closely related.

But what is the connection of electricity and magnetism to light? Well, light is produced when the outermost electrons in atoms change their position slightly and so decrease the amount of energy that they possess. The energy that electrons lose is emitted as light energy. Conversely, electric fields and magnetic fields can cause the energy of an electron in an atom to increase. In this case electromagnetic energy is converted to energy possessed by the electron. Furthermore, a moving electron generates a magnetic field and an *accelerating* electron radiates electromagnetic waves. Thus the connection between electricity, light and magnetism is both intimate and intricate. Some aspects of the relationship between light, electricity and magnetism will unfold as the chapter progresses.

Light is the name that we give to one section of the continuous range of frequencies of radiation that are called electromagnetic radiation. This radiation includes what are commonly called radio waves, television waves, microwaves, infrared rays, visible light, ultraviolet rays, X-rays and gamma rays. Visible light is the range of frequencies of electromagnetic radiation that stimulate the sensation of vision. The range of sensitivity of the human eye lies within the frequencies from about 3.9×10^{14} Hz to about 7.5×10^{14} Hz, consequently these are called the 'visible frequencies'. Stated in terms of wavelength, light is in the range from 400 nm to 770 nm (see Figure 12.1). In this book, 'light' will be used synonomously with 'visible light'.

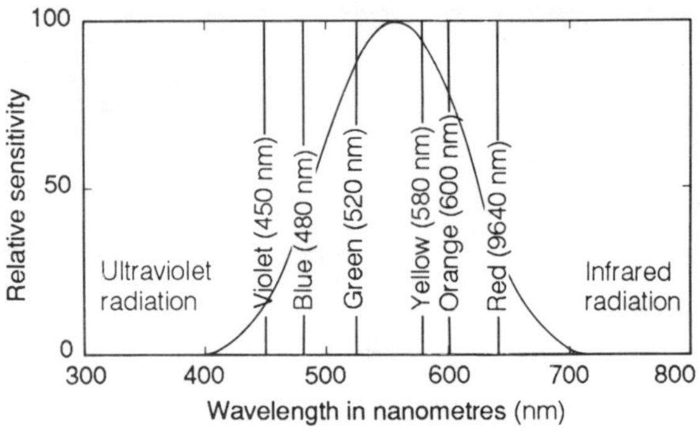

Figure 12.1 *Relative sensitivity of the human eye to various wavelengths of electromagnetic radiation. The eye is most sensitive to light between the wavelengths that produce sensations of green and yellow*

In the 1860s James Clerk Maxwell proposed that radiation was a form of energy that propagated through space as waves which arise from the oscillation of the magnitude of electric and magnetic fields. Hence it became known as electromagnetic radiation. Heinrich Hertz proved Maxwell correct in 1888 by producing electromagnetic waves in a laboratory and measuring their speed. For these achievements, the unit for frequency (the hertz, Hz) is named after him. The electromagnetic spectrum is discussed in greater detail in Section 12.6.

In air, light and all other electromagnetic radiation travel at close to 3×10^8 m/s. In other media the speed is slower. For example, in glass, light travels at about 2×10^8 m/s. Furthermore different frequencies of light travel at slightly different speeds through media. Thus red light travels more quickly through glass than violet light. This difference in speeds enables sunlight (which we call 'white light') to disperse as it passes through a prism into a spectrum of colours. These were named red, orange, yellow, green, blue and violet by Isaac Newton in about 1670. He also coined the word 'spectrum'. The colour 'spectral red' consists of those frequencies that fall within the range of (say) 4.4×10^{14} Hz and 3.9×10^{14} Hz, so is 'pure red' because it is not 'mixed in' with other frequencies. Most of the 'red' objects that we see are not pure red. Rather, they reflect a variety of frequencies to our eyes that mix together to form a colour that appears closer to red than to any other.

Since light is a wave, it exhibits all the phenomena that are characteristic of waves. That is, light refracts, reflects, diffracts, interferes, may suffer a phase change on reflection and can be polarised. Most of these will not concern us in this book, but we will spend some time discussing refraction.

12.2 Refraction of Light

Refraction is the term applied to the change in the speed of light (or any other wave!) as it leaves one medium and enters another medium which has a density different to the original medium (see Figure 12.2). For example, as light passes from air into the cornea of the eye, it slows down. Refraction is usually accompanied by a change in direction of the wave unless it enters the second medium at an angle of 90° to the boundary. That is, not only does light slow down as it enters the cornea from air, it also deviates from its previous direction.

In Figure 12.2, the **normal** is an imaginary line perpendicular to the boundary (interface) between air and the cornea (the two media being considered). The angle formed by the normal and the line of the incoming ray (the incident ray) is called the **angle of incidence**, and is labelled *i*. The angle between the normal and the reflected ray is the **angle of reflection**, and is labelled *r*, and the angle between the normal and the refracted ray is the **angle of refraction** (labelled *R*).

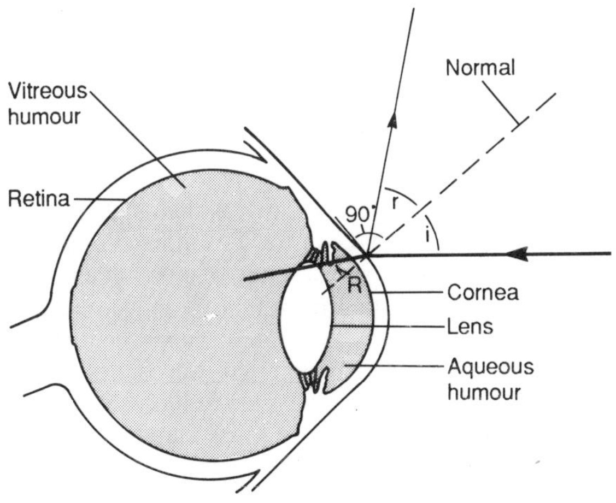

Figure 12.2 *Light undergoes its greatest refraction as it enters the cornea. The refracted ray is then deviated only slightly by the lens before it strikes the retina*

Notice

1. $i = r$, that is, the two angles are the same.
2. i will be larger than R if the ray enters a denser medium (as is the case when light passes from air into the cornea).
3. i will be less than R if the ray enters a less dense medium (passes from glass into air).
4. $d + R = i$, where d is the angle of deviation.

The refraction of light is the phenomenon responsible for producing rainbows, mirages, making pools of water seem shallower than they are, the operation of all optical instruments and for making objects partly submerged in water seem bent. Refraction of light also allows us to form images on our retina from the light that enters our pupil. The light that we see is refracted at every interface it crosses on the way to the retina. Thus refraction occurs at the air–cornea interface and also at the cornea–aqueous humour, aqueous humour–lens and lens–vitreous humour interfaces.

Willebrod Snell (in the 1610s) discovered that, for a light ray passing from air into another medium, the 'sine' of angle *i* when divided by the 'sine' of angle *R* results in a constant number (to 'take the sine of a number' is a mathematical operation that need not concern us here). This number is called the **refractive index** of the medium and has the one value, regardless of the angle *i* with which the light ray enters the medium.

$$\frac{\text{sine } i}{\text{sine } R} = n \text{ (the refractive index)}$$

The refractive indices of some common materials are given in Table 12.1. The index is useful, as the difference between the refractive indices of two media tells us how much refraction will occur. Thus between the air ($n = 1.0$) and our cornea ($n = 1.37$) quite a bit of refraction (and thus focusing) occurs but between the lens and the humours only a small amount of refraction occurs. This means that the cornea rather than the lens provides most of the focusing power of our eye. When we swim underwater, the cornea ($n = 1.37$) is in contact with water, which has a refractive index of 1.33. The two refractive indicies are very similar, so very little refraction will occur as light passes from water to the cornea. Consequently, the eye loses most of its focusing power and our sight is blurred. In order to improve vision, underwater divers keep air around their cornea by wearing a face mask.

Table 12.1 *The refractive indices of some transparent materials*

air	1.00 (the lowest)
water	1.33
aqueous humour	1.33
vitreous humour	1.33
cornea	1.37
lens of the eye	1.40
diamond	2.42 (one of the highest)

12.3 Lenses

A lens is any transparent object with a curved face. Thus both our 'lens' and our cornea are lenses. If the curve is 'outwards', making the middle of the lens fatter and the edges thin, the lens is **convex**. A lens curved in the opposite sense is called **concave** (see Figure 12.3). The functional difference between the two types of lens is that a convex lens causes rays of light to converge to a focal point, while a concave lens causes light rays to spread further apart (diverge). Consequently a convex lens can be used as a magnifying glass. The two most important quantities of a lens are the **focal length** and the **aperture**.

For a convex lens, the focal length is the shortest distance between the lens and the point where light rays converge. This point is called the 'principal focus' or the 'focal point'. If a piece of paper is held behind a convex lens, so that it is one focal length from the lens, then the light that is passing through the lens is brought to focus on the paper and an image can be seen. The human eye has a focal length of about 2 cm. The aperture refers to the size of the circular hole through which light passes to enter the lens. In a camera, the aperture of the lens is controlled by the diaphragm and is measured by the 'f stop'. As the exposed area of the lens is made larger, more light can pass through. Consequently, the greater will be the intensity of the image formed by the lens. For this reason, telescopes are built with the largest possible lens. The aperture of our eye is the black pupil. Its size may be varied from a circle of diameter about 3 mm to about 8 mm by adjusting the iris (the colourful ring of tissue that surrounds the pupil).

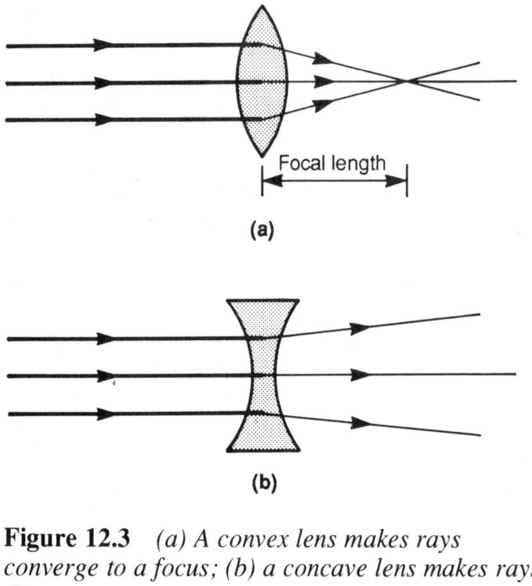

Figure 12.3 *(a) A convex lens makes rays converge to a focus; (b) a concave lens makes rays diverge*

The majority of optical instruments have more than one lens to enable more flexibility in focusing ability and also to magnify the image of the object being looked at. Our eye is also a two-lens system. Both the cornea and the eye lens have curved faces so each one of them is a lens. Together, they produce the focusing that occurs to light entering our eye. An optical instrument is able to focus on objects that are at different distances from it by altering the distance between the lenses. This adjustment changes the length of the optical tube in the instrument. Thus a lens may be screwed out to bring an image into sharp focus. The human eye has a much better system that does not depend on the distance between its lenses. It is able to 'accommodate', that is, it can alter the focal length of its lens so that light emanating from objects at any distance may be brought to a focus on the retina. The ability to accommodate our lens means that the eye can focus at any distance without altering the distance between the lens and retina.

The lens of our eye is biconvex, that is, convex on both sides, with the back of the lens more curved than the front. The degree of curvature of a lens determines its 'strength' (a term that refers to the amount of refraction that is produced). The stronger the lens, the greater the angle of deviation that it produces in rays that pass through it. Strongly curved lenses produce a large 'bend' in a light ray and cause parallel light rays to come to a focus a short distance from the lens. Thus they have a short focal length, f. A 'weak' lens is not very curved and so has a long focal length. The strength of prescription spectacles is the inverse of the focal length of the lens and is stated as a number of **dioptres**. Thus if $f = 0.1$ m, then strength, S, can be calculated as follows:

$$S = \frac{1}{f} = \frac{1}{0.1} = 10 \text{ dioptres}$$

The lens in our eye is flexible so its curvature may be lessened to cause the parallel light rays from distant objects to focus on the retina, or increased to focus the diverging light rays from closer objects. The process of refocusing at different distances is called **accommodation** (see Figure 12.4) and can alter the strength of the eye through about 5 dioptres.

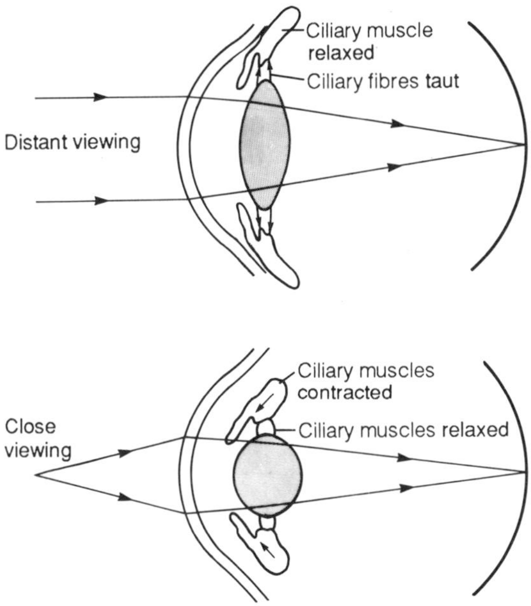

Figure 12.4 *As our gaze shifts from a close object to a distant one, our lens accommodates by decreasing its radius of curvature and so producing less deviation of the light rays*

The lens is suspended by ciliary fibres from the circular ciliary muscle. When the muscle is relaxed it forms a large circle so that the fibres are pulled taut and the lens is stretched into a thin shape. This produces a long focal length and clear images of distant objects. When the ciliary muscle contracts, it forms a smaller circle around the lens, causing the fibres to slacken off and they in turn allow the lens to 'ooze' into a more spherical shape. The increase in the lens curvature shortens its focal length and close objects come into focus.

With age, our lens loses its elasticity so is not able to ooze into the short focal lengths of a youthful lens. As a consequence, the closest point at which objects can be focused moves away to arms length or beyond, making reading difficult. The age-related deterioration in focusing ability is called **presbyopia** (old sight) and can be corrected with glasses or by bifocal lenses (which were invented by Benjamin Franklin in 1784) if glasses are already worn.

The lens is not transparent to ultraviolet radiation. This is because ultraviolet energy is absorbed by the lens. The consequence of this deposition of ultraviolet energy in the lens is the development of cataracts. These destroy the clarity of the lens. A consequence of ageing may be senile cataracts. The lens progressively loses its transparency until it becomes opaque. Such a lens can be surgically removed and replaced by an artificial substitute with additional correction added by wearing glasses.

12.4 The Eye and Defective Vision

12.4.1 *Neural Elements of the Eye*

Light enters the eye through an aperture, the size of which is altered by the **iris**. The aperture of the eye is called the **pupil**. It appears black because essentially all the light that enters the eye is absorbed inside the eye. Consequently, no light passes out of the pupil. The coloured iris can alter the diameter of the pupil, from about 3 mm in bright light to about 8 mm in the dark. This change will vary the amount of light that can enter the eye by a factor of seven. However, the eye can handle light that is 10^{10} times brighter than the minimum level in which we can see, so the retina, as well as the iris, must be able to adapt to different lighting conditions.

The **retina** is the light-sensitive part of the eye. It converts light energy into electrical nerve impulses that are sent to the brain. Visible light has enough energy to cause a reaction while infrared radiation has insufficient energy. Ultraviolet radiation has more than enough energy to produce the reaction, but is absorbed by the eye (mainly in the lens) before it reaches the retina. Individuals who have had the lens of the eye removed because of a cataract are able to see into the near ultraviolet region because the major absorber is no longer present.

The retina covers the back half of the eyeball, making us sensitive to light entering our eye over a wide angle. However, most of the time our vision is restricted to a small area called the **macula lutea** (or yellow spot) and all detailed vision takes place in a very small area of the macula lutea called the **fovea centralis** (0.3 mm in diameter). It is because of this that we turn our heads to face whatever we wish to see. By looking directly at something, we cause the light rays emanating from it to fall on the fovea. At the fovea the several layers of nerve tissue that overlie the retina are pushed aside allowing light to strike the cones directly. Thus the maximum amount of light falls on the cones, improving our vision in this area.

Rods and **cones** are the two general types of photoreceptors in the retina. The cones are primarily found in the fovea (but occur throughout the retina) and are used mainly for daylight vision and colour vision. Each of the cones in the fovea has its own nerve connection to the brain while in the rest of the retina several cones share one nerve fibre. Hence in the fovea each cone can be stimulated separately from its neighbour and this improves the acuity of our sight.

The rods are used for night vision and for peripheral vision (for seeing things out of the corner of our eye). They cover most of the retina and are much more numerous than cones. Their maximum density is at about 20° from our line of vision. This means that the best view of a faint object at night (such as a faint star) is obtained by looking towards a point some 20° to one side of it. Hundreds of rods send their information to the same nerve fibre so rods have a poor ability to resolve close sources of light.

There is a region on the retina without rods or cones. This is the **blind spot** and is the point where the nerve fibres come together and leave the eye as the optic nerve. Fortunately the image that falls on the blind spot of one eye misses the blind spot of the other so we are normally not aware of it.

Another benefit of having two eyes is stereoscopic vision. That is, we perceive three-dimensional images, so can estimate distances and the position of objects in space.

12.4.2 *Defects of Vision*

Some forms of defective vision are due to focusing problems and so can be corrected by wearing glasses.

Myopia (near-sightedness) is usually caused by excessive curvature of the cornea or by an eyeball that is longer than normal. Myopic eyes produce too much convergence in light rays, so that the image forms in front of the retina. A concave (also called negative) lens is used to diverge the rays before they enter the eye, so that the position of image formation is moved back to the retina (see Figure 12.5a).

Hyperopia (long-sightedness) is usually caused by a short eyeball or a cornea without enough curve. Hyperopic eyes produce too little refraction to focus light onto the retina, that is the rays have not converged enough to form a clear image. A convex (also called positive) lens is used to produce the necessary extra convergence to bring the image forward onto the retina (see Figure 12.5b).

Astigmatism is caused by a cornea whose surface does not form part of a spherical surface. If the cornea is less curved from left to right than it is from top to bottom, then horizontal lines will not be focused while vertical lines will. A lens with a cylindrical curve (rather than a spherical one) whose axis is vertical can provide the extra horizontal curvature to produce a focus.

Presbyopia (old-age vision) is caused by the lens losing its elasticity and consequently, light from nearby objects (for example, books) cannot be focused. Loss of accommodation usually becomes noticeable after age 40, and reading glasses, or bifocals if glasses are already worn, can correct this.

Colour 'blindness'. There is no current theory that completely accounts for all that is known about our perception of colour. It is thought that there are three different pigments (as yet undiscovered) in the cones in our retina that have their greatest sensitivity to one of red, green or blue light, but also have a lower

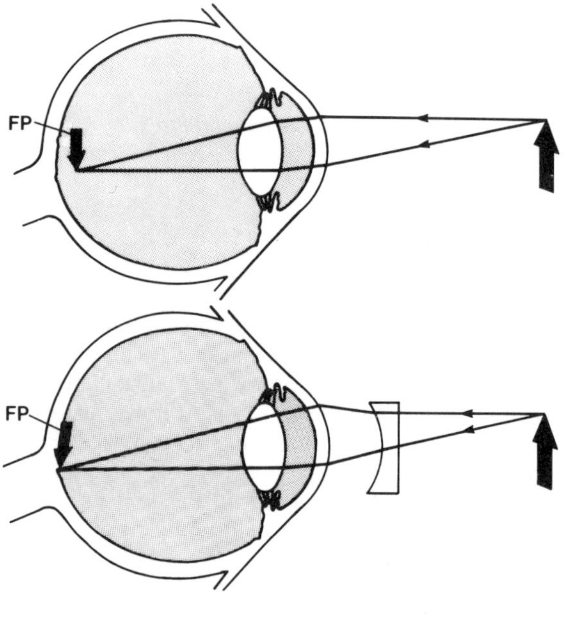

Figure 12.5a *A myopic eye*

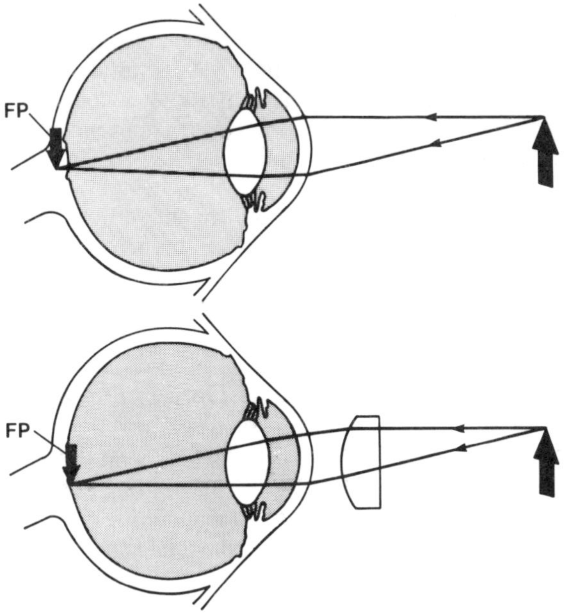

Figure 12.5b *A hyperopic eye*

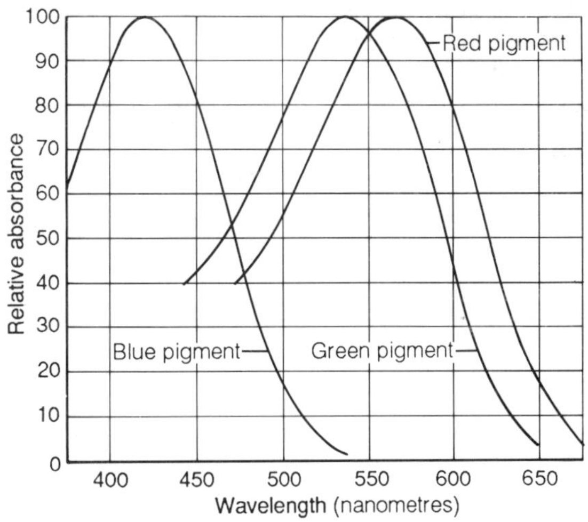

Figure 12.6 *Cones with blue pigment absorb light with wavelengths from 370 nm to 530 nm but are most sensitive to wavelengths of 420 nm. Red and green pigments are most sensitive to 560 nm and 530 nm respectively*

sensitivity to other wavelengths (see Figure 12.6). If the red-sensitive cones are missing then red light is only able to stimulate the green cones so is perceived as green. The condition is called **protanopia** (or **red-minus dichroma**). In the reverse situation, green cones are missing so green light stimulates red cones only, a condition called **deuteranopia** (or **green-minus dichroma**). However, these two names actually group together people with varying degrees of anomalous colour sensitivity and defectiveness in colour vision, so that the vision defect of one deuteranope is not necessarily the same as another. Both protanopia and deuteranopia are commonly, but misleadingly, called 'red–green' colour blindness. Neither protanopes nor deuteranopes are blind to colour. Furthermore, a deuteranope may be able to see both red and green. One of the authors (M.C.) is deuteranopic, yet can still see red and green; however, there are certain hues that people with complete colour vision perceive as different that he finds indistinguishable.

Cataracts. Ultraviolet light, neutrons and X-rays can damage the cornea causing it to become opaque. These opacities are called cataracts. The opacity can be excised and another piece of cornea may be successfully transplanted from a dead donor. The lens can also develop cataracts. The faulty lens can be removed and, since 1958, be replaced by a plastic substitute thus restoring some vision to the eye.

Glaucoma which produces 'tunnel vision' in moderate cases and blindness in severe cases is caused by increased pressure in the aqueous humour in front of the lens. Aqueous humour is continually circulating in the eye, being produced at the ciliary processes, then moving between the lens and the iris and draining into the canal of Schlemm. If the removal of aqueous humour is prevented, pressure will build up from the normal value of between 1.3 and 4.0 kPa to as much as 9.3 kPa. The increased pressure in the eyeball restricts the blood supply to the retina and this affects vision. Glaucoma can be treated with drugs if the increased pressure is detected soon enough. It is also treated by a laser technique in which the energy of the laser is concentrated at a tiny point. This very rapidly heats the fluid at that point to a plasma. The plasma expands very rapidly to produce a shock wave that tears the posterior capsule of the eye (which surrounds the space between the suspensory ligament and the iris). This allows aqueous humour to resume its circulation and drain into the canal of Schlemm.

Retinal detachment will affect vision at the place of detachment because the retina is deprived of its blood supply there. The retina can be reattached by photocoagulation by laser beam. The energy carried by the laser beam is enough to 'spot weld' the retina back to the underlying pigmented layer and hence restore the blood supply.

12.5 The Compound Light Microscope

Visual acuity (how sharp your eyes are) is also called the **resolution** of the eyes. Under optimum conditions, our eye can just barely distinguish a pattern of alternate white and black lines when there are 30 black lines per millimetre. This limit is set by the dimension of the cone cells in our retina, and roughly corresponds to a black line falling on a cone, the white line falling on the adjacent cone and the next black line falling on the cone after that. Hence two adjacent black lines stimulate the outside cones of a trio of adjacent cones. Objects of smaller dimensions cannot be resolved by our eye. However, very small objects can be made visible if they are magnified and correctly illuminated.

In order to obtain the large magnification of small objects a compound light microscope is used. This essentially consists of an objective lens system and an eyepiece lens system, together with an illumination system. The microscope is termed 'compound' because both the eyepiece 'lens' and the objective 'lens' consist of several component lenses. One type of eyepiece lens (the Ramsden type) uses two lenses while the objective used for oil immersion contains as many as 10 lenses (see Figure 12.7). Such complex lens systems are necessary to remove the various distortions and aberrations that occur as light passes through glass. They occur because light consists of a continuous range of frequencies and different frequencies are refracted by different amounts as they pass through glass. Microscope lens systems also attempt to correct for light rays that come from different portions of the object; these rays necessarily pass through a different part of the lens and so are subjected to different distortions.

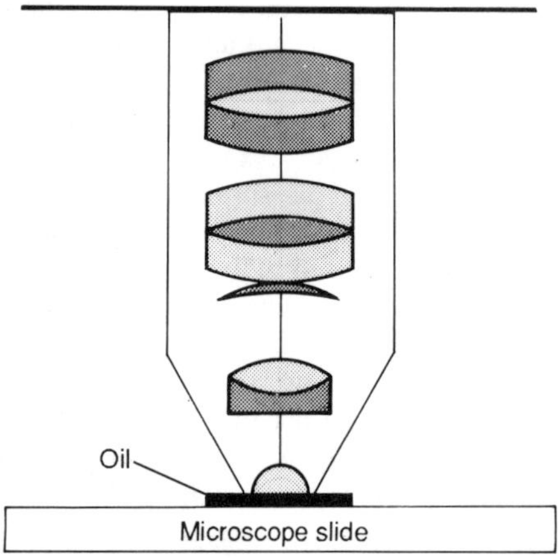

Figure 12.7 *The 10 lenses of this oil immersion objective correct so well for spherical and chromatic aberrations that the effective magnifying power is set by the diffraction effects of light rather than by the design of the objective*

12.5.1 *The Measures of Optical Quality*

The **magnification** of a particular lens combination is determined by multiplying the magnifying power of the eyepiece (say 10X) by the magnifying power of the objective (say 40X) to give the total magnification (400X in this example). Of related interest is the **resolution** of the microscope. Resolution refers to how close two small features can be while still being distinguishable as separate features (rather than the one blur). Generally speaking, resolving power increases as the magnification of the lens increases. The 4X objective of a typical student microscope can resolve two objects separated by about 3.4 μm, while the 10X objective can resolve to about 0.5 μm. If the limit of resolution of the instrument has been reached, then two very small objects that appear as the one blurred image at 400X will become a larger but still blurred image at 1000X. Thus very little has been achieved by using a higher magnification. The ability of a microscope to distinguish detail clearly is measured by a quantity called the **numerical aperture** (NA). As NA increases, the amount of detail that a lens can resolve increases. This number is usually inscribed on the objective lens and has typical values of 0.1 for 4X, 0.25 for 10X and 0.65 for 40X. Without the technique of oil immersion, the practical limit for the numerical aperture is about 0.95.

12.5.2 *Oil Immersion*

An oil-immersion objective can increase the resolution of fine details above that which can be achieved by an ordinary objective, so is used for high-power microscopy. Light that enters an ordinary objective has passed through the material on the slide, the glass of the coverslip and the air between the coverslip and the objective. When the light rays pass from the coverslip into air, they change their direction (refract) because air is much less dense than glass (air has a smaller refractive index than glass). The rays refract again as they leave air and enter the objective. This refraction of light rays as they enter different media limits the amount of light that can enter the objective and also its resolution.

Immersion oil takes the place of the air gap between objective and slide. The oil has the same refractive index (about 1.52) as the glass hemispherical lens of the objective (which is the lens in the compound oil-immersion objective that is closest to the slide). This means that light rays do not refract (or bend) when they pass from the oil into the hemispherical lens. As far as the light rays are concerned, the oil is a *continuation* of the glass lens because the refractive indices are the same. In effect, the material on the slide has been, for practical purposes, placed 'inside' a spherical 'lens' whose upper hemisphere is made of glass and whose lower hemisphere is made of oil. The result of placing the object being viewed 'inside' a spherical lens is to markedly improve on the resolution that could otherwise be achieved. Of course there is no way of placing the object inside a solid glass lens, so using oil is a convenient device for achieving increased resolution. Typically a numerical aperture of 1.25 can be achieved in student microscopes.

12.6 The Electromagnetic Spectrum

12.6.1 *The Historical Perspective*

We have discussed light as if it is a wave. However, the nature of light is not so clear cut. From about 1670, most people believed Isaac Newton's theory that light was a stream of 'corpuscles' (another name for particles) issuing forth from a source of light. The alternative theory of Christian Huygens, that light was 'undulatory' like a sound wave, was not held in such high esteem. This was because of the enormous standing of Newton in the scientific community at the time, and the inability of anyone to show that light could 'interfere' as other types of waves could.

In the early nineteenth century, Thomas Young in England and Augustin Fresnel in France collaborated on a wave theory of light. Young had earlier (about 1801) demonstrated interference between light waves, and had measured the wavelength of light to be less than one millionth of a metre. Their work culminated in 1817 with the theory that light was a *transverse* wave (rather than a longitudinal one). Their wave theory of light could explain every observed phenomenon and experimental result for light up to that time. J. B. L. Foucault conclusively ruled out Newton's corpuscular theory in 1850 when he showed that light travelled more slowly in water than in air (which was the opposite of the prediction of Newton's corpuscular theory).

Our understanding of the nature of light was considerably enhanced by James Clerk Maxwell. Maxwell, in 1864, published his mathematically correct and complete theory on electric currents, charges and magnetism. Somewhat surprisingly, he showed that electricity, magnetism and light were related phenomena. Maxwell's equations showed that light must be an 'electromagnetic' wave of some kind and that radiations of shorter and longer wavelength than light should exist. In 1888 Heinrich Hertz, using an electric circuit, generated electromagnetic waves of long wavelength (radiowaves) which could be detected electrically although they could not be seen. For his achievements, the unit for frequency (cycles per second) was renamed in his honour as the **hertz** (Hz).

Every kind of electromagnetic radiation, regardless of its wavelength, can be understood in terms of Maxwell's theory. 'Different' electromagnetic radiations differ from each other in frequency (and therefore in wavelength) but not in nature (see Figure 12.8). The differences between electromagnetic radiations may be likened to the differences between pieces of the timber from one species of tree (say, radiata pine). The pieces of timber may be of different lengths and thickness and hence are distinguishable from each other, but nevertheless they are all radiata pine. Different electromagnetic radiations have different frequencies, but they are all oscillations of electric and magnetic fields. Electromagnetic radiations without the same frequency are perceived to be different because they carry different amounts of energy. The higher the frequency is, the greater the energy carried. The effects caused by electromagnetic radiation depend on the amount of energy carried by the radiation.

All electromagnetic radiations travel with the same speed through empty space (3×10^8 m/s). When they travel through a material medium their speed is decreased due to the density of the medium. However, there is no apparent movement of the particles of the medium to mark the passage of the waves. The oscillations that do occur are in the magnitudes of the electric and magnetic fields which comprise the wave, rather than in the material medium through which the wave may happen to be passing.

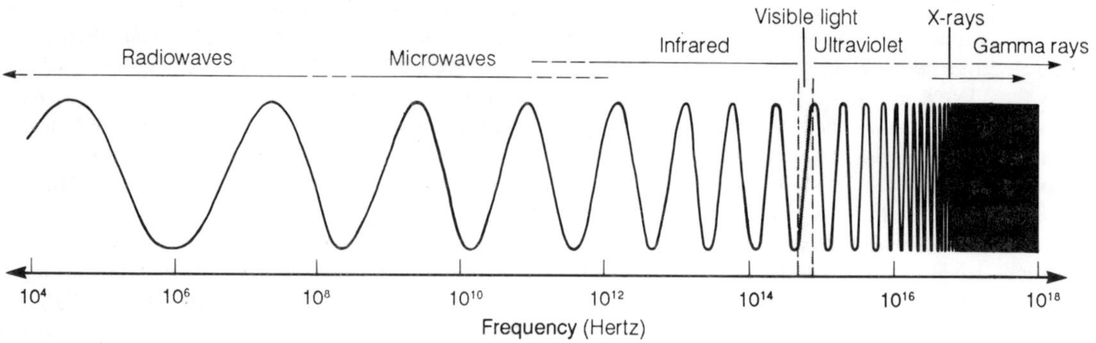

Figure 12.8 *The electromagnetic spectrum comprises a continuous range of frequencies from radio waves to gamma rays. The descriptive names for different regions are historical and do not signify actual differences in the nature of the radiation. The regions in fact overlap each other*

12.6.2 *The Sections of the Electromagnetic Spectrum*

The so-called 'forms' of electromagnetic radiation were given descriptive names based on some detail from their original discovery or on their relationship to visible light. **Gamma rays** were discovered in 1900 by Paul Villard. They have very high frequencies and originate from the rearrangements of the particles in the nucleus of an atom. Gamma rays were the third form of nuclear radiation that was detected so were given the name of the third letter of the Greek alphabet. **X-rays** were discovered in 1895 by Wilhelm Roentgen. Since the nature of these rays was unknown at the time of their discovery, Roentgen named them 'X' for unknown rays. These rays originate from the rearrangement of the innermost electrons (those closest to the nucleus) of large atoms and from X-ray machines. X-rays, like gamma rays, have extremely high frequencies.

Johann Ritter in 1801 discovered the presence of energy in the invisible portion of the solar spectrum beyond violet. These rays, now called **ultraviolet rays**, have frequencies higher than visible violet light and are 'adjacent' to visible light in the spectrum of electromagnetic frequencies. Visible light is that narrow range of frequencies that causes the retina of a normal human eye to respond. **Infrared rays** have been known since about 1800 when noticed by William Herschel. They are lower in frequency than visible red light and are 'adjacent' to red in the spectrum. Ultraviolet, visible, and infrared radiation can all be produced by the rearrangement of electrons in atoms or by raising the temperature of some material to the appropriate level.

Frequencies lower than infrared are called **microwaves** and frequencies lower still than microwaves, are called **radiowaves**. Such waves are produced by causing electrons to oscillate at the appropriate frequency in the transmitter. Certain ranges of these relatively low frequency waves are also named according to the specific use to which they have been assigned by law. Thus some are used to transmit radio and television signals such as UHF, TV, FM, radar and so on.

12.6.3 *The Continuous Nature of the Electromagnetic Spectrum*

It is important to realise that the spectrum of electromagnetic radiation is continuous and that the frequency at which the name given to the radiation changes is not rigidly set. Rather the boundaries between 'different' types of radiation are indistinct and are delimited in practice to the frequencies that the means of producing the radiation is able to supply. Thus as frequency increases, the name applied to the radiation gradually changes from (say) infrared to visible red to visible violet to 'near' ultraviolet to 'far' ultraviolet to 'soft' X-rays and so on. There is no identifiable frequency which forms the boundary between ultraviolet rays and X-rays. Nor is there any need to identify such a boundary.

Since the range of electromagnetic frequencies is continuous, the name assigned to a particular electromagnetic radiation often comes from the method used to produce the radiation, rather than the precise value of its frequency. Gamma rays are produced by some radioactive atoms, X-rays are produced in 'linear accelerators' where very fast moving (and hence high energy) electrons are stopped in a target. Thus it is possible for a 'hard' X-ray to have a higher frequency than a 'soft' gamma ray. This is indeed the case for X-rays used in radiotherapy. Electromagnetic radiation with wavelengths of a few millimetres can be produced by microwave techniques (using microwave oscillators) or by infrared techniques (a heated source).

The naming of different sections of the electromagnetic spectrum is analogous to the naming of the lifespan of humans. When we identify infancy, childhood, adolescence, maturity, middle age, senior citizens and so on, we understand perfectly well the age span in question. Yet we know that the ageing process is continuous rather than compartmentalised, and that middle age is achieved gradually rather than overnight.

Even within the range of frequencies known by their own name, there are often subranges identified by their specific name. For example, red is used to identify visible light of low frequency while blue denotes visible light of high frequency. The terms 'soft' and 'hard' are used for X-rays of lower and higher frequency respectively. 'Near' and 'far' are used to describe ultraviolet radiation of low and high frequency respectively.

12.7 Photons

It is ironical that Heinrich Hertz, while conducting experiments that established the validity of Maxwell's electromagnetic wave theory of light, also noticed an effect that would prove to be inexplicable by Maxwell's theory. Hertz had experimentally 'proved' that light was a wave. He also noticed an event (that came to be known as the **photoelectric effect**) which, on explanation, was to 'prove' that light was not a wave. In 1905 Albert Einstein provided the explanation and the photoelectric effect became evidence that light was composed of corpuscles called photons. Hence the corpuscular theory of light first espoused by Newton was revived, albeit in modified form.

What then is light? Light and all electromagnetic radiation is a non-material phenomenon, so is difficult to visualise. It may correctly be thought of as a stream of energy in the form of oscillating electric and magnetic fields which are strongly interdependent on each other. However, the stream of energy is *discontinuous* — it exists as a great many separate bundles of energy called photons. Thus a beam of light striking an object may be thought of as a 'rain' of individual photons in the same way that a jet of water from a hose is composed of individual water molecules. Ultraviolet photons possess more energy than photons of visible light because they have a higher frequency. Photons of X-radiation in turn, have more energy than ultraviolet photons.

The apparent 'size' of a photon depends on its energy. If an infrared photon is, by analogy, about the size of a cherry pip, a visible photon would be the size of a marble, ultraviolet photons would range in size from a golf ball to a tennis ball, while X-rays and gamma rays would range in size from soccer balls to large ballons. A radiowave photon of frequency 10^8 Hz carries less than one microelectron-volt of energy (about 10^{-23} J; see Section 14.4.1 for the definition of electron-volt). Photons with such small amounts of energy are impossible to detect individually so radio waves appear, for all intents and purposes, to be continuous streams of energy. They are adequately referred to as waves. On the other hand, an X-ray photon may have an energy of several million electron-volts. It is capable of wreaking bullet-like destruction to the molecules in its path. For all intents and purposes, a high-energy photon appears to be an isolated 'bullet'. The properties of electromagnetic radiation having photons with energies between these two extremes form a gradual transition between continuous extended waves and localised bullets depending on the energy they carry.

12.8 Ultraviolet Radiation, Tanning and Skin Cancer

Since sunlight contains some ultraviolet radiation and exposure to it is inevitable, we will discuss its effects on us. The normal, immediate responses of the skin to ultraviolet radiation are erythema (sunburn), delayed melanin pigmentation (suntan) and vitamin D production. In addition, the long-term effects of chronic exposure are skin ageing and skin cancer. The Anti-Cancer Foundation of South Australia reported in 1988 that two out of three Australians can expect to develop some form of skin cancer during their lifetimes.

Different parts of the ultraviolet spectrum show enormous variations in their ability to cause biological damage. Thus it is convenient to divide the near ultraviolet radiation from our sun into three regions, UV-A, UV-B and UV-C, according to wavelength (see Table 12.2).

(Note that wavelength is more easily measured than frequency so is often quoted as a wave characteristic even though frequency is the more 'fundamental' quantity. Frequency is more characteristic of a particular radiation because it does not alter as the radiation passes into different media whereas the wavelength does. In a vacuum the two quantities are related thus: frequency = $3 \times 10^8 \div$ wavelength.)

Table 12.2 *The ultraviolet spectrum*

Spectral region	Wavelengths (nm)
visible violet	420–400
UV-A	400–315
UV-B	315–280
UV-C	280–100

lengths cannot penetrate the atmosphere as readily as longer ones.

UV-C has wavelengths shorter than 280 nm so solar UV-C cannot reach us through the atmosphere. However, 'excimer' lasers, arc welders, sterilising lamps and some therapeutic sun lamps produce some UV-C so exposure to these must be carefully controlled. Short-wavelength electromagnetic radiation has a high frequency and the higher the frequency the greater the energy carried. The high energy content of UV-C produces damaging burns because of the chemical changes it causes in the skin.

UV-B wavelengths lie between 280 and 315 nm and do penetrate the atmosphere to sea level. These short wavelengths carry a greater amount of energy than UV-A and so can do more harm. It is these ultraviolet wavelengths that produce sunburn (erythema) and that sunscreen ointment preparations attempt to block out. Even with a cloud blocking the sun there is enough scattered UV-B to produce sunburn. The ability of UV-B to produce sunburn is highly dependent upon the wavelength. Erythemal effect increases very rapidly as wavelength decreases from 315 nm to 280 nm. However, the intensity of solar UV-B decreases along with wavelength. Consequently, the peak sunburning effect occurs for wavelengths close to 300 nm and it is this wavelength that sunscreens are designed to block out.

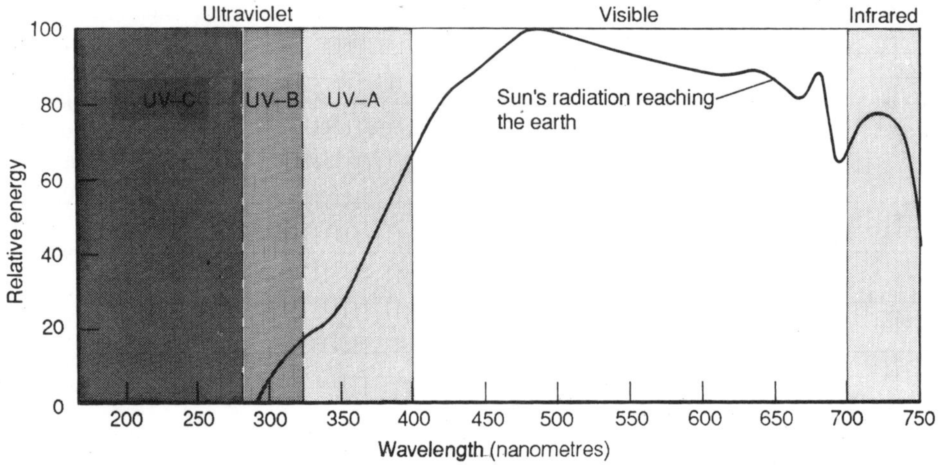

Figure 12.9 *The relative energy of different wavelengths of the sun's radiation. The earth's atmosphere is transparent to visible light but its transparency decreases as the wavelengths move further into the ultraviolet and infrared regions*

The ultraviolet radiation that reaches us from the sun lies between the wavelengths of 280 and 400 nm (nm stands for nanometre which is 10^{-9} of a metre). Shorter wavelengths than 280 nm are (mercifully) prevented from reaching us by the absorbing effect of the atmosphere. The intensity of the ultraviolet radiation that does reach the earth is greatest at 400 nm and gradually decreases to zero at a wavelength of 280 nm (see Figure 12.9). This is because the shorter wave-

UV-B, and to a lesser extent UV-A, initiate melanogenesis (tanning). Once present, melanin gives some protection against sunburn by decreasing the amount of ultraviolet radiation that can reach the lower layer of skin. Tanning is accompanied by a thickening of the outer horny layer of skin (the stratum corneum).

Laboratory experiments on mice indicate that wavelengths longer than 320 nm (UV-A) have little carcinogenic effect. However, tumour production increases rapidly as the wavelength shortens. There seems little question that squamous cell carcinomas are caused by chronic exposure to sunlight, but the cause of basal cell carcinomas (particularly melanomas) are not so clearly understood. Some aspects of melanoma incidence appear to be related to sun exposure but the connections are not clear. Nevertheless it is possible to postulate that DNA damage to melanocytes is initiated by wavelengths shorter than 320 nm, and that this may lead to melanoma.

12.9 Medical Uses of Infrared and Ultraviolet Radiation

Heating. Infrared radiation produces the sensation of warmth on our skin. The energy deposited in the skin by infrared photons causes the skin temperature to rise, capillaries to dilate and consequently peripheral circulation to increase. The increase in blood circulation promotes the healing of muscular injuries and relieves the pain of arthritis. Consequently 'heat ray' lamps are used for these purposes.

Psoriasis. Some chemicals that can be taken up by the cells of the body are photoactive. That is, they produce a photochemical modification to the nucleic acids of rapidly dividing cells when these cells are exposed to long-wavelength ultraviolet radiation. The psoralens are such drugs, and PUVA (Psoralen Ultra-Violet-A) therapy has been used to treat skin diseases such as acne and psoriasis.

Cutaneous T-cell Lymphoma. This malignancy of the white blood cells may be treated by the process called photopheresis. One unit of blood is removed from the patient and centrifuged to separate the red blood cells from the plasma and white blood cells. These last two are treated with the photoactive drug, mixed with saline and passed through a very thin but wide channel of clear plastic film. While in the film, the white blood cells were irradiated with high-intensity UV-A light. The radiation causes the photoactive drug 8-MOP (8-methoxypsoralen) to bind with the DNA in the diseased T-cells. After irradiation the red blood cells are added and the treated blood retransfused to the patient. The body's own immune system can then respond to the cancerous T-cells.

Jaundice. Neonatal jaundice is effectively treated with phototherapy using blue light of wavelength between 400 and 480 nm. Note that despite the heading to this section, these wavelengths are *not* in the ultraviolet region. Typically, standard flourescent 'daylight' tubes (spectral range 330 to 750 nm) are used but there are 'blue' lamps available which emit chiefly in the region of 400 to 500 nm. In either case an ultraviolet absorbing material is placed between the lamps and the baby to prevent irradiation with wavelengths below about 380 nm.

Sterilisation. UV-C radiation in the range 260 to 270 nm has a germicidal effect, effectively killing bacteria and preventing the growth of mould. The low-pressure mercury-discharge lamps that are used in sterilising cabinets emit strongly at 254 nm. This wavelength is damaging to the eyes and skin, so warning signs are displayed where these lamps are used. They also emit light in the visible wavelength region which gives them their characteristic pale-blue glow when in operation.

Laser Surgery. The beam of light produced by lasers may be ultraviolet or infrared. Surgical lasers use high-intensity infrared radiation to perform bloodless surgery. It is an alternative form of surgical procedure to the scalpel or diathermy. Lasers are discussed at greater length in the following section.

12.10 Lasers

In 1954 at Columbia University, USA, some scientists were able to generate microwaves without using the customary electron tube. They called their device the maser. By 1959 the range of frequency of the electromagnetic waves that could be generated had been extended to the visible region of the spectrum. The new device was, in essence, an 'optical maser' but is known as the **laser**. The word is an acronym for Light Amplification by the Stimulated Emission of Radiation. A laser is a generator of electromagnetic waves, as is a light globe, a flame, a neon tube, the sun, an electron tube and a radio transmitter. However, it is a very special source of radiation because the light it produces is almost precisely of the one wavelength (**monochromatic**), highly coherent, virtually parallel and highly focusable. The explanation of the laser mechanism lies in the abstract atomic and quantum theories, both of which are beyond the scope of this book. However, we will delve into some basic ideas in order to develop an informed layman's appreciation of the theory.

12.10.1 *The Fundamentals of Laser Action*

An atom is believed to consist of a central positively charged nucleus surrounded by a cloud of negatively charged electrons. Each electron possesses a particular amount of energy. Within the volume of the atom, electrons are arranged into 'energy levels' (or shells) according to the amount of energy they have. The electrons with greater amounts of energy are generally further from the nucleus. Each energy level can only contain a limited number of electrons before it is 'full' (see Figure 12.10). For example, the first level is full with two electrons, the second level is filled if it contains eight electrons, the third can hold eighteen, the fourth and fifth each hold thirty two. There are no elements with enough electrons to fill the sixth and seventh energy levels completely. Electrons in each energy level actually differ slightly in energy, so are further sorted into sublevels.

The most common arrangement for electrons in an atom is for them to occupy the lowest possible levels

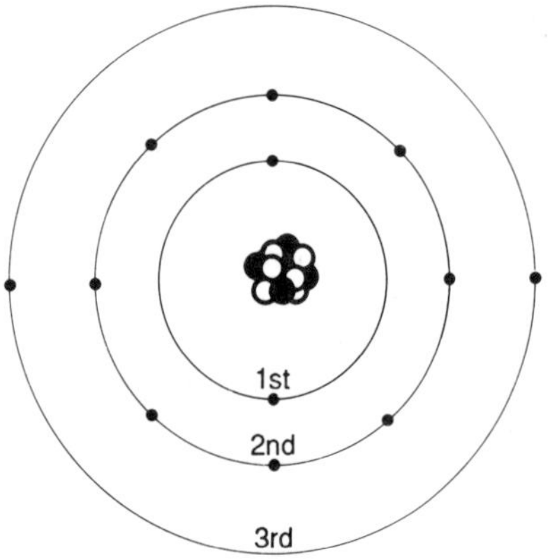

Figure 12.10 *A representation of a magnesium atom containing 12 electrons in their ground state. The first and second energy levels are filled*

of energy. That is, electrons will not be in level five if there are vacancies in levels three and four. Electrons that reside in their lowest energy state are said to be in their **ground state**. However, electrons can gain extra energy by a variety of means and so move temporarily to a higher energy level (and further from the nucleus). This leaves a vacancy in the lower level. Electrons that have reached a higher energy state are said to be in an **excited state** (see Figure 12.11).

Electrons do not remain in an excited state for long (only for about 10^{-8} seconds), but return to the ground state and emit their extra energy as a photon of electromagnetic energy (a wavetrain of a few metres in length). Because the life of the excited state is so short, an individual atom may be excited and then emit a photon in order to return to its ground state many millions of times per second. All that is required is an energy source to excite the electron. The emission of a photon as an excited electron returns to ground state is termed **spontaneous** because it occurs without any prompting. The light emitted from the white-hot filament of a globe is produced by spontaneous emission from atoms whose electrons have been excited by the heating effect of electric current. These emitted photons are totally independent of each other in direction and phase.

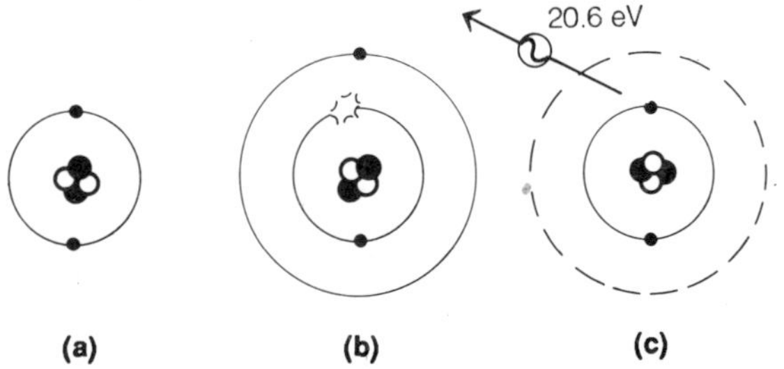

Figure 12.11 *(a) A helium atom in the ground state. (b) An electron gaining 20.6 eV of energy can 'jump' to the next energy level (an excited state). (c) It will de-excite almost immediately (by emitting a photon of energy 20.6 eV) to the ground state*

As well as spontaneous emission, the emission of a photon by an electron in an excited state can be prompted by another photon. The 'prompting photon' has to be of identical energy to the photon that would have been spontaneously emitted. Such emission is called **stimulated** emission and results in the two photons leaving the atom together. Note that the emitted photon and the prompting photon have the same direction, wavelength, frequency, energy, phase and state of polarisation. Stimulated emission is the mechanism that produces the special characteristics of laser light.

In some atoms, there are excited states that last ten thousand times longer than is usual (that is about 10^{-3} seconds) and these are called **metastable states**. Such states are crucial for the laser action. Consider a substance containing atoms with three electron energy states, the ground state A, a metastable state B (of higher energy than ground state) and a normal short-lived state C, of higher energy still. The electrons of most of the atoms will be in their ground state, perhaps a few will be in the higher metastable state (see Figure 12.12). It is possible to reverse the positions of the electrons, that is, for most of the electrons to be in the metastable state with only a few in the ground state. Such a situation is referred to as a **population inversion**.

A population inversion can be achieved by several techniques, one of which is called 'optical pumping'. This technique surrounds the lasing medium with an intense source of light which has a continuous spectrum of wavelengths. The light energy is absorbed by the atoms of the lasing medium and causes their electrons to be excited to energy state C; these electrons will lose their energy immediately and fall back into energy level B. B is a metastable state, so electrons will remain there for some time before dropping back to the ground state. In fact, the time spent in level B exceeds the time it takes for an electron to be pumped up from ground state to state C and then fall into state B. Thus a 'bottle neck' will develop at level B as electrons wait to fall back into the ground state. That is, a population inversion has been achieved.

The lasing medium, with a population inversion of electrons in the metastable state, is ready for stimulated emission. A stray photon of the correct energy will now prompt an 'avalanche' of electrons into the ground state. This avalanche is accompanied by a burst of photons (stimulated emission) with all the photons

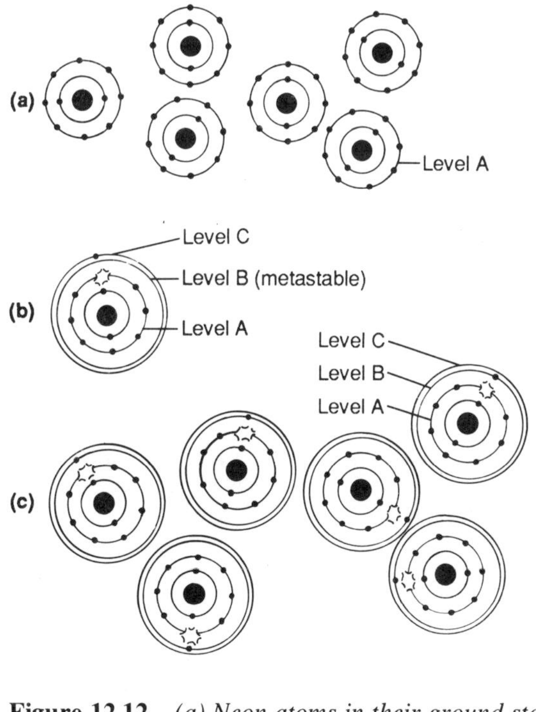

Figure 12.12 *(a) Neon atoms in their ground state. (b) Excited neon atom. An electron from the ground state (level A) has been promoted to an excited state (level C). (c) A population inversion. Neon atoms with electrons that have de-excited to a metastable energy level (level B)*

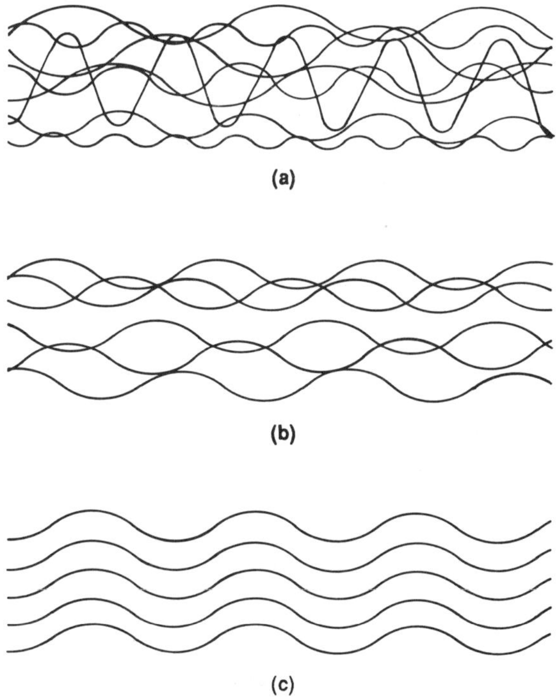

Figure 12.13 *(a) Incoherent white light. A mixture of visible electromagnetic frequencies out of phase with each other. (b) Light of a single frequency is called monochromatic. It may still be out of phase. (c) Coherent light. All the waves are identical and are in phase*

being identical to each other. If the optical pumping is continuous, then as electrons return to their ground state, they are immediately excited once more to energy level C. Electrons in C fall immediately into the metastable state where they pause briefly. That is, the metastable state will always have more electrons than either the ground state or the excited state C. Hence the laser action is continuous.

By identical photons we mean that they all have the same wavelength, are travelling in the same direction and are in phase. 'In phase' is the situation when the oscillations of the electric and magnetic fields that comprise the photons are synchronised (see Figure 12.13). Such **coherent** behaviour among photons allows enormous power densities (10^{12} W/cm^{2}) to be produced for extremely short periods (nanoseconds). The large energy available from a laser beam can be concentrated into a spot of less than a millimetre in diameter and this fact makes it a useful surgical device.

12.10.2 *The Basic Parts of a Laser*

Hundreds of materials — solids, liquids and gases — have been found to exhibit laser action, that is, to possess a metastable state. Common ones that have found applications in medicine are carbon dioxide (CO_2), argon (Ar), helium-neon (HeNe) and neodymium-yttrium-aluminium-garnet (Nd-YAG). Each different laser material produces electromagnetic radiation of different wavelength (see Table 12.3) and these wavelengths are best suited to different applications.

Table 12.3 *The wavelength (in nanometres) and radiation produced by different lasers*

Laser	Wavelength	Radiation
ArF Excimer	193	ultraviolet
KrF Excimer	248	ultraviolet
Ar	488–514	blue-green
Kr	530–680	yellow-red
HeNe	630	red
Nd-YAG	1 060	near infrared
CO_2	10 600	far infrared

A laser consists of a cylinder of the lasing medium enclosed by two concave mirrors, a pumping mechanism for producing a population inversion, and a laser delivery system. The bulk of the cabinet associated with the laser comprises the power supplies, cooling mechanism, safety devices and associated electronics.

The two mirrors cause the photons to be reflected repeatedly so as to pass through the lasing medium again and again. The repeated reflections mean that photons which are not travelling parallel to the axis of the laser will, because of their angle of travel, eventually strike the sides of the laser rather than emerging as part of the beam. Consequently, the photons that do emerge are collimated (travelling along parallel paths) to a high degree. The reflections also provide a ready supply of photons of the correct energy to stimulate emission by electrons in the metastable state. One of the mirrors (the back one) is totally reflecting, while the other (at the front) allows a small proportion of the photons that strike it to pass through and so emerge as the laser beam.

The laser beam used for surgery must be directed very precisely to the intended target and this is achieved by the **beam delivery system**. One such system is the relatively bulky articulated arm which contains mirrors and or lenses. The carbon dioxide laser beam is reflected and focused by these mirrors and lenses in the arm and so delivered to the target body site. However, the size of the arm limits its usage to the more accessible areas of the body such as the brain, nose and throat and to gynaecology. Some laser beams can be directed through optical fibres. These are narrow, flexible fibres of transparent material from which light cannot escape (except at each end). Hence optical fibres can be contained in an endoscope and the laser beam directed onto any interior body site that can be reached by an endoscope. Other beam delivery systems are the metal tip and the crystal. A metal tip can be heated by the laser beam and the hot tip delivers heat to a tumour or clears out an atheroma. A crystal (for example, sapphire) can be used to focus or defocus the heat and light of a laser beam. The effect is to form a 'scalpel' of light.

12.10.3 *The Medical Uses of Lasers*

The effect of a laser on tissue is determined by the wavelength, the power delivered per square millimetre and the duration of the pulse. Basically there are four different effects that can be achieved by laser beam. Lasers can be used for precision cutting (a photoablative effect), for massive tissue ablation (removal) and coagulation of blood vessels (photothermal effects), for stone disintegration (an electromechanical effect) and for a photochemical effect. The benefits of laser surgery are that it is relatively bloodless (because of the coagulating effect on small blood vessels), produces no electrical trauma and little mechanical trauma. Laser surgery is a relatively cheap form of surgery and patients are usually discharged sooner than those that undergo the alternative surgical procedures.

Laser beams can be focused onto a spot much less than one millimetre and deliver energy at the rate of up to 150 W. This energy is absorbed by tissue and generates enough heat to vaporise cells and so produce a 'cut'. Lower power levels produce less heat, but enough to shrink tissue and so seal small blood vessels.

The argon laser is used for photocoagulation because the blue-green light it produces is readily absorbed by blood and melanin. Thus 'port-wine stains' on skin and tattoos can be removed by the argon laser. Vascular retinal diseases, such as diabetic retinopathy and retinal branch vein occlusion, where blood vessels grow in front of the retina, are treated by photocoagulation using the argon laser or in more recent times a krypton laser.

Excimer lasers such as argon-fluorine, krypton-fluorine and xenon-chlorine produce various ultraviolet wavelengths. These lasers can operate at very high power densities (10^8 W/cm^2) in pulses lasting only nanoseconds to produce a photoablative effect. The photons from these lasers have enough energy (4–6 eV) to break the bonds within molecules. Excimer lasers can be used to sculpt the cornea (radial keratotomy) to correct vision as an alternative to wearing glasses.

For surgical procedures, the Nd-YAG or the carbon dioxide laser is used. The former is used to stop gastrointestinal bleeding and in thoracic surgery to remove bronchial and tracheal tumours. The carbon dioxide laser is most useful in the treatment of lesions of the lower genital tract in women and in neurosurgery. It should be remembered that laser surgery is still in its infancy and that many more procedures than have been mentioned can be performed with lasers. Laser surgery will undoubtedly become more common as the results of clinical trials become available, the pool of surgeons skilled in laser surgery expands and as lasers and optical fibres with different characteristics are developed.

12.10.4 *The Hazards of Laser Surgery*

The eye is the organ that is most susceptible to damage when exposed to a laser beam. Visible and near infrared radiation is focused by the eye onto the retina. The intensities of light from lasers are sufficient to cause local heating of the retina which may burn the pigment epithelium and the rods and cones. This will result in temporary or permanent loss of vision. Ultraviolet and longer infrared radiation is absorbed in the cornea, lens and vitreous humour and may result in a corneal burn or cataract formation. Since a laser can deliver a damaging amount of energy to the eye before the blink reflex has time to operate, the eye must be protected by a shield that is opaque to the laser wavelength being used but still allows the wearer to see.

The appropriate laser safety glasses must be worn by everyone (including the patient) in the room with the laser. Note that a single pair of safety goggles will not protect against all types of laser so it is usual to have at least two types available. The safety eyewear will have marked on it the wavelength for which it is suitable. It is also important to realise that lead glass, which is opaque to X-rays, is transparent to the wavelengths of surgical lasers, so afford no protection at all to observers standing behind it. Lead glass windows that open onto adjacent rooms are usually covered for the duration of the laser procedure.

A lesser but significant hazard is the damage to skin of staff or to healthy tissue in the patient that may occur when the laser beam reflects from polished metal speculae. This hazard is reduced by using plastic or matt-finished metal speculae.

Tissue that is vaporised by the laser beam will form a plume of smoke containing a plasma of cell material. This smoke plume must be extracted from the laser room at the site of its production by using a high flow rate, filtered evacuation unit. The plume interferes with clear vision and has been shown to contain viable viral DNA when warts (due to human papilloma virus) are treated.

12.11 X-rays

12.11.1 *The Discovery of X-rays*

In 1895 the German physicist Wilhelm Roentgen serendipitously discovered a radiation that caused a fluorescent screen to light up brightly. The fluoresence occurred even when the path of the new rays was blocked by materials that were opaque to visible and ultraviolet radiation. That is, most materials were transparent to these rays. In fact when a hand was held over a sealed photographic plate and the new rays allowed to fall on it, the plate showed the outline of the bones in the hand. The fact that the rays permitted one to 'see' through opaque objects caused a sensation among the public at the time. There was great consternation lest, by the improper use of these new rays, fully dressed people would be made to appear naked.

Since the rays were of unknown nature (whether they were waves or particles was not clear), Roentgen called them 'X' rays. Many people preferred to call them Roentgen-rays and in Germany an X-ray photograph is known as a 'Roentgenogram'. Charles G. Barkla and Max von Laue showed that X-rays were short-wavelength electromagnetic radiation. Barkla in 1906 correctly identified the polarisation of X-rays and in 1912 Laue demonstrated that the rays could be combined destructively into a diffraction pattern. Both of these effects are characteristic of electromagnetic radiation.

12.11.2 *The Production of X-rays*

X-rays are produced whenever electrons that have been accelerated to a high velocity by a very large potential difference are allowed to strike some material (the target). The electrons are slowed down and stopped in the target due to their electric interaction with the electrons and nuclei of the atoms of the target material. The kinetic energy of the bombarding electrons is largely converted to heat but some becomes electromagnetic energy in the form of X-ray photons. The German term *bremsstrahlung*, meaning braking radiation, is aptly used to describe the radiation produced. As the electrons slow down, they emit photons with energy equal to the kinetic energy that they have lost.

Modern radiographic X-ray 'tubes' are based on an innovation by William D. Coolidge in 1913. The **Coolidge tube** is a highly evacuated glass envelope in which electrons are produced from a tungsten filament that is heated by an electric current (the Edison effect). The heat produced by the current causes electrons to leave the filament (the cathode) and enter the evacuated tube whereupon they are accelerated and focused by a high voltage onto the target (the anode). The potential difference involved is between 20 000 and 200 000 V. Note that 20 kV would supply an electron with 20 000 eV of energy and in turn result in X-rays with a maximum energy of 20 keV as the electrons are stopped in the target.

The maximum achievable X-ray energy from a Coolidge tube is limited to below 250 keV by the problems of insulating the electrical supply cables. To produce the X-rays of 10 MeV and more that are required for deep radiation therapy in the treatment of cancer, a **linear accelerator** is used. This device accelerates electrons to energies of up to 18 MeV by using pulsed microwaves. On striking the target the electrons give up their energy to form X-rays with a maximum energy of 18 MeV.

12.11.3 *Radiographic Images*

X-rays can expose photographic film just as visible light can. Since soft tissues are more transparent to X-rays than bone is, a shadow image of bony structures can be produced on film by the transmitted rays. These X-ray photographs, or radiographs, of bones were first used in medicine within a year of Roentgen's discovery of the rays.

Although a photographic emulsion can be exposed to X-rays directly, more commonly the energy of X-rays is converted into radiation in the visible light spectrum. The direct exposure of film requires a relatively high intensity of X-rays. This would cause excessively large doses of X-ray to be absorbed in the patient. Therefore the radiographic image is converted to visible light, at some stage, by a luminescent screen. The light from the luminescent screen then exposes a photographic film (in radiography or photofluorography), or the light may be viewed directly (in fluoroscopy).

Luminescence is the emission of visible light photons by the atoms of a substance (called the phosphor) following some stimulus (such as the absorption by the atoms of an invisible photon). **Fluorescence** is that form of luminescence where the emission of light is instantaneous (**phosphorescence** is delayed emission). Recall that it was the ability of X-rays to produce fluorescence that lead to their discovery so it is not surprising that this ability is exploited in their medical use.

The fluorescent screens in use also have an intensifying effect. That is, a few X-ray photons absorbed in the screen will be converted to a lot of visible light photons. Intensifying screens are used because they reduce the X-ray dose that would otherwise be absorbed by the patient, yet still produce a properly exposed X-ray film. The ratio of X-ray intensity (number of photons) required for film exposure with a screen to X-ray intensity for direct film exposure is 1:34. Hence by using a flourescent screen, the patient is exposed to only 3% of the X-rays required to directly expose a film.

Fluoroscopic screens for direct viewing are similar to the intensifying screens used for radiography. The difference is that the light from the former has a wavelength of between 500 to 600 nm, which corresponds to the maximum sensitivity of the eye. When a fluoroscopic screen is viewed directly, the observer must be protected from any X-rays transmitted through the screen. This is achieved by using lead glass. This glass has a high proportion of lead (about 60% by weight) and is transparent to visible light but effectively absorbs X-rays of the energy used in fluoroscopy.

Photofluorography is used for projects such as mass public chest X-raying in tuberculosis screening. The image on the fluorescent screen is photographed for later examination.

12.11.4 *The Fluoroscope*

When it is necessary to view the motion of internal parts of the body, such as the action of a joint or the insertion of a catheter, a fluoroscope is used. In effect, a moving X-ray picture can be produced. The fluoroscope consists essentially of a Coolidge X-ray tube and a fluorescent screen with the patient being placed between the two. The other parts are designed to protect the patient and operator from stray radiation and to facilitate examination.

To raise the level of fluorescence to that which allows viewing to occur in a room with the lights on, X-ray image intensifiers are used. The increased brightness afforded by these intensifiers reduces the dose to the patient and allows video recording of the fluoroscopic examination and instant playback. Thus prolonged study of the recorded image is possible without prolonging the exposure.

12.12 Computed Tomography

A **tomograph** is an image of the internal structures of the body viewed as a thin slice across the axis from head to foot. Slicing a carrot into rounds produces the same effect (for a carrot). In fact the word tomograph is derived from the Greek words *tomos* which means slice and *graphos* which means written. A tomograph can only be produced with the assistance of a computer to calculate the amount of absorption or emission of electromagnetic radiation that occurs in the body slice. Hence the technique of producing a slice-image is called **computed tomography** (CT). Sometimes the technique is called computerised axial tomography or computer-assisted tomography (both abbreviated to CAT) but they are the same as CT.

The CT technique to form an image of a thin layer of the body can be used with X-rays (the so-called CAT scans), gamma rays (PET and SPECT scans) and microwaves (NMR scans). The most common tomographic images produced in Australia are CAT scans, but the other imaging modalities are increasingly being used (see Section 14.8).

12.12.1 *CAT Scans*

An 'X-ray photo' (a radiograph) of a chest shows the backbone, covered by the lungs which are themselves covered by the rib cage. That is, the radiographic image of each of these structures is obscured to some extent by the others. This masking does not occur in a CAT scan.

A CAT scanner consists of a 'barrel' along the axis of which the patient is aligned. On one side of the barrel is the X-ray source and on the opposite side is an array of detectors. The barrel rotates around the patient (while the patient lies still) so that X-rays are directed through the patient from every angle. The X-ray beam is very thin and spreads out as a fan shape (so its shape is somewhat like a sector from a pizza). The intensity of the X-rays that reach a detector is compared to the intensity of the beam before it passes through the patient. By subtracting one intensity from the other, the amount of absorption that has occurred as the X-rays pass through the body can be calculated. Since this absorption is calculated for beams that enter the body from every direction, each square millimetre is crossed by many beams. The amount of absorption that has occurred in any particular square millimetre of the slice can be determined by the computer from the amount of absorption that has occurred to each beam that crosses the square millimetre. The absorption pattern is then displayed as a two-dimensional picture.

The CAT scan provides a picture of the gross anatomy within a thin slice of the body. Detail as small as about half a millimetre can be resolved, so many pathological changes can be detected in the image.

Bibliography

Koretz, J. F. and Handelman, G. H. 'How the human eye focuses', *Scientific American*, **252**(7), 64–71, 1988.

Questions

1. Visible light waves are examples of
   J. electromagnetic waves
   K. mechanical waves
   L. longitudinal waves
   M. compressional waves
2. The quantity that is most characteristic of an electromagnetic wave is its
   J. amplitude
   K. wavelength
   L. frequency
   M. velocity
3. In the human eye the greatest refraction occurs
   J. in the lens of the eye
   K. at the retina
   L. as light passes from air into the cornea
   M. as light passes from the lens into the vitreous humour
4. Myopia may be corrected with a lens that is
   J. bifocal
   K. concave
   L. cylindrical
   M. convex
5. The change in vision that occurs with ageing is called
   J. protanopia
   K. hyperopia
   L. deuteranopia
   M. presbyopia
6. Ultraviolet radiation is damaging to the eye because
   J. the heat produced as it is absorbed distorts the cornea
   K. it causes an increase in the pressure in the eyeball which results in glaucoma
   L. the energy of the radiation destroys the cones in the fovea
   M. the energy of ultraviolet radiation is mainly absorbed in the lens, which harms the cells
7. As part of the normal ageing process, our eyes deteriorate because
   J. the ciliary muscles gradually lose their tone
   K. the lens loses its flexibility
   L. parts of the retina detach from the underlying blood vessels
   M. the distance between the lens and the retina gradually changes
8. The three pigments in the retina have their major sensitivities to light that is
   J. red, green and blue
   K. red, blue and yellow
   L. green, yellow and red
   M. green, yellow and blue

CHAPTER 13

Organic Compounds, the Basis of Life

In this chapter we take the ideas about atoms, ions and molecules set out in Chapter 2 and extend them into the realm of organic chemistry. We shall see that these ideas are a help in understanding how the body uses the organic compounds present in the food which we eat. From this food is obtained the vast array of different organic compounds which are needed for the maintenance of life and its continuation from one generation to the next.

The simple compound water accounts for 60–75% of the body's mass. Most of the remaining 25–40% consists of an enormous number of different organic compounds obtained, ultimately, from food, drink and air. We also make use of organic compounds as medicines, cosmetics, food preservatives, pesticides, plastics and in a host of other ways.

You have probably heard the saying 'we are what we eat'. This chapter should convince you that this is true to a point. We eat a mixture of protein, carbohydrate, lipid and nucleic acid. Our digestive systems dismantle all these into simpler substances which are then absorbed into our circulations and carried to all parts of the body where they are assembled into: protein, carbohydrate, lipid and nucleic acid! We are what we eat only to a point though, because there are differences between these substances in the human body and the same types of substance in the tissues of other living things. This is particularly true of protein and nucleic acid.

Learning Objectives

At the completion of this chapter you should be able to:

1. State two reasons why it is unlikely that the element silicon could serve as an alternative to carbon as the basis for life.
2. Explain, giving examples, the meaning of each of the following terms: saturated; unsaturated; radical; functional group; family of organic compounds; spot test.
3. Describe, in a general way, the basis on which different families of organic compounds are named.
4. Interpret the diagrams commonly used to represent organic molecules and use them to decide on the family(ies) to which an organic compound belongs.
5. Explain what is meant by the phrase 'alphabet of biochemistry'.
6. Distinguish between the chemical nature of proteins, carbohydrates, lipids and nucleic acids and state the main roles which each plays in the body.
7. Name the three main classes of biological macromolecules and describe, in a general way, the relationship between each class and other more simple organic compounds.

8. Distinguish between primary, secondary, tertiary and quaternary structures of proteins and account for some important aspects of protein behaviour in terms of these structures.
9. Describe the ways in which hydrogen bonds contribute to the structures of proteins and nucleic acids.
10. Describe, in a general way, the role played by nucleic acids in the synthesis of proteins.

13.1 Silicon, an Alternative to Carbon for Living Things?

In the jargon of science fiction, human beings are described as 'carbon-based life forms', a description which implies the existence of life forms based on elements other than carbon. Such life forms often feature prominently in the plots of science fiction novels and films with the element which serves as the alternative to carbon usually being **silicon**. This is the element of atomic number 14 and it is found immediately below carbon in Group IVA of the Periodic Table.

Silicon atoms account for 21% of the atoms making up the earth's crust, a proportion second only to oxygen which accounts for 60%. Being a member of the same group of the Periodic Table as carbon, silicon has a number of similar properties. For example, both elements exist as non-molecular substances having very high melting points and both elements form four covalent bonds when they combine with other elements. Furthermore, silicon is one of the essential elements and appears to play a role in the growth of bone and cartilage. Given these properties of silicon, it is not surprising that science fiction writers should imagine the existence of life forms based on silicon rather than carbon. However, such life forms exist only in the imagination of these writers and other factual evidence suggests that carbon is the only element capable of serving as the basis for life.

In Section 2.7.1 we saw that carbon is able to form more compounds than any other element, this being mainly due to the ability of its atoms to form covalent bonds with each other and create long chains. There seems to be no limit to the length of these chains and they are usually very stable. Thus, the organic compound polyethylene, which is a plastic used to manufacture many common products such as bottles, pipes and sheets, consists of molecules which contain as many as 50 000 carbon atoms joined together. Polyethylene is a very stable compound and it can be heated, exposed to sunlight and held in contact with other chemicals for extended periods without undergoing much change.

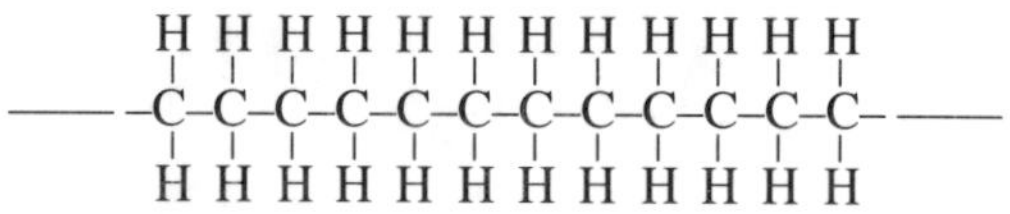

Figure 13.1 *Structural formula for polyethylene. Only a small section of the molecule is represented*

Silicon atoms can also join with each other to form chains but silicon–silicon bonds are weaker than their carbon counterparts. For this reason the length of silicon chains in which the silicon atoms are linked directly to one another is limited to about six atoms and compounds which contain such chains are very unstable. Thus, the compound Si_4H_{10}, when exposed to oxygen, ignites spontaneously and explodes, forming silicon dioxide, SiO_2, and water. The corresponding carbon compound, C_4H_{10} (butane), is quite stable in contact with air and it requires a source of ignition such as a flame or a spark to make it burn.

While the silicon–silicon bond is weaker than the carbon–carbon bond the reverse is true for the bonds which carbon and silicon form with oxygen. This allows silicon to form very long chains in which silicon and oxygen atoms alternate. One of these chains is represented in Figure 13.2.

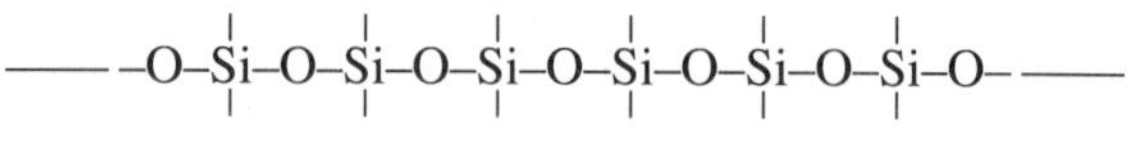

Figure 13.2 *Representation of a silicate chain*

The question which now arises is: 'Why can't we have a collection of silicon compounds built upon silicon–oxygen chains and comparable in number and diversity to the organic compounds which are built upon carbon–carbon chains?' Part of the reason is that in a silicon–oxygen chain half the atoms making up the chain (the oxygen atoms) have, simply by forming the chain, entirely used their capacity to join with other atoms (remember that oxygen atoms normally form only two bonds with other atoms). Thus, any diversity in compounds obtainable using silicon–oxygen chains must come entirely from the silicon atoms. These cannot join with each other to anywhere near the same extent as carbon atoms can and so this severely limits the diversity which can be achieved.

Furthermore, the silicon–hydrogen bond is much weaker than the carbon–hydrogen bond and this makes compounds which contain significant numbers of silicon–hydrogen bonds unstable. This is not the case with carbon, and most organic compounds contain many carbon–hydrogen bonds. Since hydrogen is by far the most abundant atom in the earth's oceans, rivers and lakes, as well as being the fourth most abundant (after oxygen, silicon and aluminium) in the earth's crust, the low stability of compounds containing silicon–hydrogen bonds further restricts the number and diversity of compounds which silicon may form.

If we compare some properties of silicon dioxide with those of carbon dioxide we see yet another reason why it is unlikely that silicon could serve as an alternative to carbon in living things. Silicon dioxide has a melting point of 1700 °C while carbon dioxide is a gas at room temperature; silicon dioxide is, for all practical purposes, completely insoluble in water, while carbon dioxide has a low, but significant, solubility.

Carbon dioxide, being a gas which is soluble in water, can cycle readily among different living creatures and among soil, air and water. In this way, the carbon content of the tissues of most living creatures remains available after they have died, and can be used to form the tissues of creatures in later generations. In contrast to this, silicon, which has formed silicon dioxide, is effectively 'locked up' for all time as a high melting, insoluble solid and so is prevented from participating in the natural cycles upon which living things depend (see Section 2.7.2).

It is quite clear from considerations of this sort that silicon is not capable of forming a set of compounds which compares in number and diversity with that formed by carbon. Nevertheless, silicon compounds are made important by their great abundance in the earth's crust and by the useful properties which certain synthetic silicon compounds possess. A good example of compounds in this latter category is the **silicones**, sometimes called the **siloxanes**. These are compounds with molecules consisting of long silicon–oxygen chains. Usually, the silicon atoms are also joined to carbon atoms and most of the diversity which these compounds display is due as much to the carbon which they contain as it is to the presence of silicon. The structural formula for the particular silicone **dimethylpolysiloxane** is shown in Figure 13.3.

Dimethylpolysiloxane is insoluble in water and is water repellent. It has a very low toxicity, virtually no

$$\begin{array}{c} \mathrm{CH_3\ \ CH_3\ \ CH_3\ \ CH_3\ \ CH_3\ \ CH_3} \\ \mathrm{|\ \ \ \ |\ \ \ \ |\ \ \ \ |\ \ \ \ |\ \ \ \ |} \\ \mathrm{-\!-O\!-\!Si\!-\!O\!-\!Si\!-\!O\!-\!Si\!-\!O\!-\!Si\!-\!O\!-\!Si\!-\!O\!-\!Si\!-\!O\!-\!-} \\ \mathrm{|\ \ \ \ |\ \ \ \ |\ \ \ \ |\ \ \ \ |\ \ \ \ |} \\ \mathrm{CH_3\ \ CH_3\ \ CH_3\ \ CH_3\ \ CH_3\ \ CH_3} \end{array}$$

Figure 13.3 *Structural formula for dimethylpolysiloxane*

physiological activity of any sort and is non-irritant when applied to the skin. This combination of properties makes the substance very desirable as a component of protective skin creams and lotions.

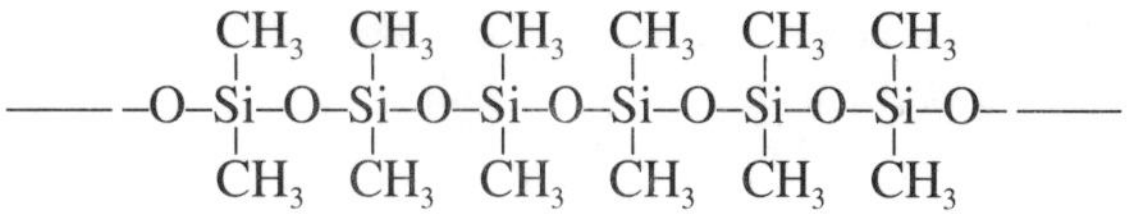

The molecular structures of silicones can be altered by changing the length of the silicon–oxygen chain and by attaching different groups to the silicon atom in place of the methyl groups (CH_3) found in dimethylpolysiloxane. These changes provide new materials having different properties and, in particular, different viscosities and solubilities. At the same time the new materials often remain non-toxic and non-irritant and so they can still be safely applied to the skin. For example, silicones having high viscosities (viscosity is the ease with which a material flows; the higher the viscosity the less readily it flows) are used in cosmetic and protective lipsticks.

The simplest naturally occurring compound of silicon is **silicon dioxide**, SiO_2, commonly called **silica**. In this compound chains of silicon–oxygen atoms are joined together by oxygen atoms to form a three-dimensional structure. Silicon dioxide occurs in several different forms but the best known is **quartz**. This form

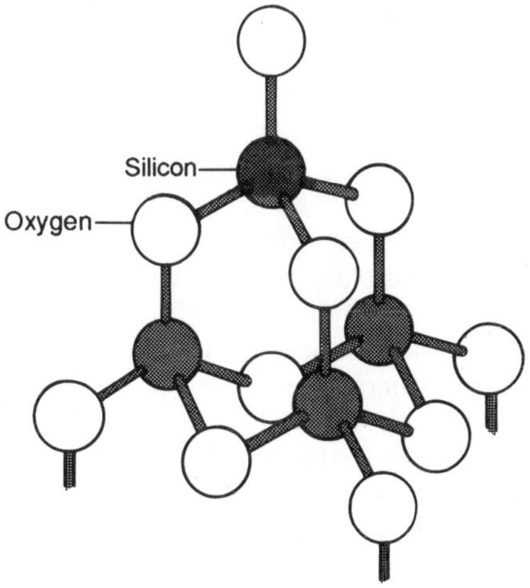

Figure 13.4 *Structure of silicon dioxide*

of silicon dioxide is the main component of sand and is used in the manufacture of glass.

Although silicon dioxide is an inert substance it does produce a biological response on prolonged contact with living tissue. When lumps of the substance are implanted into tissue the response is formation of a thick, fibrous capsule which encloses the lump but does not adhere to it. Finely divided silicon dioxide is toxic to living tissue and prolonged contact with lung tissue leads to the disease known as **silicosis** in which deposits of the fibrous protein **collagen** form on the surface of the lungs. These deposits impair lung function and increase the incidence of lung infections including **tuberculosis**. An association between lung disease and the inhalation of silicon dioxide dust by mine and quarry workers was recognised in the Middle Ages and silicosis remains an important occupational disease even today.

In spite of the toxic nature of silicon dioxide, it has proved possible to use the compound to prepare other substances which are not toxic and which can be left in contact with living tissue for an indefinite period. The usefulness of some of these materials is due to their ability to form chemical bonds with living tissue thereby becoming a permanent part of it. For example, when silicon dioxide is combined with varying proportions of calcium oxide (CaO) and diphosphorus pentaoxide (P_2O_5) it forms a series of different glasses and some of these are capable of bonding to tissue without causing any toxic effects. These glasses can also be machined into precise shapes and they show great potential for use in the manufacture of **prosthetic** devices (artificial substitutes for a missing body part). They are already being used to construct middle ear replacements. Other uses include tissue and bone supplementation in plastic and orthopaedic surgery.

The main limitation of silicate glasses in prosthesis manufacture is their lack of mechanical strength. This prevents them from being used to replace load-bearing parts of the body such as teeth and joints. However, even in these applications, silicate glasses may have some application as coating materials on metal prostheses. The advantage would be that the glass would allow the prosthetic device to bond chemically to the surrounding tissue rather than being cemented or fixed mechanically in place.

In this brief excursion into the chemistry of silicon compounds we have seen that the element is essential for human life and that it forms many different compounds, including some which are capable of being incorporated into living tissue. Even so, there is no prospect of life based on silicon rather than carbon. Silicon is not capable of forming a sufficient variety of molecular compounds and there is no simple compound of silicon which can play a role analogous to that played by carbon dioxide in the carbon cycle. Carbon is the only element on which life can be based and in the following sections we go on to consider its properties in more detail.

13.2 Bonding Patterns for the Carbon Atom

In organic compounds carbon atoms are joined to one another, and to atoms of other types, by covalent bonds. In most organic compounds the atoms other than carbon which are present are **hydrogen** and one or more of the elements **oxygen**, **nitrogen**, **sulphur**, **phosphorus**, **fluorine**, **chlorine**, **bromine** and **iodine**. The atoms of all these elements form covalent bonds in accord with the ideas set out in Section 2.6.4.They share electrons and the number shared in each case can be predicted by comparing the number of electrons which atoms of that element have with the number which an inert gas atom has. If you are not sure about this you should turn back to Section 2.6.4 and read it once more. In Table 13.1 the numbers of covalent bonds formed by atoms of each of the elements commonly found in organic compounds are listed.

Table 13.1 *Numbers of covalent bonds formed by atoms in organic compounds*

Element	Number of covalent bonds
carbon	4
hydrogen	1
oxygen	2
nitrogen	3
sulphur	2 (6)
phosphorus	3 (5)
fluorine, chlorine bromine, iodine	1

Note: Sulphur and phosphorus often form 6 and 5 covalent bonds respectively.

Although carbon is invariably tetravalent (forms four bonds) in organic compounds it may form its four bonds in several different ways. These are specified below:

1. four single bonds (saturated);
2. two single bonds, one double bond (unsaturated);
3. one single bond, one triple bond (unsaturated);
4. two double bonds (unsaturated).

Carbon atoms which have formed four single covalent bonds will be joined directly to four other atoms. This is the maximum number of atoms to which a carbon atom can be bound and so such atoms are said to be **saturated**. The term conveys the meaning that the carbon atom has fully exploited (saturated) its capacity to join to other atoms. Where a carbon atom is participating in a double or triple bond it must be joined to less than four other atoms and such carbon atoms are said to be **unsaturated**.

The terms, saturated, unsaturated and **polyunsaturated** are commonly encountered in discussions of edible fats used for cooking. A saturated fat is an organic compound in which all, or nearly all, of the carbon atoms present in its molecules are saturated. Polyunsaturated cooking fats are composed of molecules in which many of the carbon atoms are unsaturated. Fats obtained from animal sources are predominantly saturated and they are usually solids at room temperature. Polyunsaturated fats are obtained from plant sources. As the degree of unsaturation of fats increases their melting points become less. Most polyunsaturated fats are liquids at room temperature and because of this they are often called **oils**. The nature and amount of fat which is present in our diets is a topical issue because of the now widely held view that large quantities of saturated fat can contribute to the occurrence of serious diseases affecting the heart and circulatory system. This is why the manufacturers of table margarine and cooking oils usually display the proportion of unsaturated fat which their product contains on the product container.

13.3 Families of Organic Compounds and Functional Groups

There appears to be no limit to the number of different organic compounds which may exist. Each year thousands of new compounds are prepared in laboratories, or are isolated from some natural source such as a plant or an animal. If it was necessary to study each compound individually then organic chemistry would be an impossibly complex field. In fact, in its early days, many scientists avoided the study of organic chemistry because they regarded it as an 'impenetrable thicket' of seemingly unrelated compounds and reactions which was best left alone. Today, though, the 'impenetrable thicket' has been transformed into a well-organised field of study which has the enthusiastic attention of thousands of chemists. It is a field which continues to produce a stream of remarkable compounds for use in the treatment of disease, in food production, plastic manufacture and for many other purposes.

There are a number of ways in which it has been possible to simplify the study of organic chemistry and one of the most effective of these is the organisation of organic compounds into 'families'. These 'families' contain organic compounds with closely related molecular structures and for this reason they behave in a similar fashion to each other. Usually the knowledge that an organic compound belongs to a particular family is sufficient to predict the way in which it will behave. Conversely, when a new organic compound is discovered, or made, its properties can be compared to those of members of various families. In this way the molecular structure of the new compound can be determined.

13.3.1 *Hydrocarbons, the Simplest Organic Compounds*

Hydrocarbons are organic compounds which contain only the elements hydrogen and carbon (hence the name 'hydrocarbon'). There are several families of hydrocarbons.

Alkanes (Sometimes Called Paraffins). All the members of this family are saturated compounds. The simplest member of the alkanes is **methane** which has the formula CH_4. Every member of the alkane family has a molecular formula which conforms to the general formula C_nH_{2n+2} (n is a simple whole number, 1, 2, 3 . . .). Other members of the family differ from methane by the addition of $-CH_2-$ units to the methane molecule. The first five members of the alkane family are listed in Table 13.2.

The alkanes are quite familiar compounds. Methane is the main component of natural gas which is burned in many Australian homes. **Propane** and **butane** are the fuels used in portable gas bottles. The petrol which is burned in motor vehicles is a mixture of hydrocarbons which includes **pentane** and other alkanes having between six and ten carbon atoms in their molecules. The alkanes are relatively unreactive and the small number of chemical reactions which they do undergo

Table 13.2 *Names, molecular formulae, structural formulae and boiling points for the first five alkanes*

Name	Molecular formula	Structural formula	Boiling point (°C)
methane	CH_4	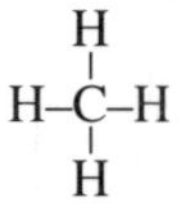 H–C(H)(H)–H	−160
ethane	C_2H_6	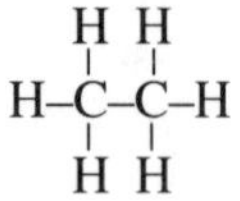 H–C(H)(H)–C(H)(H)–H	−88
propane	C_3H_8	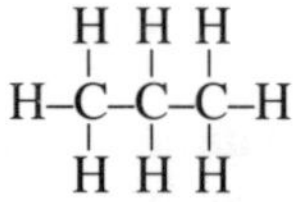 H–C(H)(H)–C(H)(H)–C(H)(H)–H	−41
butane	C_4H_{10}	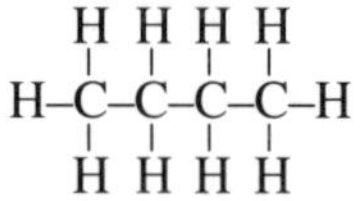 H–C(H)(H)–C(H)(H)–C(H)(H)–C(H)(H)–H	−1
pentane	C_5H_{12}	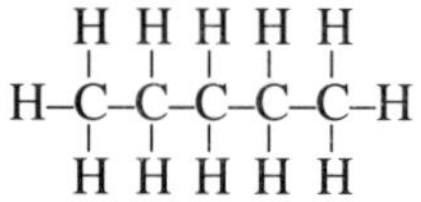 H–C(H)(H)–C(H)(H)–C(H)(H)–C(H)(H)–C(H)(H)–H	38

are difficult to control. For this reason their main uses are as **fuels** and **solvents**.

You will notice that the boiling points of the alkanes increase as the size of their molecules increase and this is a trend observed with all other families of organic compound.

Alkenes (Sometimes Called Olefins). These are hydrocarbons containing a carbon–carbon double bond in their molecules. The simplest member of the family is **ethene**, C_2H_4, and, as was the case with the alkanes, other members of the alkene family are related to ethene by the addition of $-CH_2-$ units to the ethene molecule. The general formula for this family is C_nH_{2n}. The first five alkenes are listed in Table 13.3. The first three are often referred to by common names and these are given in parentheses in Table 13.3.

The alkenes undergo a much wider range of chemical reactions than the alkanes do and many of these reactions can be controlled to yield useful quantities of new organic compounds. For example, ethene reacts with chlorine to form dichloroethane and this compound can then be converted to vinyl chloride which is used to make the familiar plastic known as polyvinyl chloride (PVC). Ethene is also used to make alcohol, ethylene glycol (used as anti-freeze in car radiators), lead tetraethyl (the petrol additive), polystyrene (another plastic) and many other useful compounds.

At first sight there does not seem to be much difference between an alkane molecule and an alkene molecule and so the question arises: 'What causes the two families to behave so differently?' The answer is that there *is* a difference between an alkane and an alkene and it is that in an alkane all the bonds are single bonds whereas in an alkene molecule there is a double bond between two of the carbon atoms (alkanes are saturated, alkenes are unsaturated) This is shown in Figure 13.5 for the two substances pentane and pentene.

All parts of the pentane molecule are much the same as one another. Any reaction that involves modifying the structure of the molecule at one point is

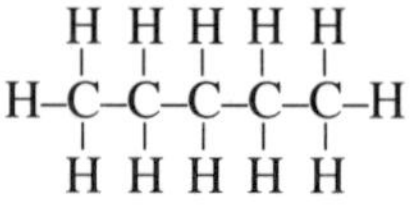

```
H H H H H                    H H H H H
| | | | |                    | | | | |
H-C-C-C-C-C-H              H-C=C-C-C-C-H
| | | | |                        | | |
H H H H H                        H H H
  pentane                        pentene
```

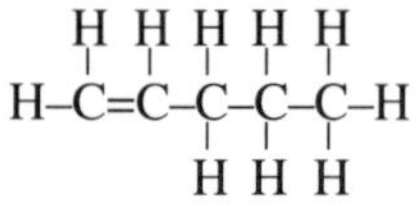

Figure 13.5 *Structural formulae for pentane and pentene*

Table 13.3 *Names, molecular formulae, structural formulae and boiling points for the first five alkenes*

Name	Molecular formula	Structural formula	Boiling point (°C)
ethene (ethylene)	C_2H_4	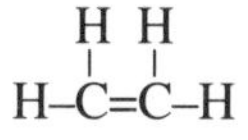	–104
propene (propylene)	C_3H_6	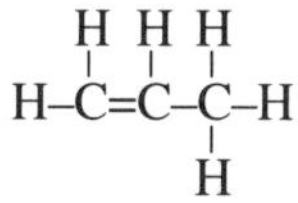	–48
butene (butylene)	C_4H_8	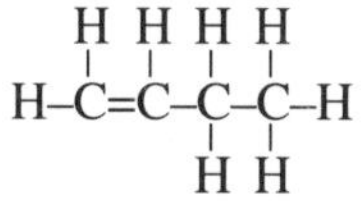	–6
pentene	C_5H_{10}	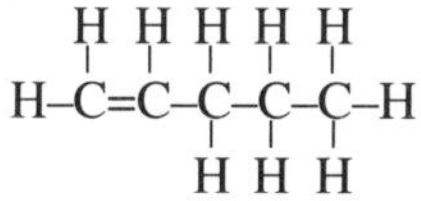	30
hexene	C_6H_{12}	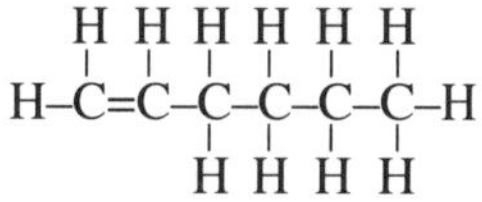	64

Note: The names in parentheses are the common names.

very likely to cause the same modification at other points. The result will be the formation of several slightly different compounds. If a pure substance is required, as is usually the case, it will have to be separated from all the others. In many instances the increase in difficulty and cost which this involves is prohibitive and it is better to choose another route to the desired compound.

The different parts of a pentene molecule are not the same as each other. The two carbon atoms which form the double bond are quite different to the other three. Because of this difference there are many reactions in which modifications can be made to the molecule at the position of its double bond without the same modifications occurring elsewhere in the molecule at the same time. These reactions, therefore, lead to the formation of mainly one new compound which is often obtained in large amount and which can be easily purified.

To illustrate this point let us consider two ways in which the substance vinyl chloride could be obtained.

Method A: Ethene is allowed to react with chlorine in the absence of light and under these conditions the chlorine molecules, Cl_2, add on to the ethene molecule converting it to the saturated compound, dichloroethane. Thus:

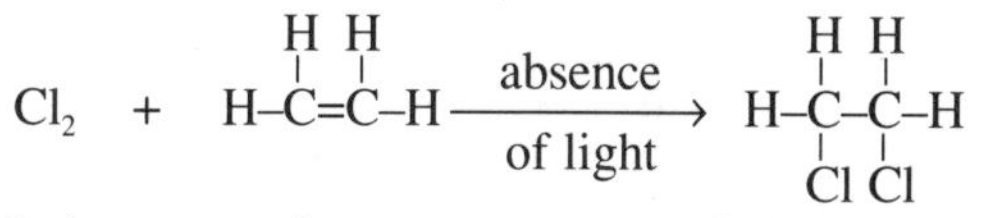

chlorine ethene dichloroethane

This type of reaction, in which two molecules simply add together, is called an **addition** reaction and the alkenes undergo addition reactions with many different substances. Once one chlorine molecule has added to the ethene no further reaction occurs because the dichloroethane is saturated and no additional atoms can attach to it. Consequently, dichloroethane is the only compound formed in any significant quantity. It can be easily purified and then, when it is heated in the presence of a catalyst, it forms vinyl chloride and hydrogen chloride.

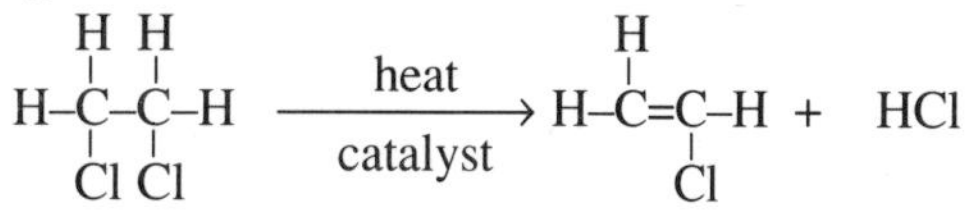

dichloroethane vinyl chloride hydrogen chloride

Hydrogen chloride and vinyl chloride are both gases but hydrogen chloride has a high solubility in water while the solubility of vinyl chloride is very low. This makes the two compounds easy to separate and allows vinyl chloride to be obtained as a pure substance.

Method B: Ethane will react with chlorine in the presence of sunlight. The products which form from this reaction correspond to a one-at-a-time replacement of the hydrogen atoms of ethane by chlorine atoms and this type of reaction is called a **substitution** reaction. Most of the reactions undergone by alkanes are of this type. In this particular case, each time a chlorine atom replaces a hydrogen atom in the ethane molecule, the hydrogen atom which has been replaced ends up joined to another chlorine atom in a molecule of hydrogen chloride. Unlike the addition of chlorine to ethene, this substitution reaction can take place several times in the same molecule. At first sight this seems fortunate because, in order to obtain dichloroethane from the reaction, we need two chlorine atoms to replace one hydrogen atom on each of the two carbon atoms present in the ethane molecule.

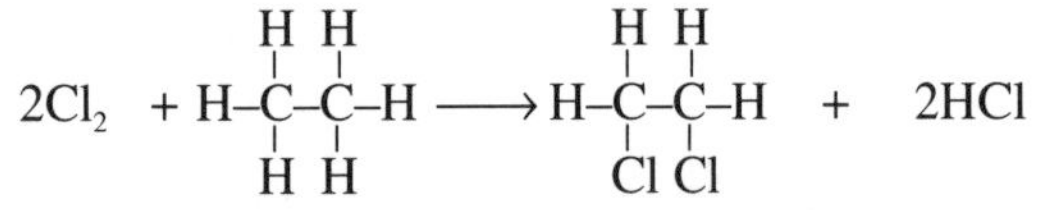

chlorine ethane dichloroethane hydrogen chloride

This reaction does occur, but there are many additional ways in which chlorine atoms can replace hydrogen atoms in ethane and so the compound which we need to make our vinyl chloride is just one component of a mixture containing many other similar compounds. This makes Method B quite impractical for the production of vinyl chloride and Method A is the one preferred.

Alkynes (Sometimes Called Acetylenes). The compounds in this family of hydrocarbons contain a carbon–carbon triple bond in their molecules. The simplest member is **ethyne**, C_2H_2. This compound is better known by its common name, **acetylene**, and it is used as a fuel in the high-temperature oxy-acetylene torch. The other members of the alkyne family correspond to the addition of $–CH_2–$ units to the ethyne molecule and the general formula for the alkynes is C_nH_{2n-2}. Some details about the first five members of the alkynes are presented in Table 13.4.

The alkynes resemble the alkenes in that they undergo a wide variety of reactions, most of which are addition reactions.

Aromatic Hydrocarbons. This is a diverse group of compounds with molecules which contain *sets of unsaturated carbon atoms arranged to form cyclic structures.* The compounds are called aromatic because

Table 13.4 *Names, molecular formulae, structural formulae and boiling points for the first five alkynes*

Name	Molecular formula	Structural formula	Boiling point (°C)
ethyne (acetylene)	C_2H_2	H–C≡C–H	–84
propyne	C_3H_4	H H–C≡C–C–H H	–23
butyne	C_4H_6	H H H–C≡C–C–C–H H H	8
pentyne	C_5H_8	H H H H–C≡C–C–C–C–H H H H	27
hexyne	C_6H_{10}	H H H H H–C≡C–C–C–C–C–H H H H H	40

Note: The name in parentheses is a common name.

many of the first examples discovered had distinctive odours. This name has stuck even though many of the compounds made available since those early days have turned out to have no odour at all. Today, the term aromatic simply signifies that a compound consists of molecules which include certain sets of unsaturated carbon atoms arranged in cyclic fashion. The most commonly encountered aromatic hydrocarbon is **benzene**, C_6H_6. The compound is an important industrial chemical and its annual world-wide production is measured in millions of tonnes. Benzene is known to be **carcinogenic** (cancer-causing) and strict controls apply to its use in industry.

The molecular structure of benzene is shown in Figure 13.6. In textbooks it is quite rare to encounter the molecular structure of benzene written out in full. Instead, it is usually represented in shorthand fashion by a hexagon containing either a circle or a set of three straight lines which occupy alternate sides of the hexagon. These shorthand representations have been included in Figure 13.6.

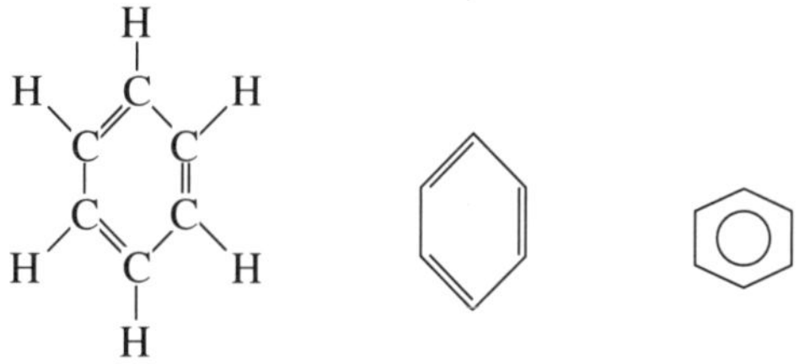

Figure 13.6 *Structural formula for benzene and its shorthand representations*

At first sight benzene might appear to be simply an alkene which contains three carbon–carbon double bonds. This is not so and the cyclic arrangement of the three double bonds is a very stable one which gives benzene properties that are quite different from those of the alkenes. In particular, benzene does not participate readily in addition reactions. The reason is that addition reactions necessarily involve loss of at least one of these three carbon–carbon double bonds of benzene and, therefore, loss of its stability. Instead, benzene undergoes substitution reactions more readily because these allow benzene to retain the stable arrangement of three carbon–carbon double bonds.

As an illustration of the difference in behaviour between benzene and the alkenes we can compare the behaviour of benzene with that of another compound, **cyclohexene**, when each is mixed with chlorine under different conditions. Cyclohexene has the molecular formula C_6H_{10} and its structural formula is given in Figure 13.7. Like benzene, it contains a cyclic arrangement of six carbon atoms but only one carbon–carbon double bond instead of three. The prefix 'cyclo' in the name of cyclohexene simply indicates that the double bond is part of a system of six carbon atoms organised as a cyclic structure.

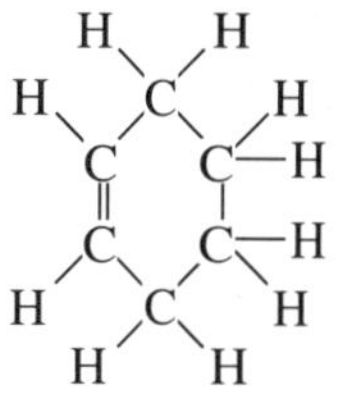

Figure 13.7 *Structural formula for cyclohexene*

If Chlorine is bubbled into a solution containing cyclohexene the two substances react in an addition reaction and form dichlorocyclohexane.

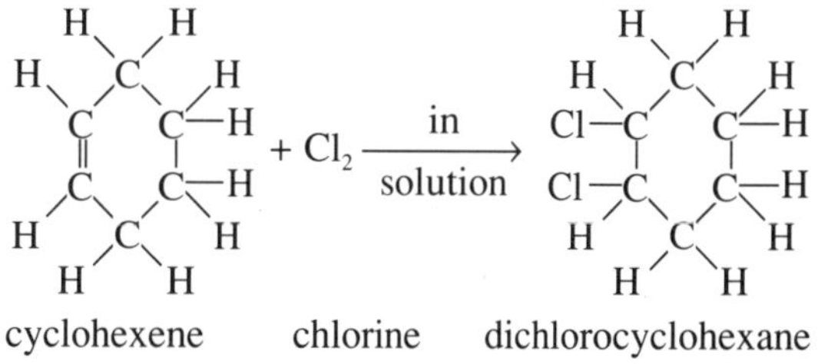

Under the same conditions there is no reaction between chlorine and benzene. However, if benzene is heated with chlorine at about 60 °C in the presence of an iron catalyst it undergoes a substitution reaction to form chlorobenzene. Under these conditions the main reaction undergone by cyclohexene is still the addition reaction outlined above.

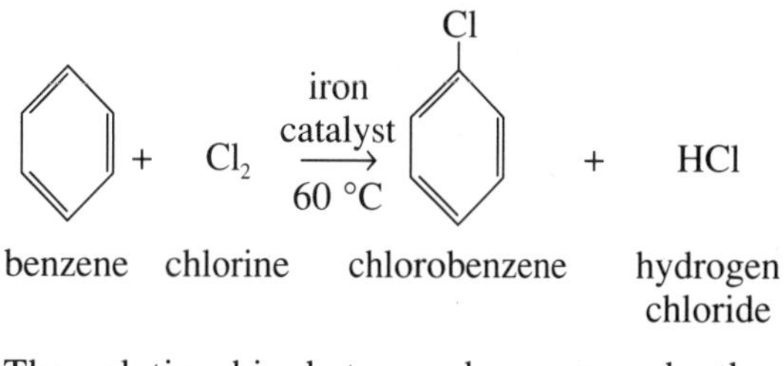

The relationship between benzene and other aromatic hydrocarbons is not as straightforward as that which exists between the members of the other three classes of hydrocarbons that we have considered.

An aromatic hydrocarbon related to benzene may consist of molecules which have a set of saturated carbon atoms attached to a single benzene ring, or it may consist of molecules in which benzene rings are joined to each other along one edge (benzene rings joined in this way are said to be **fused** together). Some examples are presented in Table 13.5.

Table 13.5 *Names, molecular formulae, structural formulae and boiling points for some aromatic hydrocarbons*

Name	Molecular formula	Structural formula	Boiling point (°C)
benzene	C_6H_6	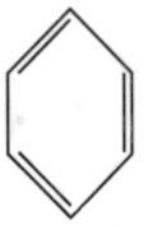	80
methylbenzene (toluene)	C_7H_8	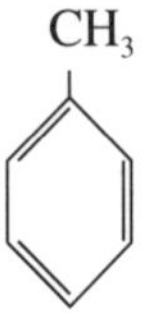	111
ethylbenzene	C_8H_{10}	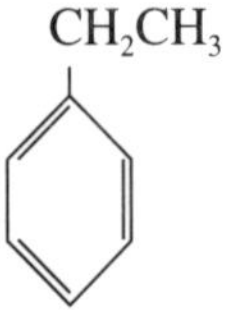	136
naphthalene	$C_{10}H_8$	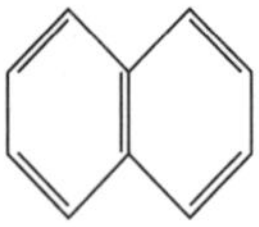	218
benzopyrene	$C_{20}H_{12}$	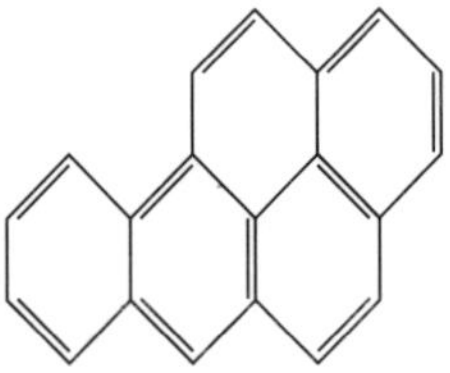	177*

* Melting point.
Note: The name in parentheses is a common name.

Naphthalene and benzopyrene are examples of **polycyclic aromatic hydrocarbons** (PAHs). Naphthalene is found in the form of mothballs in many homes. This would suggest that it is harmless to humans but there are some people for whom naphthalene is very toxic. These are people who have an hereditary deficiency of the enzyme **glucose-6-phosphate dehydrogenase** (see Section 13.8.5 for discussion of enzymes and their functions). This deficiency occurs with greater frequency in some populations than in others and people from the Mediterranean countries are at an increased risk.

The absence of glucose-6-phosphate dehydrogenase allows naphthalene to cause the destruction of red blood cells (haemolysis). This releases haemoglobin which precipitates from the plasma and blocks the renal capillaries. At the same time, serious neurological damage usually occurs. These toxic effects of naphthalene may occur following ingestion or inhalation of the substance. Blankets which have been stored in contact with naphthalene and then used without adequate airing have caused the deaths of many young children and even the occasional adult.

Benzopyrene is a proven and powerful carcinogen. It is prone to form whenever organic material is burned and it is present in all kinds of soot and smoke. It has been detected in cigarette smoke, in car exhaust fumes and in charcoal-cooked steak. Benzopyrene is now known to be the causative agent in the first clearly identified occupational cancer. This was cancer of the scrotum observed in London chimney sweeps more than 200 years ago by the surgeon Percivall Pott. These unfortunate children spent their short lives climbing through chimneys and getting covered in soot which remained in permanent contact with their bodies. The soot contained benzopyrene and its prolonged close contact with the scrotum produced cancer in many chimney sweeps. The disease usually appeared at puberty and death came soon after.

13.3.2 *Functional Groups*

In the previous section we saw that the alkenes and alkynes behave quite differently to the alkanes even though all three classes of compound are hydrocarbons. In particular, they undergo addition reactions whereas the alkanes cannot. The ability of the alkenes and alkynes to undergo addition reactions is due to the presence in their molecules of carbon–carbon double bonds and carbon–carbon triple bonds respectively. The carbon atoms involved in these bonds are unsaturated and so other atoms are able to attach to them. In any alkane molecule all the carbon atoms are saturated and cannot attach to additional atoms unless one of the hydrogen atoms already present in the molecule is removed first.

In other words, the difference in behaviour of these families of organic compounds can be attributed to particular collections of atoms within their molecules. As long as a molecule contains a carbon–carbon double bond its chemical behaviour will closely resemble that of all other molecules in which the same system is present. Likewise, all molecules which contain a carbon–carbon triple bond will display similar chemical behaviour. This relationship between chemical behaviour and molecular structure is observed with all families of organic compounds and is described by the two equivalent terms **characteristic group** and **functional group**. *A functional group or characteristic group is a group of atoms within an organic molecule which is responsible for most of its chemical and physical properties.* This idea of the functional group is very useful in understanding the behaviour of organic compounds.

It is usual to regard the alkanes as not containing a functional group and this is consistent with the fact that they display very little chemical behaviour which is not also displayed by many other families. In other words they display very little characteristic behaviour. For example, the alkanes burn readily in air to form carbon dioxide and water, but so do most other families of organic compounds; the alkanes are good solvents for non-polar substances, but so are many other families and so on. However, every other family of organic compounds has its own functional group and as we consider some of these other families we shall, in each case, specify its functional group.

13.3.3 *Radicals*

The term radical is used to describe the part(s) of an organic molecule other than the functional group. By way of illustration let us take a close look at the structural formulae of pentene and pentyne (Figure 13.8). In Figure 13.8 the functional group in each of the molecules of pentene and pentyne has been enclosed in a box and named. What remains of each molecule is the group of atoms C_3H_7. This is referred to as the **radical portion** of the molecule and in this particular case the radical is given the name **propyl radical**. This name is derived from propane which is the name for the alkane containing the same number of carbon atoms as the radical. The relationship between propane molecules and propyl radicals is that the radicals correspond to propane molecules which have lost one hydrogen atom (Figure 13.9).

Looking at Figure 13.9 and the structural formulae for the alkanes presented in Table 13.2, you will see that there is a radical of this type corresponding to every member of the alkane family. These radicals are known collectively as **alkyl radicals** and they are defined as **alkane molecules minus one hydrogen atom**. The name for an alkyl radical is obtained by replacing the ending 'ane' in the name of the corresponding alkane with the ending 'yl'.

Exercise 13.1
What are the names for the alkyl radicals corresponding to the last two alkanes listed in Table 13.2?

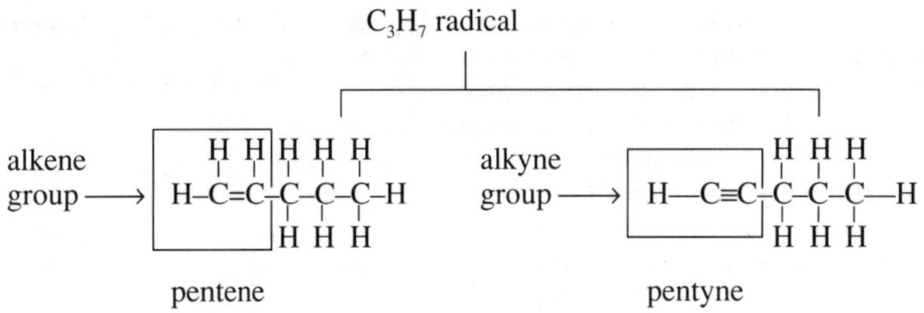

Figure 13.8 *Structural formulae for pentene and pentyne*

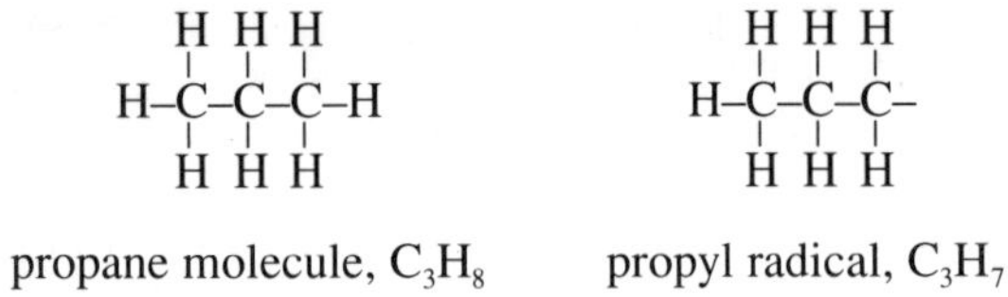

Figure 13.9 *Comparison of the propane molecule and the propyl radical*

As the alkyl radical attached to the alkene, or any other functional group, changes from methyl, to ethyl, to propyl and so on, there is virtually no effect on the chemical properties of the substances. Only small changes in physical properties such as melting point and boiling point occur.

The small effect which radicals have on the behaviour of organic compounds might make you wonder why they are called radicals. After all, in ordinary language, the term radical has about it the sense of drama, excitement, being spectacularly different and so on. Well, take a look back at the structural formula for the propyl radical which is presented in Figure 13.9. You will notice that one carbon atom in the propyl radical is only participating in three bonds rather than the four which is normal for carbon, and so one of the four electrons which it normally uses for bonding to other atoms is not being used for this purpose. Because of this, propyl radicals (and all other alkyl radicals) are inherently unstable and they cannot exist in significant numbers for very long. If there were large numbers of propyl radicals

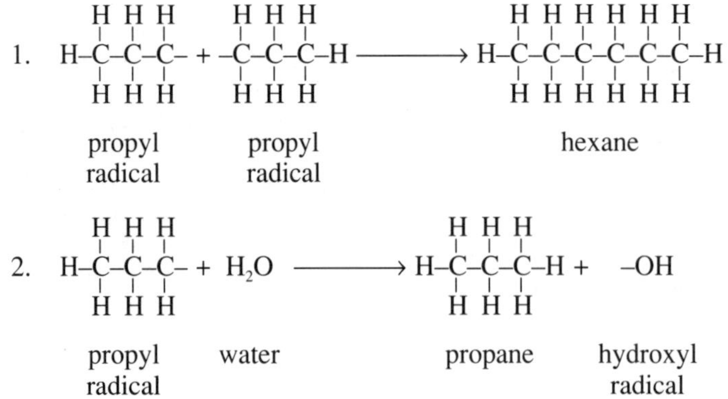

Figure 13.10 *Reactions which destroy alkyl radicals. The hydroxyl radical formed in reaction 2 goes on to react with some other particle in its vicinity*

which came into existence in the same place then they would quickly be destroyed by combination with each other or with other molecules in their vicinity. Two examples of these radical-destroying reactions are presented in Figure 13.10.

In this way, chemical radicals are forced to conform to the rules which are obeyed by most other groups of atoms. They can exist as independent entities for a brief time but are inevitably destroyed by themselves and their surroundings. This is the fate which awaits all radicals and it provides a connection between use of the term radical in ordinary language and its use in chemical language.

There is a radical derived from the benzene molecule by the loss of one hydrogen atom and it is given the name **phenyl radical**. You might have expected it to have the name **benzyl radical** but this name is used for a different aromatic radical in which there is a $-CH_2-$ group attached to the benzene ring. Structural formulae for these two radicals are presented in Figure 13.11.

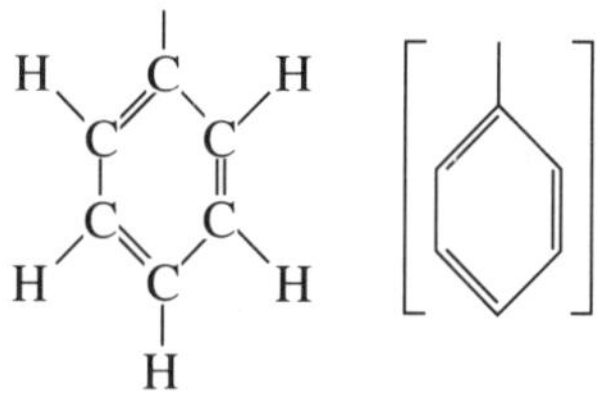

phenyl radical

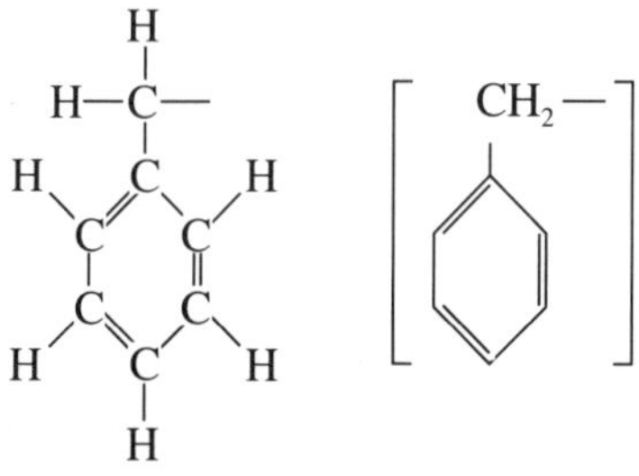

benzyl radical

Figure 13.11 *Structural formulae and their shorthand representations for phenyl and benzyl radicals*

13.4 Systematic Names for Organic Compounds

In this section we provide only a very brief outline of the method which is used to name organic compounds and some quite important aspects of the method are ignored. However, as we consider other families of organic compounds in later sections, you will see that the outline given is sufficient to allow the successful interpretation of the names for most of the compounds which we encounter.

You have probably noticed that the names for the alkanes, alkenes and alkynes are all quite similar. For the members of each family, the first part of the name refers to the length of the carbon chain present in molecules of the compound. Thus, the alkane with four carbon atoms is **butane**, the alkene with four carbon atoms is **butene** and the alkyne with four carbon atoms is **butyne**. The second part of the name distinguishes each family from the others. Thus, all the alkanes have names which end in 'ane', all the alkenes have names which end in 'ene' and all the alkynes have names which end in 'yne'. You will see this pattern maintained as we deal with other families of organic compound which are not hydrocarbons but which bear a close structural relationship to the alkanes. These families always have names in which the first part is derived from the name of the alkane which has the same number of carbon atoms. The ending of the name is determined by the functional group which is present.

In Chapter 3, 'Learning to Speak Chemistry', we saw that numbers played a prominent role in the systems used to name some inorganic compounds. For example, the compound of formula $FeCl_2$ was named iron(II) chloride. So far, in our naming of organic compounds, we have not used numbers at all, but they are very necessary. To demonstrate this we need only look at the two structural formulae in Figure 13.12. Both of these structural formulae show five carbon atoms joined in a chain and both show that two of the carbon atoms in the chain are joined by a double bond. Thus each formula represents an alkene in which there are five

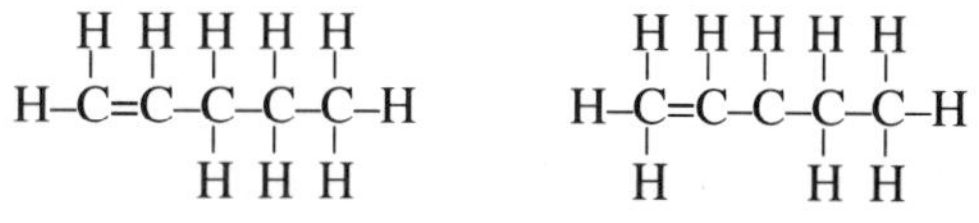

Figure 13.12 *Structural formulae for two pentene molecules*

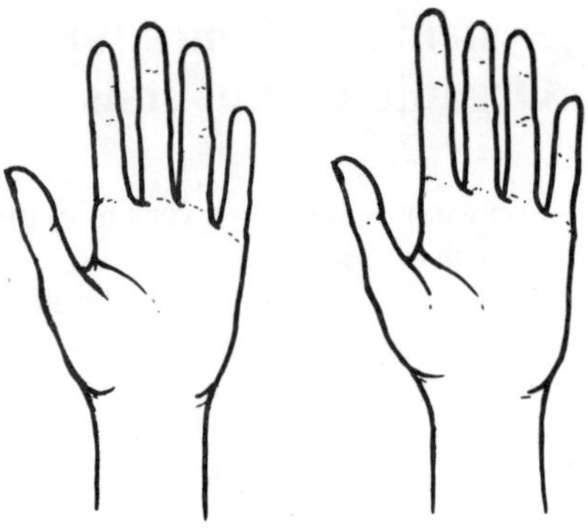

Figure 13.13 *Left hands with the fingers occupying different positions*

carbon atoms present and so could be called pentene. However, the two molecules which are represented in Figure 13.12 are not identical because their double bonds occupy different positions in the carbon chain. They differ from each other in much the same way as the two left hands which have been drawn in Figure 13.13 differ from one another.

The two pentenes of Figure 13.12 are distinguished from each other using numbers written before their names as follows:

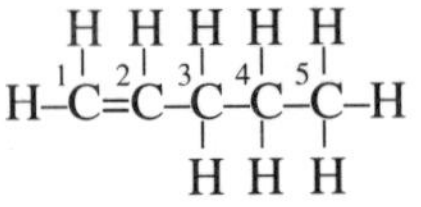
1-pentene

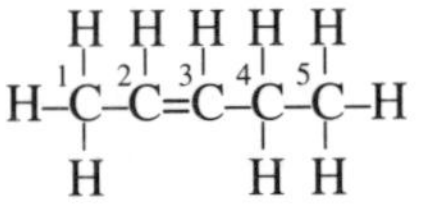
2-pentene

These numbers are obtained by counting along the carbon chain from the end closer to the alkene functional group. The number appearing in the name is the number of the first carbon atom encountered which is part of the functional group. The same approach is used to specify the location of radicals within organic molecules. The name of the radical and its accompanying number are written at the front of the name for the compound. This is illustrated for two compounds in Figure 13.14.

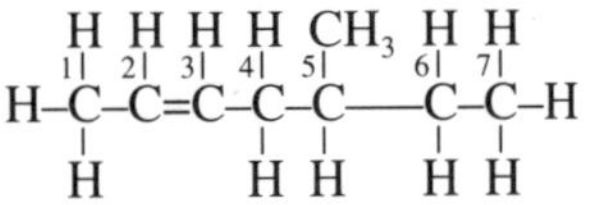
5-methyl-2-heptene

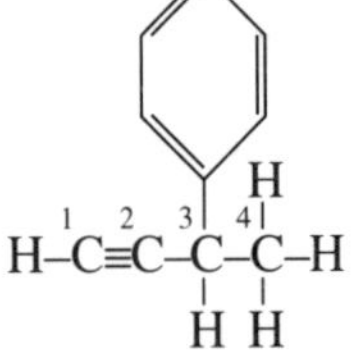
3-phenyl-1-butyne

Figure 13.14 *Structural formulae and systematic names for two hydrocarbons containing radicals attached to the chain of carbon atoms which includes the functional group*

Numbers are also used in the naming of aromatic compounds whenever there is more than one radical or functional group attached to the aromatic ring. These numbers specify the positions which the groups occupy relative to one another. Two examples of the use of numbers in the naming of aromatic compounds are given in Figure 13.15. The benzene ring is always numbered in the direction which gives numbers with smaller values.

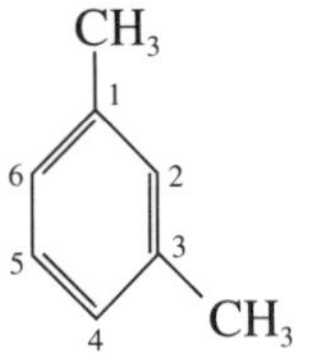
1,3-dimethylbenzene

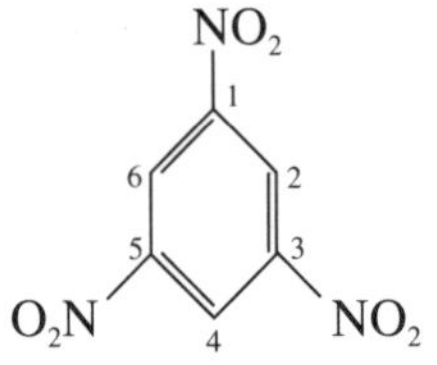
1,3,5-trinitrobenzene

Figure 13.15 *Structural formulae and systematic names for two aromatic compounds*

To summarise, we can say that the systematic name for an organic compound will generally consist of at least a **root** and a **suffix**. In addition, it may contain one or more prefixes. The root portion of the name is derived from the name of an alkane or of some cyclic structure such as benzene. The suffix portion of the name corresponds to a functional group present in the molecule, and the prefixes to radicals or other functional groups which are also present. The locations of radicals and functional groups within an organic molecule are shown by the use of numbers in association with their names.

13.5 Representation of Complex Organic Molecules

In the previous section, use was made of a shorthand method for the representation of the benzene molecule. This was a line diagram containing no atomic symbols. The diagram was a hexagon which had alternate single and double lines as its sides. Use of this diagram, or something similar to it, is much more convenient than use of the full structural formula, and in most textbooks you will find the diagram used almost exclusively. Benzene is by no means the only common organic compound having a structural formula which is sufficiently complex to warrant its representation in a shorthand, diagrammatic fashion. As a matter of fact, such representations are more the rule than the exception and they are used in all texts where the structural formulae of organic molecules are considered to be important.

Structural formulae for organic molecules are simplified by omitting the symbols for some of the carbon and hydrogen atoms present in the molecule. This is hardly surprising because carbon and hydrogen atoms often make up a large majority of all the atoms present in an organic molecule. Consequently, their omission offers the greatest opportunity for reducing the complexity of the structure. All the diagrams used in this text to represent organic molecules can be interpreted fully in terms of the following rules.

1. Carbon atoms are located at all positions in the diagram where a line ends or changes direction.
2. If a molecule contains atoms other than carbon or hydrogen their locations are shown by writing in the symbol for the atom at the appropriate location in the diagram.
3. If a carbon atom is not shown directly in the diagram any hydrogen atoms attached to it may also be omitted. The number of hydrogen atoms located at one of these positions is simply the number which must be located there in order to ensure that the carbon atom is participating in four covalent bonds as carbon atoms always do.

In Figure 13.16 a shorthand representation of the structural formula for penicillin is shown and compared with the full structural formula. If you compare each position in the full formula with the corresponding position in the shorthand formula you will see that the rules set out above do apply. You should also be able to see that the nitrogen, oxygen and sulphur atoms present in the molecule all form the numbers of covalent bonds expected from their positions in the Periodic Table.

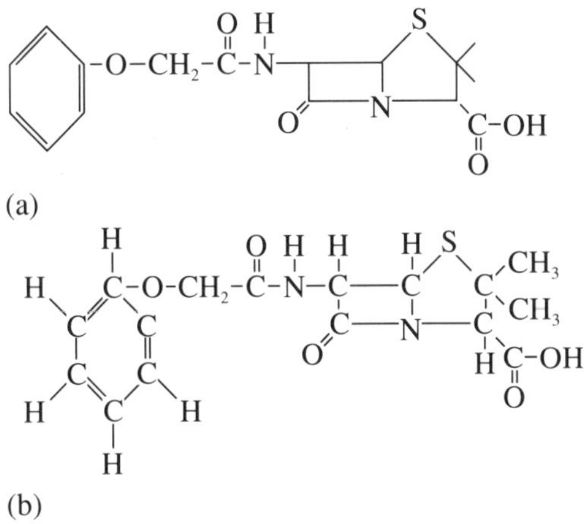

Figure 13.16 *Representations of the structural formula of penicillin: (a) shorthand structural formula; (b) full structural formula*

13.5.1 *The Shapes of Organic Molecules*

The representations of organic molecules which we have so far used can easily create some false impressions about their shapes. For example, in Table 13.2 the methane molecule is represented as:

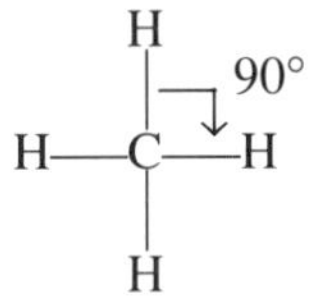

This creates the impression that the methane molecule has a planar (two-dimensional) shape in which the carbon atom is at the centre of a square with one hydrogen atom at each corner. On paper the angle between adjacent carbon–hydrogen bonds is 90°. In fact, the methane molecule is tetrahedral (three-dimensional) in shape. The carbon atom is at the centre of the tetrahedron, there is one hydrogen atom at each corner and the angle between all carbon–hydrogen bonds is about 109°. The diagram in Figure 13.17 is a more faithful representation of the methane molecule.

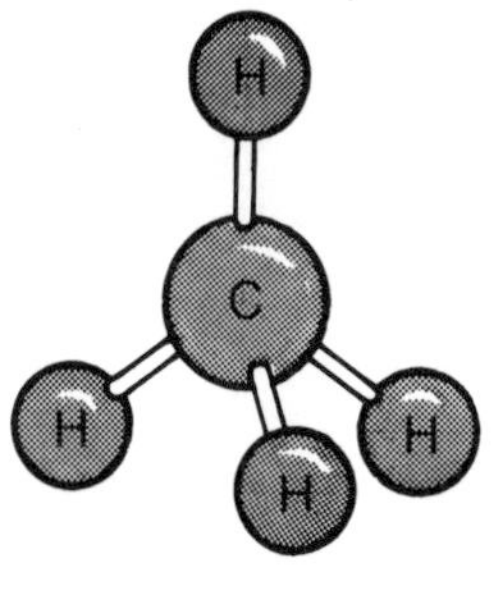

Figure 13.17 *A representation of the three-dimensional shape of the methane molecule*

The structural formulae for propane and all the compounds listed below it in Table 13.2 also create the false impression that the carbon atoms in the corresponding molecules lie along a straight line. They do not. The angle between adjacent carbon–carbon bonds in all these molecules is 109° and so the carbon atoms lie along a zig-zag line. This is shown in Figure 13.18.

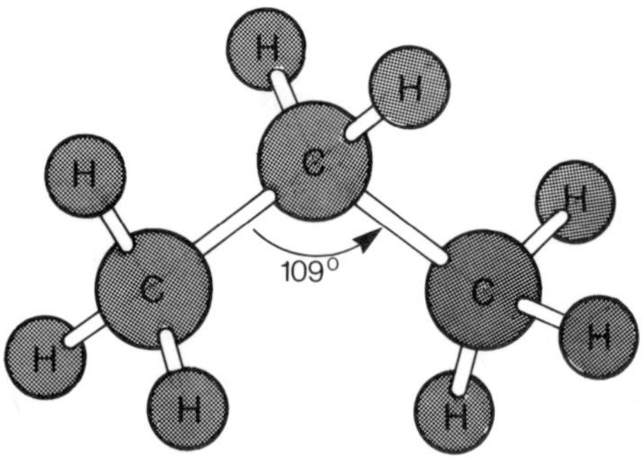

Figure 13.18 *Zig-zag arrangement of carbon atoms in an organic molecule*

Look at the two structural formulae written in Figure 13.19. On paper they are different, but do they represent different molecules? The answer is no. Both structural formulae in Figure 13.19 represent a molecule of butane. The reason for this is that every carbon atom in a simple chain of carbon atoms held together by single bonds is constantly rotating as illustrated in Figure 13.20.

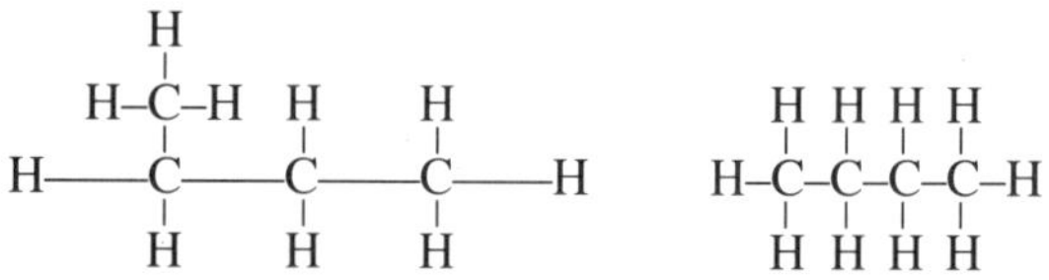

Figure 13.19

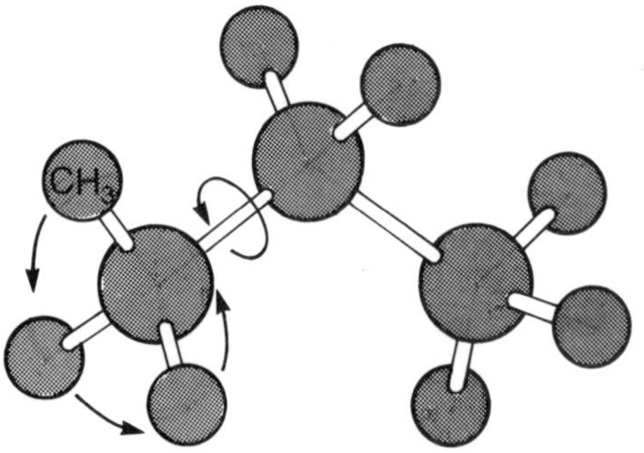

Figure 13.20 *Rotation around carbon–carbon single bonds*

As a result of the rotation around carbon atoms held together by single bonds, every atom attached directly to each carbon passes through a complete circle many times every second. This makes all the different positions which they adopt equivalent and structural formulae which show the atoms occupying positions which differ only in this way are also equivalent. The main exception to this occurs with compounds known as optical isomers (see Section 13.8.2).

Rotation around bonds does not occur when the bond is a double bond or when it is part of a ring structure. In these situations structural formulae which differ from each other in much the same way as the structural formulae of Figure 13.19 differ from each other may actually represent different substances. This is the case for the two structural formulae drawn in Figure 13.21.

In Figure 13.21 the structural formulae (a) and (b) represent different substances having properties which are different in at least some respects. The carbon–carbon double bond and the atoms attached directly to it all lie in the one plane and the structural formulae have been drawn so that this plane is perpendicular to the plane of the paper. In (a) the two hydrogen atoms both project out of the plane of the paper towards you while in (b) one of them projects towards you and one projects away from you. There is no free rotation around the carbon–carbon double bond, and in each molecule these two hydrogen atoms are 'stuck' permanently in these different orientations. The substance represented by (a) is known as **oleic acid** and is an important component of fat.

The molecules represented by the two formulae in Figure 13.21 are said to be **stereoisomers**. This is the name given to molecules which contain the same set of atoms joined in the same sequence but having permanently different arrangements in space. There are several different types of stereoisomerism and that which arises because there is no free rotation around carbon–carbon double bonds is called **geometrical isomerism**. Geometrical isomers are often distinguished from one another using the prefixes **cis** and **trans**. The isomer is designated 'cis' if it has two identical atoms or groups of atoms projecting towards the same side of the double bond and 'trans' if they

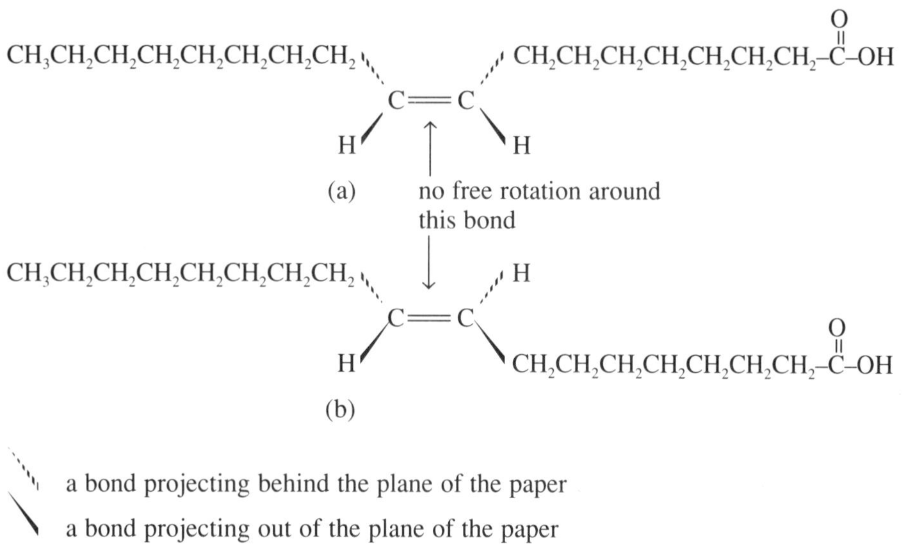

Figure 13.21

project towards opposite sides of the double bond. Thus, oleic acid is a cis isomer.

13.6 More Families of Organic Compounds

13.6.1 *Alcohols*

These are organic compounds which contain the –OH group of atoms joined to an alkyl radical. The –OH group is the functional group for the alcohol family and it is referred to as the **alcohol group** or, sometimes, as the **hydroxy group**. Several members of the alcohol family are listed in Table 13.6.

From Table 13.6 you can see that systematic names for alcohols are obtained, as the names for alkenes and alkynes are, by modifying the name of the alkane which contains the same number of carbon atoms. In this case the ‘e’ on the end of the name of the alkane is removed and replaced by ‘ol’. The position which the alcohol group occupies within the molecule is specified by using numbers in much the same way as they were used in the names for alkenes and alkynes. The chain of carbon atoms in the molecule is numbered starting from the end closer to the alcohol group. The number of the carbon atom to which the alcohol group is attached is written immediately before the name. Whenever the name of an organic compound has the ending ‘ol’ it is bound to be an alcohol. For example, the much talked about compound **cholesterol** is an alcohol although the radical attached to its alcohol functional group is not a simple alkyl radical (see Figure 13.22).

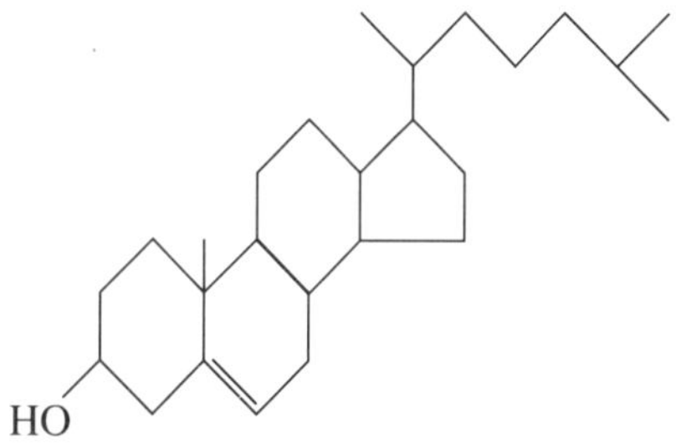

Figure 13.22 *Structural formula for cholesterol*

All the alcohols listed in Table 13.6 are frequently referred to by their common names. This is due to the fact that the compounds have been used widely for many years and so have common names which are firmly entrenched.

You will notice that the boiling points of the alcohols display a similar trend to those displayed by the alkanes, alkenes and alkynes, but the actual boiling point of each alcohol is much higher than that of the simple hydrocarbon which contains the same number of carbon

Table 13.6 *Names, structural formulae, boiling points and solubilities in water for a series of simple alcohols*

Name	Structural formula	Boiling point (°C)	Solubility (% w/w)
methanol (methyl alcohol)	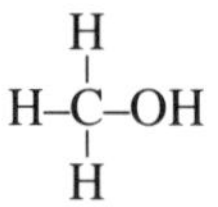	65	∞
ethanol (ethyl alcohol)	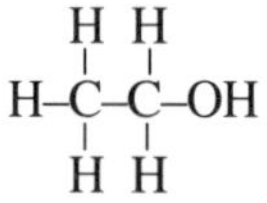	78	∞
1- propanol (propyl alcohol)	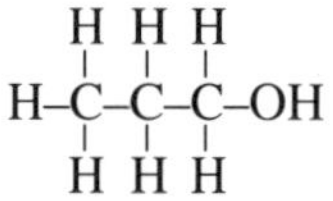	97	∞
2-propanol (isopropanol)	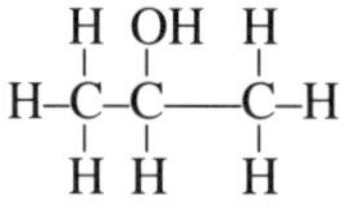	82	∞
1-butanol (butyl alcohol)	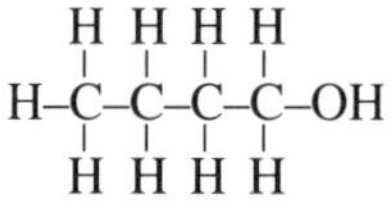	117	8
1-pentanol (pentyl alcohol)	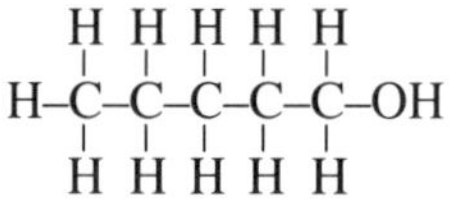	138	2.3

Notes: 1. The names in parentheses are common names.
2. The symbol ∞ means infinity and is used here to signify that the alcohol mixes completely with water.

atoms. Thus, the boiling point of ethanol is 78 °C while the boiling points for ethane, ethene and ethyne are –88, –105 and –84 °C respectively. Alcohols owe their relatively high boiling points to hydrogen bonding. This occurs between the –OH groups of different alcohol molecules in much the same way as it occurs between different water molecules (see Figure 13.23).

The first few members of the alcohol family have high solubilities in water and this is also due to the ability of alcohol molecules to participate in hydrogen bond formation. However, as the size of the alkyl radical in the alcohol molecule increases, the compound's solubility in water decreases. This is due to the low polarity of carbon–carbon and carbon–hydrogen bonds which are present in alkyl radicals. The low polarity of these bonds prevents the alkyl radical portion of the alcohol molecule from forming bonds with the polar water molecules among which they must become dispersed if the alcohol is to dissolve.

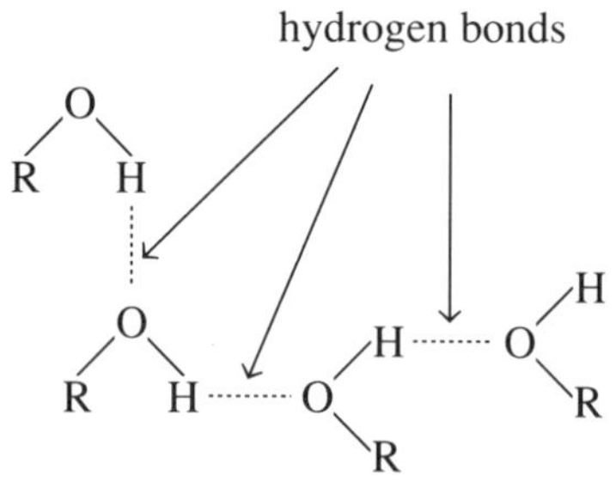

Figure 13.23 *Hydrogen bonds acting between alcohol molecules. R stands for any radical*

As long as the radical is small, then the alcohol group's ability to form hydrogen bonds with water molecules is sufficient to take the entire molecule into solution. Eventually, however, the increasing size of the radical overwhelms this ability and the compound is prevented from dissolving to any significant extent. Alcohols which have radicals containing more than about eight carbon atoms usually have very low solubilities in water.

13.6.2 *Clinical Uses for Specific Alcohols*

Ethanol. This alcohol is a component of **elixirs**, a use reflecting its ability to dissolve compounds which are not readily soluble in water. Ethanol is also a central nervous system depressant and clinical use is made of this by employing alcoholic beverages to cause sedation and sleep. The compound is sometimes administered intravenously for preoperative or postoperative sedation in cases where alternative methods of sedation cannot be employed or are ineffective.

Ethanol is also used externally. Its good solvent properties make it suitable for washing the skin when it is contaminated with various toxic chemicals. For example, it is effective in removing the chemical responsible for the effects of ivy poisoning. It is also effective in removing phenol from the skin. This compound (phenol) if left in contact with the skin will produce severe chemical burns. Aqueous solutions of ethanol are used for a number of different purposes. At a concentration of 25% (v/v) it is used to bathe the skin for the purpose of cooling. Solutions in the concentration range 60–90% (v/v) have useful germicidal properties and so are used as disinfectants on the skin and on clinical instruments.

2-Propanol. This alcohol is also called **isopropyl alcohol** and **rubbing alcohol**. This latter name came into use because a solution of 2-propanol (70% w/v in water) was once used as a rubbing agent. When rubbed into the skin it disinfects and cools the region to which it has been applied. It also assists in keeping the skin dry and causes contraction of the underlying tissues. The cooling effect of rubbing alcohol makes it effective in fever reduction and its other effects assist in the prevention of bed-sores. However, 2-propanol is no longer used as a rubbing agent, because in some cases the harm done to damaged tissue by the mechanical action of rubbing it into the skin outweighs any beneficial effects.

A mixture of 2-propanol and acetic acid is used for the treatment of 'swimmer's ear', an inflammation of the ear canal caused by retention of water in the canal and the associated growth of microorganisms there. The alcohol acts as a drying agent and germicide. The acid increases the acidity of the environment in the ear canal and this combination of actions severely inhibits the growth of most of the microorganisms involved in the condition.

Glycerol. This alcohol, often called **glycerine**, is different from the others we have considered in that it contains three alcohol functional groups in the one molecule. Glycerol is completely soluble in water and has the very high boiling point of 290 °C. Both of these properties are consistent with the presence of three alcohol groups in the glycerol molecule and its consequent capacity to form hydrogen bonds with itself and with water. Glycerol's structural formula is shown in Figure 13.24.

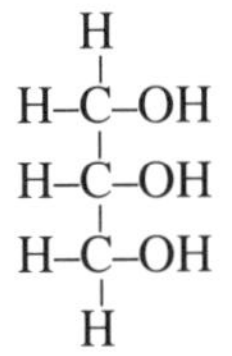

Figure 13.24 *Structural formula for glycerol*

Glycerol is present in many clinical preparations and its widespread use is due to a combination of useful properties which it possesses. These include:

1. having a sweet taste;
2. having a low toxicity;
3. being a good **emollient** (a substance which softens the skin or soothes some irritated internal surface of the body);
4. being a good solvent;
5. being hygroscopic, which means that it absorbs water from the atmosphere.

The combination of sweet taste, low toxicity and being a good solvent makes glycerol a useful ingredient for many medications which must be taken orally. Its hygroscopic and emollient properties make it suitable for the preparation of skin lotions and suppositories.

Phenol. In molecules of this compound the alcohol functional group is attached directly to a benzene ring. The structural formula for phenol is presented in Figure 13.25.

Phenol has a high toxicity and in concentrated form is capable of producing severe burns to the skin. Not surprisingly, it has few clinical uses. It deserves a mention though because it is an effective germicide and under the name 'carbolic acid' it was the original surgical antiseptic used by Joseph Lister in 1867 (see Figure 13.26). Today its use as a germicide is restricted mainly to dilute solutions in water which are sold as household cleaning fluids.

It is quite common to consider phenol as the simplest member of a distinct family of alcohols called the **phenols**. All members of this family have at least one alcohol functional group attached directly to a benzene ring. The reason for considering this set of compounds as a family, distinct from other alcohols, is that it exhibits quite a few properties which the other alcohols do not. For example, phenols are more acidic than ordinary alcohols; phenols react with solutions of iron(III) chloride and produce characteristic colours whereas the simple alcohols do not. These differences in behaviour are due to the fact that the alcohol functional group is attached directly to the benzene ring. Thus the alcohol, **benzyl alcohol** (Figure 13.27), in which a benzene ring is present but not attached directly to the alcohol functional group, behaves as a simple alcohol and not as a phenol. Because the differences in behaviour make it possible to distinguish readily between a phenol and a simple alcohol it is sensible to consider the two groups of compounds as separate families even though each contains the alcohol functional group.

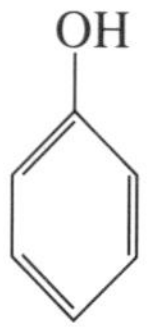

Figure 13.25 *Structural formula for phenol*

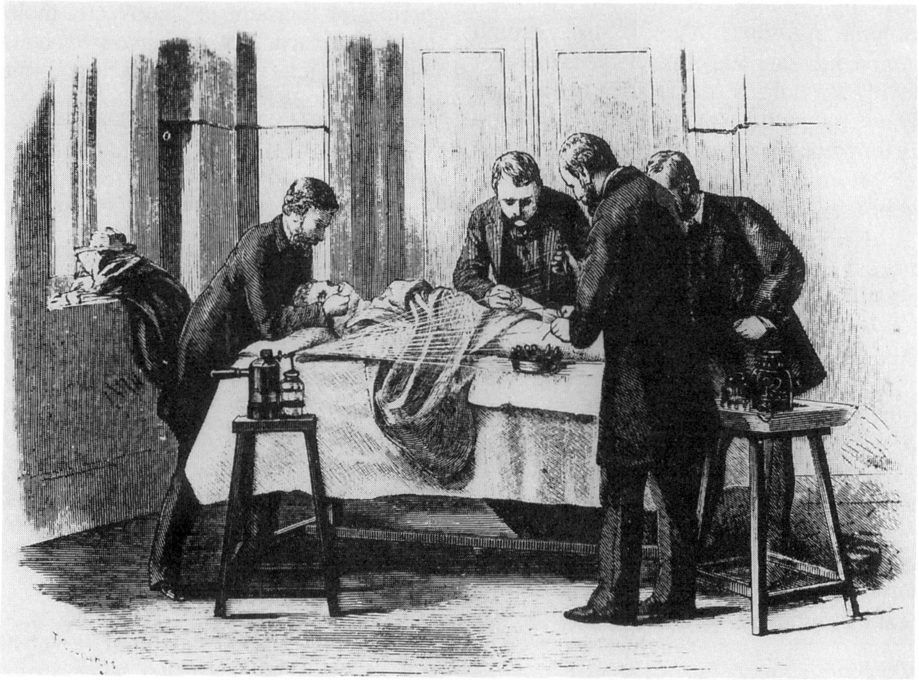

Figure 13.26 *Use of phenol (carbolic acid) as a surgical antiseptic*

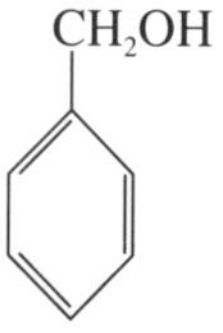

Figure 13.27 *Structural formula for benzyl alcohol*

13.6.3 *Ethers*

The functional group for the ether family is –O– and in all ether molecules this oxygen atom has two alkyl radicals joined to it. An ether is named by stating the word 'ether' after the names of the alkyl radicals which are present in its molecules. If the two radicals are identical then the prefix 'di' is used to indicate this. However, some writers will omit this prefix and simply use the name for the radical, leaving their readers to assume that the ether contains two radicals having the same identity.

The boiling points and solubilities in water of the simple ethers are much lower than those of the corresponding alcohols (see Table 13.7). This is due to the absence of the –OH group from their molecules and their reduced ability to exert forces of attraction on each other or on water molecules.

Table 13.7 *Names, structural formulae, boiling points and solubilities in water for three ethers*

Structural formula	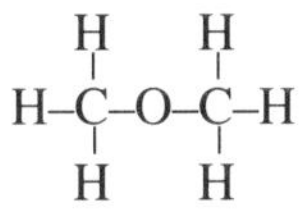	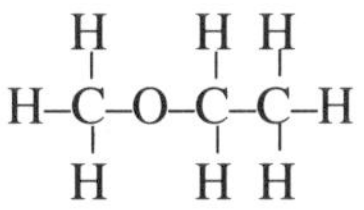	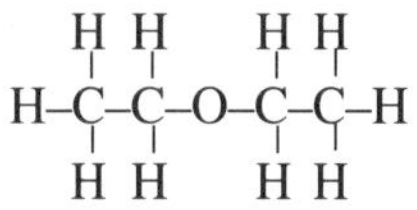
Systematic name	dimethyl ether	ethyl methyl ether	diethyl ether
Common name	—	—	ether
Boiling point (°C)	–24	11	35
Solubility in water (% w/w)	7	11	8

13.6.4 *Clinical Uses for Ethers*

The best known example of a clinically useful ether is **diethyl ether** which has made a great contribution to the relief of human suffering through its use as an anaesthetic. It was the first chemical anaesthetic and its initial use was in the United States about the middle of the nineteenth century. At first its use was restricted to dental surgery where its main benefit was the avoidance of pain. It soon became widely used for general surgery where it extended the range of surgical procedures which could be attempted, and allowed improvements in many of those already being carried out. Ether continues in use even today, although it has now been largely replaced by other anaesthetic agents.

Diethyl ether is easy to administer, is capable of producing a very deep anaesthesia and it is very safe in the sense that there is a large gap between the dose needed to produce anaesthesia and the fatal dose. These advantages have, until recently, far outweighed some disadvantages, which include flammability and nauseous after-effect. The contribution to human welfare made by diethyl ether and other chemical anaesthetics is described in more detail in Chapter 15, 'Commercial Chemicals and Human Health'.

Diethyl ether also finds some use as a component of expectorant coughing mixtures. These are used to promote the coughing up and spitting out of material from the respiratory tract.

13.6.5 *Aldehydes, Ketones and Carboxylic Acids*

We shall consider these three families together because the functional group of each includes the pair of atoms C , O joined by a double covalent bond (–C=O). This pair of atoms is often called the **carbonyl group**. The three families differ from each other in the nature of the two groups of atoms which are attached to the carbon atom of the carbonyl group.

Aldehydes. Members of this family have an alkyl radical and a hydrogen atom attached to the carbonyl group. The one exception to this is the first member of the family which simply has two hydrogen atoms attached. The aldehyde functional group is the group of atoms –C(H)=O. Aldehydes are named by taking the name of the alkane with the same number of carbon atoms, removing the 'e' and replacing it by 'al'. The aldehyde group must always be located at the end of a carbon chain and so it is never necessary to use numbers to specify its position within a molecule. The first three aldehydes are represented in Table 13.8.

Ketones. Members of this family have two alkyl radicals attached to the carbonyl group. The compounds are named by replacing the 'e' ending of the name of the corresponding alkane by 'one'. The functional group in ketones is simply the carbonyl group itself, and its location within the molecule is specified using numbers in the usual way. However, it does not become necessary to use numbers to specify the position of the ketone group until there are at least five carbon atoms in the chain containing it. Three ketones are represented in Table 13.9.

Carboxylic Acids. This family of compounds has an alkyl radical and a hydroxy group attached to the carbonyl group. The only exception is the first member of the family which has a hydrogen atom in place of the alkyl radical. The carboxylic acid functional group is the set of atoms –C(=O)–OH. The compounds are named by replacing the ending 'e' in the name of the alkane having the same number of carbon atoms with 'oic'

Table 13.8 *Names, structural formulae, boiling points and solubilities in water for three aldehydes*

Structural formula	H–C(=O)–H	H–CH₂–C(=O)–H	H–CH₂–CH₂–C(=O)–H
Systematic name	methanal	ethanal	propanal
Common name	formaldehyde	acetaldehyde	—
Boiling point (°C)	–21	20	48
Solubility in water (% w/w)	high	∞	16

Table 13.9 *Names, structural formulae, boiling points and solubilities in water for three ketones*

Structural formula	H–CH₂–C(=O)–CH₂–H	H–CH₂–CH₂–C(=O)–CH₂–H	H–CH₂–C(=O)–CH₂–CH₂–CH₂–H
Systematic name	propanone	butanone	2-pentanone
Common name	acetone	methyl ethyl ketone	—
Boiling point (°C)	56	80	102
Solubility in water (% w/w)	∞	26	6

Table 13.10 *Names, structural formulae, boiling points and solubilities in water for three carboxylic acids*

Structural formula	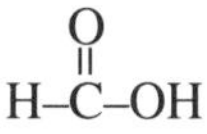	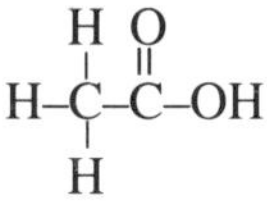	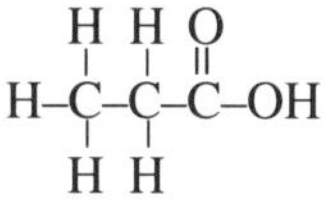
Systematic name	methanoic acid	ethanoic acid	propanoic acid
Common name	formic acid	acetic acid	propionic acid
Boiling point (°C)	101	118	141
Solubility in water (% w/w)	∞	∞	∞

and then adding the separate word 'acid'. Table 13.10 gives information for three carboxylic acids.

Aldehydes and ketones have lower boiling points than the corresponding alcohols or carboxylic acids. The reason for this is that aldehyde and ketone molecules contain no –OH groups and so are unable to form hydrogen bonds with one another as alcohol and carboxylic acid molecules can. The presence of –OH groups in alcohol and carboxylic acid molecules is also responsible for them being generally more soluble in water than aldehydes and ketones. This raises the question of why the simplest aldehydes and ketones have such high solubilities in water? After all, they contain no –OH groups with which to form hydrogen bonds. The answer to this question is that the carbonyl group has quite a high polarity in its own right and this allows any molecule containing the group to interact quite strongly with water molecules. The interaction of aldehyde and ketone molecules with water molecules is illustrated in Figure 13.28.

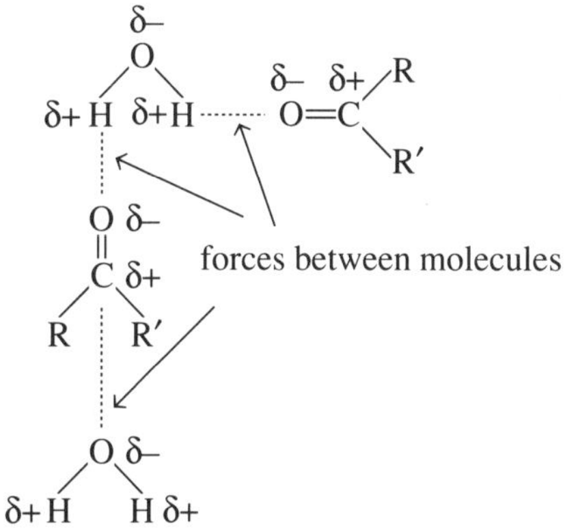

Figure 13.28 *Forces acting between aldehyde or ketone molecules and water molecules. R stands for any radical and R′ stands for a radical in the case of ketones, but a hydrogen atom in the case of aldehydes*

The carboxylic acids are weak acids. They react with water to produce a small proportion of hydronium ions and they are neutralised by bases to form salts. Aldehydes and ketones have no significant acidic properties.

13.6.6 *Clinical Uses for Aldehydes, Ketones, Carboxylic Acids*

The compounds making up the first few members of each of these families have relatively few important clinical uses. However, in later sections of this chapter and in other chapters we shall see that there are many examples of more complex aldehydes, ketones and carboxylic acids which are used clinically or which play an important role in body function. For the time being there are a few clinical uses for some simple members of these families which may be described.

Methanal. This compound is used in the form of an aqueous solution (37% w/w in water) to disinfect biological material and inanimate objects. Solutions of methanal, usually referred to as **formalin**, are used to preserve cadavers. Methanal is also used in the form of **paraformaldehyde** which is a solid formed by the joining together of many methanal molecules. This is an example of a process known as **polymerisation** and paraformaldehyde is a polymer of methanal. When the polymer is heated it releases gaseous methanal which is very effective in disinfecting surfaces with which it makes contact. Paraformaldehyde is sometimes sold in the form of candles. When they are placed in a room and lit, the heat produced converts the paraformaldehyde to methanal which then disinfects the room.

Methanal is present in specialised toothpastes which are used to relieve the discomfort of sensitive teeth. The compound is also used in dental surgeries as a fixative (a preserving agent which maintains the normal structure of a biological specimen) for tissue samples taken for close examination.

Propanone. This compound, which is often referred to by its common name, **acetone**, is used as a mixture with dry ice (solid carbon dioxide) to remove warts and other growths from the skin. Dry ice sublimes at –78 °C and when it is mixed with the propanone it evaporates rapidly, cooling the propanone to this very low temperature. Propanone has a melting point of –95 °C and so remains a liquid at the temperature of dry ice. This makes the mixture easy to apply in small portions to the areas of skin needing treatment.

A word of caution is needed about handling propanone because the compound is highly flammable and volatile. Although the cold mixture of dry ice and propanone will not produce sufficient vapour to constitute a fire hazard it is a different story when the compound is at room temperature. For this reason bottles of propanone should always be sealed tightly after each portion of the compound is withdrawn for use. Also, they should only be used in locations where smoking is prohibited and there are no other sources of ignition, such as flames or bar radiators. If a bottle of propanone is left unsealed at room temperature it can produce enough vapour to form a flammable mixture with air. If, at the same time, there happens to be a source of ignition present, then the mixture will ignite and the flame produced may flash back to the poorly sealed bottle causing it to explode.

Propanone is also used as a solvent for some preparations used to treat skin infections. Two examples are **Castellanis Paint**, which contains phenols and boric acid as its active ingredients, and **Mercurochrome**, in which the active ingredient is a compound of mercury.

Ethanoic Acid. This compound, which is usually referred to by its common name, **acetic acid**, is used in the form of aqueous solutions of various concentrations. These solutions are **bacteriostatic** which means that they inhibit the growth of microorganisms. They owe this property to their ability to lower the pH in regions where they are applied. Acetic acid is more effective in doing this than a dilute solution of a strong inorganic acid such as hydrochloric acid because it is better able to penetrate cell membranes and reach the inside of cells. This is due to the presence of low-polarity methyl radicals in molecules of acetic acid. They allow the acetic acid to dissolve more readily in the low-polarity lipid material of which cell membranes are composed.

Acetic acid is present in a preparation known as 'Aci-Jel'. It is a vaginal jelly used to used to restore and maintain the acidity of the vagina. It is also present in 'Phytex', a preparation used in the treatment of tinea.

13.6.7 *Amines*

This family of organic compounds is so named because its members are related to the simple compound **ammonia** (NH_3). They have structures which correspond to the replacement of one or more of the three hydrogen atoms of ammonia by alkyl radicals. The functional group for the amine family is $-\overset{|}{N}-$. They are classified as being primary, secondary or tertiary amines when there is one, two or three alkyl radicals respectively attached to the nitrogen atom of the amine.

Amines are named by specifying the alkyl radicals present in their molecules and adding the ending 'amine'. When two or three identical radicals are present the prefixes 'di' and 'tri' are used. These prefixes must not be omitted otherwise the name will represent a different amine containing just one of these radicals. Some characteristics of three amines are given in Table 13.11.

Hydrogen bonds operate between molecules of primary and secondary amines with the result that they have boiling points which are much higher than the corresponding alkanes. This is also why the simple amines have high solubilities in water.

Amines are weak bases and they react with water in much the same way as ammonia does. The reaction of any amine with water may be represented as follows (R = alkyl radical or hydrogen atom):

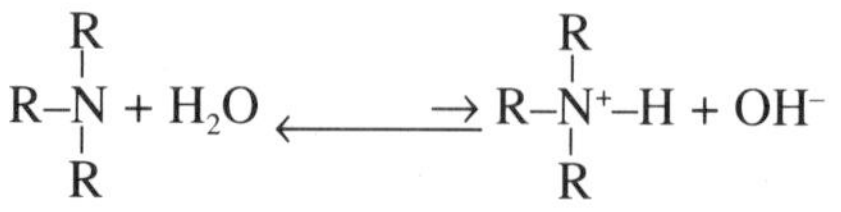

Table 13.11 *Names, structural formulae, boiling points and solubilities for three amines*

Structural formula	$H{-}N(H){-}CH_3$	$H{-}N(CH_2CH_3){-}CH_2CH_3$	$N(CH_2CH_3)(CH_2CH_3){-}CH_2CH_3$
Class of amine	primary	secondary	tertiary
Systematic name	methylamine	diethylamine	triethylamine
Boiling point (°C)	−6	55	89
Solubility in water (% w/w)	high	high	1.5

When amines are mixed with acids they undergo neutralisation and form salts. An equation for the neutralisation of methylamine by hydrochloric acid is shown below.

$$\underset{\text{methylamine}}{CH_3NH_2} + \underset{\text{hydrochloric acid}}{H_3O^+_{aq} + Cl^-_{aq}} \rightleftharpoons \underset{\text{methylammonium chloride}}{CH_3NH_3^+Cl^-} + H_2O$$

Amines are often used in the form of salts because, in this form, amines which would not otherwise dissolve in water can be made soluble (remember, salts are ionic compounds and ionic compounds are usually soluble in water). Another useful property of salts is that they are usually solids with high melting points. This makes them easy to store and reduces losses due to evaporation.

The simple amines have unpleasant, fishy odours and they are responsible for the odour which stale fish often produce. One of the reasons why vinegar is so often used on meals of fish is that the acid which it contains (acetic acid) neutralises the amines in the fish, converting them to salts. In this form they have a very low volatility and so their odour is much less noticeable.

13.6.8 *Clinical Uses for Amines*

Most of the amines which are clinically useful have complex structures and one example is the substance **morphine**. The salt form of morphine has already been referred to in Section 7.11.3 where its long-standing use as an **analgesic** (pain reliever) was described.

Another well-known and clinically useful amine is **amphetamine** which is usually administered as amphetamine sulphate. It is a stimulant which is used in the treatment of narcolepsy (excessive desire to sleep) and some forms of depression. Strangely enough, it is also effective in reducing the activity of hyperactive children. Structural formulae for morphine and amphetamine are given in Figure 13.29.

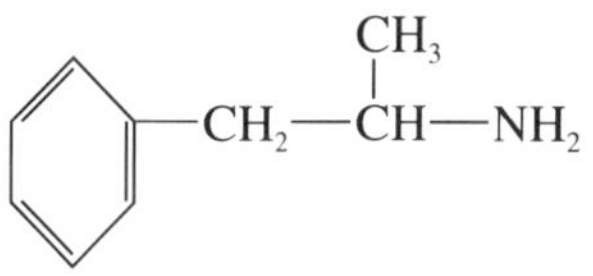

amphetamine

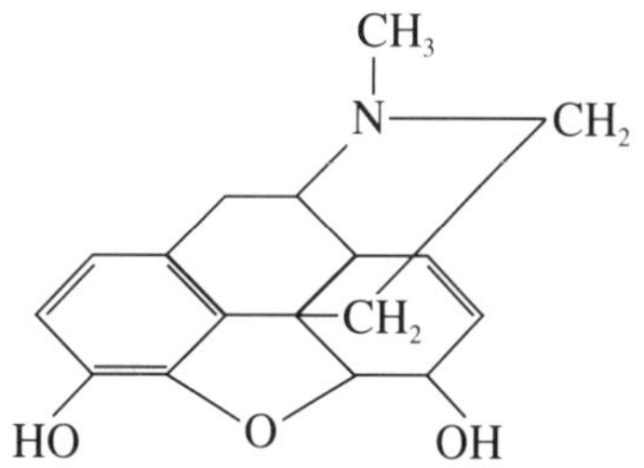

morphine

Figure 13.29 *Structural formulae for amphetamine and morphine*

13.6.9 *Esters*

Esters form when acids react with alcohols. If the acid involved is a carboxylic acid (and it usually is) then the equation for this reaction can be written as follows (R, R′ stand for any radical):

$$\underset{\text{carboxylic acid}}{R\text{–}\overset{\overset{O}{\|}}{C}\text{–}OH} + \underset{\text{alcohol}}{H\text{–}O\text{–}R'} \rightleftharpoons \underset{\text{ester}}{R\text{–}\overset{\overset{O}{\|}}{C}\text{–}O\text{–}R'} + \underset{\text{water}}{H_2O}$$

When an ester forms in this way the set of atoms $R\text{–}\overset{\overset{O}{\|}}{C}\text{–}$ is provided by the carboxylic acid and the set of atoms –OR′ is provided by the alcohol. This fact can be used, in conjunction with the structural formula for an ester, to decide which carboxylic acid and which alcohol could be used to make it.

Exercise 13.2
Give the systematic names for the carboxylic acid and alcohol from which the following ester could be made.

$$CH_3CH_2\overset{\overset{O}{\|}}{C}\text{–}O\text{–}CH_2CH_3$$

There are two parts to the name of an ester and they correspond to the alcohol and carboxylic acid from which it can be formed. The first part of the name is obtained from the name for the alcohol by removing the ending 'ol' and replacing it with 'yl' (this is equivalent to simply stating the name for the radical which is present in the alcohol). The second part of the name for an ester is obtained by removing the ending 'ic' from the name of the carboxylic acid and replacing it with 'ate'. Thus the ester which can be obtained from the reaction of ethanol with ethanoic acid is named **ethyl ethanoate**. If the common name for ethanoic acid (acetic acid) is used (and it usually is) then the ester would be called **ethyl acetate**.

Exercise 13.3
What is the systematic name for the ester in Exercise 13.2?

Although most esters are formed using carboxylic acids they are also obtained when alcohols react with strong inorganic acids such as nitric acid and sulphuric acid. An equation for the formation of an ester of this type is written below. You will see, from the name given to the ester, that names for esters of inorganic acids are obtained in much the same way as the names for esters of carboxylic acids.

$$\underset{\text{nitric acid}}{HNO_3} + \underset{\text{ethanol}}{HO\text{–}CH_2CH_3} \longrightarrow \underset{\text{ethyl nitrate}}{NO_2\text{–}O\text{–}CH_2CH_3} + \underset{\text{water}}{H_2O}$$

13.6.10 *Clinical and Other Uses for Esters*

There are very few significant clinical uses for the esters of simple carboxylic acids and alcohols. However, many of the compounds responsible for the sweet smell of fruits are simple esters and large quantities of some of these are manufactured for use as artificial flavourings and perfumes. For example, **ethyl butanoate** contributes to the odour of apricots and peaches; **octyl acetate** contributes to the odour of oranges.

One interesting example of a simple ester having clinical importance is **glyceryl trinitrate** also known as **nitroglycerine**. This is the ester of glycerol and nitric acid and it is best known as the explosive component of dynamite! However, it is also effective in providing relief from the pain of **angina pectoris** which is a throttling pain in the chest associated with a restricted blood supply to the heart.

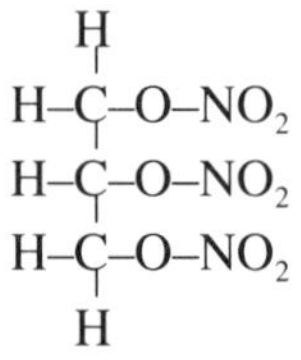

Figure 13.30 *Structural formula for glyceryl trinitrate*

13.6.11 *Amides*

The functional group for members of the amide family is $\text{–}\overset{\overset{O}{\|}}{C}\text{–}\overset{|}{N}\text{–}$. Members fall into three different classes according to the number of radicals which are attached to the nitrogen atom. These classes are **primary**, **secondary** and **tertiary** when the number of radicals attached to the nitrogen is zero, one and two respectively. Primary amides are named by replacing the 'oic' ending of the name of the corresponding carboxylic acid by the ending 'amide'. For secondary and tertiary amides the names of the alkyl radicals attached to the nitrogen atom are written in front of the main part of the name with the symbol 'N' being used to signify that the radicals are attached to the nitrogen atom of the amide. This method of naming is illustrated by the examples below.

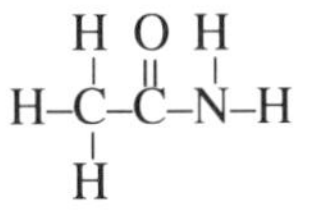

ethanamide

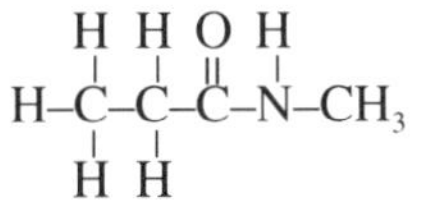

N-methylpropanamide

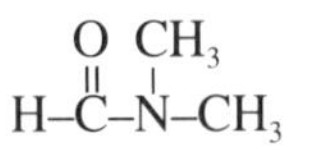

N, N-dimethylmethanamide

There are few clinical uses for simple amides but the amide family is very important in living systems because it includes the proteins which are discussed in considerable detail in Section 13.8.3. An interesting example of a complex amide is **N, N-diethyllyserg-amide**, usually called **lysergic acid diethylamide (LSD)**. This compound, which has the structural formula shown in Figure 13.31, produces dramatic effects on the perceptions of all people who are exposed to it. Its potency is very high and a dose of 100–250 μg is sufficient to cause dramatic changes in a person's perceptions of self and surroundings. A common experience reported by those who have taken LSD is **synesthesia**, in which a stimulus of one sense is perceived as a sensation of another sense. For example, sounds may be perceived as colours. Another common report of LSD takers is of a tactile illusion in which the person feels as if ants are crawling under the skin. These strange perceptual effects have attracted many seekers after unusual experiences. As a result, LSD is an important illicit drug sold under the name **acid**.

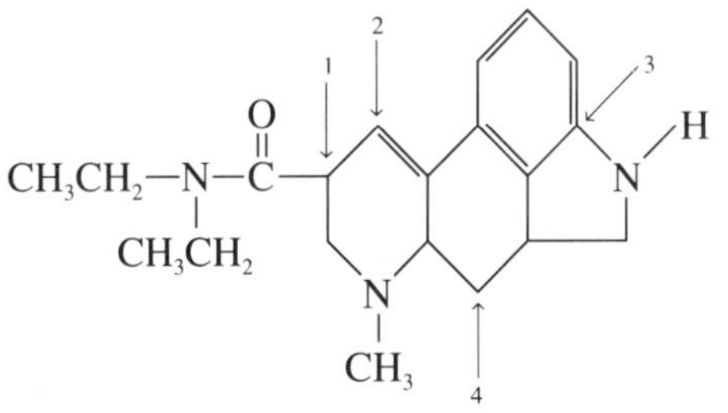

Figure 13.31 *Structural formula for lysergic acid diethylamide*

Exercise 13.4
In the diagram in Figure 13.31 what is the type and number of atoms present at the positions labelled 1–4?

LSD has no established therapeutic uses but it is a compound of considerable interest to researchers because it appears to produce states of mind which are very similar to those experienced in **schizophrenia**. There are also some clinicians who consider that LSD might eventually prove useful for the relief of pain in some cases of terminal cancer.

13.6.12 *Multifunctional Organic Compounds*

So far in our discussion of different families of organic compounds we have mainly considered compounds in which only one functional group is present. However, there are many compounds which are **multifunctional**, meaning that they contain more than one functional group in their molecules and belong to more than one family of organic compounds. This is very common among the compounds which occur naturally in living things and among compounds used as medicines. For example, cholesterol (Figure 13.22) contains both an alcohol group and an alkene group; morphine (Figure 13.29) contains alcohol, alkene, ether and amine functional groups. Some more examples are provided by the three analgesic (pain-relieving) substances represented in Figure 13.32.

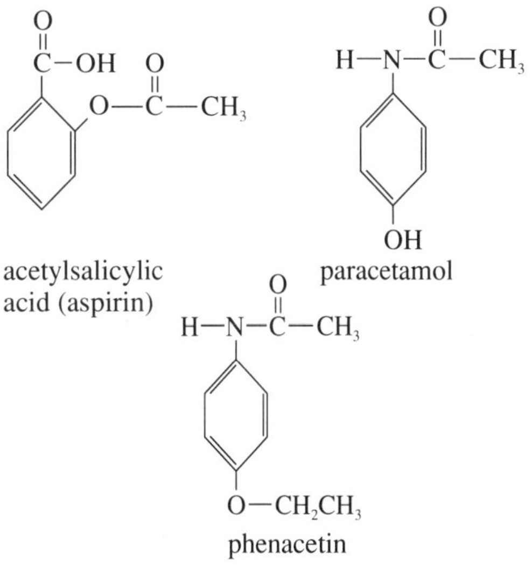

Figure 13.32 *Structural formulae for three analgesics*

Generally speaking, multifunctional organic compounds exhibit a set of behaviours which is the sum of the behaviours exhibited by all the different families to which they belong. The main exceptions to this occur when two or more functional groups are located very close to one another within the molecule. In such cases the substance may exhibit some property which is not exhibited by any compound in which just one of the functional groups is present.

13.7 Spot Tests for Functional Groups

When molecules of an organic compound contain a particular functional group, then the substance will behave in a predictable way and display chemical properties which correspond to that functional group. The functional groups present in molecules of an organic compound can be detected using chemical tests. These tests involve mixing the organic compound with a particular combination of other chemicals and looking for a visual result such as a colour change or the release of a gas (effervescence). These simple tests are called **spot tests** and they have proven very useful in medical technology for determining if a particular compound is present in a body fluid. In addition, they often provide the means for determining a compound's concentration from the magnitude of the effect which is produced. Some examples of spot tests are described below.

13.7.1 *Iron(III) Chloride Test for Carboxylic Acids and Phenols*

Iron(III) chloride ($FeCl_3$) forms a pale yellow solution when dissolved in water. The colour of the solution is due to the ion $Fe(H_2O)_6^{3+}$ in which six water molecules have become associated with the Fe^{3+} ion as shown in Figure 13.33.

Two classes of organic compound may be detected using iron(III) chloride solution: phenols and carboxylic acids which have either an alcohol or ketone group located adjacent to the carboxylic acid group. When one of these classes of organic compound is mixed with iron(III) chloride some of the water molecules around the Fe^{3+} ion are replaced by molecules of the organic compound. This causes a change in colour of the solution and, in this way, the presence of the phenol or carboxylic acid is revealed. Depending on the particular phenol or carboxylic acid involved, the colour produced may vary from green to purple.

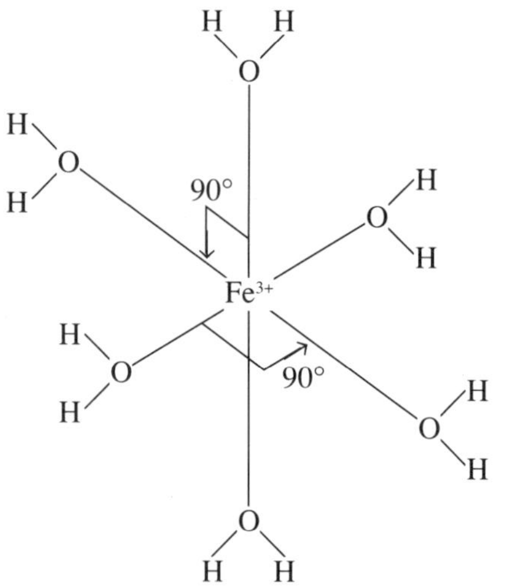

Figure 13.33 *The ion $Fe(H_2O)_6^{3+}$ which is responsible for the yellow colour of iron(III) chloride solutions*

Iron(III) chloride is used in the clinical chemistry laboratory to detect **salicylic acid** in blood or urine in cases where salicylate poisoning is suspected. The most common cause of such poisoning is ingestion of aspirin by children.

Iron(III) chloride also provided the first means for early detection of the potentially catastrophic condition known as **phenylketonuria** (PKU). This is an inherited condition which occurs once in every 10 000–20 000 births. The child affected does not possess an enzyme needed for the conversion of one amino acid, **phenylalanine**, into another, **tyrosine** (Figure 13.34). If the deficiency is not detected soon after birth the accumulation of phenylalanine leads to

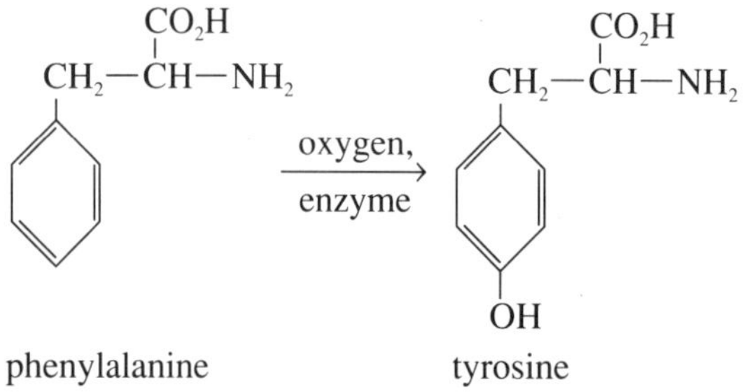

Figure 13.34 *The conversion of phenylalanine to tyrosine*

irreversible brain damage and a life of severe mental retardation.

About 50 years ago the Norwegian physician Asbjörn Fölling noticed that the urine of two mentally retarded siblings produced a blue-green colour when mixed with iron(III) chloride solution. He correctly concluded that the compound causing this colour change was related to the children's mental retardation and he was also able to establish that it was **phenylpyruvic acid**. This compound forms in the kidneys from phenylalanine as shown in Figure 13.35. In its molecules a ketone group is located adjacent to a carboxylic acid group and this causes it to produce a characteristic colour with iron(III) chloride.

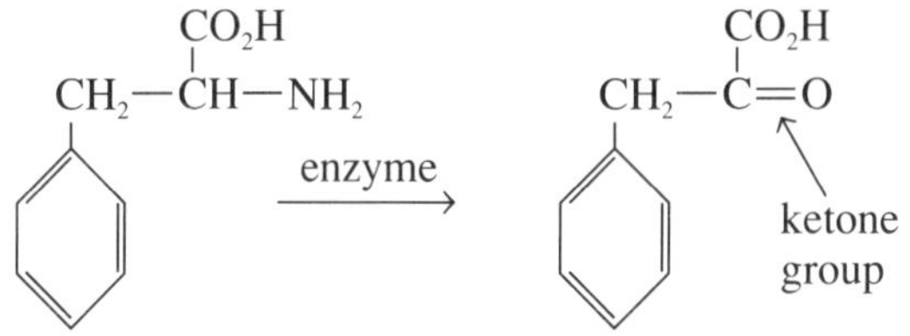

phenylalanine phenylpyruvic acid

Figure 13.35 *Conversion of phenylalanine to phenylpyruvic acid*

From the time of Fölling's discovery until the mid-1950s iron(III) chloride solution was the means used to diagnose phenylketonuria. A small sample of the test solution was simply applied to the child's wet nappy. Where the disease was detected in the first few days after birth a child could be saved from its usual consequences by being fed a diet supplemented with tyrosine but containing just the minimum amount of phenylalanine needed for normal growth and development. This strict dietary control must be maintained for about the first 10 years of life by which time most brain growth and development is complete. After this time the diet may be somewhat relaxed. The iron(III) chloride test has now been replaced by other procedures which are more sensitive and more reliable, but its use over the years has saved many children and their families from the tragic consequences of PKU.

Another clinically significant compound which produces a colour with iron(III) chloride is **lactic acid**. In this compound an alcohol group is located adjacent to a carboxylic acid group as shown in Figure 13.36 and the substance produces an intense yellow-green colour with iron(III) chloride.

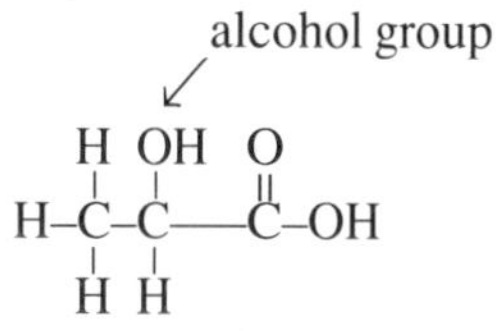

lactic acid

Figure 13.36 *Structural formula for lactic acid*

Iron(III) chloride solution is used to detect the presence of lactic acid in gastric juice. The clinician will be interested in this information where carcinoma of the stomach is a possibility. This disease is often accompanied by elevated levels of lactic acid in gastric juice.

13.7.2 *Benedict's Test for Glucose*

Benedict's reagent is a clear blue solution obtained by dissolving copper(II) sulphate ($CuSO_4{\cdot}5H_2O$) in a strongly basic solution. It is an oxidising agent and, on warming, is capable of oxidising many, but not all, aldehydes to carboxylic acids. As it does, it is itself reduced to copper(I) oxide which appears as a reddish precipitate. An equation for this reaction is written below.

$$\mathrm{R{-}\overset{H}{\overset{|}{C}}{=}O} \quad + \quad 2Cu^{2+} + 4\,OH^- \longrightarrow$$

aldehyde — Benedict's reagent (clear, blue solution)

$$\mathrm{R{-}\overset{O}{\overset{\|}{C}}{-}OH} \quad + \quad Cu_2O\downarrow + 2H_2O$$

carboxylic acid — copper(I) oxide (red precipitate)

Glucose is an aldehyde and Benedict's reagent has been used for many years for its detection in urine. Significant levels of glucose in urine indicate very high levels in the blood and this occurs in *diabetes mellitus*.

The Benedict's reagent used clinically is in the form of tablets which contain copper sulphate and sodium hydroxide. These are dissolved in the urine sample and, as they dissolve, the sodium hydroxide, as well as ensuring that the mixture is strongly basic, produces enough heat to raise the temperature to the required value without additional heating being necessary.

Benedict's reagent is now being replaced by a more specific and more convenient technique in which an enzyme is used for oxidation.

13.7.3 *Sodium Bicarbonate Test for Carboxylic Acids*

Carboxylic acids may be recognised by their reaction with sodium bicarbonate ($NaHCO_3$) solution. In this reaction carbon dioxide gas forms and bubbles from the solution. The reaction is a neutralisation reaction and the carboxylic acid ends up in the form of a salt.

$$R{-}\overset{\displaystyle O}{\overset{\|}{C}}{-}OH + NaHCO_3 \longrightarrow$$

carboxylic acid   sodium bicarbonate

$$R{-}\overset{\displaystyle O}{\overset{\|}{C}}{-}O^-Na^+ + CO_2\uparrow + H_2O$$

salt   carbon dioxide

This type of reaction is responsible for the effervescing action of some solid mixtures sold as health drinks. The mixtures often contain a carboxylic acid and a bicarbonate but they do not react with each other in the solid state as long as the mixture is kept dry. However, when added to water they do react, carbon dioxide forms rapidly and produces the effervescent effect as it bubbles from solution.

13.8 Organic Compounds in Living Things

13.8.1 *The Alphabet of Biochemistry*

Biochemistry is that branch of science which is concerned with the compounds found in living things, and with the reactions which they undergo in those living systems. There are thousands of different compounds present in even simple life forms and many of these undergo a range of different chemical reactions. Science is sometimes described as 'a search for simplicity in the midst of complexity' and biochemistry is an area of science which illustrates this very well. There are countless thousands of different compounds in the human body and most of them are very complex, but the biochemist's search for simplicity in the midst of this complexity has revealed that most of these compounds are built from a small number of simple substances. These simple substances make up the **alphabet of biochemistry**. This phrase is used to describe them because their number is about 30, which is close to 26, the number of letters in the English alphabet. Furthermore, like the letters of the English alphabet, they can be joined in an unlimited number of different ways. We shall take the alphabet of biochemistry to consist of:

20 amino acids	glycerol
3 pyrimidine bases	choline
2 purine bases	palmitic acid
glucose	phosphoric acid
ribose	

13.8.2 *Amino Acids*

The biggest group of compounds in the alphabet of biochemistry is the **amino acids**. There are about 20 of these and, as the name suggests, they are organic compounds which contain both the amine group and the carboxylic acid group. Structural formulae and names for these compounds are presented in Table 13.12.

If you look carefully at the structural formulae in Table 13.12 you will notice that each amino acid listed has an amine group attached to the carbon atom immediately alongside the carboxylic acid group. This relationship between the positions in the molecule occupied by the amine and carboxylic acid functional groups is often specified by calling the amino acid an α–amino acid. This name is part of an old system used for the naming of organic compounds in which letters of the Greek alphabet, rather than numbers, are used to specify the positions which functional groups and radicals occupy within a molecule. For carboxylic acids the carbon atom immediately adjacent to the carboxylic acid group is designated **alpha**, the carbon atom one position further away is designated **beta** and so on. This is shown below.

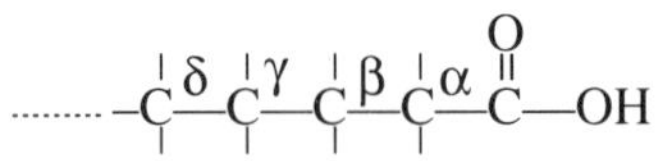

The overwhelming majority of amino acids used in the human body are α-amino acids but other types of amino acid may play very important roles in the biochemistry of other life forms. For example, there is the amino acid known as **p-aminobenzoic acid** (PABA) which is essential for the growth of many bacteria. The amino group of p-aminobenzoic acid is located on the fourth carbon atom away from the carboxylic acid group and so it is an example of a δ-amino acid (see Figure 13.37).

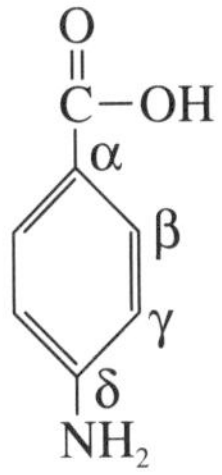

p-aminobenzoic acid (PABA)

Figure 13.37 *Structural formula for p-aminobenzoic acid, an example of a δ-amino acid*

Amino Acids and Stereoisomerism. We are all familiar with the fact that there is a difference between our left and right hands. Left-handed people are particularly conscious of this difference because they often find themselves in difficulty trying to use a hand-held device which has been made for a right-handed person. Some common examples of such devices are scissors, golf clubs, baseball gloves and pistols.

Although it is obvious that left and right hands are different it is not so easy to express what the difference is. The relationship which exists between our right and left hands is the same as that which exists between any object and its image in a mirror. Quite often two objects which are related in this way can be made to occupy the same space (but not simultaneously, of course). In other words they are perfectly superimposable. One object can be lowered onto the other so that all their corresponding parts coincide. Such objects are identical. Now, left and right hands are mirror images of each other but they are not capable of occupying the same space. They are not superimposable. You cannot take your right hand and lay it down on top of your left hand so that the thumb and fingers on each hand coincide. We are made aware that our left and right hands are not identical every time we attempt to place a right-handed glove on our left hand or vice versa. So, we can say that right and left hands are different objects related in the sense of being *non-superimposable mirror images of one another.*

Many organic molecules also exist in forms which are non-superimposable mirror images of each other. The most common examples of this are molecules in which a carbon atom is joined to four *different* groups of atoms. Such carbon atoms are said to be **asymmetric** and, with the exception of glycine, there is an asymmetric carbon atom present in all the amino acid molecules listed in Table 13.12. If you look carefully at the two representations of the alanine molecule which are drawn in Figure 13.38 you will see that they represent molecules which are non-superimposable mirror images. No matter how you imagine the two drawings being rotated or tilted you will not find a way of superimposing them, that is, you will not find a way of lowering one onto the other so that all the corresponding parts of each molecule coincide.

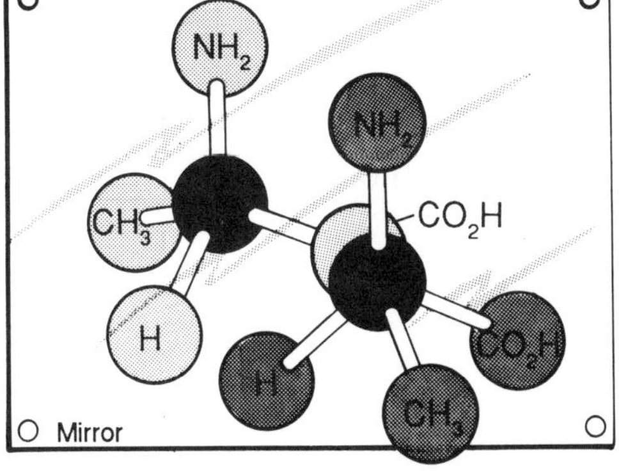

Figure 13.38 *Stereoisomers of alanine*

Table 13.12 *Structural formulae, names and abbreviations for amino acids used in the body*

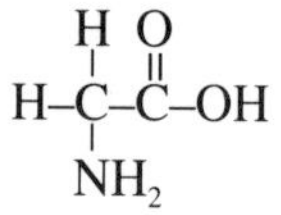
glycine (Gly)

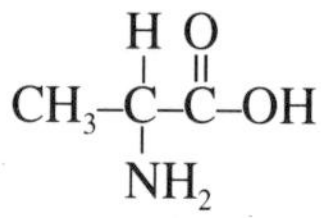
alanine (Ala)

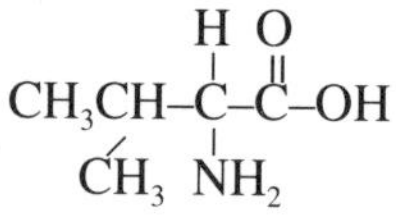
valine (Val)*

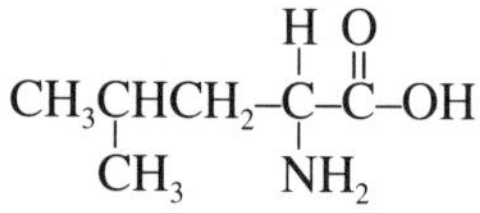
leucine (Leu)*

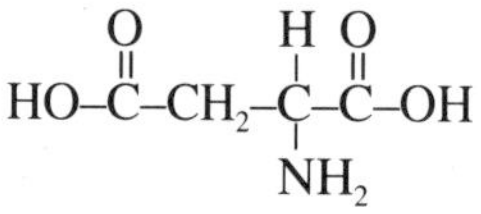
aspartic acid (Asp)

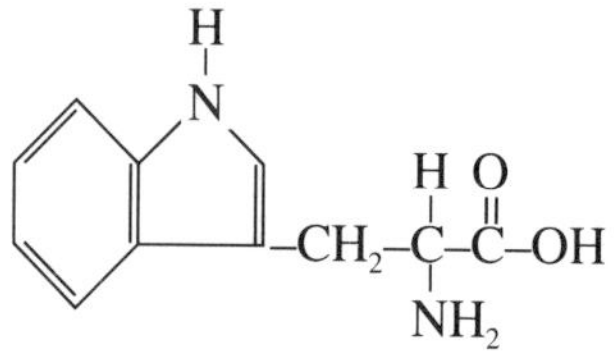
tryptophan (Trp)*

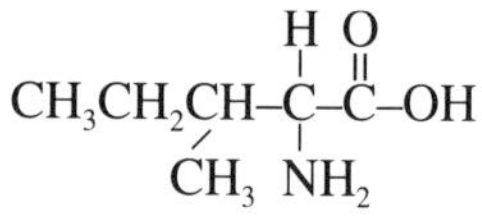
isoleucine (Ile)*

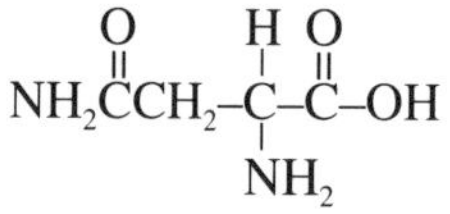
asparagine (Asn)

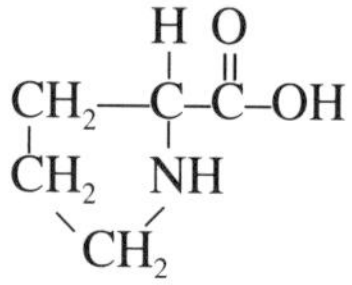
proline (Pro)

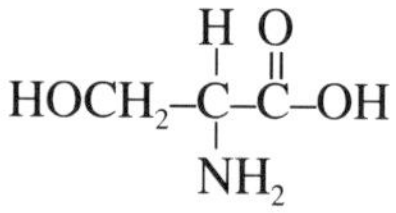
serine (Ser)

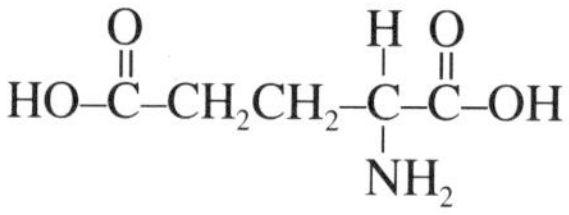
glutamic acid (Glu)

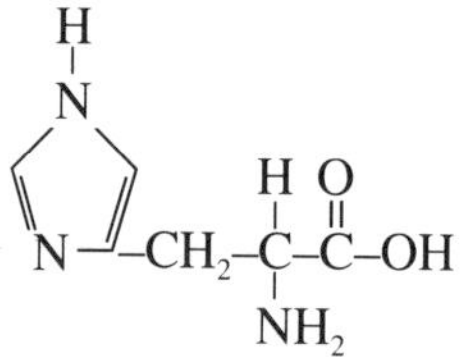
histidine (His)*

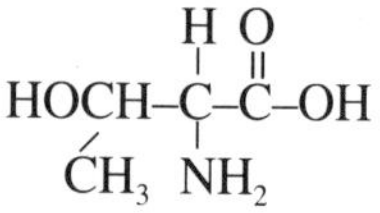
threonine (Thr)*

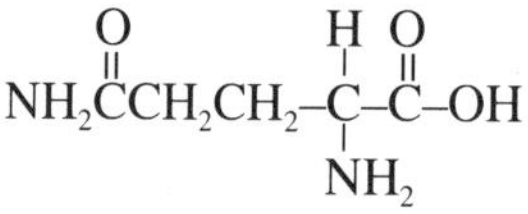
glutamine (Gln)

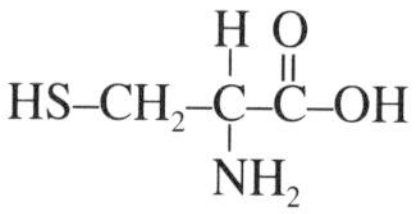
cysteine (Cys)

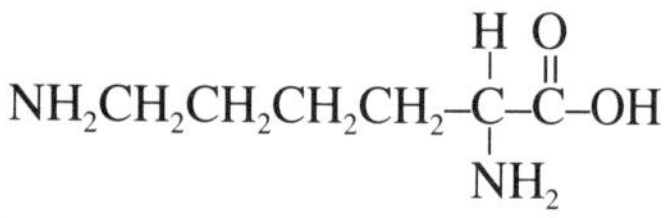
lysine (Lys)*

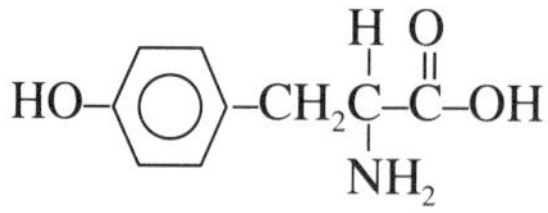
tyrosine (Tyr)

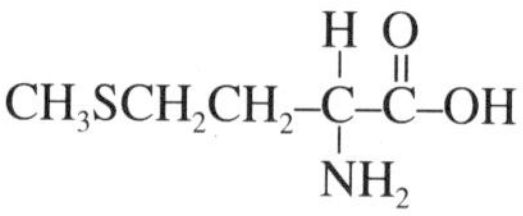
methionine (Met)*

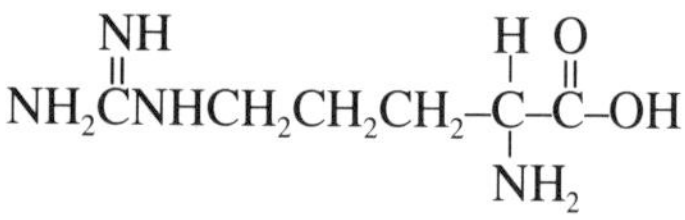
arginine (Arg)*

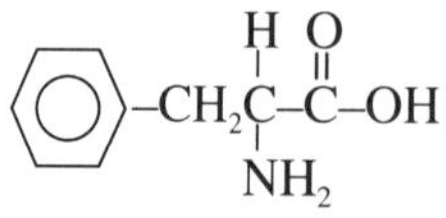
phenylalanine (Phe)*

* An essential amino acid.

The two molecules represented in Figure 13.38 contain the same set of atoms joined in the same sequence but their orientations in space are different. Thus, they are **stereoisomers**. This type of stereoisomerism is usually called **optical isomerism**. The reason for this is that the isomers differ from each other in the effect which they have on a certain type of light (polarised light) when it passes through solutions which contain them.

Optical isomers are often distinguished from each other by being designated as D or L. To decide whether a molecule of one of the amino acids listed in Table 13.12 is a D or an L isomer it is necessary to view a diagram of the molecule as illustrated in Figure 13.39.

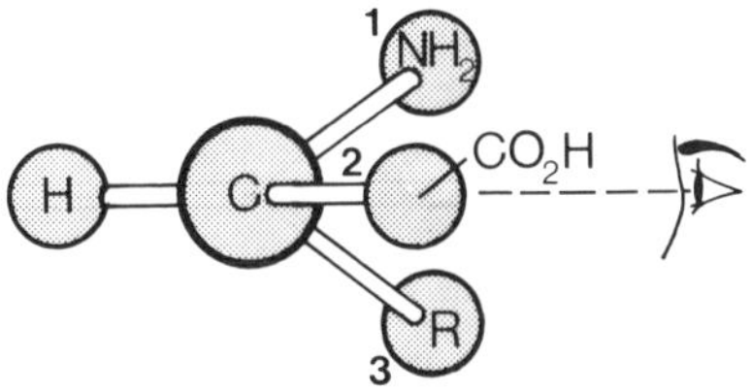

Figure 13.39 *L isomer of an amino acid*

The line of sight must be along the carbon–hydrogen bond from the side opposite the hydrogen atom. The other three groups attached to the carbon atom are numbered 1 (NH_2 group), 2 (CO_2H group) and 3 (the remaining group). Now move around the three groups in the order 1, 2, 3. If the direction taken is clockwise then the amino acid is a D isomer. If the direction is anticlockwise then the amino acid is an L isomer.

Optical isomerism is very important in living systems. Many of the substances which the human body uses are able to exist as optical isomers but the body normally uses only one of these. For example, all the human body's essential amino acids are L isomers. Most of the carbohydrates which the body uses are D isomers. Many medicines are also capable of existing as optical isomers and it is very common to observe that different isomers have different potencies. A good example of this is provided by the medicine **isoproterenol** which is used in the treatment of bronchial asthma. It is effective because it acts as a **bronchodilator**, increasing the size of the bronchial passages and making it easier to breathe. A structural formula for isoproterenol is shown below and the asymmetric carbon atom is marked with an asterisk.

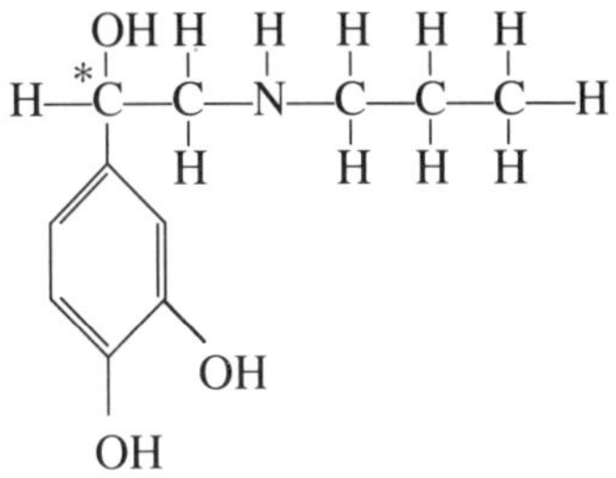

The D isomer of isoproterenol is about 800 times more effective as a bronchodilator than the L isomer. Large differences in the potency of optical isomers are quite common and the reason is that the substances exert their effects by attaching to biological molecules using three of the groups attached to the assymetric carbon atom. Only one optical isomer will be capable of doing this (see Figure 13.40).

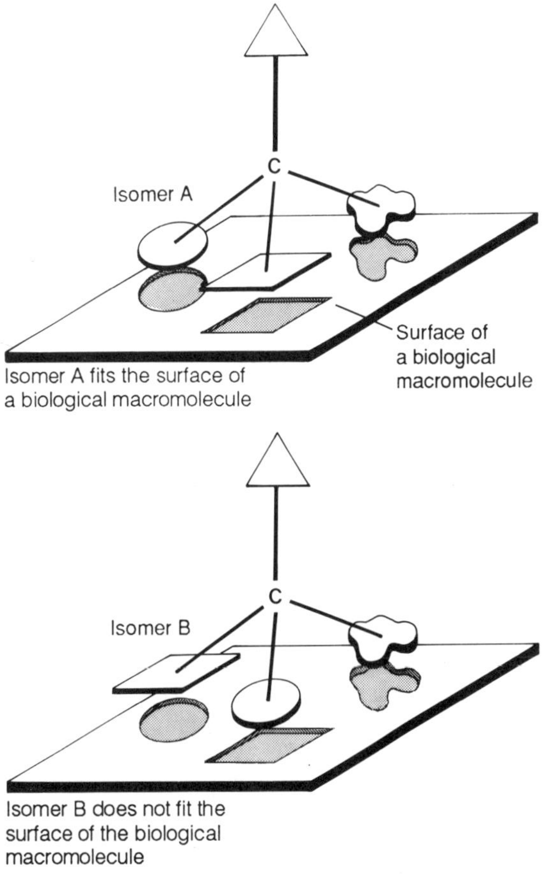

Figure 13.40 *Biological action of an optical isomer*

Acid–Base Nature of Amino Acids. Amino acids are capable of behaving both as acids and as bases. They owe this ability to the presence in their molecules of at least one acidic group (the carboxylic acid) and one basic group (the amine). When an amino acid is added to water these groups can react to form hydronium and hydroxide ions. This is shown below using alanine as an example.

$$\text{H}_2\text{N}-\underset{\underset{\text{H}}{|}}{\overset{\overset{\text{CH}_3}{|}}{\text{C}}}-\text{CO}_2\text{H} + \text{H}_2\text{O} \longleftrightarrow \text{H}_2\text{N}-\underset{\underset{\text{H}}{|}}{\overset{\overset{\text{CH}_3}{|}}{\text{C}}}-\text{CO}_2^- + \text{H}_3\text{O}^+$$

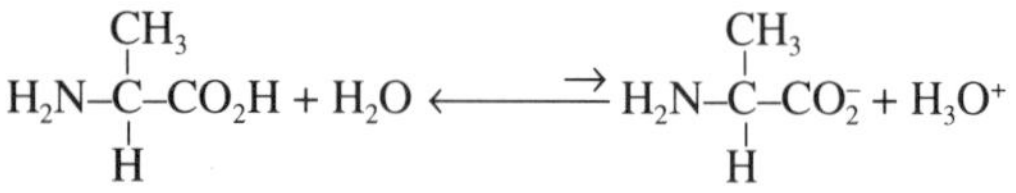

alanine acting as an acid

$$\text{H}_2\text{N}-\underset{\underset{\text{H}}{|}}{\overset{\overset{\text{CH}_3}{|}}{\text{C}}}-\text{CO}_2\text{H} + \text{H}_2\text{O} \longleftrightarrow \text{H}_3\text{N}^+-\underset{\underset{\text{H}}{|}}{\overset{\overset{\text{CH}_3}{|}}{\text{C}}}-\text{CO}_2\text{H} + \text{OH}^-$$

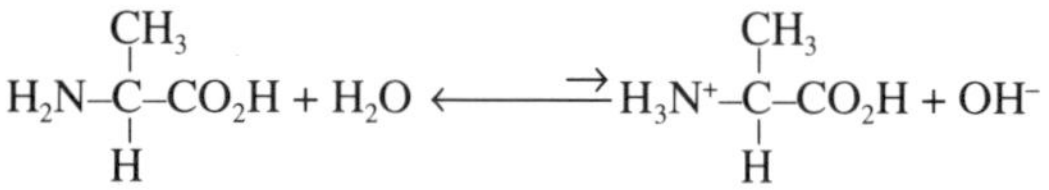

alanine acting as a base

Although in Table 13.12 all the amino acids listed are shown as neutral molecules their dual acid–base nature ensures that they rarely exist in this form. In the solid state, and in solutions having pH values close to 7, they exist as particles in which the amine group and carboxylic group are both ionised. This type of particle, containing both a positive and a negative charge, is known as a **dipolar ion** or as a **zwitterion**. The structural formula for the zwitterion of alanine is shown below.

$$\text{H}_3\text{N}^+-\underset{\underset{\text{H}}{|}}{\overset{\overset{\text{CH}_3}{|}}{\text{C}}}-\text{CO}_2^-$$

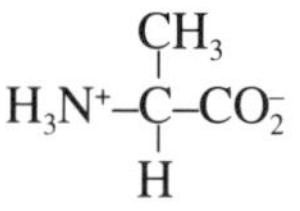

zwitterion of alanine

In solutions where the pH is far below or far above 7 an amino acid will exist either as a positive ion (pH well below 7) or as a negative ion (pH well above 7) and so we see that under all conditions of solution pH, and in the solid state, amino acids exist as particles in which full electrical charges are present on at least one group of atoms within the particle. In effect, we may say that amino acids nearly always exist in an ionic form or, in other words, as salts. This explains the observation that amino acids usually have melting points which are far higher than simple carboxylic acids containing the same number of carbon atoms (see Table 13.13). It also explains why amino acids which contain large non-polar sections within their molecules are still often quite soluble in water.

Essential Amino Acids. Most of the amino acids listed in Table 13.12 can be manufactured in the body from other compounds present in the diet. However, there are a few for which this is not true and, for a person to enjoy good health, it is essential that their diet contain adequate supplies of these particular amino acids. For this reason they are called **essential amino acids** and they are marked with asterisks in Table 13.12. For the case of children born with the disease phenylketonuria the list of essential amino acids must be extended to include tyrosine. These children are not able to manufacture tyrosine from phenylalanine and so all the tyrosine that they require must be made available in the diet.

In Section 2.7.5 we saw that a dietary deficiency of some trace elements could cause disease and there are also deficiency diseases associated with the inadequate supply of essential amino acids. The best known of these diseases is **kwashiorkor**, which is common among children in underdeveloped countries. The name kwashiorkor originated in the African country of Ghana where it means 'first-second' and it came into use because the disease is most likely to affect the first born child of a mother who soon afterwards has a second child. The reason for this pattern is that the first child is fed on breast milk which provides an adequate supply of protein (we shall see presently that protein is the form in which most amino acids occur in living material). However, when the second child is born, the first child is often switched to a diet of cereal in which the protein (and, therefore, amino acid) content is poor. Consequently, the first child, who is still very young, is deprived of an adequate supply of amino acids at a stage of life where these are particularly important for healthy growth and development.

13.8.3 *Proteins*

Proteins are compounds in which large numbers of amino acid molecules have joined together to form one very large protein molecule. The process of protein formation is one in which a simple chemical process occurs over and over again. This simple process is outlined in Figure 13.41 using the two amino acids phenylalanine and glycine as examples.

The process represented in Figure 13.41 involves one amino acid molecule losing one of the hydrogen atoms of its amine group while the other amino acid molecule loses the hydroxy group of its carboxylic acid group. These hydrogen and hydroxy fragments combine to form water. As they leave their respective amino acid molecules the nitrogen atom of the amine group in one molecule forms a bond with the carbon

Table 13.13 *Melting points of amino acids compared with those of carboxylic acids*

Name	Structural formula	Melting point (°C)
glycine	$CH_2–CO_2H$ NH_2	262
ethanoic acid	$CH_3–CO_2H$	16
alanine	$CH_3–CH–CO_2H$ NH_2	314
propanoic acid	$CH_3–CH_2–CO_2H$	–21
phenylalanine	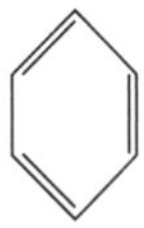 $–CH_2–CH–CO_2H$ NH_2	283
3-phenyl propanoic acid	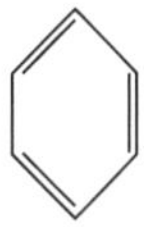 $–CH_2–CH_2–CO_2H$	49

atom of the carboxylic acid group in the other molecule, thereby joining the two molecules together and forming a larger molecule. This larger molecule is known as a **dipeptide** and if you look closely at its structural formula shown in Figure 13.41 you will see that in its molecule it still has a carboxylic acid group and an amine group. So, it is still an amino acid but now the amine and carboxylic acid groups are further apart and it is no longer an α-amino acid. Being an amino acid though, it remains capable of having additional α-amino acids join to its amine group and to its carboxylic acid group in the same way as phenylalanine and glycine are shown joining in Figure 13.41. In this way, a chain of α-amino acid molecules

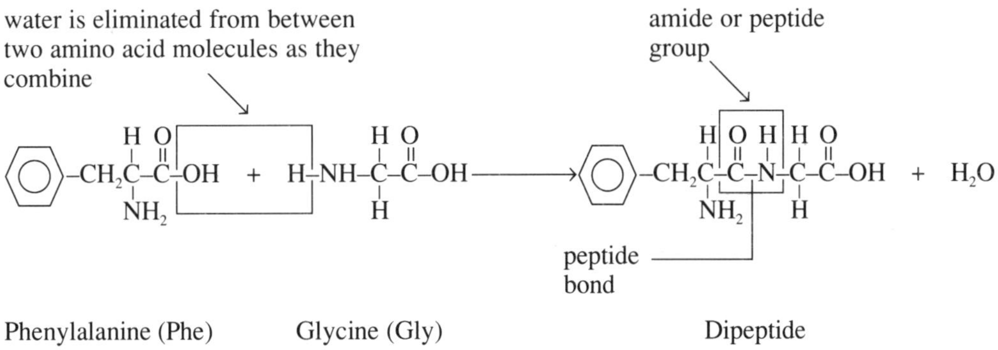

Figure 13.41 *Combination of two amino acid molecules to form a dipeptide*

can grow longer and longer. The term **peptide** is used to describe all molecules which form in this way by the joining of α-amino acids. When three α-amino acid molecules have joined the molecule formed is called a **tripeptide**, if four have joined, a **tetrapeptide** and so on. The word peptide is also used in the terms **peptide group** and **peptide bond**. The term peptide group is used to describe the group of atoms $-\overset{\overset{O}{\|}}{C}-\overset{|}{N}-$ which joins each amino acid unit in a peptide chain to the next. However, if you go back to Section 13.6.11 which dealt with the family of organic compounds called the amides you will see that this same set of atoms makes up the amide functional group and so peptide group is simply another name for the amide group. The term peptide bond is used to describe the covalent bond between the nitrogen and carbon atoms in the peptide group.

It is a simple matter to make a dipeptide. All that one need do is take any two amino acids and mix them under the right conditions. Two dipeptides will form because an amino acid may join to another amino acid either by making use of its amino group or its carboxylic acid group. This is illustrated in Figure 13.42 using the amino acids glycine and alanine as examples. The names given to the two dipeptides deserve a brief comment. They have been obtained by noting which amino acid unit in the dipeptide still has its carboxylic acid group unreacted. The name of this amino acid is written in full and given a prefix obtained from the name of the other amino acid by replacing the ending 'ine' with 'yl'. The same system is used for higher peptides which will have an additional prefix for every additional amino acid unit which is present.

Rather than go to all the trouble taken in Figure 13.42 to represent the structures of alanylglycine and glycylalanine we can (and will) simply represent them as:

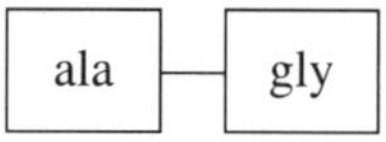

| ala | — | gly | or ala—gly, alanylglycine

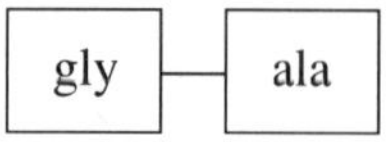

| gly | — | ala | or gly—ala, glycylalanine

With this simple method, which is widely used, it is understood that the amino acid on the right-hand end of the sequence is the one in which the carboxylic acid group is unreacted. This means of course that the amino acid unit on the left-hand end of the sequence has its amine group unreacted.

Dipeptide formation is the first step in the formation of a protein. A complete protein molecule contains many (perhaps thousands) α–amino acid molecules joined together and so they are often called **polypeptides** or **polyamides** (the prefix 'poly' means 'many'). A section from a protein molecule is represented in Figure 13.43. The line of atoms which forms as the amine and carboxylic acid groups join with each other is called the **backbone** of the protein. The remaining portions of each amino acid unit, which in Figure 13.43 are designated 'R', and shown as projecting upwards from the backbone, are referred to as **side chains**.

Other terms which may be used to describe proteins are the terms **polymer** and **macromolecule**. The name 'polymer' means 'many (poly) parts (mer)' and this description fits proteins because they consist of many α–amino acid units joined together. The name 'macromolecule' means 'large (macro) molecule' and protein molecules are very large in the sense that they contain a large number of atoms. Of course, protein molecules are not large in the ordinary sense of the word, being far smaller than the tiniest grain of sand. In Table 13.14 the numbers of atoms present in the molecules of various substances are listed for comparison.

$$H_2N-\underset{\underset{H}{|}}{\overset{\overset{H}{|}}{C}}-\overset{\overset{O}{\|}}{C}-OH + H-NH-\underset{\underset{H}{|}}{\overset{\overset{H_3C}{|}}{C}}-\overset{\overset{O}{\|}}{C}-OH \longrightarrow H_2N-\underset{\underset{H}{|}}{\overset{\overset{H}{|}}{C}}-\overset{\overset{O}{\|}}{C}-NH-\underset{\underset{H}{|}}{\overset{\overset{H_3C}{|}}{C}}-\overset{\overset{O}{\|}}{C}-OH$$

glycine   alanine   glycylalanine

$$HO-\overset{\overset{O}{\|}}{C}-\underset{\underset{H}{|}}{\overset{\overset{H}{|}}{C}}-NH-H + HO-\overset{\overset{O}{\|}}{C}-\underset{\underset{H}{|}}{\overset{\overset{CH_3}{|}}{C}}-NH_2 \longrightarrow HO-\overset{\overset{O}{\|}}{C}-\underset{\underset{H}{|}}{\overset{\overset{H}{|}}{C}}-NH-\overset{\overset{O}{\|}}{C}-\underset{\underset{H}{|}}{\overset{\overset{CH_3}{|}}{C}}-NH_2$$

glycine   alanine   alanylglycine

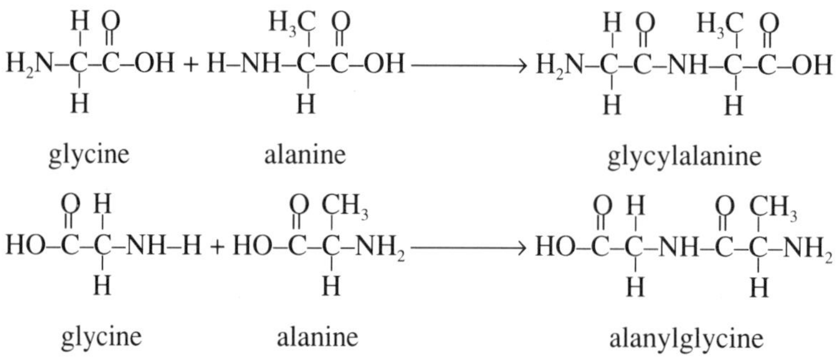

Figure 13.42 *Two dipeptides formed by combination of glycine and alanine*

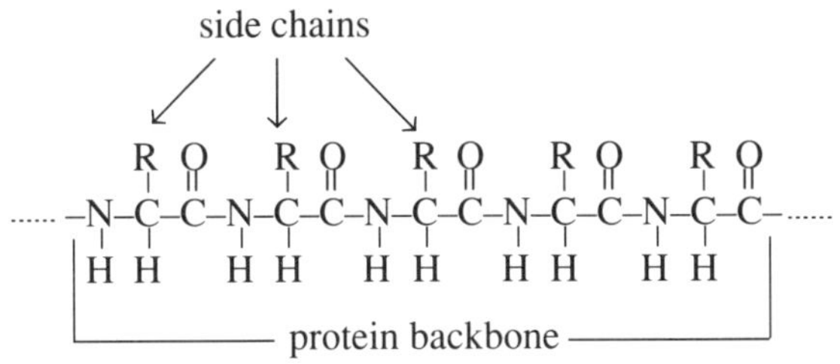

Figure 13.43 *Section of a protein molecule showing the protein backbone and side chains*

Table 13.14 *Numbers of atoms present in molecules of various substances*

oxygen	2
water	3
glucose	24
cholesterol	64
a simple protein	>5000

Proteins make up about 15% of the body's total mass and about 50% of its dry mass. Just on this basis they can be seen to be important, but the *quantity* of protein in our bodies is much less impressive than the *quality* of the functions which they perform while we live. The word protein comes from the Greek word *proteiros* which means 'primary' or 'of first importance' and in the next section we shall see that the proteins have been very aptly named.

13.8.4 *Structure of Proteins*

All proteins have at least three levels to their structure and these are called the **primary structure**, **secondary structure** and **tertiary structure**. There are some proteins which have a fourth level of structure called the **quaternary structure**.

Primary Structure. This is the *number and sequence of amino acid units* in the protein molecule. The primary structure is maintained by the peptide bond which is a strong covalent bond. Consequently, the primary structure is a very robust aspect of protein structure and the most difficult to disrupt. A protein molecule will usually contain more than 50 amino acid units and so a particular amino acid will appear at several different positions in the molecule. Proteins with quite different properties may be very similar in terms of the numbers and types of amino acid which are present in their molecules. This is possible because the properties of a protein depend on the sequence in which amino acid units join to each other. An analogy can be made here with the sequencing of letters in words. One sequence of the letters d, e, o, p and t produces the meaningful sequence 'depot' while another produces the equally meaningful, but quite different, sequence 'opted'.

Primary structure is determined by using chemical reagents and enzymes which break the protein chain at known locations. For example, a chemical procedure called the 'Edman Degradation' removes only the amino acid at that end of the protein chain where the $–NH_2$ group of an amino acid remains free. This procedure allows the amino acid units of a protein chain to be removed from one end of the protein, one at a time. As each amino acid is removed, it is identified and the sequence of the amino acid units in the protein chain (that is, the primary structure) is revealed. The enzymes **trypsin** and **chymotrypsin** are also useful in primary structure determination. Trypsin breaks protein chains only at positions where either arginine or lysine is present. Chymotrypsin breaks the chains only where phenylalanine or tyrosine is present.

A protein's primary structure determines what its secondary and tertiary structures will be and the functions which it will be able to perform. In some cases a protein may be largely unaffected by small changes in its primary structure and this is so with insulin which has the primary structure shown in Figure 13.44. The insulin molecule consists of two amino acid chains which are joined together by –S–S– (disulphide) 'bridges' between cysteine units in each chain. In Figure 13.44 the two chains are labelled A and B and within each chain the amino acids are numbered from one end of the chain to the other.

Insulin is a **hormone** (a substance having a regulatory effect on the activities of cells or organs) produced in the **pancreas**. It regulates the concentration of glucose in blood by facilitating its transport into cells where it can be used, and by promoting its conversion to glycogen which can be stored in the liver and in muscle tissue. *Diabetes mellitus* is caused by the failure of a person's pancreas to produce sufficient insulin. Prior to 1921 the disease was always fatal, but in that year the Canadian scientists Frederick Banting and Charles Best discovered insulin in extracts obtained from the pancreatic tissue of dogs. They were able to show that pancreatic extracts from several domestic animals could be used to control *diabetes mellitus* in humans. This was very fortunate because a large quantity of these extracts could be obtained using the

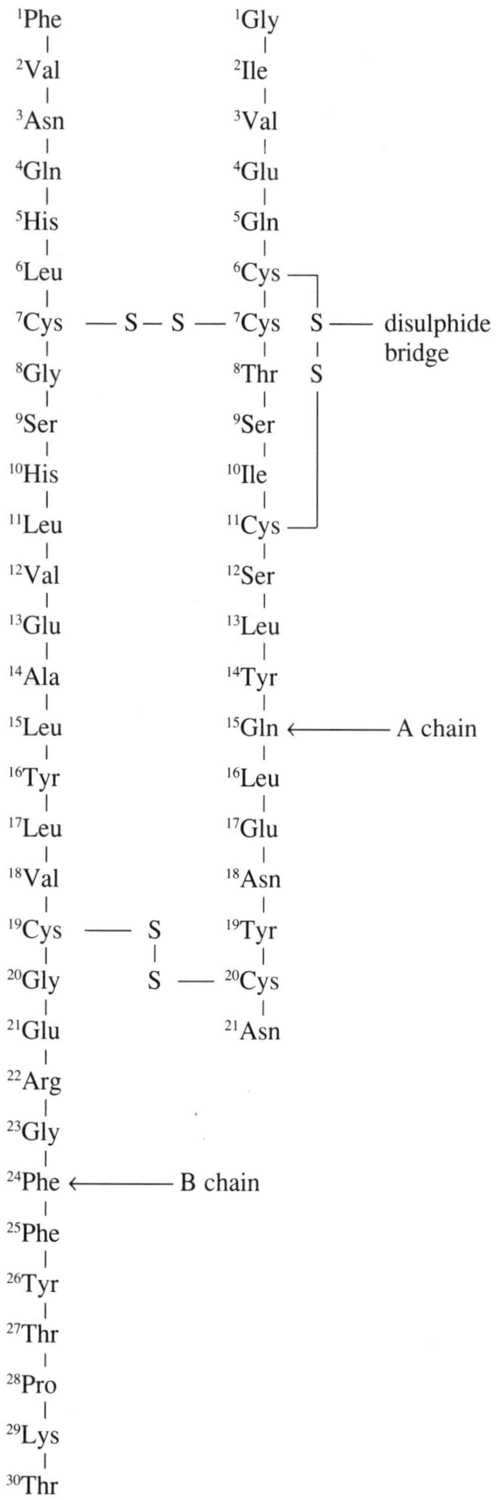

Figure 13.44 *Primary structure of insulin (human)*

pancreatic tissue of the millions of domestic animals which were being slaughtered each year for food. For his work on insulin, Banting shared the 1923 Nobel Prize in Medicine and Physiology with another scientist, John Macleod. In a controversial decision, Best was not included in the award.

Insulin was used for the control of *diabetes mellitus* for many years prior to the determination of its primary structure by Frederick Sanger. Although insulin is a relatively simple protein the task occupied Sanger and his co-workers for 10 years and earned him the Nobel Prize for Chemistry in 1958. It is now known that animal insulins differ slightly from each other, and from human insulin, in their primary structures. The differences, which occur at positions 8–10 in chain A and position 30 in chain B, are summarised in Table 13.15.

Table 13.15 *Differences in primary structure between human and animal insulins*

Type of insulin	Chain A 8	Chain A 9	Chain A 10	Chain B 30
human	Thr	Ser	Ile	Thr
cattle	Ala	Ser	Val	Ala
pig	Thr	Ser	Ile	Ala
sheep	Ala	Gly	Val	Ala

Animal insulins are not quite as effective as human insulin and some people become allergic to insulin from one type of animal but can then switch to insulin of another type without suffering the same allergic response. These observations show that the differences in primary structure do have some effect on the properties of animal insulins but not enough to prevent them from being useful in the treatment of *diabetes mellitus*. This is very fortunate because chemical synthesis of human insulin could not have been attempted until its primary structure had been determined. This would have delayed the availability of an effective therapy for years while the structure was worked out and a synthetic method devised. In any event, therapy based on synthetic insulin would have been far more expensive and, therefore, less readily available to many diabetics.

Small differences in protein structure are not always as benign as those which exist between the different types of insulin. The human protein

haemoglobin, which plays a vital role in oxygen transport in the body, contains 574 amino acid molecules joined in four chains. Some people have an inherited condition causing them to produce haemoglobin in which the amino acid valine replaces glutamic acid at just two positions in the haemoglobin molecule. This small change in primary structure has the effect of causing red blood cells to change shape when the oxygen concentration in the blood falls. The change in shape alters the flow characteristics of blood and leads to the blockage of small blood vessels. The cells blocking these vessels are destroyed by the body's defense mechanisms and **anaemia** (reduced number of red blood cells) results. The consequences of this anaemia, and other effects associated with the condition, are severe and people affected have a dramatically reduced chance of living into adulthood. The disease is called **sickle cell anaemia** because the red blood cells have a sickle shape rather the normal doughnut shape (see Figure 13.45).

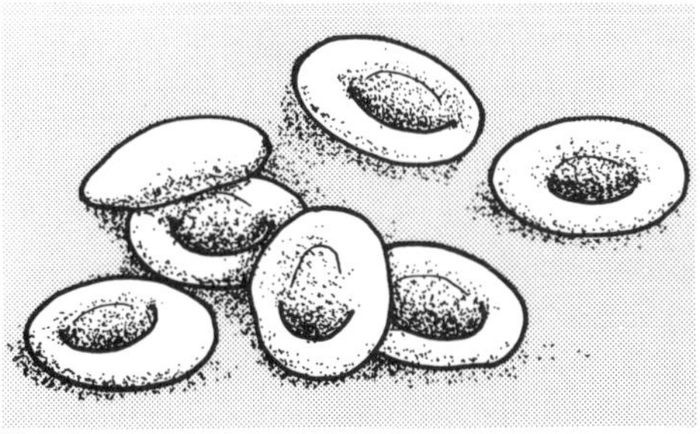

(a)

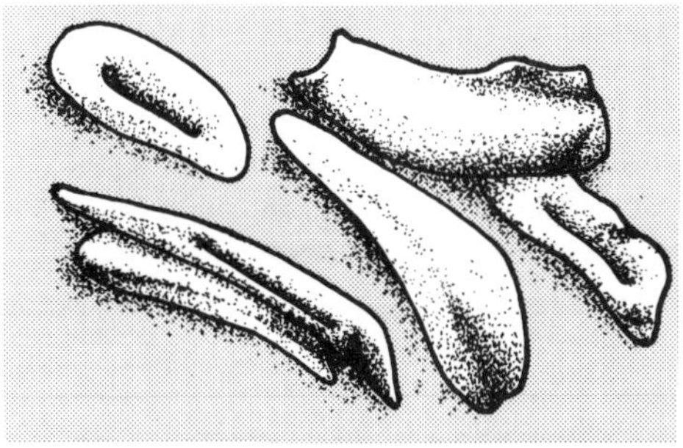

(b)

Figure 13.45 *(a) Normal and (b) sickle red blood cells*

Secondary Structure. Protein molecules are so large that different parts of the same molecule are capable of interacting with each other. When these interactions produce a repeating pattern in some sections of the protein chain it is said to have a secondary structure. The most common type of repeating pattern is the ***α*–helix** which is illustrated in Figure 13.46.

A secondary structure may not exist in some sections of a protein molecule. These sections are called **random coils** and the diagram in Figure 13.46 shows a random coil section of a protein molecule adjacent to a section having the *α*–helix structure.

In those sections of a protein molecule where the *α*–helix structure exists it is maintained by hydrogen bonds which form between $-\overset{|}{N}-H$ groups in amino acid units in one coil of the helix and $-\overset{O}{\overset{\|}{C}}-$ groups in the adjacent coils. These groups are found in nearly every amino acid unit along the protein molecule and so it is possible for a large number of hydrogen bonds to exist between adjacent coils.

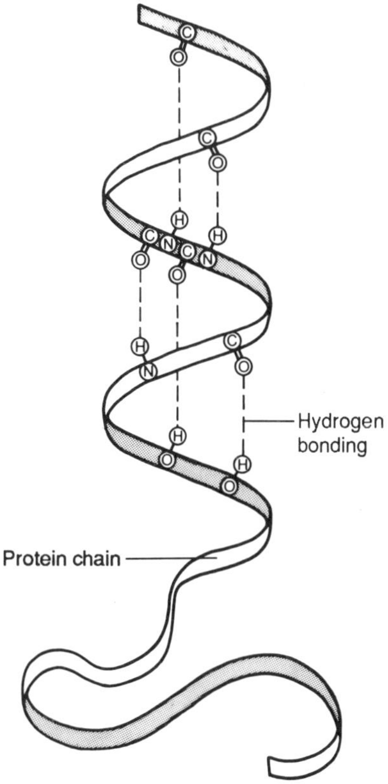

Figure 13.46 *Secondary structure of a protein: α–helix and random coil*

Hydrogen bonds are nowhere near as strong as covalent bonds and so the secondary features of protein structure are much more delicate and more prone to disruption than the primary structure. This is an important point to remember when we consider the function of proteins.

Even when we have specified the primary and secondary structures of a protein we have not said all that there is to say about its structure. Knowing the primary and secondary structure of a protein only permits us to say how a particular section of the protein molecule is related to other sections nearby. For example, in insulin we know from the primary structure that in chain B, at position 8, we will find the amino acid unit glycine sitting between cysteine in position 7 and serine in position 9. We can be confident that these amino acid units will always be very close to the glycine unit since each is held tightly to it by a peptide bond. However, as we move further away from position 8 in chain B we know less and less about the position which amino acid units occupy relative to the glycine unit. The proline unit at position 28 in chain B may be a long way away or it might be quite close if the chain of amino acid units has looped back upon itself.

If we know that a protein has a region of α–helix as its secondary structure then we know something about the way in which any sequence of several amino acids is positioned in relation to the sequences located on either side in the primary structure. Such sequences will be part of adjacent coils of the α–helix. However, it is once again the case that we cannot say much about the way in which amino acid units widely separated in the primary structure are located in relation to each other. This brings us to the next aspect of protein structure.

Tertiary Structure. This refers to the folding and bending of the protein's amino acid chain due to interactions between amino acid units which may be quite widely separated in the protein's primary structure. The tertiary structure of a protein is a complete three-dimensional description of the spatial arrangement of all its amino acid units.

The interactions which maintain the tertiary structure of a protein are: **covalent bonds, hydrogen bonds, ionic bonds** and **hydrophobic bonds.** The most common type of covalent bond contributing to the tertiary structure of a protein is the disulphide bond (–S–S–). It forms between the –SH (thiol) groups of cysteine (see Table 13.12 for the structural formula of cysteine) as shown in Figure 13.47.

If you look back to Figure 13.44 you will see that disulphide bonds hold the two chains of the insulin molecule together. This severely restricts their ability to move independently of each other and increases the opportunity for hydrogen bonds to form within and between them.

The hydrogen bonds contributing to tertiary structure are different to those involved in secondary structures in the sense that they operate between polar groups of atoms in side chains of the amino acid units rather than between the –N–H and –C=O groups in the backbone of the protein molecule. For example, the side chains of serine, glutamic acid and lysine contain the alcohol, carboxylic acid and amine groups respectively. All of these are capable of forming hydrogen bonds with each other.

The ionic bonds which contribute to the maintenance of a protein's tertiary structure arise as a result of the ionisation of amine and carboxylic acid groups in the side chains of the protein. This is shown in Figure 13.48. The oppositely charged groups which form attract each other and this helps maintain the protein's tertiary structure. The proportion of amine and carboxylic acid groups which are ionised is very much dependent on the pH of the protein's environment. As pH rises more carboxylic acid groups and fewer amine groups will be ionised. As pH falls the reverse applies.

Some amino acids have side chains which are distinctly non-polar. These include alanine and valine

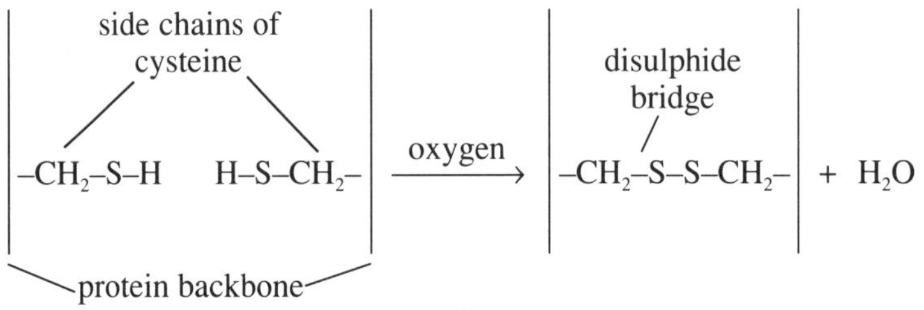

Figure 13.47 *Formation of the disulphide bond in proteins*

$$-NH_2 + H_3O^+ \rightleftarrows -NH_3^+ + H_2O$$

$$-\overset{\displaystyle O}{\overset{\|}{C}}-OH + OH^- \rightleftarrows -\overset{\displaystyle O}{\overset{\|}{C}}-O^- + H_2O$$

Figure 13.48 *Ionisation of amino and carboxylic groups in protein side chains*

in which the side chains are the methyl (CH_3–) and 2-propyl ($CH_3\overset{|}{C}HCH_3$) radicals respectively. These side chains are incompatible with water (**hydrophobic**) and when a protein contains many of them it adopts a tertiary structure in which they are tucked away inside the space occupied by the protein molecule. This takes them out of contact with the surrounding water and puts them in contact with other similar groups of atoms. We may describe this situation by saying that the protein's tertiary structure is influenced by **hydrophobic bonds** which can be regarded as **forces of repulsion** between the protein's non-polar side chains and the polar water molecules in its environment. Hydrophobic bonds are weaker than hydrogen bonds but in a protein which contains many non-polar side chains their total effect can be very significant in determining the protein's tertiary structure.

The dependence of tertiary structure on the operation of relatively weak hydrogen and hydrophobic bonds ensures that this, like the secondary structure, is a very fragile aspect of protein structure.

Quaternary Structure. Some proteins consist of several polypeptide chains which are not joined by covalent bonds but which, nevertheless, achieve a close association with each other and act as a single unit. Each polypeptide chain has its own primary, secondary and tertiary structures and the relationship which the different polypeptide chains have with each other is called the protein's quaternary structure. An example is haemoglobin, the oxygen transport protein. It contains four polypeptide chains and these must maintain a close association with each other if the protein is to perform its normal functions. Hydrophobic bonds often play a very important role in the maintenance of quaternary structures.

In Table 13.16 a summary is presented of the types of bonds which make a contribution to the different levels of protein structure.

Information about the secondary, tertiary and quaternary structures of proteins cannot be obtained by chemical means. The reason is that these aspects of protein structure are too easily disrupted. The main technique used for the study of secondary, tertiary and quaternary structure is **X-ray crystallography** in which a solid sample of the protein interacts with X-rays. The pattern which the X-rays form as a result of their interaction with the protein can be used to determine the spacing between atoms in the protein molecule.

Table 13.16 *Bonding at different levels of protein structure*

Structure type	Dominant bond types and their origins
primary	covalent bonds between adjacent amino acid units
secondary	hydrogen bonds operating between parts of the protein backbone
tertiary	hydrogen bonds, ionic bonds and hydrophobic bonds operating between side chains of the protein
quaternary	hydrophobic bonds operating between different polypeptide chains

13.8.5 *Functions of Proteins*

Proteins are the most versatile of all the body's chemical components. They play vital roles in maintaining the structure of tissues and in the regulation of the chemical reactions which proceed constantly within tissues.

Proteins and Tissue Structure. The best example of a protein which contributes to tissue structure is **collagen**. This is an insoluble protein which does not become dispersed in water. It makes up about 30% of the protein in the human body and it is found in skin, bone, teeth, cartilage and the tissue making up the large blood vessels. It provides these tissues with strength and elasticity. The effectiveness of collagen as a structural material can be substantially explained by reference to its primary, secondary and tertiary structures.

In the primary structure of collagen about half the amino acid units present are either glycine or proline. If you look back at the structural formulae for these two amino acids in Table 13.12 you will notice that each has a non-polar side chain. In proline this is the set of atoms $-CH_2CH_2CH_2-$ which completes the ring containing the amine group. In glycine it is simply a hydrogen atom. The high proportion of non-polar side chains in collagen reduces its solubility in water, and the ease with which it can be dispersed in water.

The high proportion of proline units in collagen also has an influence on the protein's secondary structure. This influence is due to the fact that proline is the only common amino acid which has its amine group locked into a ring system (see Table 13.12). This restricts the flexibility of protein chains in those regions where proline units are located and the relatively large number of these units which are present in collagen chains prevent the formation of the α–helix secondary structure. Instead, collagen adopts a secondary structure in which three polypeptide chains wind round each other to form what is called a **triple helix**. The three chains are held in position by hydrogen bonding between their backbones as shown in Figure 13.49.

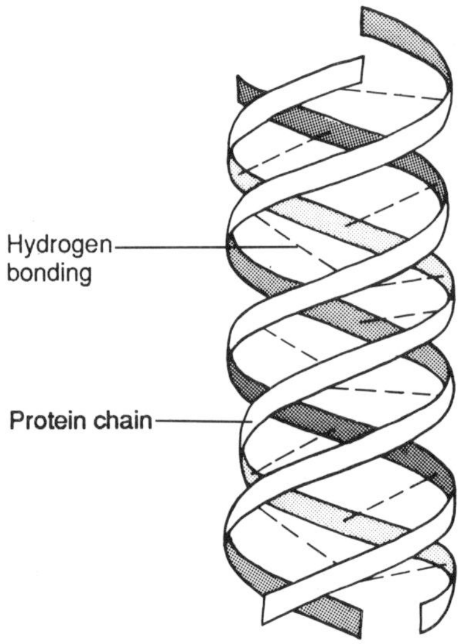

Figure 13.49 *Secondary structure of collagen*

This secondary structure gives collagen a certain amount of elasticity. When a sample of collagen is subjected to a deforming force the hydrogen bonds acting between its polypeptide chains lengthen allowing the collagen molecules, and the sample, to stretch. When the force is removed the hydrogen bonds restore the collagen molecules, and the sample, to their original conditions.

To explain the strength of collagen we must refer to its tertiary structure which consists of triple helices joined together by covalent bonds. However, these are not disulphide bonds. Collagen contains no cysteine and therefore cannot form disulphide bonds. Instead, covalent bonds form between the side chains of lysine units. This creates a structure which is able to withstand the effects of quite strong deforming forces without being torn apart or permanently deformed.

Collagen and Ageing. As a person grows older,the extent of covalent bonding between triple helices of the collagen molecule increases. This leads to a more and more rigid tertiary structure for the protein and less and less flexibility for the tissues of which it is a part. This contributes to the steady deterioration, with age, of skin, blood vessels, ligaments and tendons.

There are other structural proteins and they include **myosin** which is a component of muscle tissue and **keratin** which is found in hair and nails.

Proteins and Chemical Change in the Body: Enzymes. One of the most remarkable things about the human body is that it is the site of seething chemical activity. This chemical activity is remarkable first for its complexity: hundreds of different reactions proceed simultaneously without interfering with one another. It is also remarkable for the fact that it proceeds at 37 °C (body temperature) and at pH = 7.4 which is very close to neutral. These conditions are mild when compared to those which must often be used to bring about the same chemical change outside the body. A good illustration of this point is provided by the conversion of **starch** into **glucose**. Outside the body, this requires the starch to be heated with a strong acid solution, but the same change begins to occur as soon as starch is placed in the mouth and makes contact with saliva.

$$\text{Starch outside the body} \xrightarrow[\text{high temperature}]{\text{strongly acidic solution}} \text{glucose}$$

$$\text{starch in the mouth} \xrightarrow[\text{body temperature (37 °C)}]{\text{weakly acidic solution}} \text{glucose}$$

The great ease with which chemical reactions occur in the body is due to the action of **enzymes**. These are proteins (or partly proteins) which act as **catalysts** for the reactions. *A catalyst is a substance which alters the rate of a chemical reaction without being permanently affected itself.* The substance which the catalyst causes to undergo a chemical reaction is called the **substrate**.

Catalysts are very common outside living things and are widely used to increase the rates of chemical reactions used for synthesis of new chemicals, or to obtain energy. These catalysts differ from enzymes in that they are far less selective. For example, a catalyst often used for chemical synthesis is finely divided platinum metal. It facilitates the addition of hydrogen (H_2) to alkenes.

$$\underset{\text{alkene}}{\text{R–CH=CH–R}} \quad + \quad \underset{\text{hydrogen}}{H_2} \quad \xrightarrow[\text{catalyst}]{\text{platinum}} \quad \underset{\text{alkane}}{\text{R–CH}_2\text{–CH}_2\text{–R}}$$

However, platinum metal will not just facilitate the addition of hydrogen to alkenes. It also facilitates addition to ketone, aldehyde and other unsaturated functional groups. Platinum metal also acts over very wide ranges of temperature and solution composition. This tendency to facilitate a reaction for a wide range of different substrates and act over a wide range of conditions is typical of many catalysts found in the non-living world and they are said to be **non-specific** catalysts. In contrast to this, enzymes, the catalysts of the living world, are highly specific. Each enzyme catalyses the reaction of only one substrate, or a limited range of similar substrates, and it will only function effectively within restricted ranges of temperature, pH and solution concentration.

Just as we were able to explain the effectiveness of collagen as a structural protein by referring to its structure, so the characteristics of enzymes may also be accounted for in terms of protein structure.

Mechanism of Enzyme Action. The proteins which act as enzymes are usually **globular proteins**. In these proteins significant numbers of both polar and non-polar side chains are present. This causes them to adopt tertiary structures in which the non-polar side chains are tucked away inside the space which the protein occupies while the polar side chains sit on the outside of this space. The tertiary structure of a globular protein is illustrated in Figure 13.50.

When globular proteins are present in aqueous systems their polar side chains are able to exert forces of attraction on water molecules and this allows the protein to dissolve or become dispersed throughout the system. This in itself is useful because it allows an enzyme to be transported throughout the body via the circulation. However, the critical feature of protein structure as far as enzyme action is concerned is that every enzyme has an active site. This is a region within the protein where some set of atoms adopts a very

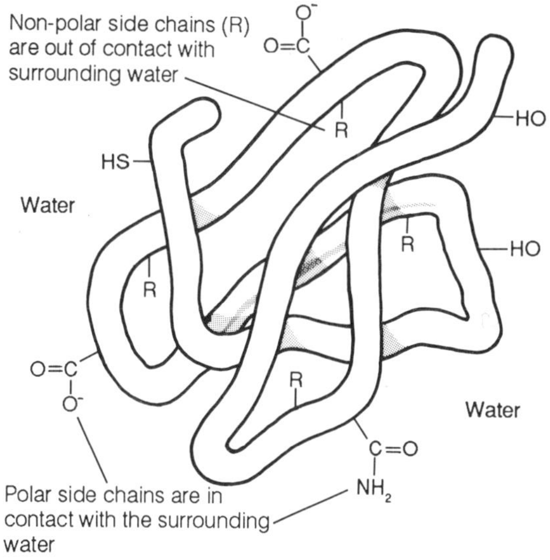

Figure 13.50 *Tertiary structure of a globular protein*

precise spatial arrangement. This spatial arrangement matches the shape of substrate molecules for the enzyme. Furthermore, atoms at the active site exert forces of attraction on the substrate molecules, causing them to become closely associated with that region of the protein. This combination of substrate and protein is referred to as the **enzyme–substrate complex** and its formation is illustrated in Figure 13.51.

Once an enzyme–substrate complex has formed, the substrate becomes very prone to conversion into

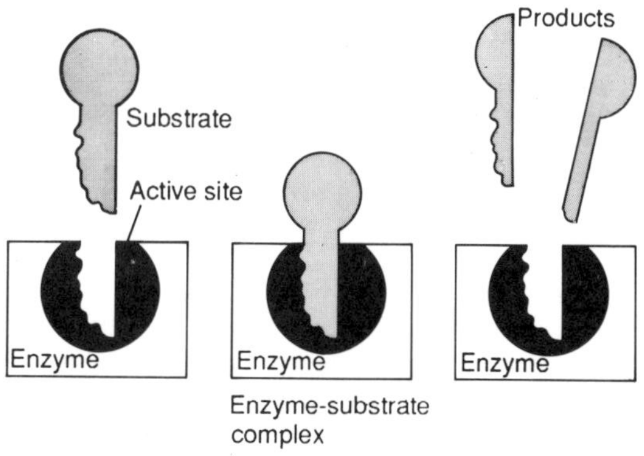

Figure 13.51 *Formation of an enzyme–substrate complex*

products. This is usually explained by saying that the substrate's interaction with the enzyme has the effect of stretching and weakening crucial bonds within the substrate molecule which then break, leading to the formation of the product. Once formed, the product moves away from the active site of the enzyme, making it available for another substrate molecule. All of this has no permanent effect on the enzyme itself which simply goes on converting one substrate molecule after another into product.

This account of the way in which enzymes work is known as the **lock and key theory** of enzyme action. The lock is the active site of the enzyme and the key is the substrate molecule. Just as a key must have the right shape to fit the lock which it opens, so the substrate must have the right shape to fit the active site of its enzyme. Another related, but more sophisticated, model of enzyme action is the **induced fit** or **hand-in-glove** model. According to this model, the active site has a flexible shape which alters during formation of the enzyme–substrate complex in much the same way as the shape of a glove alters to that of the hand on which it is worn (see Figure 13.52)

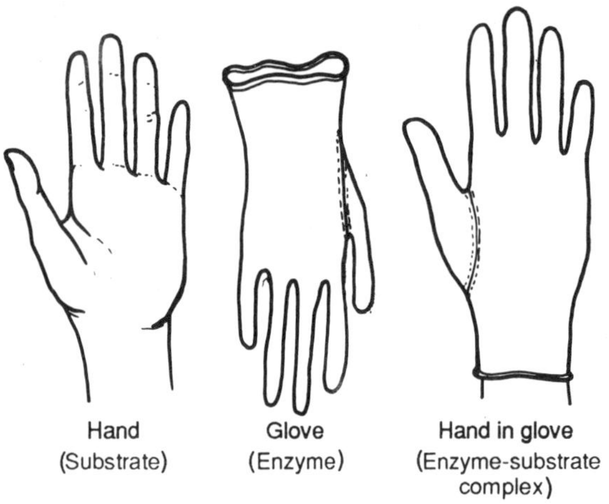

Figure 13.52 *Hand-in-glove model of enzyme action*

The essential feature of both these models of enzyme action is that an active site exists within the protein molecule. This idea requires some set of atoms within the protein to be maintained in a well-defined relationship to each other. It is an idea n very nicely with our knowledge that e well-defined tertiary structures in which many parts of the protein chain are held in close proximity to each other.

Cofactors and Coenzymes. While some proteins are capable of acting as enzymes entirely in their own right, others can only do so if they join with other molecules or ions. These other molecules or ions are called **cofactors**. Some cofactors are simple metal ions such as Fe^{2+} or Mg^{2+}. Other cofactors may be quite complex organic molecules and these are called **coenzymes**. Coenzymes are often vitamins. For example, the vitamins thiamine, riboflavin and niacin are all coenzymes.

Naming of Enzymes. Some enzymes are known by names given to them by their discoverers. These common names usually say nothing about the function of the enzyme and some examples are trypsin, rennin and pepsin. All these enzymes catalyse the hydrolysis of peptide groups in proteins and they differ from one another in that they hydrolyse peptide groups formed by the combination of different pairs of amino acids.

Most enzymes are named systematically and these names always have the ending 'ase'. The rest of the name is derived from the type of reaction which the enzyme catalyses or the identity of the substrate on which it acts. For example, the enzymes **urease** and **sucrase** act upon the substrates urea and sucrose respectively. The enzyme **monoamine oxidase** catalyses the oxidation of amines. The enzymes trypsin, rennin and pepsin are all **peptidases** if named on this basis.

13.8.6 *Denaturation of Proteins*

When a protein loses its capacity to perform its normal biological function it is said to have been **denatured**. The common agents responsible for denaturation are:

heat
change in pH
presence of detergents
presence of heavy metal salts
presence of hydrogen bonding compounds

The proteins most susceptible to denaturation are those which are dissolved or dispersed in water and this includes many proteins which act as enzymes. Denaturation is another phenomenon which is readily understood in terms of protein structure. Its cause is always disruption of the protein's secondary, tertiary or quaternary structures and each of the denaturing agents listed above achieves this disruption in ways which are quite easily understood.

Denaturation by Heat. In any system, as the temperature increases, the constituent atoms and molecules move more and more violently. The secondary, tertiary and quaternary structures of proteins are substantially maintained by relatively weak hydrogen and hydrophobic bonds. Once the temperature of a system which contains proteins has been raised to a temperature of about 50–60 °C the increase in motion of the atoms and molecules in the system is more than sufficient to disrupt the structures of most of the proteins present.

Denaturation by pH Change. Proteins usually have many side chains which are ionised. Carboxylic acid side chains ionise to form negative ions and amine side chains form positive ions. Forces of attraction between these oppositely charged ions are important in the maintenance of tertiary structures. As pH increases the proportion of ionised carboxylic acid side chains will increase and the proportion of ionised amine side chains will decrease. As pH decreases the proportions change in the reverse directions. It is clear that such changes must affect the magnitude of attractive forces acting between many sections of the protein chain and lead to disruption of its tertiary structure.

Denaturing by Detergents. The long non-polar tails of detergent molecules (see Section 6.6 for a description of the nature and mode of action of detergents) interact with the non-polar side chains of protein molecules and disrupt the hydrophobic bonds which help maintain its tertiary structure.

Denaturation by Heavy Metal Salts. Heavy metals may be defined as those having a density in excess of 4 g/ml and they include many of the elements found between Groups IIA and IIIA of the Periodic Table. The best known examples are lead, mercury and cadmium which have notorious reputations as toxic contaminants of the environment. But iron, gold, silver, copper and many other well known and 'respectable' elements are also heavy metals.

In heavy metal salts the metal atoms exist in the form of positively charged ions and in this form they bind tightly to the –SH (thiol) group in the side chain of the amino acid cysteine. They generally bind to more than one cysteine unit and this can have the effect of disrupting a protein's tertiary or secondary structure as cysteine units are pulled out of the positions which they normally occupy.

Denaturation by Hydrogen Bonding Compounds. Many proteins are denatured by the addition of ethanol or urea. These two compounds, which are quite different from each other, do have in common an ability to participate in hydrogen bond formation because of the presence in their molecules of –OH and $-NH_2$ groups respectively.

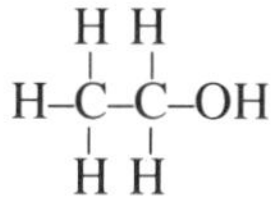

ethanol

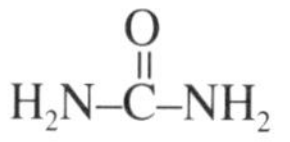

urea

Ethanol and urea (and many other hydrogen bonding compounds) denature protein by forming hydrogen bonds with sections of the protein molecule already participating in the hydrogen bonds responsible for the maintenance of its secondary and tertiary structures. These additional hydrogen bonds are disruptive and so cause denaturation.

No matter which of these agents is responsible for denaturation the most common visual change which occurs is **coagulation**, in which the previously soluble protein precipitates as a solid mass. For example, the protein in an egg coagulates when the egg is boiled or fried. Coagulation occurs because the amino acid chains of the denatured protein unfold and instead of bonds acting within each chain to create the secondary and tertiary structures they act between different chains causing them to form a large, insoluble mass.

Clinical Significance of Protein Denaturation. All the agents of denaturation listed above can be used to destroy or inhibit the growth of microorganisms. Heat, for example, is an infallible disinfectant because at the temperature of a steam autoclave (about 120 °C) all proteins are denatured and no microorganism may live.

The disinfectant properties of ethanol are due to its ability to denature proteins upon which many microorganisms depend for their viability. In desperate situations urine is used to sterilise wounds and its effectiveness is due to the urea which it contains. Very few microorganisms are able to survive in the stomach because the low pH there denatures proteins upon which they depend. The disinfectant properties of soaps and detergents are partly due to protein denaturation.

Heavy metal salts are used as the active ingredients of antiseptic ointments and their effectiveness is due to their ability to denature proteins. However, these preparations must be used with care because they are toxic if absorbed into the circulation. This toxicity is due to denaturation of human proteins.

The denaturation of protein is the basis of the first aid procedure used in cases of acute heavy metal poisoning. In this procedure the person affected is made to drink milk or swallow egg white, both of which are rich in protein. Vomiting is induced soon afterwards. This technique is effective because the protein of the milk or egg white is denatured by the heavy metal salt and coagulates in the stomach. The heavy metal salt is itself deposited from solution as part of the coagulated protein mass and this slows its absorption from the stomach. Vomiting removes the protein mass from the stomach and with it most of the heavy metal salt. This is an important part of the technique because in the absence of vomiting the coagulated protein is digested and the heavy metal salt is released to exert its toxic effects.

13.8.7 *Where Do Proteins Come From?*

Making a dipeptide would seem to be a simple matter. We could just mix two amino acids under the right conditions However, the situation is not as simple as it looks to be at first sight. First of all, two different amino acid units may join in two different ways. So, from glycine and alanine we could get glycylalanine, [gly]–[ala], and alanylglycine, [ala]–[gly]. We could also get [gly]–[gly] and [ala]–[ala]. Even this is not the end of the possibilities because once there is some dipeptide present in the system it could react to form a tripeptide, then a tetrapeptide and so on.

If we wished to prepare a particular tripeptide by simply mixing three amino acids and letting them react there would be many more possibilities for the formation of peptides other than the one in which we were interested. So, we see that making even quite simple peptides is not a simple matter for a chemist forced to work with non-living materials.

These considerations serve to highlight the marvellous control which living tissue is able to exert over the formation of peptide chains. For example, in pancreatic tissue, some mechanism operates to arrange 51 amino acid units in the one particular sequence which occurs in human insulin. It also operates in bone marrow to arrange hundreds of amino acid units in the exact sequences needed for the formation of haemoglobin. At every step in the development of these sequences there is ample opportunity for something to go wrong because a growing polypeptide chain will be in contact with many amino acids in addition to the one which it needs for the next step in its growth. How does a growing protein 'know' that the next amino acid which it needs is (say) lysine and not (say) phenylalanine and how does it stop phenylalanine from 'butting in' in place of lysine when both amino acids are nearby? These questions bring us to consider another great class of biological polymers known as the nucleic acids.

13.9 Nucleic Acids, the Compounds of Inheritance

The body's ability to construct proteins from the jumble of amino acids present in the cytoplasm of cells is rather like the ability of an architect to transform a jumble of wood, masonry, steel and plastic into a great building. Of course, we all know that to do this the architect must have a plan. Likewise, the human body (as well as every other living system) must have a 'plan' for the construction of its proteins. This plan is drawn up in the form of the chemical structures of a class of biological polymers known as the **nucleic acids**. They have this name because they are **acidic** substances found in the **nuclei** of all cells. They are the most important component of the material from which chromosomes and genes are made.

13.9.1 *Nucleic Acids and the Alphabet of Biochemistry*

The alphabet of biochemistry includes three pyrimidine bases, two purine bases, phosphoric acid and ribose. These are the simple units from which nucleic acid polymers are built. There is one additional compound which is a component of many nucleic acids and this is **deoxyribose** which is formed from ribose by the removal of one oxygen atom from its molecule. Ribose and deoxyribose are both members of a class of organic compounds called the **carbohydrates** or **sugars** (see Section 13.10). No nucleic acid contains both ribose and deoxyribose. Likewise, nucleic acids do not contain all three of the pyrimidine bases. If thymine is present then uracil will be absent and vice versa. More will be made of this later when the different classes of nucleic acid are described. Structural formulae for all the simple components of the nucleic acids are shown in Figure 13.53.

In the next few paragraphs we shall simplify the discussion by using the collective term 'base' for all the pyrimidine and purine bases and the collective

Pyrimidine bases

Purine bases

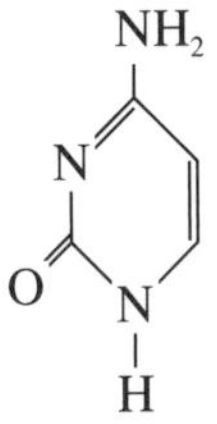

cytosine (C)

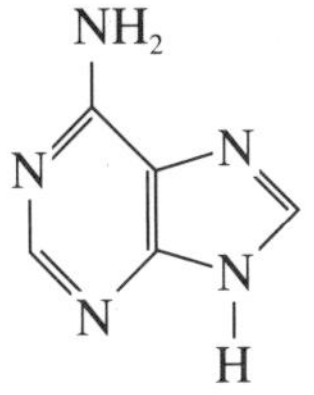

adenine (A)

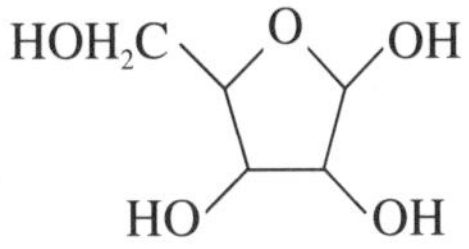

ribose

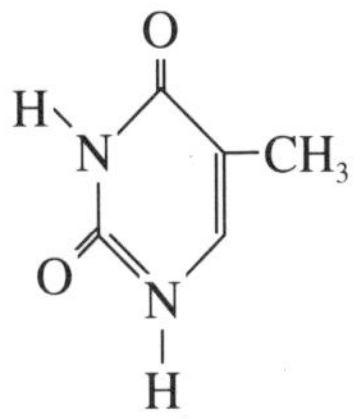

thymine (T)

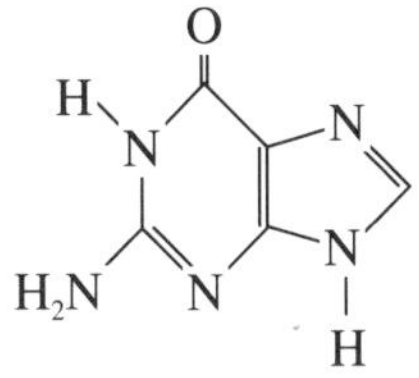

guanine (G)

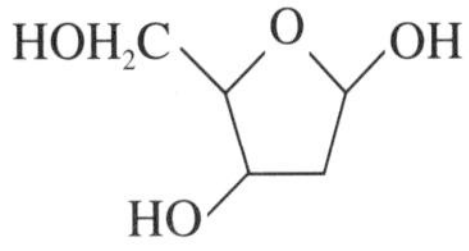

deoxyribose

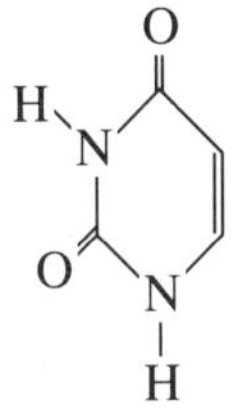

uracil (U)

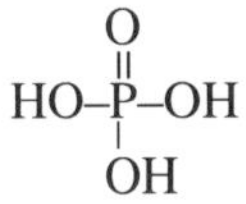

phosphoric acid

Figure 13.53 *Structural formulae for the components of nucleic acids*

term 'sugar' for both ribose and deoxyribose. We shall also make use of the simple diagrams set out in Figure 13.54 to represent base and sugar molecules. It is important to realise that these diagrams do not conform to the rules for writing shorthand representations of structural formulae which have been set out in Section 13.5.

The formation of nucleic acid polymers from base, sugar and phosphoric acid units may be considered to take place in the following stages.

Nucleoside Formation. In this first stage a sugar unit and a base unit join to form a **nucleoside**. This involves the elimination of a water molecule from between the two combining molecules (see Figure 13.55).

Nucleotide Formation. In this next stage nucleosides combine with phosphoric acid via an alcohol group of their sugar component. Once again water is eliminated from between the two combining molecules (see Figure 13.56).

Nucleic Acid Formation. This final stage involves the joining together of many nucleotides. As each nucleotide joins the growing chain a water molecule is eliminated from between a phosphoric acid group in one molecule and an alcohol group in another (see Figure 13.57).

The structure of a nucleic acid may be described by saying that it has a primary structure in which the backbone consists of sugar units joined to each other by phosphoric acid units and in which the side chains consist of base units joined to the sugar units of the backbone. Most of the nucleic acid found in the nuclei of cells contains deoxyribose in its backbone and is called **deoxyribonucleic acid** (DNA).

The secondary structure of DNA consists of two strands of nucleic acid entwined to form a double helix and held in that arrangement by hydrogen bonds which

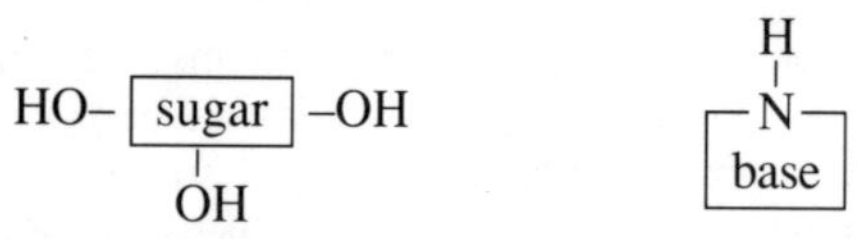

Figure 13.54 *Simple representations for the sugar and base components of nucleic acids*

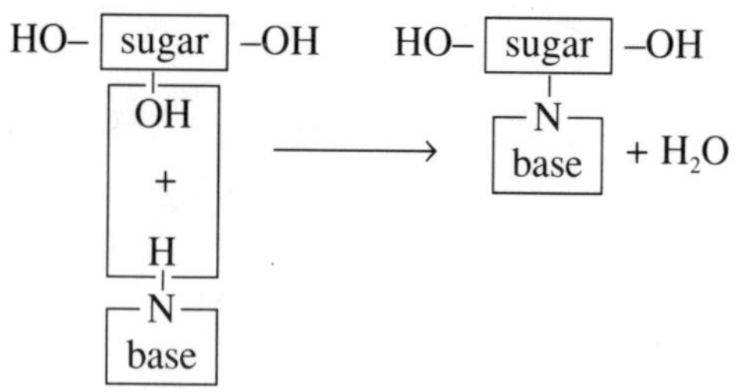

Figure 13.55 *Formation of a nucleoside*

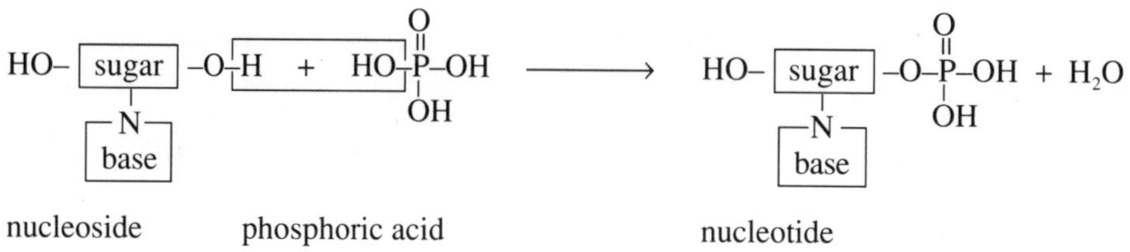

Figure 13.56 *Nucleotide formation*

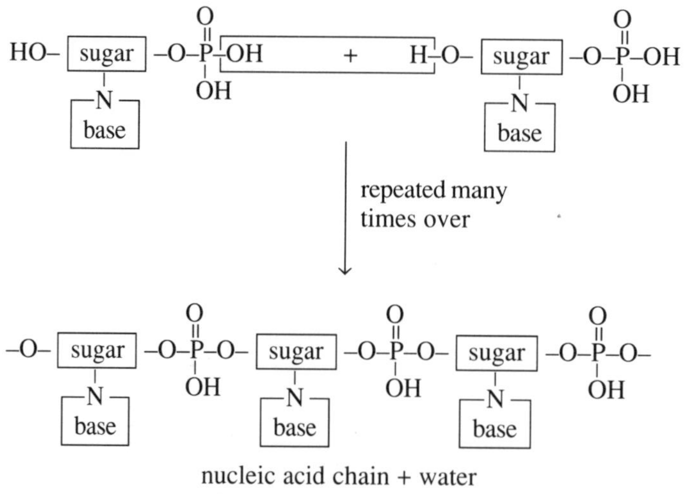

Figure 13.57 *Formation of a nucleic acid chain by combination of nucleotides*

operate between the base side chains of each strand. The double helix structure for DNA (Figure 13.58) was first proposed by James Watson and Francis Crick in 1953. Watson and Crick were led to their famous proposal by the following pieces of evidence:

1. In all DNA the bases thymine and adenine are present in equal numbers and so are cytosine and guanine.
2. DNA molecules are all very long and of the same thickness.
3. The base pairs thymine–adenine and cytosine–guanine are able to form a very effective set of hydrogen bonds with each other. Hydrogen bonding between other base pairs is much less effective.
4. The widths of hydrogen-bonded thymine–adenine pairs and hydrogen-bonded cytosine–guanine

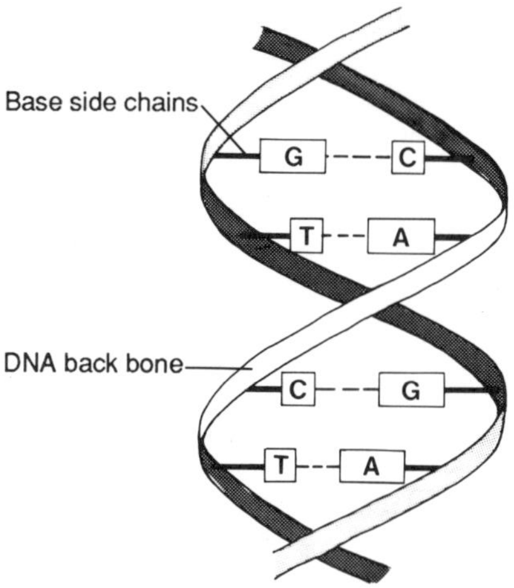

Figure 13.58 *The double helix of DNA*

pairs are about the same as the width of the DNA molecule.

The double helix structure was consistent with all these observations but most important of all it provided an explanation for the ability of DNA to carry the information which an organism needed to reproduce itself and, in particular, to synthesise the thousands of different proteins which it needed. Before Watson and Crick, the great puzzle with DNA was that the compound always consisted of molecules of very similar dimensions. How could such similar molecules carry information so different that in one instance it was used to produce a bacterium while in another it was used to produce a human being?

The answer which Watson and Crick gave to this question was that DNA molecules differed from each other in the *sequencing of base units* along the backbones of the molecules. They proposed that the only restriction on this sequencing was that wherever there was a cytosine unit in one strand of the helix there must be a guanine unit in the corresponding position in the other strand and likewise for the pair of bases thymine–adenine. Alterations in sequencing would make no difference to the general shape of the DNA molecule as long as these restrictions held.

The pairing of bases in the two strands of DNA means that a knowledge of the sequence in one strand can be used to work out the sequence in the other strand and this relationship between the base sequences in the two strands is described by saying that they are **complementary**. This feature of the DNA helix provides the insight needed to understand how organisms are able to reproduce themselves. A DNA molecule may unwind from its double helix structure to form two separate nucleic acid strands. Each of these then serves as the template for the formation of a complementary strand by the combination of individual nucleotides which are available in the vicinity. Each of the original strands and its newly formed complement then wind round each other to form two new DNA molecules which are exactly the same as the original molecule. In this way a new set of DNA molecules becomes available to provide the plan needed to construct another cell and another organism.

The Genetic Code. This is the sequence of base units along the backbone of the DNA molecule. The component parts of the code consist of sequences of three bases and these sequences are called **codons**. There are 64 possible codons (four objects can be lined up in 64 different sequences of three) and the genetic code makes use of all of them. Sixty-one of the codons code for the 20 amino acids found in protein and the other three code for termination of the growing protein chain. Since there are only 20 amino acids and 61 codons it is clear that a particular amino acid may have more than one codon and this feature of the genetic code is described by saying that it is **degenerate**. However, there is no single codon which codes for more than one amino acid and so there is no ambiguity in the code. A DNA molecule always knows what it is supposed to do next!

A complete list of the codons of the genetic code is given in Table 13.17. You will notice that thymine (T) is not part of any codon and this is explained below.

DNA is located inside the nucleus and yet protein synthesis occurs outside the nucleus in structures called **ribosomes**. Clearly, there must be some way in which the information needed to construct a protein is carried from DNA in the nucleus to the ribosomes. This involves a nucleic acid in which deoxyribose is replaced by ribose. This nucleic acid is called **ribonucleic acid** (RNA). As well as containing ribose instead of deoxyribose, RNA also contains uracil in place of thymine and it is a single-stranded molecule. RNA synthesis is controlled by DNA. The DNA strands separate and serve as a template for the synthesis of complementary RNA strands. In this way the RNA acquires the information contained in the section of DNA from which it formed. However, where thymine units were present in the DNA molecule uracil units will appear in the corresponding positions of the RNA molecule. Since it is RNA and not DNA which has a direct role in protein synthesis amino acid codons include uracil but not thymine.

Table 13.17 *Codons of the genetic code*

Codon	Amino acid	Codon	Amino acid	Codon	Amino acid	Codon	Amino acid
UUU	Phe	UCU	Ser	UAU	Tyr	UGU	Cys
UUC	Phe	UCC	Ser	UAC	Tyr	UGC	Cys
UAA	Leu	UCA	Ser	UAA	Stop	UGA	Stop
UUG	Leu	UCG	Ser	UAG	Stop	UGG	Trp
CUU	Leu	CCU	Pro	CAU	His	CGU	Arg
CUC	Leu	CCC	Pro	CAC	His	CGC	Arg
CUA	Leu	CCA	Pro	CAA	Gln	CGA	Arg
CUG	Leu	CCG	Pro	CAG	Gln	CGG	Arg
AUU	Ile	ACU	Thr	AAU	Asn	AGU	Ser
AUC	Ile	ACC	Thr	AAC	Asn	AGC	Ser
AUA	Ile	ACA	Thr	AAA	Lys	AGA	Arg
AUG	Met	ACG	Thr	AAG	Lys	AGG	Arg
GUU	Val	GCU	Ala	GAU	Asp	GGU	Gly
GUC	Val	GCC	Ala	GAC	Asp	GGC	Gly
GUA	Val	GCA	Ala	GAA	Glu	GGA	Gly
GUG	Val	GCG	Ala	GAG	Glu	GGG	Gly

There are three different types of RNA. **Messenger RNA** (mRNA) carries the information needed for the synthesis of proteins to the ribosomes which are the sites of protein synthesis. The ribosomes consist of 35% protein and 65% RNA. This RNA is simply called **ribosomal RNA** (rRNA) and, of all nucleic acids, its function is least well understood. Finally, there is **transfer RNA** (tRNA) each molecule of which has a particular amino acid attached to it. Each molecule of tRNA also carries a set of three bases which are complementary to those making up the codon for its amino acid on molecules of mRNA. This set of bases on the tRNA molecule is called an **anticodon** and it is located in such a position within the tRNA molecule as to facilitate its attachment to molecules of mRNA.

The synthesis of a protein involves the following steps.

1. In the nucleus, that section of a DNA molecule which contains the information needed to construct the protein unwinds from the double helix arrangement and serves as a template for synthesis of a mRNA molecule in which the information is copied as a complementary base sequence. In ordinary language the process of making a copy of something is called **transcription** and the term is also used for this first stage of protein synthesis.
2. The mRNA molecule diffuses out of the nucleus and arrives at a ribosome.
3. At the ribosome tRNA molecules attach themselves to mRNA molecules in a sequence governed by the sequence of bases present in the mRNA molecule. These tRNA molecules are carrying amino acid units and in every case the amino acid unit is the one which is coded for at that position on the mRNA molecule. In this way amino acid units are lined up in accord with the 'instructions' laid down in the DNA of the nucleus. Another way of describing this situation is to say that tRNA is responsible for 'translating' the language of DNA into the language of proteins. Consequently, this stage of protein synthesis is called **translation**.
4. Amino acid units attached to adjacent tRNA molecules join together and the protein forms.

These different stages in protein synthesis are represented diagrammatically in Figure 13.59.

13.10 Carbohydrates

These compounds contain only the elements carbon, hydrogen and oxygen. Many of them have hydrogen and oxygen atoms present in their molecules in the ratio 2 : 1 which is the same as the ratio of these atoms in water. This is the origin of the term carbohydrate which literally means 'hydrate of carbon'. The formulae for glucose ($C_6H_{12}O_6$) and sucrose ($C_{12}H_{22}O_{11}$) conform to this definition of carbohydrate but there are

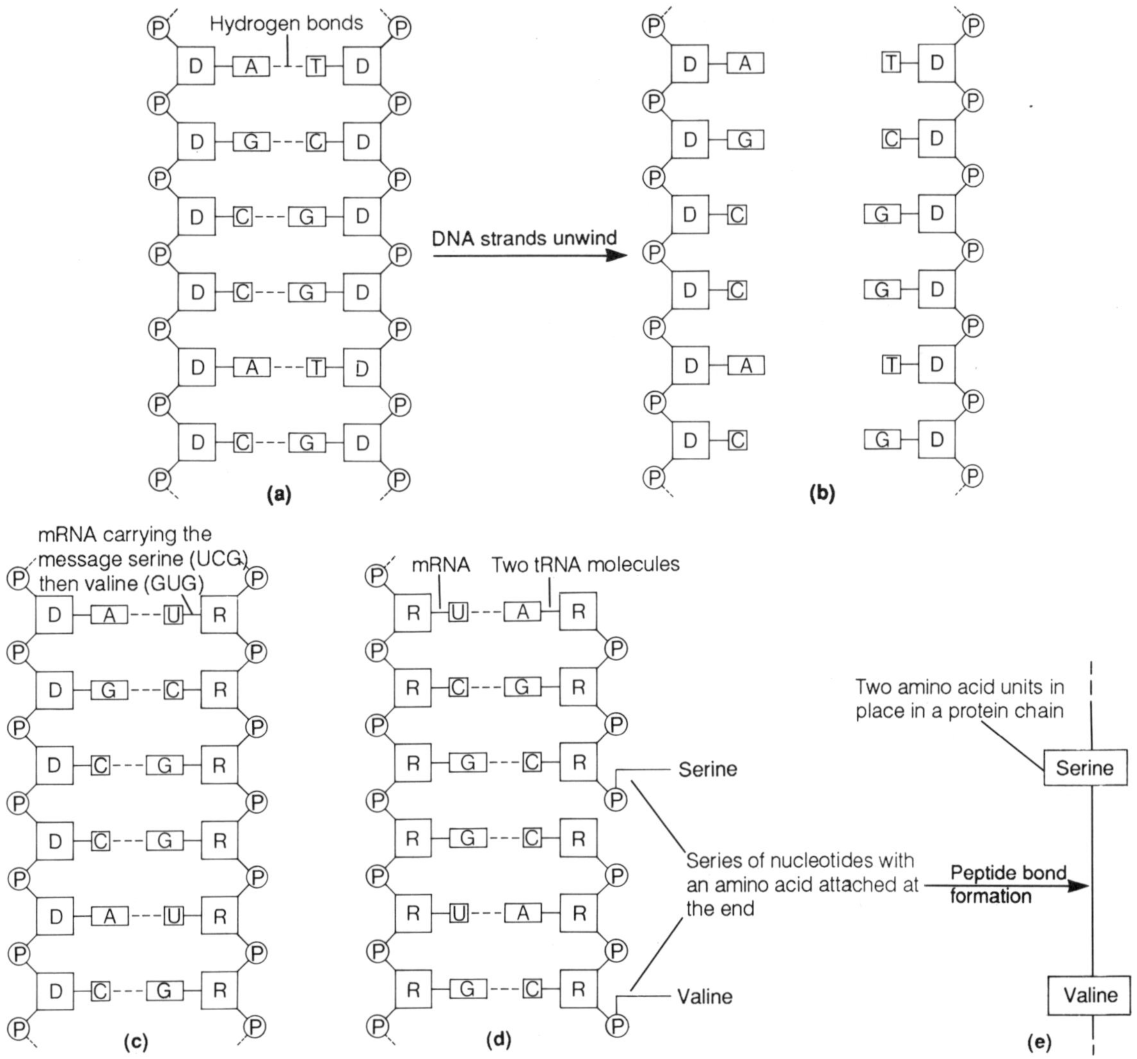

(a) ⟶ (b) The unwinding of complementary strands making up the gene for synthesis of a particular protein.

(b) ⟶ (c) **Transcription**. A single DNA strand serves as the template for formation of mRNA.

(c) → (d) → (e) **Translation**. tRNA molecules line up in position alongside the mRNA molecule. Each tRNA carries an amino acid and, in this way, amino acids are lined up in the sequence required for the formation of the protein which was coded for in the DNA represented in (a).

Figure 13.59 *DNA and protein synthesis*

compounds which do not contain hydrogen and oxygen atoms in the ratio 2:1 which, nevertheless, behave like carbohydrates. An example is the compound **rhamnose**, which has the formula $C_6H_{12}O_5$. There are also compounds which are certainly not carbohydrates which do contain hydrogen and oxygen atoms in the ratio 2:1. An example is acetic acid, $C_2H_4O_2$.

A more satisfactory definition for the carbohydrates is that they are *polyhydroxy aldehydes or ketones or substances which form these compounds on hydrolysis.* By looking at the structural formulae for glucose and fructose in Figure 13.60 you will be able to see that glucose and ribose are polyhydroxy aldehydes while fructose is a polyhydroxy ketone (if you can't then you should refer back to Section 13.6.5 in which aldehydes and ketones are described).

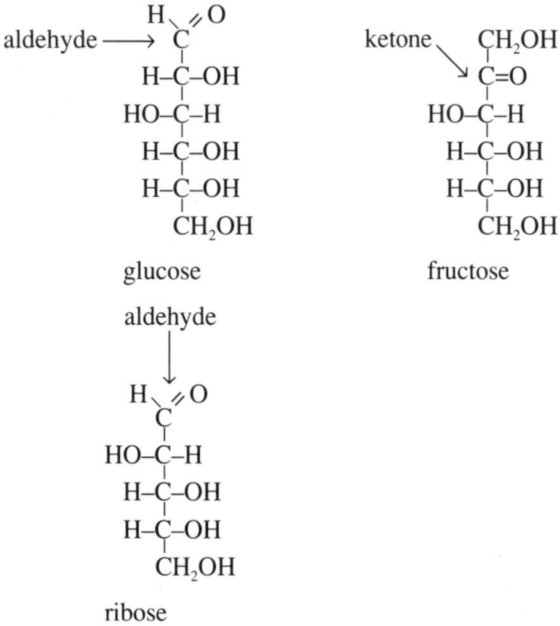

Figure 13.60 *Structural formulae for glucose, fructose and ribose*

You may have noticed that the structural formula given in Figure 13.60 for ribose is different to that given in Figure 13.53 where it was represented as a cyclic molecule. The cyclic structure forms as a result of a reaction between the aldehyde portion of the molecule and one of its alcohol groups. This is actually very common among carbohydrate molecules and many of them exist in cyclic form. In solution this form is in equilibrium with the open chain form. It is usually the cyclic form which predominates.

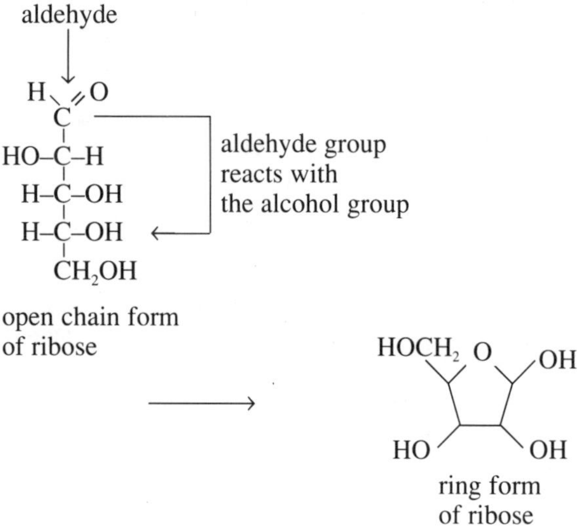

Figure 13.61 *Open chain and ring form of ribose*

The definition of carbohydrates includes compounds which can be converted into polyhydroxy aldehydes or ketones by hydrolysis. This is necessary because carbohydrate molecules commonly join with each other, by the elimination of water, to form more complex molecules in which the aldehyde and ketone groups are no longer present. This combination is reversed by hydrolysis. Thus, the compound sucrose does not have either an aldehyde or ketone group in its molecule but when subjected to hydrolysis it produces both glucose and fructose and so is a carbohydrate in terms of the definition given above.

$$\underset{\text{sucrose}}{C_{12}H_{22}O_{11}} + H_2O \longrightarrow \underset{\text{glucose}}{C_6H_{12}O_6} + \underset{\text{fructose}}{C_6H_{12}O_6}$$

13.10.1 *Classes of Carbohydrates*

There are three main classes of carbohydrates and they differ from each other in the complexity of their molecules. In order of increasing complexity, these are known as **monosaccharides**, **disaccharides** and **polysaccharides**.

Monosaccharides are carbohydrates which cannot be converted into simpler forms by hydrolysis. They are often called **simple sugars** and the most important examples are glucose, fructose and ribose. The importance of glucose and fructose is due to their involvement in **glycolysis**, the process by which the body obtains its energy. Glucose is a component of many solutions used in intravenous therapy. Ribose is important because it is a component of the nucleotides from which nucleic acids are constructed.

Disaccharides are carbohydrates formed when two monosaccharide molecules join together. This joining occurs by the elimination of water from between the two monosaccharide molecules. The most important disaccharides are **maltose**, **sucrose** and **lactose**. In maltose two molecules of glucose are joined together. Sucrose forms by the combination of glucose and fructose, while lactose is formed from the combination of galactose and glucose. Sucrose is one of the most commonly occurring carbohydrates and it is produced commercially from the sugar cane and sugar beet plants. Lactose is a component of breast milk of which it constitutes about 5% by weight.

Properties of Monosaccharides and Disaccharides. These compounds usually have high melting points and high solubilities in water. This is consistent with them being compounds which have large numbers of hydroxyl groups in their molecules. These groups allow them to participate in extensive hydrogen bond formation with water and with themselves.

Many monosaccharides and some disaccharides are sweet tasting. For this reason, as well as for their intrinsic food value, they are consumed in great quantities in food and drink. Common table sugar is pure sucrose while many sweets and soft drinks contain glucose.

An important difference between monosaccharides and disaccharides is that monosaccharides are able to pass through biological membranes whereas disaccharides cannot. The monosaccharides present in food and drink can be absorbed immediately into the circulation but disaccharides must first of all be broken down by hydrolysis.

In polysaccharides there are many (up to a million) monosaccharide units joined together. As was the case with proteins and nucleic acids, these carbohydrate polymers form as a result of the repeated joining of simple units. The process is represented in simplified fashion in Figure 13.62. Monosaccharide units are represented by boxes to which several hydroxyl groups are attached.

The most important polysaccharides for human beings are **starch** and **glycogen**. Both of these are

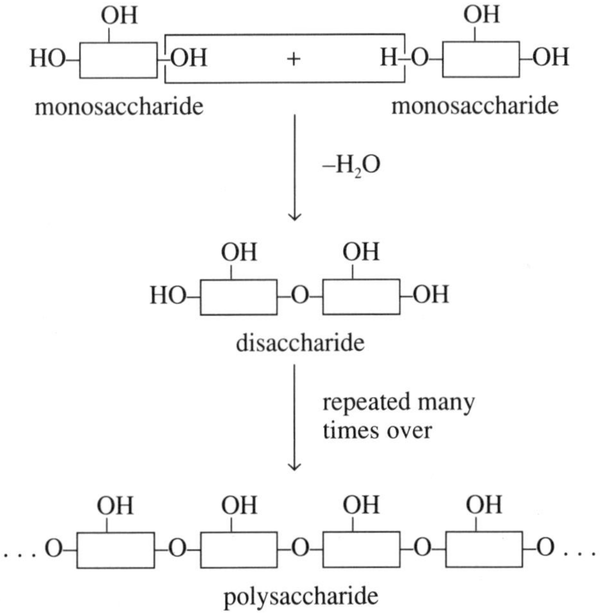

Figure 13.62 *A simple representation of polysaccharide formation*

polymers of glucose and can be converted to glucose by hydrolysis. Their function in living tissue is to serve as a means of storage for glucose. Starch serves this purpose in plant tissue; glycogen in animal tissue. Starch and glycogen differ mainly in the extent to which the chains of glucose units are branched. This branching is made possible by the fact that glucose contains many hydroxyl groups per molecule.

Another important polysaccharide is **cellulose**. This is also a polymer of glucose which differs from starch and glycogen in the way in which its glucose units are joined. It is the dominant material in plant tissue where its main role is structural.

Most of the body's glucose requirement is met by polysaccharides which are part of the plant and animal tissue which we eat. The polysaccharide molecules are far too large to pass across biological membranes and must be broken down by hydrolysis into glucose before absorption can occur.

The human diet contains all three of cellulose, glycogen and starch, but cellulose is treated quite differently from the other two. Human beings are not capable of hydrolysing cellulose due to a lack of the required enzymes and so cellulose simply passes straight through the human digestive tract to be eliminated in faeces. Nevertheless, cellulose is an important component of the human diet and it makes up what is normally described as the **fibre** content of the diet. Its role is to provide bulk to the contents of the intestine and, by keeping it filled, to stimulate peristalsis so that regular elimination of faeces can occur. This is considered to be important in the prevention of cancer of the lower portions of the gastrointestinal tract.

Starch and glycogen are both hydrolysed in the human gastrointestinal tract. The glucose released is absorbed and used to supply energy through glycolysis. The normal level of glucose in the blood is 65–95 mg/100 ml. In a healthy person when the level rises above this range the excess glucose is converted to glycogen which is deposited in muscle and liver tissue where it acts as a store of glucose to be used if blood glucose levels fall below the normal range. The conversion of glucose into glycogen is called **glycogenesis** while the reverse process in which glucose is formed by hydrolysis of glycogen is called **glycogenolysis**.

$$\text{glucose} \underset{\text{glycogenolysis}}{\overset{\text{glycogenesis}}{\rightleftarrows}} \text{glycogen}$$

From this description of carbohydrates it is clear that glucose deserves its place in the alphabet of biochemistry. In its monosaccharide form it provides the body with its energy, and it is also present in more complex carbohydrates which serve not only as glucose stores (sucrose, starch and glycogen) but as structural materials (cellulose).

13.11 Lipids

The name **lipid** refers to any component of living tissue which is soluble in non-polar solvents (such as the alkane hydrocarbons) but insoluble in water. In terms of chemical structure the lipids are a diverse group of compounds but they all do share the structural feature of having a large, non-polar section in their molecules. This is why they all have low solubilities in water.

Lipids perform two main functions in the body. They make up the membranes of cells, and they are the form in which the body stores most of the energy which is not required for immediate use. The ability of lipids to form membranes is due to their low solubility in water and they are used as the means of storing energy because on combination with oxygen they provide over twice as much energy per gram as either carbohydrate or protein.

13.11.1 *Classes of Lipid*

Lipids are categorised according to their chemical structures.

Simple Lipids. These are esters (see Section 13.6.9). If the alcohol component of the ester is glycerol then the simple lipid is referred to as a **fat** if it is a solid at room temperature, or an **oil** if it is a liquid. These compounds are often also referred to as **glycerides**. The carboxylic acid component of most fats and oils usually consists of one or more of the compounds **palmitic acid**, **stearic acid** and **oleic acid**. This relationship between fats and carboxylic acids is why the carboxylic acids are often referred to as the **fatty acids**. If all three alcohol groups of glycerol combine with a carboxylic acid the compound is known as a **triglyceride**. In Figure 13.63 structural formulae for palmitic, stearic and oleic acids are presented together with a general formula for a triglyceride. You can see that all three carboxylic acids contain a long chain of carbon atoms and this is responsible for the acids themselves and the glycerides in which they are present having low solubilities in water and high solubilities in non-polar solvents such as the hydrocarbons.

Simple lipids make up a relatively high proportion of adipose (fat) tissue which is found mainly below the skin, around the kidneys, around the joints, and on the surface of the heart and at its base. These tissues, through the lipid which they contain, serve as the body's main store of energy. They also provide support and protection for organs and they help reduce heat loss from the body.

$CH_3(CH_2)_5CH=CH(CH_2)_7CO_2H$
oleic acid

$CH_3(CH_2)_{14}CO_2H$
palmitic acid

$CH_3(CH_2)_{16}CO_2H$
stearic acid

$$\begin{array}{l} CH_2-O-\overset{\overset{O}{\|}}{C}-R \\ | \\ CH-O-\overset{\overset{O}{\|}}{C}-R \\ | \\ CH_2-O-\overset{\overset{O}{\|}}{C}-R \end{array}$$

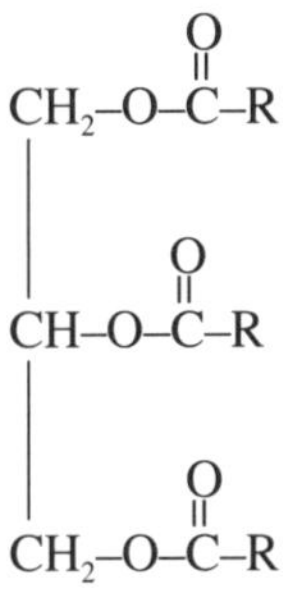

a triglyceride

Figure 13.63 *Structural formulae for fatty acids and a fat. R is a long chain radical*

Simple lipids also include **waxes** which differ from fats and oils in that the alcohol present is not glycerol but a long chain, simple alcohol. Examples of waxes are **spermaceti**, which is obtained from the oil of the sperm whale; **beeswax**, which is the substance from which bees build their honeycombs; and **carnauba wax** which is obtained from the leaves of a Brazilian palm and used as an ingredient in car and floor polishes.

Compound Lipids. These are also esters of carboxylic acids and alcohols but they contain other groups as well. In **phospholipids** glycerol uses two of its alcohol groups to form esters with carboxylic acids and the remaining group forms an ester with phosphoric acid which is also connected to another alcohol. The structural formula for a typical phospholipid is shown in Figure 13.64.

Phospholipids are important components of most cell membranes and this is due to the presence in their molecules of highly polar or charged groups of atoms. They form membranes by arranging themselves in a layer which is two molecules thick. The long, non-polar sections of the molecules are on the inside of the layer where they participate in hydrophobic bond formation with one other. These hydrophobic bonds

$$\begin{array}{l} CH_2-O-\overset{\overset{O}{\|}}{C}-(CH_2)_{16}-CH_3 \\ | \\ CH-O-\overset{\overset{O}{\|}}{C}-(CH_2)_7-CH=CH-(CH_2)_5-CH_3 \\ | \\ CH_2-O-\overset{\overset{O}{\|}}{P}-O^- \\ | \quad\quad\quad + \\ O-CH_2CH_2-N(CH_3)_3 \end{array}$$

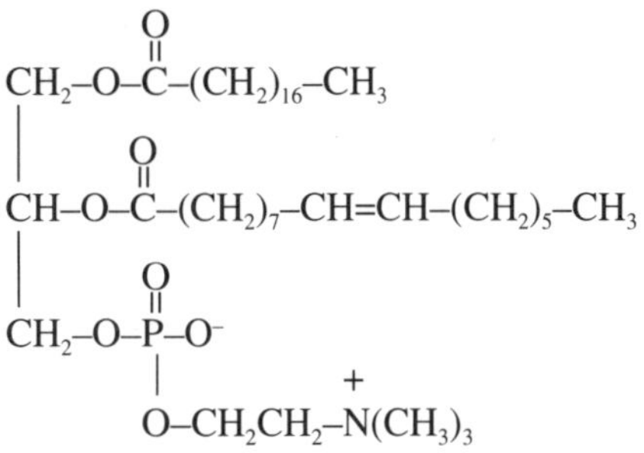

Figure 13.64 *Structural formula for a phospholipid*

hold the two layers of the membrane together. The ionic portions of the molecules are at the outsides of the layer where they make contact with the aqueous environments on either side of the membrane. This picture of membrane structure is called the **lipid bilayer** and it is illustrated in Figure 13.65.

Non-polar tails in contact with each other   Polar heads in contact with water

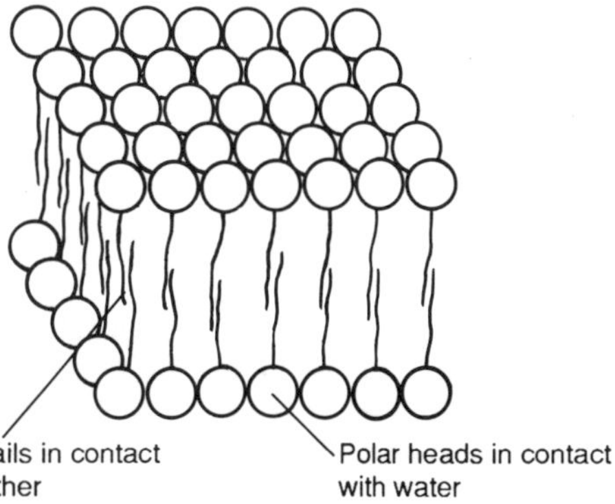

Figure 13.65 *The lipid bilayer structure of cell membranes*

Other types of compound lipid include **glycolipids** which contain carbohydrate portions in their molecules. These constitute about 7% of the solid matter of the brain and they form an insulating sheath around many nerve fibres in the central and peripheral nervous systems.

Derived Lipids. These are so named because they are obtained (derived) by hydrolysis of simple or compound lipids but still have the general physical characteristic of being soluble in non-polar solvents but insoluble in water.

An example of a derived lipid would be any one of the long chain carboxylic acids found in simple lipids. They can be obtained by heating a simple lipid with strong sodium hydroxide solution. This breaks the lipid up into glycerol and carboxylic acid. The carboxylic acid, once formed, is neutralised by the sodium hydroxide and converted to a sodium salt. The process is often called **saponification** (see Figure 13.66) because the sodium salts of long chain carboxylic acids obtained in this way are used as soaps. Knowing that this is the origin of soap it is not too surprising to learn that it is sometimes used as bait to catch yabbies.

Another example of a derived lipid is cholesterol which is an alcohol having the structural formula shown

$$\begin{array}{c} CH_2-O-\overset{O}{\overset{\|}{C}}-R \\ | \\ CH-O-\overset{O}{\overset{\|}{C}}-R \\ | \\ CH_2-O-\overset{O}{\overset{\|}{C}}-R \end{array} \xrightarrow[NaOH]{heat} \begin{array}{c} CH_2-OH \\ | \\ CH-OH \\ | \\ CH_2-OH \end{array} + 3\ RCO_2^- Na^+$$

triglyceride → glycerol + soap

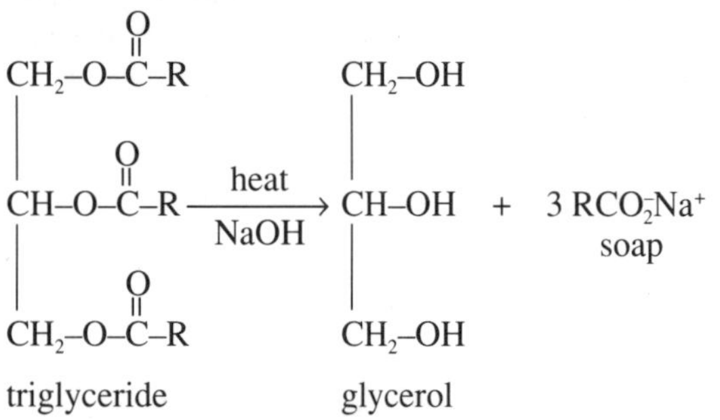

Figure 13.66 *An equation for saponification*

in Figure 13.22. This lipid has acquired a sinister reputation in recent years due to its association with diseases of the circulatory system. We are constantly urged by health authorities to have our cholesterol levels checked regularly and to limit our intake of the substance. However, cholesterol is essential for good health and is normally produced in significant quantities by the liver. It is used as the starting material for the synthesis of the **steroid hormones**. These compounds include sex hormones (**testosterone** and **estradiol**), hormones involved in carbohydrate metabolism (**cortisol**) and hormones involved in the regulation of ion concentrations in body fluids (**aldosterone**).

Cholesterol is also used for the synthesis of **bile salts**. These compounds are synthesised in the liver and stored in the gall-bladder. They pass into the intestine through the bile ducts. Their role is to assist in the digestion of fats and they do this because they are soap-like substances which are able to emulsify fat and break it into very small globules. These small globules are much more susceptible to the action of fat-digesting enzymes (**lipases**).

Structural formulae for some steroid hormones are given in Figure 13.67 and, by comparison with Figure 13.22, you can see that they all contain the characteristic set of rings which is present in cholesterol. This set of rings is often referred to as the **steroid nucleus**.

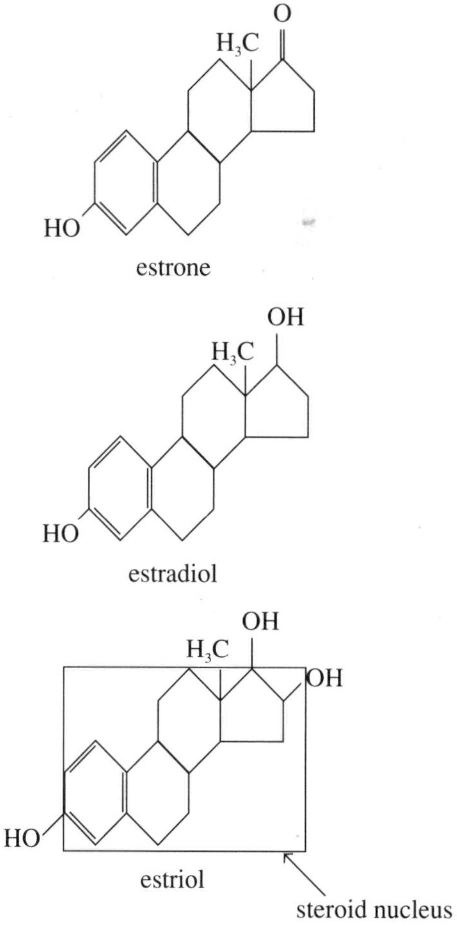

Figure 13.67 *The steroid nucleus and structural formulae for several steroid hormones*

13.11.2 Lipids and the Alphabet of Biochemistry

The members of the alphabet of biochemistry which are used to build lipids are glycerol, choline and acetic acid. From the preceding discussion the roles played by glycerol and choline in lipid structure are obvious. This is not so for acetic acid (ethanoic acid) which received no mention in that discussion. However, if you look back at the structural formulae for the carboxylic acid components of simple lipids presented in Figure 13.63 you will notice that each of the acids listed contains an even number of carbon atoms. This is true of all the carboxylic acid components of simple fats and the reason is that the body builds them all from acetic acid units which contain two carbon atoms per molecule.

13.11.3 *Digestion of Food*

Our food consists mainly of tissue or tissue extracts from plants or animals. It contains protein, carbohydrate, nucleic acids and lipids. Except for monosaccharides and some lipids none of these substances can be absorbed directly from the gastrointestinal tract. They must first of all be broken down into their simplest components. This process of breaking down is called **digestion**. In the build-up of protein, carbohydrate, nucleic acid and lipid from their simpler components a water molecule was eliminated from between two combining molecules at every stage in the process. This elimination involved loss of a hydrogen atom by one of the combining molecules and loss of an hydroxyl group (–OH) by the other. In digestion the reverse process occurs and at each stage one hydrogen atom and one hydroxyl group is re-inserted into the molecule thus breaking it down into its simpler components.

Bibliography

Albert, A. *Selective Toxicity: The Physico-chemical Basis of Therapy* (sixth edition). Chapman and Hall, London, 1981.

Bettelheim, F. A. and March, J. *Introduction to General, Organic and Biochemistry*. Saunders College Publishing, Philadelphia, 1984.

Brown, W. H. *Introduction to Organic Chemistry* (second edition). Willard Grant Press, Boston, 1978.

Everard, D. and O'Connor, M. (eds) *Silicon Biochemistry*. John Wiley, Chichester, 1986.

Hoover, J. E. (ed.) *Remington's Pharmaceutical Sciences* (fifth edition). Mack Publishing Company, Pennsylvania, 1975.

Noll, W. *Chemistry and Technology of Silicones*. Academic Press, New York, 1968.

Solomon, Sally. *Introduction to General, Organic and Biological Chemistry*. McGraw-Hill, New York, 1987.

Thomas, J. (ed.) *Prescription Products Guide*. Australian Pharmaceutical Publishing Company, Melbourne, 1989.

Questions

1. Which one of the following formulae represents a saturated organic compound?

   J. CH_3CH_2OH

   K. $CH_3CH_2\overset{\overset{O}{||}}{C}-OH$

   L. $CH_3CHCHCH_3$

   M. $CH{\equiv}CH$

2. Only one of the following patterns of bonds is ever displayed by carbon atoms in organic compounds. Which is it?

   J. $-\overset{|}{\underset{|}{C}}=$

   K. $-\overset{||}{\underset{|}{C}}-$

   L. $-\overset{|}{C}=$

   M. $-\overset{|}{C}\equiv$

3. The major component of cell membranes is

   J. polysaccharide

   K. protein

   L. lipid

   M. nucleic acid

4. Which of the following carbohydrates is *not* digestible by human beings?

   J. cellulose

   K. glycogen

   L. maltose

   M. sucrose

5. The sequence of amino acids in a protein chain is known as its

   J. primary structure

   K. secondary structure

   L. tertiary structure

   M. quaternary structure

6. Enzymes are members of which class of biological compounds?

   J. amino acids

   K. lipids

   L. nucleic acids

   M. proteins

7. Which of the following is the name for a class of biological macromolecules?

   J. lipid

   K. nucleoside

L. nucleotide
M. protein

8. The main genetic material of cells is
J. carboxylic acid
K. fatty acid
L. amino acid
M. nucleic acid

9. Which aspect of the structure of a protein is *least* affected by denaturation?
J. primary structure
K. secondary structure
L. tertiary structure
M. quaternary structure

10. Which of the following is the name of an enzyme?
J. maltose
K. glycine
L. dextrose
M. urease

11. Explain the meaning of the following terms as they are used in organic chemistry:

(a) functional group	(b) alkyl radical
(c) aromatic	(d) saturated
(e) spot test	(f) general formula

12. The structural formulae for a number of organic compounds which are used as drugs are shown below. Nominate the families of organic compound to which each belongs.

(a)
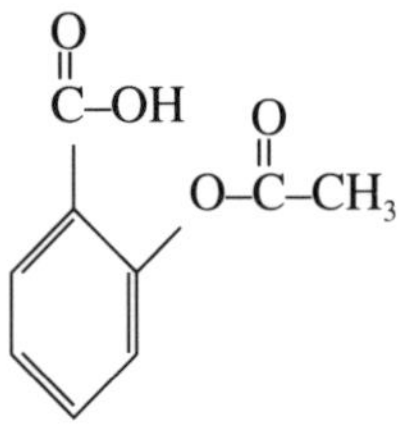

acetylsalicylic acid (aspirin)

(b)
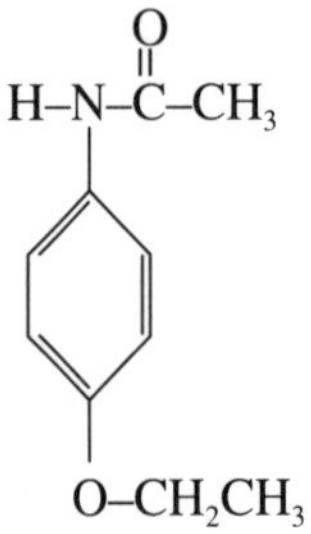

phenacetin

(c)
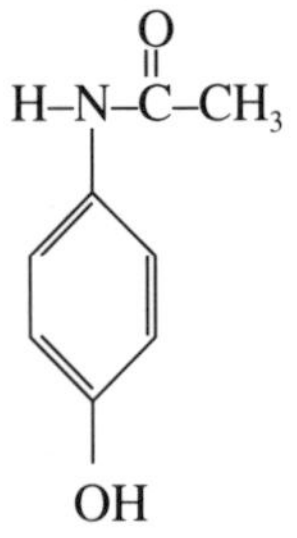

paracetamol

(d)
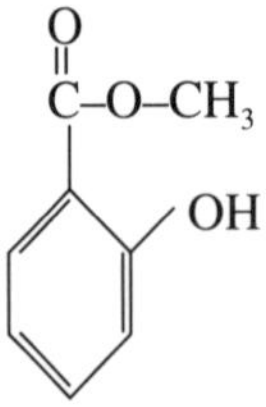

methyl salicylate

13. Set out below are structural formulae for a number of **estrogens**: compounds which are female sex hormones influencing the development of the egg and the maintenance of secondary sex characteristics.

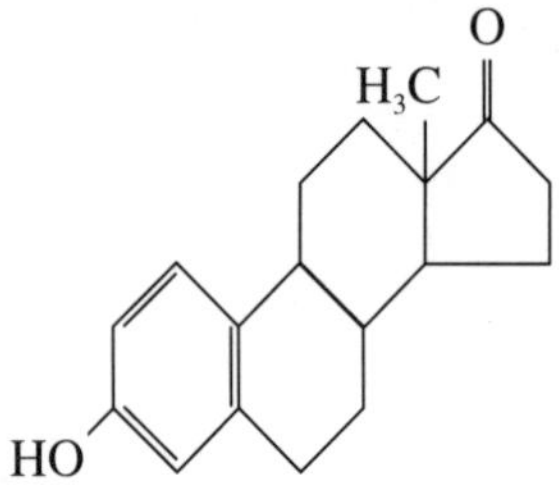

estrone

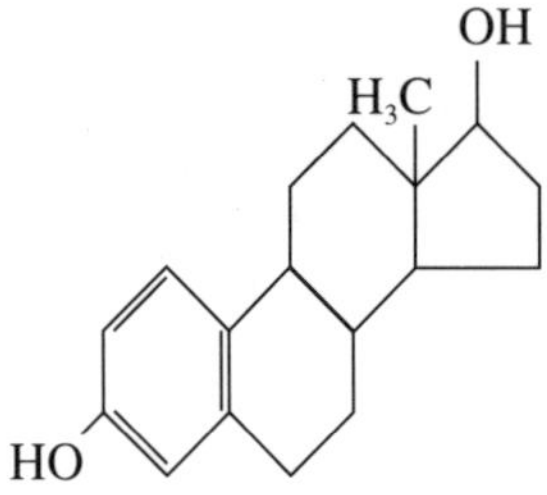

estradiol

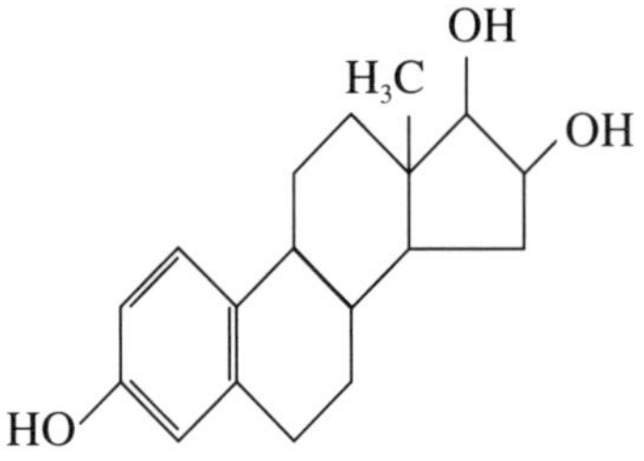

estriol

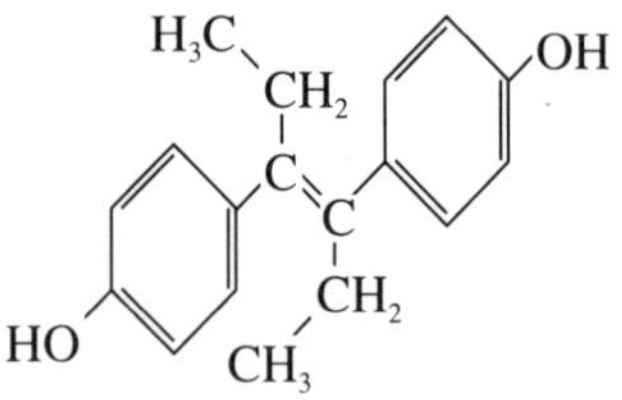

diethylstilbestrol

(a) What is the difference in chemical structure between estrone and estradiol? How is this difference reflected in the names of the two compounds?
(b) What is the difference in chemical structure between estradiol and estriol? How is this difference reflected in the names of the two compounds?
(c) One of the estrogens listed is synthetic (not

produced by the body itself). Which compound do you think this is?

(d) To what family of organic compounds do all four of these compounds belong?

14. Name the families to which each of the following compounds belongs.

(a) 2-methylbutane	(b) cyclohexene
(c) 1,3-dimethylbenzene	(d) pentanol
(e) methyl ethanoate	(f) propanal

15. Write structural formulae for the compounds listed in Question 14.

16. What property do all lipids have in common and what feature of their molecular structures is responsible for this?

17. Hydrogen bonds are aptly described as 'threads in the fabric of life'. What basis is there for describing hydrogen bonds in this way?

18. The protein insulin is used for the control of *diabetes mellitus* but it cannot be taken orally. Why do you think this is?

19. When a fresh egg is broken and dropped into a dish containing alcohol the effect observed is very similar to that seen when an egg is fried or poached. Why should this be?

20. What are the main features of the behaviour of enzymes? Account for these features of behaviour in terms of the structure of enzymes.

21. In the descriptions given of the role played by nucleic acids in the synthesis of proteins the following terms and abbreviations are usually encountered. Write an account of protein synthesis in which the meaning of each term is made clear and distinguished from the others.

(a) genetic code	(b) codon
(c) anticodon	(d) DNA
(e) RNA	(f) mRNA
(g) tRNA	(h) transcription
(i) translation	

22. By reference to the proteins, nucleic acids, polysaccharides and lipids explain the basis of the expression 'alphabet of biochemistry'.

CHAPTER 14

Nuclear Medicine

The possibility of exposure to radiation can easily produce fear and anxiety in people who know little about radiation. Large doses will produce a sensation of burning and the skin will become red. However, lower but quite significant doses of nuclear radiation are undetectable by any of our senses during the exposure period. Hence humans have no way of knowing when they are being exposed to it. Furthermore, any adverse symptoms may take some time to become apparent, and indeed may not show up until children are born. By having an understanding of what radiation is, and how exposure to it can be minimised, genuine fears and anxieties may be placed in the appropriate context.

To this end we will discuss the basic physics of the nucleus of the atom that is needed to understand nuclear radiation, before going on to discuss the role that nuclear medicine plays in diagnosis and therapy in hospitals. An historical discussion of how the structure of the atom was discovered appears in Chapter 2. The last part of this chapter deals with radiation safety and the strategies for minimising exposure to ionising radiation.

Learning Objectives

At the completion of this chapter you should be able to:

1. Define radioactivity and distinguish between alpha, beta and gamma radiation.
2. Define isotope, radioisotope and radiopharmaceutical.
3. Distinguish between gamma radiation and X-radiation.
4. Know the units of energy used, the joule and the megaelectron-volt.
5. Define half-life and know the implications of a short half-life compared to a long one.
6. Know that the ability of gamma rays and X-radiation to penetrate a given thickness of material depends on the energy of the radiation.
7. Know why radioisotopes that emit low-energy gamma rays are preferred for *in vivo* diagnosis.
8. Outline the effect of ionising radiation on living tissue.
9. Understand why radiation therapy is effective in treating cancer.
10. Know the SI units used to measure exposure and the ones that they replaced.
11. Recognise that statements about radiation safety depend on the amount of exposure, the reliable measurement of exposure and which parts of the body are exposed.
12. Explain why keeping one's distance, using shielding and minimising exposure time are the three most useful strategies for keeping the absorbed dose as small as possible.

14.1 Radioactivity, Protons, Neutrons and Isotopes

The word 'radioactivity' was coined by Marie Curie at the start of this century to refer to the spontaneous emission of a particle or of electromagnetic radiation from the nucleus of an atom. Radioactivity was first discovered by Henri Becquerel in 1896 in salts of the element **uranium**. New knowledge of the phenomenon and additional radioactive elements were discovered very rapidly thereafter. Ernest Rutherford in 1897 showed that the radiation was of two types which he called alpha (α) and beta (β). His discovery led to an intensive experimental effort aimed at determining just what the radiations were.

In 1899 Becquerel found that the beta rays could be deflected by a magnetic field and also by an electric field. He went on to find that their 'charge to mass ratio' was similar to that of cathode corpuscles (which are now known as electrons) as determined by Joseph Thomson two years earlier. Since it was not possible to measure the amount of charge or mass separately, the charge to mass *ratio* was used as a convenient means to compare different particle radiations. Paul Villard found a third radiation in 1900, more penetrating than the other two. It was known as gamma (γ) radiation. Madame Curie deduced from their absorption in materials that alpha rays were particles with mass (and not electromagnetic radiation). In 1903 Rutherford succeeded in deflecting the alpha rays with a magnetic field, thereby showing that alpha rays were particles with a positive charge of electricity.

Note that alpha, beta and gamma are just the first three letters of the Greek alphabet and were first used as a convenient way of referring to the emanations from radioactive materials. We now know that alpha rays are helium atoms that have lost their two electrons (and hence are charged with positive electricity), that beta rays are negatively charged electrons, and that gamma rays are very high frequency electromagnetic radiation, that is, are photons. In the 1930s it was discovered that some radioactive isotopes emitted 'electrons' that had a positive charge, so these particles came to be known as positrons. The term 'beta particle' is now used to refer both to electrons and positrons of nuclear origin; the two are also called 'beta minus' and 'beta plus' respectively.

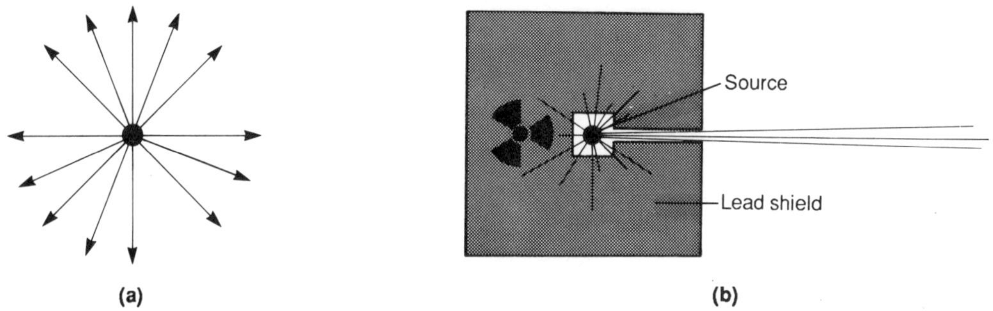

Figure 14.1 *(a) A radioactive source will emit radiation in every direction in an analogous manner to the way that an incandescent light globe will shine light in every direction. (b) A beam of radiation can be formed by shielding the source*

Radioactivity was amazing to the scientists who first worked with it, because it seemed to violate the well-established law of conservation of energy. Radioactive sources produced a steady stream of high-energy rays for an indefinite period of time with no input of energy. As exciting as the discovery of X-rays was, just months earlier, they required the input of electrical energy for their production. Radioactivity, on the other hand, occurred spontaneously, with no indication of where the energy came from.

Rutherford (and his research students) used the high-energy alpha particles to 'bombard' very thin foils of metal elements in an attempt to discover more about the atoms making up the foil (Figure 14.2). The highly unexpected result of these famous 'alpha scattering experiments' was the discovery (circa 1911), of the existence of a very small (even compared to the size of an atom), almost inconceivably dense, **nucleus** within the atom. This nucleus seemed to contain all the positive charge of the atom and almost all of the mass. Negatively charged electrons 'orbited' around the nucleus, occupying the bulk of the volume of the atom.

Since it was known that the intensity of the radiation from uranium was proportional to the concentration of uranium, regardless of the variation in its temperature, pressure, chemical composition or the presence of electric and magnetic fields, the radioactive properties of uranium were attributed to its newly discovered nucleus. Nothing that was done to a radioactive sample could prevent the emission of its radiation and there is still no way to prevent a radioactive nucleus from emitting.

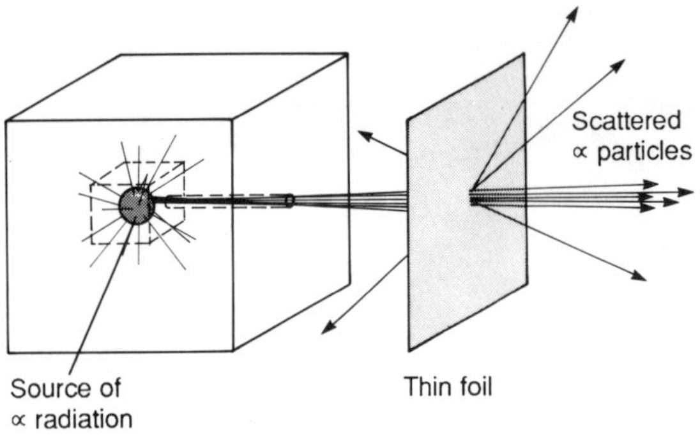

Figure 14.2 *A narrow beam of alpha particles being used to bombard very thin (10^{-4} mm) metal foil. Most blast straight through but some bounce back*

Inside the nucleus there are two types of particles of about the same size: **protons** with a positive charge of the same magnitude as the charge on electrons (protons were discovered by Rutherford in 1919); and **neutrons** with no electric charge. Neutrons were discovered by James Chadwick in 1932 but their existence had been suspected ever since about 1920 when it was thought that a proton in combination with an electron could exist as a neutral particle in the nucleus. That view, however, was an oversimplification.

The number of protons present in the nucleus is called the atomic number and determines the name given to the element. Thus if there are 92 protons in the nucleus, the element is uranium. All atoms of uranium have 92 protons in their nucleus and no other element has 92 protons. However, the number of *neutrons* is not such a fixed characteristic. Atoms of different elements may have the same number of neutrons in their nucleus. For example, technetium 99 and molybdenum 98 each have 56 neutrons. Conversely, atoms of the same element may have different numbers of neutrons. Naturally occurring uranium atoms may have 142, 143 or 146 neutrons. Atoms of the one element which have different numbers of neutrons, such as the uranium atoms, are called **isotopes** (a term coined by Frederick Soddy in 1911). Isotopes are chemically identical atoms because they have the same atomic number although they have a different atomic mass. To distinguish these different isotopes of uranium they are written as, ^{234}U, ^{235}U, ^{238}U and called 'uranium 234', 'uranium 235' and so on.

Note:

1. More than 99% of uranium is ^{238}U.
2. 238 (the mass number of the nucleus) = 92 (the number of protons) + 146 (the number of neutrons).
3. Many more isotopes of uranium have been artificially produced in nuclear reactors.

Most of the 90 elements that exist naturally in the environment have more than one isotope, and all elements (both those isolated from the earth's crust and those produced artificially) have had additional isotopes — often in excess of 10 — formed when subjected to bombardment by neutrons in a nuclear reactor.

Some isotopes are naturally radioactive, that is, they exist naturally in our environment alongside non-radioactive isotopes of the same element. Thus in any sample of, for example, potassium (symbol K) obtained from the earth's crust, 93.1% will be ^{38}K, 6.88% will be ^{41}K and less than 0.012% will be radioactive ^{40}K. The metabolism of the human body cannot distinguish between a radioactive atom and a non-radioactive atom of the same element because they are chemically identical. Thus atoms of potassium 40 exist in the human body and perform the same functions as the much more numerous atoms of potassium 39. The artificially produced radioactive isotope, potassium 42, may be used in body electrolyte determinations because its presence in the body can be detected from the radiation it emits, and the body uses it in exactly the same way as natural potassium. Radioactive isotopes are also called **radioisotopes** while non-radioactive isotopes are termed **stable**.

14.2 Stability and Instability

14.2.1 *Why are some Isotopes Stable while Others are Radioactive?*

All elements whose atoms have more than 83 protons are radioactive. They have too many protons in the nucleus to be stable. Recall that protons carry a positive charge and that 'like' charges repel each other. When

84 or more protons are confined to a tiny sphere (radius 10^{-15} m) the size of a nucleus, the repulsive electric force between them is too great for all the particles to stay together. They literally fly apart, that is, they 'decay'. One way to reduce the repulsive force acting between protons in the nucleus is to decrease the number of protons. This occurs when two protons and two neutrons are emitted as an alpha particle. Eventually, radioactive decay reduces the amount of positive charge in the nucleus to a stable level.

14.2.2 *Why don't Atoms with less than 84 Protons Decay?*

Some do! There are no stable isotopes of elements number 43 and 61 (technetium and promethium). Furthermore many radioactive isotopes of elements with less than 84 protons in their nucleus do exist in the earth's crust (or atmosphere) alongside the stable isotopes, for example $^{3}_{1}H$, $^{40}_{19}K$, $^{50}_{23}V$ and $^{115}_{49}In$. The particles in these nuclei fly apart too because of the excess of repulsive forces over attractive forces. However, most of the naturally occurring isotopes of smaller elements *are* stable. To bind the nucleus together there must be a strong attractive force of a totally new kind (that is, not gravity, electricity or magnetism). It must be strong enough to overcome the repulsive electrical force acting between the positively charged protons and must act to bind both protons and neutrons into the tiny nuclear volume. Experiments have shown that this **strong nuclear force**, as it is called, operates between any two nuclear particles, whether they are protons or neutrons, as long as they are *very* close together.

14.2.3 *Why do Nuclei Fall Apart at all then?*

The strong nuclear force has a *very short range*. This means that the attractive force between two nuclear particles is effectively zero if they are separated by more than 10^{-14} m (which is the approximate diameter of a nucleus). Consequently protons and neutrons are only strongly attracted to their *nearest* neighbours, not to all the particles in the nucleus. At the same time *all* protons electrically repel *all other* protons in the nucleus because the electric force is relatively long range (see Figure 14.3). As long as the strong nuclear force can hold the nucleus together against the disruptive influence of the electric force, the atom is stable.

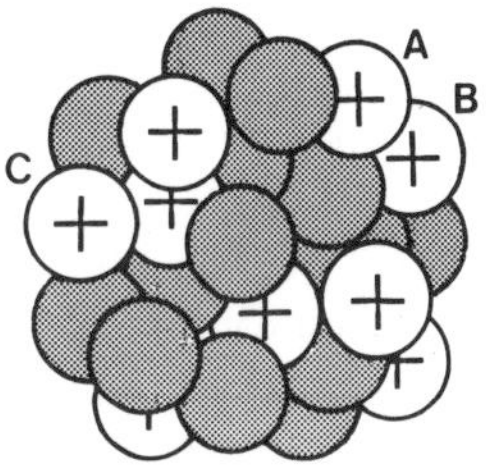

Figure 14.3 *Protons A and B are attracted by the strong nuclear force as well as being repelled from each other by their electrical charge. Proton C only feels electrical repulsion from A and B. It is held in by the strong nuclear attraction to the nucleons immediately adjacent to it*

It is important to realise that the *attractive* strong nuclear force is an effective 'glue' only between *adjacent particles* (no matter whether they are protons or neutrons) and that the *repulsive* electric force acts between *all protons*. This means that if an additional proton is included in the nucleus, it will increase the repulsion on all the other protons. If there are enough protons, their repulsion will be strong enough to overcome the 'glue' of the strong nuclear force and the nucleus will be unstable.

14.2.4 *Why are there more Neutrons than Protons in the Nucleus?*

To some extent, the disruptive influence of a large number of protons can be overcome if they are spaced further apart from each other by increasing the number of neutrons in the nucleus. This is so because electric repulsion decreases as the square of the distance between protons. Thus, elements having atoms that contain large nuclei always have more neutrons than protons in their nuclei. Making a bigger nucleus by adding a neutron will increase the attractive strong nuclear force on nearby particles without increasing the repulsive electric force. The excess of neutrons over protons is not necessary in small atoms because there are not enough protons to make the total repulsive electric force great enough to exceed the strong nuclear force. In fact many of the first 20 or so elements have equal numbers of neutrons and protons (for example,

$^{40}_{20}Ca$, $^{16}_{8}O$) but the largest atoms have a neutron:proton ratio of up to 1.6:1. For example, bismuth 209 is stable and has 126 neutrons and 83 protons, a ratio of 1.52:1.

However, there is a limit to the number of neutrons that can be added to a nucleus. Too many neutrons will also produce instability and radioactive decay. This is because one of the neutrons will transform into a proton while emitting a beta particle (an electron) and another type of particle called an antineutrino. Thus for stable atoms, there is an optimum ratio of neutrons to protons. The optimum ratio changes according to the size of the atom (it increases as the number of protons increases). If the ratio is too high or too low the isotope will be radioactive and hence decay. In the case of stable cobalt 59, it has a neutron:proton ratio of 1.19:1, while radioactive cobalt 60 has the higher neutron:proton ratio of 1.22:1. In the decay process, the neutron:proton ratio will change to a value closer to the optimum value for that element.

14.2.5 *Where Does the Energy Come From?*

This was the question asked by the early nuclear physicists. Albert Einstein gave us the answer in about 1905, but we didn't realise it at the time. Nuclear energy comes from converting some of the *mass* of the nucleus into energy. If the mass of a uranium nucleus is compared to the combined masses of the daughter nucleus (see Section 14.3) and the emitted alpha particle it is found that the parent nucleus has *more mass* than the products. However, the nuclear fragments that are produced have more *kinetic energy* than the parent uranium nucleus. The differences in mass and energy are reconciled in Einstein's famous equation which quantifies the equivalence of mass and energy,

$$E = m \times c^2$$

energy produced = mass loss × speed of light squared

In nuclear reactions, energy *alone* is not conserved, but the combination of mass and energy (mass energy) is. Since the speed of light squared is such a large number (90 000 000 000 000 000 m^2/s^2), even tiny amounts of mass produce large amounts of energy.

14.3 Nuclear Reactions

A nuclear reaction is the process that occurs when a nucleus changes into a different nucleus or to a different energy state of the same nucleus. Such a reaction often results in the production of radiation. Some nuclear reactions are also referred to as a nuclear 'decay', or, if a particle is ejected from the nucleus, as a nuclear 'disintegration'. The description of the process as a disintegration is apt. After the emission of an alpha or beta particle, the remaining nuclear fragment is part of the atom of a different element from the one that existed before the nuclear reaction. The process where one element is changed to another is called **transmutation**. In the example of Figure 14.4, uranium has transmuted into thorium by emitting an alpha particle (note that the atomic number of an element may precede its symbol ($^{4}_{2}He$) or follow it ($^{4}He_{2}$). Thus the isotope uranium 238 'decays' by alpha emission. That is, two protons and two neutrons are ejected, leaving the remaining nuclear fragment (called the 'daughter' nucleus) with 90 protons and 144 neutrons. An atom with 90 protons is an atom of the element thorium (in particular, thorium 234 because 90 + 144 = 234). Thorium 234, having more than 83 protons, is also radioactive and decays by the emission of a beta

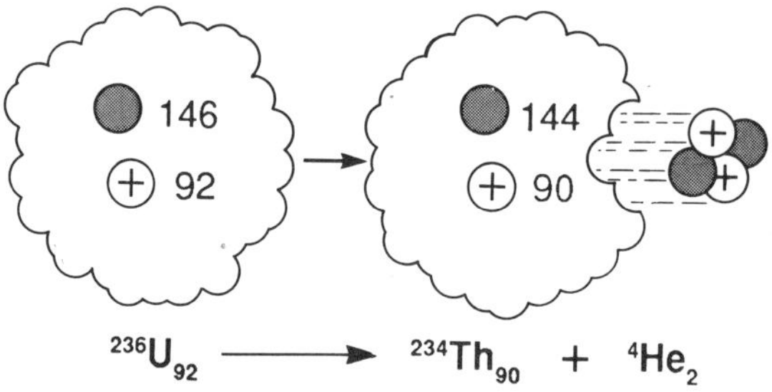

Figure 14.4 *A uranium nucleus changes into a nucleus of thorium by emitting an alpha particle*

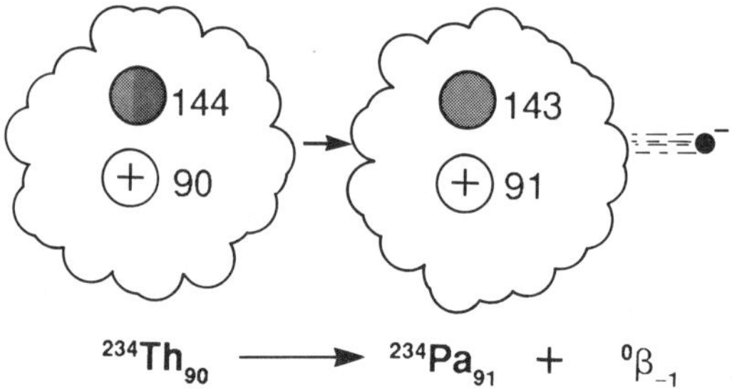

Figure 14.5 *A thorium nucleus decays into a protoactinium nucleus when one of its neutrons changes into a proton while emitting an electron*

particle (Figure 14.5). The 'granddaughter' nucleus, protoactinium 234, is also radioactive. The line of decay from 'parent' to 'daughter' to 'granddaughter' to 'great granddaughter' and so on, is called a **radioactive series**; the example above is from the uranium series.

Note:

1. The beta particle is the result of a neutron decaying into a proton and an electron, thus the net amount of electric charge has not been altered.
2. The number of protons in the nucleus has increased to 91 from 90.
3. Nuclear reactions will continue, and new daughter nuclei will be formed from the old, until a stable daughter, having less than 84 protons and a balanced neutron:proton ratio is produced.
4. An antineutrino is one of the many sub-atomic particles that we will not discuss here.

Uranium 238, thorium 234 and protoactinium 234 all emit gamma radiation as well as particles. The emission of a gamma photon may be thought of as a means by which a nucleus can rid itself of excess energy without transmuting to a new element.

14.4 Radioactivity Units, Energy, Half-life

14.4.1 *The Energy of Radiation*

Radiation presents a danger to living things because of the energy that is deposited in the organism when radiation is absorbed, and the changes that this energy causes. Thus a measure of the energy carried by radiation is useful in appreciating the risks involved.

The metric unit for energy is the joule, but this is too large for the energies of alpha and beta particles and of gamma photons. A much smaller unit with the rather strange name **electron-volt** (symbol eV) is used. One electron-volt is the amount of kinetic energy gained by an electron that has accelerated across a potential difference of one volt. Hence the name. One electron-volt = 1.6×10^{-19} J. A photon of visible light only carries about 1.5 eV of energy, but a few of these are enough to stimulate a reaction in the human retina and produce the sensation of vision. Photons with energies of more than about 4.1 eV are called ultraviolet photons and these are energetic enough to produce sunburn. Alpha, beta and gamma rays can all carry energies of several million electron-volts (MeV) so can cause far greater damage than a touch of sunburn. Cobalt 60, a gamma ray source used in cancer therapy, produces photons of energy 1.17 MeV. Gamma ray sources that are chosen for internal human administration produce photons in the range of energy 100–250 keV.

14.4.2 *Unit of Radioactivity*

The SI unit of radioactivity is the **becquerel**, Bq (after the discoverer of radioactivity). One becquerel = one nuclear disintegration per second. However, the previous unit, the curie (Ci), may still be encountered; 1 Ci = 3.7×10^{10} disintegrations per second. Another old unit which did not gain wide acceptance is the rutherford; one rutherford = one million becquerel.

The number of nuclear disintegrations that occur per second in a sample of a radioisotope is proportional to the number of atoms of radioisotope that are present. That is, if you halve the number of atoms present, then the radioactivity will be one half of the former value (Table 14.1). As the atoms of a given amount of radioisotope decay, the number of atoms of that radioisotope decreases, hence the radioactivity of the given amount of material also decreases.

Table 14.1 *The radioactivity of an isotope is proportional to the number of atoms present*

Number of atoms	Radioactivity (Bq)
4 000 000	40
2 000 000	20
1 000 000	10
500 000	5

14.4.3 *The Concept of Half-life*

The probability of decay within a certain time interval for a given radioactive nucleus is known. In the case of radium 226 there is a probability of 0.5 (one chance in two) that a particular nucleus will decay within 1600 years. The fixed probability of radioactive decay means that a constant fraction of the number of nuclei will decay in equal time intervals. The amount of time it takes for *half* of the existing nuclei to decay is called the **half-life**. In other words after a time interval of one half-life, half of the nuclei will have decayed. Furthermore, the radioactivity of a particular sample is exactly half of what it was at the start of the time interval we have called the half-life. The length of the half-life varies enormously between different isotopes.

It can be less than one thousandth of a second (for polonium 214); in this case the probability of decay of a given nucleus is very high and the material is extremely radioactive. Conversely, a half-life can be thousands of millions of years (for uranium 238), making the probability of decay very low, and the material only slightly radioactive.

Mathematically, decay with a fixed probability is described by the exponential decay equation

$$N = N_0 e^{-kt}$$

lives, the radioactivity would be 100 Bq and 600×10^{20} atoms would remain. The elapse of a further half-life would see 300×10^{20} atoms of the radioisotope still in existence and producing radioactivity of 50 Bq.

Note:

1. After three half-lives there would still be 2400×10^{20} atoms present, but only 300×10^{20} of them would be atoms of the *original* radioisotope. The rest (2100×10^{20}) would be atoms of the decay product(s) and atoms of the daughter's decay products.

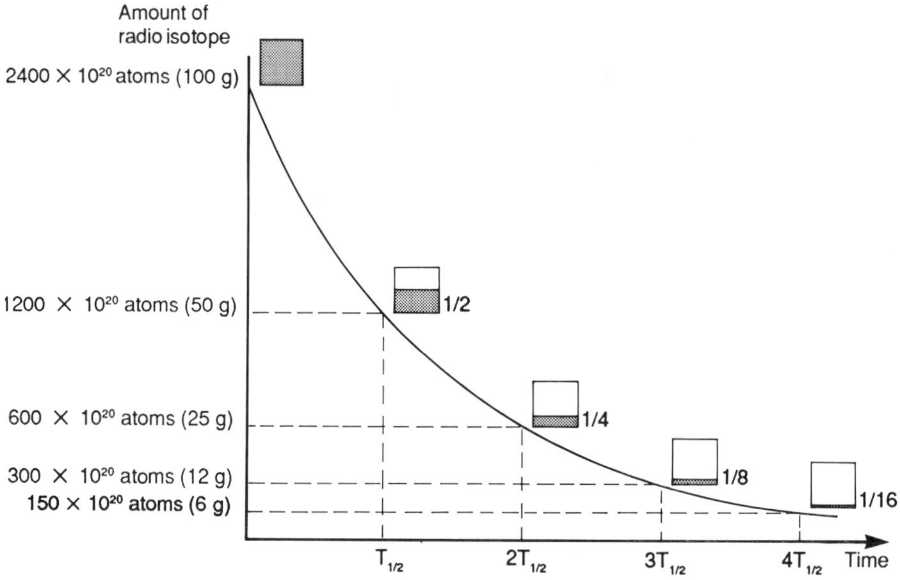

Figure 14.6 *Radioactive decay. The typical graph of 'amount of radioisotope' (in grams and in atoms) versus time (in half-lives). How much of the original isotope remains after five half-lives?*

N_0 is the number of nuclei initially present; this number reduces to N after a time interval t (k is the 'decay constant' and e is the number 2.718). The equation is 'exponential' because $-kt$ is an exponent, and the equation describes a *decay* because the exponent is negative. If a graph of N (on the vertical axis) is plotted against t (on the horizontal axis), a smooth curve like the one in Figure 14.6 results.

We will illustrate the concept of half-life with an example (see Table 14.2). If 2400×10^{20} atoms of a particular radioisotope were present when a pure sample (with mass 100 g and radioactivity 400 Bq) was removed from a nuclear reactor, one half-life later only half of them, 1200×10^{20}, would remain (and their radioactivity would be 200 Bq). After two half-

2. The decay products themselves will usually be radioactive so the radioactivity of the sample will not decrease exponentially, but the portion of the radioactivity *due to the atoms of the original radioisotope* will decrease exponentially.

3. The total mass of all the isotopes in the sample will decrease slightly from the original 100 g due to the emission of some of the mass as alpha and beta particles with kinetic energy and as electromagnetic radiation.

4. After seven half-lives 19×10^{20} atoms of the original radioisotope remain. This is less than 1% of the number of nuclei we started with.

5. It would take about 78 half-lives for all 2400×10^{20} atoms of the original radioisotope to decay.

Table 14.2 *The amount of a fictitious radioisotope remaining after successive intervals of one half-life*

Number of atoms left	Fraction	Elapsed half-lives	Mass (g)	Radioactivity (Bq)
2400×10^{20}	1.0	0	100	400
1200×10^{20}	0.5	1	50	200
600×10^{20}	0.25	2	25	100
300×10^{20}	0.125	3	12.5	50
150×10^{20}	0.0625	4	6.25	25
75×10^{20}	0.0313	5	3.13	12.5
38×10^{20}	0.0156	6	1.56	6.3
19×10^{20}	0.0078	7	0.78	3.2

6. Any particular atom has a chance of 'living' much longer than one half-life.

Radioisotopes that are suitable for human administration must have a short effective half-life (T_{eff}). The effective half-life depends on the 'physical' half-life (T_{phys})defined above and on the 'biological' half-life (T_{biol}). The biological half-life is the amount of time it takes to eliminate half of the internally administered radioisotope by metabolic means regardless of whether the isotope has decayed or not. The biological half-life is independent of whether or not the element is radioactive. T_{eff} may be calculated by the formula

$$\frac{1}{T_{eff}} = \frac{1}{T_{phys}} + \frac{1}{T_{biol}}$$

Thus the effective half-life will be shorter than either the physical half-life or the biological half-life.

14.5 The Penetration of Radiation

The ability of radiation to pass through material depends on the density of the material and the charge, mass and energy of the radiation. Alpha particles have a relatively large mass and two units of positive charge. These two factors ensure that alpha particles interact strongly with the electrons in the matter into which they enter. The interaction results in considerable energy being transferred to the electrons in the path of the alpha particle. This loss of energy means that alpha particles are stopped very easily by placing matter in their path. Their maximum range in air is about 10 cm. Alpha particles are not suitable for radiation therapy because their range in the human body is less than a tenth of a millimetre. Beta particles have a relatively small mass and one unit of negative charge so can penetrate further (up to about 1 cm in body tissue) than alpha particles, but are still regarded as short-range radiation in the body. Nevertheless an electron beam is used in the treatment of skin cancers.

Both alpha and beta particles interact with the electrons of the atoms of the material through which they pass. Since the kinetic energies of alpha and beta particles is much much more than the energy with which electrons are held to their atoms, a collision results in the electron being removed from its atom, leaving an ion. Alpha and beta particles lose a small amount of energy in each of a large number of collisions with electrons. Each encounter removes a little kinetic energy from the alpha or beta particle, until, after a certain well-defined distance, there is none left. It is easy to shield the body from charged radioactive particles because they do not penetrate very far into solid material (Figure 14.7). The atoms of a solid are so densely packed that encounters with electrons are very frequent and all the energy of the radiation is used up in a small distance.

Isotopes emitting alpha and beta radiation present a danger to humans if they are ingested or inhaled. In this case all of their energy will be deposited in the body as the radiation is not penetrating enough to escape from the body. The mining and crushing of uranium ore liberates radon gas, a product of the decay of uranium which emits alpha particles. Since radon is inert, it cannot be chemically separated from inhaled air by a gas mask. Those who work with radioactive ores will breathe the gas unless it is swept away by a very active ventilation system. Once inside the lungs radon is very destructive and may produce lung cancer. Hence the maximum permissible safe concentration of radon in the atmosphere is about 1×10^{-15} of 1% by volume.

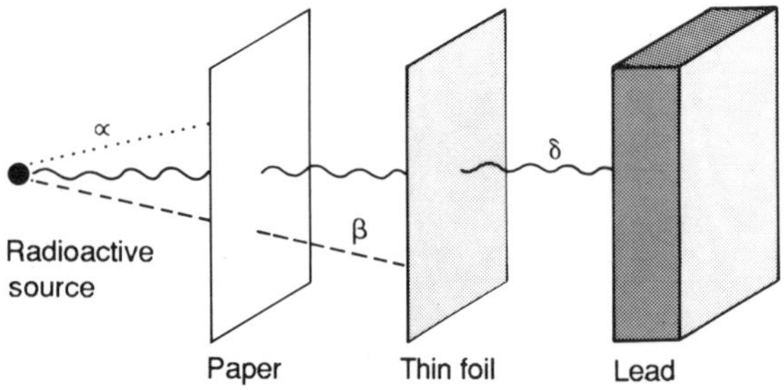

Figure 14.7 *Gamma rays are very penetrating. Some of the gamma rays will penetrate quite thick shielding. Alpha and beta rays, being charged particles, may be completely stopped by even very thin shielding* (see Errata)

Gamma radiation, being electromagnetic radiation, has no mass and no charge so is very penetrating. When a gamma ray does collide with an electron its loss of energy is catastrophic rather than gradual. That is, after one or two collisions, the energy of the gamma ray photon is completely consumed. The energy has transferred to an electron and a residual X-ray photon, both of which are deviated through a large angle to the original gamma direction. The number, N, of photons that penetrate an absorber depend exponentially on the thickness, x, of the absorber. The thicker the material (of a given density), the fewer gamma ray photons that can pass through it. The exponential law is:

$$N = N_0 e^{-ax}$$

where N_0 is the number of photons that enter the absorber, a is the absorption coefficient of the absorber and e is the number 2.718.

In body tissue, the intensity of a beam of gamma rays with energy 0.5 MeV drops by half for every 7.2 cm traversed. A high penetrating ability is diagnostically useful because once a gamma emitter is inside an organ, most of the emitted gamma rays pass easily through the body and can be detected externally by the appropriate means. Conversely, a highly penetrating external beam of X-rays or gamma rays is therapeutically useful. Gamma emitters outside the body can be used to irradiate tumours deep within the body because gamma rays are not necessarily stopped by the surface layers. Hence the energy they carry can be deposited deep within the body.

Teletherapy grade cobalt 60, used in the gamma ray treatment of cancer, is enclosed in stainless steel containers for secure containment, but also because the container absorbs the unwanted beta particles that are emitted from cobalt 60. The desirable gamma rays can easily penetrate the stainless steel container. Because of their intense radioactivity, and the penetrating ability of gamma rays, teletherapy sources must be transported in containers lined thickly with lead and having a mass of several tonnes. They are inserted into hospital teletherapy units by remote handling equipment.

14.6 Producing Isotopes for Nuclear Medicine

Nuclear medicine is the application of the techniques of nuclear physics to medicine. Most applications involve the use of artificially produced radioisotopes from nuclear reactors. These first became readily available in the USA in about 1945. Australia has had the capacity to produce radioisotopes since 1960 when the Australian Nuclear Sciences and Technology Organisation's (ANSTO) research reactor at Lucas Heights near Sydney began operation. The radioactive substances that occur naturally in the earth have little application in nuclear medicine as they are too long-lived (that is, are not radioactive enough), are difficult to extract, emit radiation of an unsuitable energy, or are not suitable for internal administration. In 1991 the National Medical Cyclotron Facility at Royal Prince Alfred Hospital in Sydney started producing the short-lived positron-emitting radioisotopes that cannot be made in a reactor.

When material is placed in a nuclear reactor it is subjected to intense irradiation by neutrons. These arise from the fission of nuclear 'fuel' (uranium 235 or plutonium 239 nuclei) into smaller nuclear fragments and several neutrons. Neutrons will enter the nuclei of the normally stable 'target' atoms and be 'captured' by the strong nuclear force, thus altering the ratio of neutrons to protons away from the optimum ratio. This makes the irradiated nuclei radioactive, as beta emitters (because they have an *excess* of neutrons). These artificial radioisotopes, or their decay products, can then be processed in the laboratories of ANSTO to make the desired product.

Target material placed in a 'compact' cyclotron is subjected to an intense but low-energy beam of charged particles such as protons or deuterons (a nucleus consisting of one proton and one neutron). The nuclear reactions that occur on collision with the target elements produce radioisotopes. These are different from the radioisotopes produced in a nuclear reactor because they are *deficient* in neutrons. Hence they are most likely to decay by emitting a positron.

The most useful radiation by far, and the one preferred for *in vivo* diagnostic techniques, is low-energy gamma radiation. Daughter isotopes that emit gamma radiation may be the result when a reactor or cyclotron-produced radioisotope decays. The ideal energy of gamma radiation is about 150 keV as this enables present-day instruments to record most clearly the distribution of the radioisotope in the patient.

Even the diagnostic use of radioisotopes involves the patient in exposure to ionising radiation, so the justification for such exposure should be a matter for concern to the physician. The question to be resolved is whether there is greater risk in submitting a patient to a test than in not having the test performed. In some cases the very sick could not tolerate the alternative forms of examination such as exploratory surgery.

14.7 Radiopharmaceuticals

Radiopharmaceuticals are radioactive substances which may be administered to humans for diagnostic or therapeutic purposes. The chemical properties of the radioisotope of a particular element in a radio-pharmaceutical are virtually identical to those of the stable non-radioactive forms of the element. The radioactive form, therefore, is handled by the body in the same manner as the stable form and the sequence of metabolic events is identical in either case.

The radioisotope selected for inclusion in radiopharmaceuticals must satisfy several criteria:

1. It should have a short half-life.
2. It should not emit alpha or beta particles.
3. It should emit gamma rays in the range 100 to 250 keV.
4. All the atoms should be radioactive. In this case the actual mass of radioisotope would be insignificantly small and would present neither toxicity problems nor interfere with normal metabolic processes.
5. It is advantageous if the radioisotope has multiple valency states so that a wide variety of compounds can be prepared from it.

The foregoing considerations reduce the existing field of approximately 1300 radioisotopes to only one, technetium 99m (^{99m}Tc). Technetium is element number 43 in the periodic table but does not occur naturally. It was first named in 1937 by Perrier and Segré but its medical significance was not realised until the 1960s. Technetium 99m emits gamma rays of energy 140 keV with a half-life of six hours (short, but long-lived enough for medical procedures). Six hours is much longer than the usual half-life for such a decay, so the radioisotope is called 'metastable'. Hence the 'm' alongside its mass number. Technetium has a radio-activity of 2×10^{17} Bq per gram, which is very high, so only very small amounts need be administered.

Technetium 99m is the daughter nucleus that results from the beta decay of the parent isotope, molybdenum 99. ^{99}Mo, produced in a nuclear reactor, has a half-life of 67 hours so can be transported thousands of kilometres by air to users remote from the reactor. ^{99m}Tc can then be 'milked' from the mixture of parent and daughter nuclei in the generator for the next few days as required. After emitting a gamma ray, each ^{99m}Tc nucleus becomes ^{99}Tc which in turn decays by beta emission to ruthenium 99 (see Figure 14.8). ^{99}Tc has a half-life of 212 000 years so is eliminated from the body, along with any undecayed ^{99m}Tc, before an appreciable number of beta particles have time to be emitted.

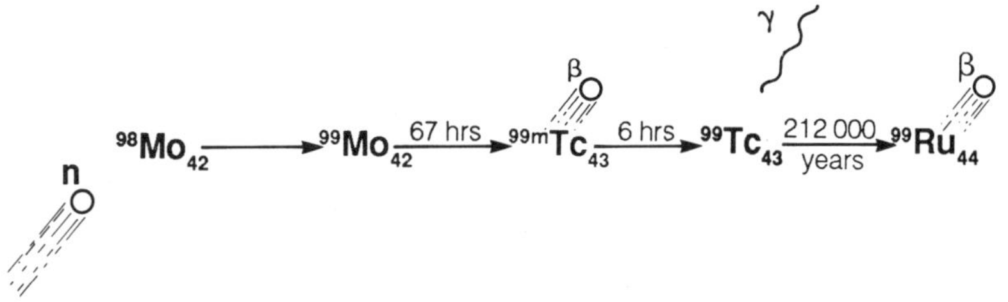

Figure 14.8 *The conversion of molybdenum 98 to radioactive molybdenum 99 in a nuclear reactor begins a series of decays with a variety of half-lives* (see Errata)

Each radiopharmaceutical can be divided into two components, the radioisotope 'label' and a combination of non-radioactive chemical compounds called the 'chelator'. The chelator is attached to technetium 99m to give it the specific biological properties that are required for the desired procedure. Together the label and the chelator are called the 'tracer'. The non-radioactive chelator compounds may be considered as the 'carriers' which transport the radioisotope to the target area in the human body. Each target area requires a highly specific carrier. For example, technetium-bromo-benzimidazole-imino diacetic acid (technetium-BIMIDA) is most suitable for imaging the liver, bile and gall-bladder.

The non-radioactive carrier compounds are supplied to the physician as a single-dose vial containing the appropriate freeze-dried chemicals. An injectible radiopharmaceutical results when the radioisotope is added to the vial.

14.8 Diagnostic Use of Radioisotopes

In diagnostic use, very small amounts of radioisotope can be used to trace metabolic pathways, so the radiation produced has a minimal effect on the patient and even less on the staff. Radioactive decay is independent of the chemical compound in which the radioisotope is carried. Furthermore the emission of a gamma ray leaves the chemical properties of the atom containing the daughter nucleus unchanged from the parent. That is, technetium is still technetium after the emission of a gamma ray. So it is possible to 'label' or 'tag' convenient molecules with a gamma-emitting radioisotope without affecting the way that the molecules are used in the body.

The radiopharmaceutical is injected intravenously (or inhaled) and moves to the target area. The emitted gamma rays are detected as they leave the body and their place of origin can be determined. In this way the location and concentration of the radioisotope, and the compound containing it, can be traced. The images produced may be obtained via a gamma ray 'camera' or by the PET technique (see below).

14.8.1 *The Nuclear Medicine Scan*

The gamma rays are detected by a sensitive and quite sophisticated gamma ray 'camera' developed by Hal O. Anger in 1958. The image (called a scan) produced by the 'camera' is a computer-generated display on the screen of a cathode ray tube. The screen displays the scintillations (flashes of light) produced when a gamma ray is absorbed in one of the large clear crystals of sodium iodide in the 'camera'. The origin of the gamma ray can be determined from its direction of travel so a reasonably good image of the organ that has accumulated the tracer can be obtained. Abnormal concentrations of radioisotope can be seen easily and indicate unusual functioning. Note that the difference between a nuclear medicine scan and a radiograph or scan using X-rays is that the former provides information on the way the body is *functioning*, while the latter provides information on *anatomical changes* in the body. Hence the two imaging modalities are complementary rather than alternatives.

Although ^{99m}Tc is used for most radiopharmaceuticals, other radioisotopes are sometimes used because of their unique physical or chemical properties. Some of them are listed in Table 14.3.

Table 14.3 *Radioisotopes used for certain procedures*

Isotope	Procedure
calcium 47	evaluating bone metabolism
chromium 51	survival time of red blood cells
cobalt 57	diagnosis of pernicious anaemia
gallium 67*	mapping certain tumours, hidden infection
indium 111*	monoclonal antibodies, abscess
iodine 123*	thyroid, brain, kidneys
iodine 125	*in vitro* thyroid studies
iodine 131 or 132	thyroid function studies, blood volume studies
iron 59	metabolism of iron, anaemia studies
mercury 195m*	paediatric heart studies
phosphorus 32	metabolic processes
potassium 42	body electrolyte determination
rubidium 81*	lung ventilation
sodium 24	body electrolyte determination
thallium 201*	monitoring heart muscle function

* Cyclotron produced, therefore very short half-life.

14.8.2 *The PET Scan*

Positron emission tomography (PET) was not available in Australia until 1991 when the facility at Royal Prince Alfred Hospital (Sydney) was completed. PET is a non-invasive investigative procedure that is used for the study of regional tissue physiology, biochemistry and pharmacology. The very short lived radioisotopes necessary for a PET scan can only be produced in a cyclotron. A cyclotron is an electrical machine that is capable of accelerating charged particles (such as protons, deuterons and mesons) to very high speeds. These very energetic particles produce a nuclear reaction when they collide with a nucleus in the target. The target nucleus loses neutrons which renders it radioactive. The radioisotopes are chemically extracted from the target and then converted to the appropriate pharmaceutical formulation and administered to the patient.

Cyclotron-produced radioisotopes will decay with a very short half-life by emitting a positron. A positron is a positively charged electron. It travels only a few millimetres in tissue before it is attracted to a negatively charged electron. The two annihilate each other leaving two gamma photons, each of energy 511 keV, which leave the point of annihilation in opposite directions. The patient is surrounded by a ring of detectors, so that the emitted gamma photons are detected simultaneously by detectors on opposite sides of the ring. The photons must have originated on the line joining the two detectors (see Figure 14.9). Computers record the relative intensities of many such lines, identify the position where the annihilation occurred and construct an image of the distribution of radioisotope.

The PET technique produces an image of the location of the positron-emitting radioisotope. The picture reflects the functional status of the organ or tissue that has absorbed the radiopharmaceutical. The radioisotopes suitable for PET are listed in Table 14.4; they are all cyclotron produced. These are the radioactive counterparts of the normal oxygen, nitrogen, carbon and hydrogen in organic molecules. Notice that their half-lives are very short, ranging from 2 to 110 minutes, thus it is necessary to locate the PET facility adjacent to a cyclotron. Such short half-lives mean that the chemical conversion to a radiopharmaceutical must be very rapid and that transport of them to distant locations is not possible.

PET is used to study glucose metabolism and oxygen metabolism. It is useful in the study of several neurological conditions and is the best method for selecting those epileptic patients that would benefit

Table 14.4 *Radioisotopes suitable for PET*

Isotope	Half-life (min)	Use
carbon 11	20	brain
fluorine 18	110	epilepsy, glucose metabolism
nitrogen 13	10	heart
oxygen 15	2	oxygen metabolism

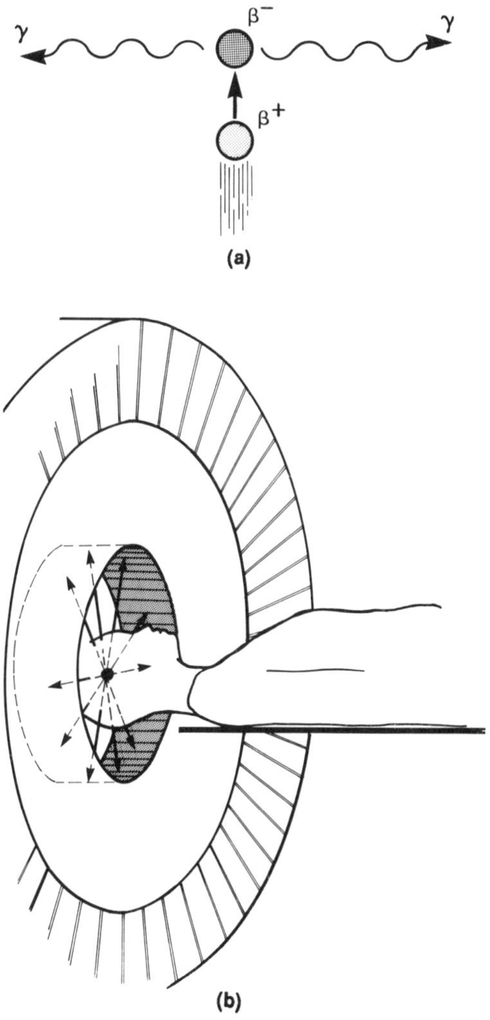

Figure 14.9 *Positron emission tomography. (a) The ejected positron combines with an electron whereupon both particles disappear and are replaced by two identical gamma photons. (b) These photons are detected by a ring of detectors when they arrive at opposite sides of the ring at the same time*

from surgery. It can also contribute to the management of heart disease, stroke and cancer. PET can relate brain chemistry to mental function so promises to be useful for the care of psychiatric patients.

14.9 The Effect of Ionising Radiation on Tissue

Ionising radiation is any radiation that produces ions when it interacts with matter. Such radiation includes alpha particles, electrons, positrons, protons and high-frequency electromagnetic radiation (ultraviolet, X- and gamma rays). Their effect on tissue is the same, differing only in the amount of energy delivered per millimetre of penetration. The mechanisms of tissue destruction are not completely understood, but have their origins in intracellular effects. Radiation seems to inhibit cell division in those cells whose normal function is to reproduce themselves (stem cells). The atomic effects of radiation on tissue are well understood. When a gamma ray or X-ray photon enters tissue it can give up energy in one of three ways: by the photoelectric effect, the Compton effect or by pair production. The method of energy loss depends on how much energy the photon had to start with.

1. If the photon has less than 1 MeV of energy, all of it may be used to eject an electron from an atom or molecule (this is called the **photoelectric effect**), thus creating a gap in the electron 'cloud' of the molecule. The gap will be filled by a nearby electron, which emits an X-ray photon in the process. The X-ray photon released by the 'gap-filling' electron is called a secondary photon.
2. Photons of all energies may find part of their energy used to eject an electron, while the remainder becomes a lower-frequency photon (this type of interaction is called the **Compton effect**). The new lower-frequency photon then repeats process 1, 2 or 3. Again the gap left by the Compton electron will be filled by a nearby electron, which emits an X-ray photon in the process.
3. If the photon has more than 1.022 MeV, **pair production** can occur. The photon imparts its energy to a nucleus, which produces and ejects an electron and a positron (a pair of beta particles). The positron annihilates with a nearby electron to produce a pair of photons, each of energy 0.511 MeV and travelling in opposite directions.

In all cases the ejected electrons and new photons have very high energy and will go speeding on to crash into other molecules to produce many more ions. The result of ionisation may be the formation of broken and altered molecules along with chemically active ions and free radicals (unbonded, electrically neutral, very chemically active fragments of molecules). The chemical reactions that are produced by free radicals also produce damage in the irradiated tissue. A reaction which occurs in some cases is that two hydroxyl radicals, HO·, combine to form hydrogen peroxide, H_2O_2, which is toxic. An hydroxl radical can also react with a biomolecule R to produce an organic free radical, R·. This could just recombine with an electron to reform the original biomolecule. However, in the presence of oxygen, R· can form a peroxiradical ROO·. This prevention of the recombination of the original biomolecule in the presence of oxygen is called the 'oxygen effect'. If the original biomolecule is no longer present, the metabolic function of the cell is impaired.

Cells are able to repair most of the molecular damage if the radiation is not too intense and there is sufficient time between exposures. If the damage can not be repaired the cells may die and be replaced by new healthy ones. Sometimes a cell will survive but have a damaged DNA molecule (a mutation) which will be inherited by the new cells when the old cell divides. The result may be insignificant, in rare cases it may be an improvement, but usually the cell will not function as well as the unmutated one.

A genetic change could be the cause of cancer in the tissue at a later time. If the mutated cell is a gamete (sperm or egg), then the embryo formed by fertilisation may be unviable or may develop to be an impaired individual. About one in ten live-born children carry some form of genetically related defect. On the other hand, small mutations selected by nature for their survival value have resulted, after hundreds of thousands of years, in the evolution of some interesting forms of life, including ourselves!

14.10 Therapeutic Use of Radiation

X-rays and gamma rays have proved to be useful in the treatment of cancer because they can kill cancerous cells just as they can kill healthy cells. The basis of radiation therapy is to expose the cancer to such a high dose of radiation that all the cancerous cells are killed. At the same time, the damage caused to normal tissue must be kept to a level from which it can recover. To achieve a high level of tumour damage, as much of the radiation energy as possible must be deposited in the cancer rather than in the normal tissue, and the normal tissue must be given time to recover from the irradiation. Too little radiation does not kill all the cancer, too much can produce serious complications in normal tissue. A number of factors make irradiation a suitable treatment for cancer:

1. Undifferentiated cells and rapidly dividing cells are more sensitive to radiation than differentiated and slowly reproducing cells. Since cancerous cells are dividing rapidly, they are more susceptible to radiation than most normal cells. Normal cells that do have a high susceptibility to radiation are white blood cells, red blood cells, gametes and the cells of the intestinal membrane because they are rapidly dividing. The inevitable damage to the membrane produces 'radiation sickness' and damage to the blood cells must be monitored carefully.

2. Normal tissue recovers faster and more completely than cancerous tissue, especially if the radiation dose is given at intervals which allow normal tissue to recover. Thus a total dose of 50 grays (see Section 14.13) may be received by a skin cancer in smaller doses of one or two grays, given four or five times a week for up to six weeks. The repair of radiation damage to normal tissue results from the multiplication of surviving normal cells and the migration and multiplication of normal cells from outside the irradiated region.

3. The presence of oxygen in tissue increases the production of free radicals in the irradiated area and hence the damage to tissue. This 'oxygen effect' was discovered by Louis Gray in England in about 1955. He found that oxygenated tissue is more susceptible to radiation damage than hypoxic tissue. Large cancers often contain hypoxic areas in their centre where the blood supply is not good, so are less sensitive to radiation than the surrounding normal oxygenated tissue. Thus small tumours with a good blood supply are more likely to be cured. If the oxygen supply to tumour cells can be increased at the time of irradiation, then their sensitivity to radiation is increased as is the efficacy of therapy.

Electromagnetic radiation is by far the most common form of radiation used in therapy; however, electrons (or beta particles) are also used for some applications. Linear accelerators are able to direct a beam of electrons as well as X-rays onto a skin cancer. The electrons, because they do not penetrate deeply, deposit all of their energy at the body surface so that large amounts of energy may be delivered to superficial tumours without affecting underlying tissues. A technique for treating arthritis using beta radiation is in the experimental stages of development. The treatment involves injecting a compound containing dysprosium 165, a beta emitter with a half-life of two hours, directly into the knee joint. The radioisotope diffuses throughout the synovial fluid and the beta particles that are emitted destroy some of the membrane that produces the fluid. In this way, production of fluid is depressed which reduces the swelling in the joint. Dysprosium 165 has such a short half-life that the radioactivity decreases to acceptable levels very quickly.

14.11 Methods of Irradiation

14.11.1 *External Beam Therapy (Teletherapy)*

Most skin cancers are treated with an external beam. The penetration of radiation is dependent on its energy, the higher the energy the deeper the penetration. Thus for superficial therapy, low-voltage X-ray units are used, while thicker lesions require a deep therapy (orthovoltage) unit, electron therapy, or caesium 137 treatment.

As the energy of radiation increases, not only does it penetrate further, but the absorbed dose will be highest several centimetres below the skin rather than at the skin surface; that is, for high-energy radiation there is a 'skin sparing' effect. For tumours below the skin, X-radiation of very high energy that is produced by a **linear accelerator** is used. Alternatively, gamma rays from cobalt 60 may be used. Recall that X-rays and gamma rays are both electromagnetic radiation so that a high-energy X-ray photon will be *exactly* the same thing as a low-energy gamma ray photon if their frequencies is the same. Only the method of production differs, the gamma ray arising from the nucleus of a radioisotope and the X-ray from the deceleration of very energetic (and therefore high-speed) electrons. To limit the dose received by the healthy overlying tissues, the beam of radiation is rotated so that its entry point to the body varies. The tumour is always in the beam so it receives a higher dose than the tissues closer to the surface which spend less time in the beam (see Figure 14.10).

The cobalt 60 source emits gamma radiation (of energies 1.17 and 1.33 MeV) uniformly in all directions so a beam must be created by shielding the source with lead or depleted uranium (which is much denser than lead) in every direction except the one desired. A gamma ray source has the advantage of not needing an electrical supply and requiring very little maintenance.

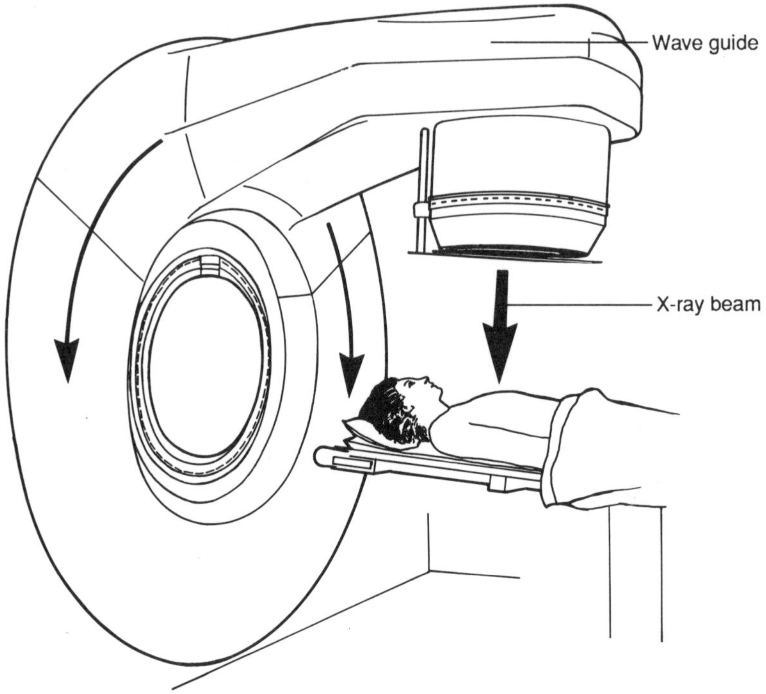

Figure 14.10 *External beam radiation therapy using a linear accelerator. The patient lies along the axis of the circle through which the accelerator turns so that the wave-guide can direct X-rays at the tumour from any angle*

Hence gamma ray therapy is used in hospitals where little technical backup is available; however, it is limited to the gamma energies stated above. X-rays are produced from an area smaller than a cobalt source so that the edge of the beam is better defined. Consequently the beam may be contoured to concentrate it onto the target area so that less of the surrounding tissue is irradiated. Since 1970, the availability of compact linear accelerators has meant that X-rays of very high energy (4 MeV, 10 MeV and higher), and hence of deeper penetration than that available from radioactive sources, can be produced. For this reason the linear accelerator is replacing radioisotopes in external beam therapy.

Patients receiving external beam therapy absorb massive (albeit localised) doses of radiation but do not become radioactive themselves. The source of radiation is external to them so once the beam is turned off it is safe to care for them as for other patients. However, during the therapy no one apart from the patient should be in the room. The therapy is monitored by closed-circuit television from the nursing station which is shielded from the linear accelerator by the walls of the therapy room which are more than a metre thick.

14.11.2 *Brachytherapy*

In this therapy, the radioisotope is surgically implanted inside the body. To reduce the exposure of staff the radioactive source may be loaded into its receptacle after the receptacle has been implanted. Caesium 137 and cobalt 60 are used in the **intracavitary** treatment of carcinoma of the cervix and vagina. The sources are inserted in the vagina for several days or for four or five hours a day for about a week.

Sometimes radioisotopes are encapsulated into structures called 'seeds', 'needles', 'grains' or 'wires' and implanted directly into the tumour. Such **interstitial** implantation ensures the maximum radiation intensity from a source of given strength and that radiation to the surrounding normal tissue is of lower intensity than to the tumour. A teletherapy beam usually has to pass through normal tissue to reach a tumour, but the radiation from an implanted source must pass through the tumour to reach normal tissue. Thus most of the energy is deposited in the tumour. Normal tissue, being further from the source, receives a lower dose, and is also shielded to some extent by the cancerous tissue.

14.12 Radiation Safety

Some of the somatic effects (those harmful to the person being irradiated) of radiation became evident soon after the discovery of X-rays. In 1896, twenty three cases of radiodermititis were reported in the world literature. The first American radiation fatality was Clarence M. Dally, an assistant to Thomas Edison, who died of cancer in 1904. However, it was not until 1921 that the British X-ray and Radium Protection Committee was set up to investigate methods for reducing exposures.

In order to reduce exposures it is necessary to measure how much exposure is occurring. Furthermore, in order to measure exposure it is necessary to know exactly what constitutes exposure and the effects it has. Neither of these tasks is straightforward as radiation cannot be detected by any of the human senses and its effects are often not apparent until a considerable time has elapsed. The detection of radiation is by indirect means and is technologically sophisticated. Different forms of radiation need different forms of detection for accurate measurement. These complications make the measurement of radiation a sophisticated procedure. The British Committee was further frustrated in their efforts by the lack of a suitable unit of radiation measurement.

In 1928 the Second International Congress of Radiology appointed a committee to install the roentgen as a unit of exposure. This became the accepted unit even though it was not accurately defined. The first recommended maximum permissible dose was set in 1931 by a group of American scientists. Since then, the recommended maximum dose has been lowered several times as our experience of radiation increases and committees have become more cautious (see Table 14.5, where the dose is stated in the SI unit, the sievert, abbreviated to Sv).

The recommended maximum permissible dose applies to people exposed to radiation through their work. The recommended maximum dose for an individual not exposed to radiation through their work is one tenth of the work-related figure (that is, 0.005 Sv/year). Furthermore the average dose for the general population as a whole is recommended as one third of this (0.0017 Sv/year). This last value cannot be further reduced as it is approximately equal to the dose from the natural background radiation. The implication in setting maximum doses is that radiation workers can receive relatively 'large' doses without significant genetic impact on the total population. This is because the genetic impact of the small number of radiation workers on the gene pool of the general population is low, when the 'dilution' effect of the large numbers in the general population is considered, provided of course that the dose to the general population is low.

Table 14.5 *Maximum permissable doses for radiation workers — the decrease in allowed dose over time*

Date	Maximum dose (sieverts/year)
1931	0.5
1936	0.3
1948	0.15
1958	0.05
? 1991	0.015

14.13 Radiation Units

There are many units in use to measure radiation and its complex interaction with humans, so we need to explain carefully the difference between them. The most important SI unit for us is the **sievert** (Sv), named after the person who in 1932 first proposed a unit to measure absorbed doses of radiation. To appreciate the significance of the sievert we need to work through the steps used to arrive at this unit.

X-rays and nuclear radiation carry energy and produce molecular ionisation events that can be accurately measured. Consequently the radiation measurements we make are in terms of the amount of ionisation produced in, and the amount of energy absorbed by, the tissue.

Recall that the becquerel measures the radioactivity of a source of radiation. One becquerel is one nuclear decay per second. The becquerel does not distinguish between alpha, beta and gamma rays and does not apply to X-radiation (as X-rays do not result from nuclear decays). Nor does the becquerel refer to the energy of the radiation, or its effect on tissue. Furthermore an external radioactive source emits its radiation in all directions, that is, away from as well as towards the patient. In addition, if radiation passes through the body, it has not been absorbed. We need a measure of the energy *actually absorbed by the tissues of the body.* The becquerel is not suitable for this.

The **roentgen** (R) is the amount of X- or gamma radiation that produces, in one cubic centimetre of air, ions carrying 3.3×10^{-10} coulombs of charge. That is, the roentgen applies to ionisation in air rather than energy absorbed in the body. The exposure of soft tissue to 1 R of X-rays results in the absorption of slightly less than 0.01 J/kg, but this absorption varies for different body tissues. Because of this inaccuracy, the roentgen was discarded in favour of the 'gray' which states the amount of energy absorbed per kilogram of *any* absorbing material.

The **gray** (Gy) is the SI unit of 'absorbed radiation dose', and was named after Louis Harold Gray (1905–1965), a Briton who, among other achievements, discovered the 'oxygen effect'. A previous unit was the **rad** (100 rad = 1 Gy). A dose of 1 Gy means that one joule of energy would be deposited in each kilogram of absorbing material. Note that the gray refers to the dose that is actually *absorbed.* A gamma ray that passes through the body without being absorbed does not add to the dose.

A radiation treatment for cancer may be stated as a 3 Gy dose to a specific area (3 mJ/g of tissue). However, a 3 Gy dose of alpha radiation has a different effect on tissue than a 3 Gy dose of gamma rays, even though the same amount of energy is absorbed. In order to compare the biological effect of a 3 Gy dose of one type of radiation to the same dose of another type of radiation, we state their effect relative to a 3 Gy dose of X-rays of energy 200 keV. Hence the biological effect of radiation is stated *relative* to 200 keV X-rays.

Consider a type of radiation having a **relative biological effect** (abbreviated as RBE) of five. This means that 200 keV X-rays would have to be administered at five times the dose of the radiation type in question to produce the same effect on tissue. The difference in 'relative biological effectiveness' depends on the amount of energy deposited in the tissue *per millimetre of distance travelled through the tissue.* Alpha particles are less penetrating than gamma rays, so the energy carried by a beam of 1 MeV alpha particles is deposited along a much shorter path than is the case for a beam of 1 MeV gamma photons. Consequently the biological effect of alpha radiation is quite different from the effect of gamma radiation. The RBE for several radiations are compared in Table 14.6.

Table 14.6 *Relative biological effectiveness of different radiation*

Radiation	RBE
beta	1
gamma	1
X	1
slow neutrons	4–5
fast neutrons	10
alpha	10–20

The sievert is a unit designed to measure the absorbed radiation dose in terms of its biological effect on humans, taking into account the different effects of radiation on tissue. Thus the sievert measures the **absorbed radiation dose equivalent**. Hence a 1 Sv dose of alpha radiation is equivalent (as far as possible) to a 1 Sv dose of gamma radiation. Note that a 1 Sv dose of alpha radiation would deposit all of its energy in the skin and would not affect the internal organs. However, a 1 Sv dose of gamma rays would affect internal organs because gamma rays are far more penetrating than alpha particles. Thus even with RBE values, there are inescapable differences between the types of radiation. A previous unit was the **rem** (100 rem = 1 Sv). The dose equivalent (in Sv) is calculated from the absorbed dose (in Gy) by multplying by the RBE:

$$\text{dose equivalent (Sv)} = \text{absorbed dose (Gy)} \times \text{RBE}$$

Note that because the RBE of beta, gamma and X-rays is one, the situation is simplified. For these types of radiation the sievert and the gray are the same unit. Hence for the electromagnetic radiation and electrons used in cancer therapy:

$$\begin{aligned} 1 \text{ sievert} &= 1 \text{ gray} = 100 \text{ rads} \\ &= 100 \text{ rems} = \text{(approx.) } 100 \text{ roentgen} \end{aligned}$$

The calculation of radiation absorbed doses (radiation dosimetry) is undertaken by specialist staff using computer-drawn maps of dose distribution. The software takes into account the dose equivalent, the X-ray intensity (or radioactivity of source), the energy of radiation, the tissues passed through and the exposure time. A typical radiotherapy dose would be 60 Sv (a large dose) while the dose for diagnostic radiography and scans using technetium would be 0.002 Sv (a very small dose).

14.14 Radiation Dose and the Body

Various parts of the body differ in their sensitivity to radiation. The hands and feet can receive a much larger dose without permanent damage than any other part. The most susceptible parts are the lens of the eye (cataracts), the bone marrow (leukemia), the gonads (sterility and mutation) and the unborn foetus (death). Lymphoid and epithelial tissue are among the most susceptible cells. If we consider the *whole body* being exposed to radiation for a time ranging from a few seconds to hours (acute exposure) then no somatic effects are detectable for doses below about 0.25 Sv. If the dose equivalent is about 1 or 2 Sv the debilitating effects are significant but temporary and full recovery can be expected. Above 5 Sv, the exposure can be expected to lead to death in 50% of cases.

In radiation therapy only certain organs or parts of the body are exposed and the dose that most organs can tolerate is considerably higher than that stated above, as long as the rest of the body is not exposed. For example, a localised skin dose of 55 Sv leads to a 5% chance of some deleterious effect after five years. The same tolerance, to a 40 Sv dose, is shown by the heart.

A radiation dose, if accumlated over many years (chronic exposure), is decidedly less damaging than if received as an acute exposure. An estimate of the average dose equivalent received by a human in his or her lifetime is about 0.16 Sv. This is due to the background radiation caused by the unavoidable exposure to naturally occurring radioisotopes (particularly the radon gas released from building materials) and cosmic rays. It also includes the effect of the nuclear power industry and weapons testing. The figure doubles if medical X-rays are taken into account.

The genetic effects of exposure to radiation are difficult to identify for humans, but we do know that DNA is readily damaged. The amount of damage is reduced by the subsequent repair reactions. Most of these reactions usually lead to complete recovery, that is, they are 'error free'. However, some are 'error prone' and lead to mutagenic repair. The radiation level at which the mutation rate becomes significant is not known. Furthermore, for low-level, long-term radiation exposure, it has not been proven that there is a threshold exposure level below which no harm is done, so it is best to assume that any dose is potentially harmful. Hence steps must be taken to minimise the exposure to ionising radiation at all times.

As long as cosmic rays, radiotherapy, diagnostic radiography, high-altitude air travel, nuclear weapons and nuclear power exist, some people will receive more radiation exposure than others. The maximum annual exposure from occupational duties was set at 0.05 Sv/year (over and above the exposure from background and medical radiation) by the International Commission for Radiological Protection in 1965. However, there is an obligation to reduce the dose to staff in accord with the 'ALARA' principle, which requires that radiation exposures be kept 'as low as reasonably achievable'. The level of exposure of workers who are in the vicinity of radiation is easily monitored by 'film badges' or by a thermo-luminescent dosemeter worn on the body. For the general population, exposure should be kept below 0.002 Sv/year.

14.15 Minimising Exposure to Radiation

Alpha and beta radiation are not extensively used in radiotherapy and are absorbed readily in the patient, so present little hazard to staff. Linear accelerators are used to irradiate patients with electrons, but these are readily stopped by matter, producing X-rays in the process. Thus we will concern ourselves with minimising exposure to X- and gamma rays. The minimum dose will be absorbed if the **time** spent near radiation sources is the minimum possible, if the **distance** between the source and staff is kept as large as practicable, and if **effective shielding** is used to absorb as much radiation as possible.

Diagnostic radioisotope investigations of the skeleton using technetium 99m result in a dose of about 8 mSv to the bone marrow of the patient. The dose is halved if other organs are investigated. In any case the dose is comparable to, if not less than, the dose from diagnostic X-rays. The potential dose to staff from the isotope inside the patient is even less because of the low energy of the gamma rays emitted, the small amount of radioisotope involved, the short half-life of technetium 99m and the short time that the isotope remains in the patient. Thus the hazard to staff is slight and decreases rapidly with the passage of several hours. Nevertheless precautions are routine and should be strictly observed. The nuclear medicine department in a hospital has a 'hot lab' with appropriate security and monitoring systems. Radioactive materials are kept there and prepared for administration. The radiopharmaceutical is loaded into the syringe by using forceps inside a fume cupboard behind a screen while the operator is shielded by a lead-glass window. The syringe containing the radiopharmaceutical is transported to the patient inside a holder made of lead. Nevertheless by keeping your distance from the patient and limiting the time spent near the patient, staff exposure outside the hot lab can be minimised. In addition, a lead-rubber apron provides effective shielding from the low-energy gamma rays (only 150 keV) involved.

Protection of staff during external beam therapy is relatively simple. Before and after treatment the radiotherapy device is turned off (for X-rays) or well shielded (for gamma rays) so presents no hazard. The patient and surrounds do not become radioactive as a result of the treatment so patient care can be carried on as normal. While teletherapy is proceeding only the patient remains in the room, which is shielded by concrete walls which are over a metre thick, so no one else should receive an appreciable dose.

Brachytherapy, however, does require special precautions. Staff treating patients implanted with radioactive sources may be exposed to radiation from quite strong sources. The energy of gamma radiation from these sources is high enough (0.66 MeV for cesium 137) to allow most of it to emerge from the patient and it will irradiate persons in the vicinity.

Fortunately, the intensity of gamma radiation decreases very rapidly with distance from the source (Figure 14.11). Since the rays spread out in all directions, their intensity decreases as the inverse square of the distance. In fact the dose received at 1 m from the source is a quarter of the dose at 0.5 m, and at 2 m the dose is one sixteenth of that at 0.5 m (an 'inverse square' relationship). Clearly, placing distance between the source and yourself is a most effective protection against large dosage. The effect of distance on dose rate is clarified in Table 14.7.

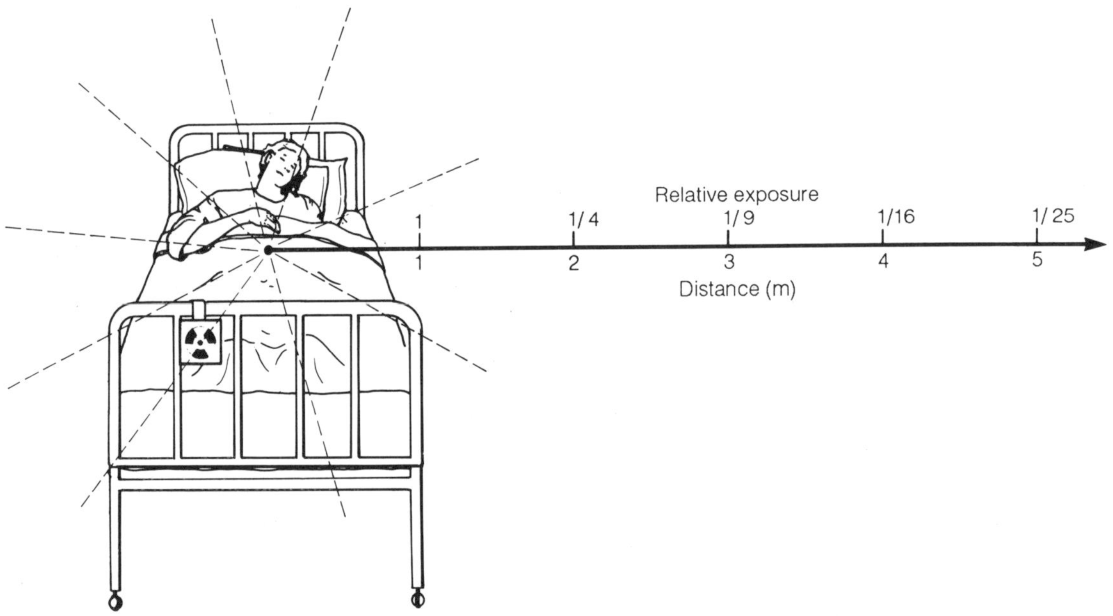

Figure 14.11 *Exposure to radiation decreases as the inverse square of the distance. Thus if you move to a distance of three metres after being one metre from the source, your distance has tripled, but your exposure has decreased to one ninth*

The less time that is spent near the patient, the smaller the dose received. The maximum permissible dose for staff is 50 mSv per year. Such a dose could be received by spending 250 hours at 1.5 m from the source. Conceivably, a nurse attending to patients in a radiotherapy ward without afterloading equipment (see Section 14.16) could receive this dose over a period of a year if not for the fact that staff are rotated.

Table 14.7 *Dose rates for an hour exposure to a typical cesium 137 source of activity 4.6 × 10^9 Bq at different distances*

distance (m)	dose per hour (mSv)
0.3	5
0.6	1.25
1	0.46
1.5	0.2
2	0.11
3	0.05
4	0.03
6	0.013
10.0	0.005

The dose to staff can be reduced further if shielding is used when working close to the patient. Although air absorbs a negligible amount of gamma radiation, solid absorbing material causes an exponential drop in gamma ray intensity with thickness (Figure 14.12). The distance that a particular gamma photon will travel through matter before it interacts cannot be predicted. We can, however, determine the thickness of an absorber through which a photon with a particular energy must pass to have a 50% chance of interacting. This is called the **half-value layer** for that energy. For a 0.5 MeV gamma photon it is 0.42 cm of lead. That is, half the number of original photons would emerge after passing through the lead, and only one quarter would penetrate 0.84 cm (that is, two half-value layers would absorb 75% of the photons of 0.5 MeV energy).

It is important to realise that *some* photons will still penetrate even very thick lead. For example, about 1% of 0.5 MeV photons will penetrate lead almost seven half-value layers (3 cm) thick. Photons of greater energy are even more penetrating; 5 MeV photons require more than 10.5 cm of lead to decrease their intensity to 1%. Even so, 1% may not be an acceptably low level if the original intensity was very high. The ultimate lower limit to the level of radiation exposure is the background radiation. If the exposure to staff is comparable to that received from the natural background then the work environment can be considered safe.

Clearly, the use of shielding alone is not an effective protection against high-energy electromagnetic radiation. Teletherapy rooms and isolation rooms that contain patients undergoing brachytherapy have walls, floors and ceiling that are heavily shielded by concrete and lead and no one but the patient is in the room during the therapy. Limiting the exposure time of staff and maximising the distance between the patient and the staff provides the necessary additional radiation protection.

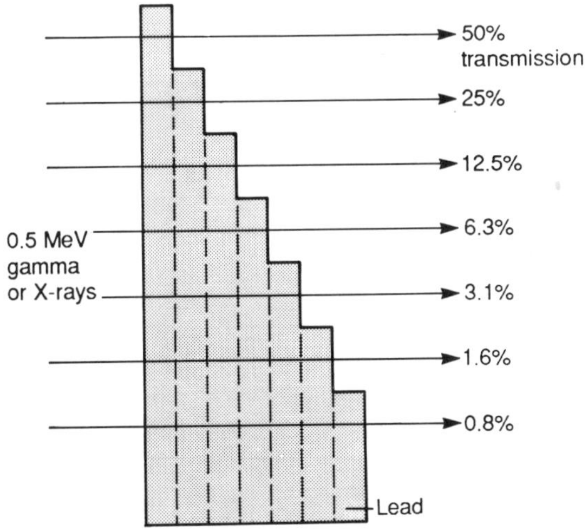

Figure 14.12 *Effect of shielding. The intensity of X-ray and gamma photons decreases exponentially with the thickness of the absorber. Seven 'half-value layers' of lead will reduce the intensity of the transmitted radiation to less than 1% of the original intensity of 0.5 MeV photons*

14.16 Afterloading to Minimise Exposure

The technique of **afterloading** in brachytherapy automatically reduces staff exposure to the minimum possible. In this technique, the tubes that will contain the radioactive beads or pellets are inserted, under general anaesthetic, into the appropriate cavity, without the radioisotope in place. That is, the tubes are empty and staff involved in the operating theatre are not exposed to any radiation. The radioactive sources are loaded afterwards either manually by one operator, or by remote control. In the brachytherapy isolation room, the remote afterloading equipment is programmed automatically to insert radioactive pellets and non-radioactive 'dummy' pellets into the tubes in the appropriate pattern to achieve the desired dose. The pellets are forced by compressed air from their well-shielded storage area in the machine, along delivery tubes connected to the patient's previously inserted tubes. Someone entering the room will cause the afterloading equipment automatically to return the pellets, by compressed air, to their shielded storage area. In this way, brachytherapy is occurring only when the patient is alone, and never when anyone else is in the room. Thus no staff, or visitors, are exposed to any appreciable dose whilst dealing with the patient.

14.17 Nursing Strategies

With the advent of afterloading techniques, radiation safety procedures have been considerably simplified. Brachytherapy is usually carried out at one centre so staff can be expertly trained, sources do not need to be transported and are always accounted for. The precautions that are taken are to:

- isolate the patient(s) in a room that is shielded;
- display radiation warning signs in the prescribed manner;
- monitor staff for radiation exposure;
- allow only persons licensed to handle radioactive sources to do so.

If sealed sources placed into a patient are not afterloaded or if a radioisotope is taken orally as a solution, additional precautions must be taken:

- nursing duties should be divided among staff;
- staff should not remain in the vicinity of the patient longer than necessary;
- staff should work at the maximum practicable distance from the source;
- a mobile lead shield should be available for protection of staff while attending the patient;
- time and distance limitations should be applied to visitors;
- pregnant nurses must not be used for patient care;
- staff of child-bearing age should be used as little as possible if at all;
- a source that slips out of a patient must be placed in a lead box using long-handled forceps, both of which should be at the bedside. The radiation safety officer should then be notified;
- dressings, bed linen and bedpans should be checked with a radiation meter before disposal to ensure that the source is not lost.

Bibliography

Coghlan, A. 'Irradiated food: too hot to handle?', *New Scientist*, **125**(1704), 14–15, 1990.

Upton, A.C. 'The biological effects of low-level ionising radiation', *Scientific American*, **246**(2), 29–37, 1982.

Questions

1. In the nuclear reaction, ${}^{238}_{92}\text{U} \longrightarrow \text{X} + {}^{4}_{2}\text{He}$, one of the products (${}^{4}_{2}\text{He}$) is an alpha particle. The other product (X) is
   J. ${}^{234}_{90}\text{Th}$
   K. ${}^{234}_{91}\text{Pa}$
   L. ${}^{236}_{91}\text{Pa}$
   M. ${}^{236}_{90}\text{Th}$
2. In an experiment to determine the half-life of a radioactive isotope, measurements of the mass of the isotope are made. If masses of 8 μg and 2 μg are recorded at intervals 8 days apart, what is the half-life of the isotope?
   J. 8 days
   K. 6 days
   L. 4 days
   M. 2 days
3. The half-value layer for gamma rays of 0.5 MeV is 0.42 cm of lead. What percentage of the original ray would penetrate four half-value layers?
   J. 50%
   K. 25%
   L. 12.5%
   M. 6.25%
4. Which one of the following radiations, all of 1 MeV energy, is the least penetrating?
   J. alpha rays
   K. beta rays
   L. gamma rays
   M. X-rays
5. Which one of the following beams is the most penetrating?
   J. 2 MeV gamma rays
   K. 2 MeV X-rays
   L. 3 MeV X-rays
   M. 5 MeV X-rays
6. The sievert is the unit of
   J. radioactivity
   K. absorbed radiation dose
   L. absorbed radiation dose equivalent
   M. energy of radiation
7. Keeping one's distance from a source of radiation is effective in minimising exposure because
   J. exposure is inversely proportional to distance
   K. exposure decreases as the inverse square of distance
   L. exposure decreases exponentially with distance
   M. electromagnetic radiation is absorbed by air
8. X-rays for radiation therapy are produced by
   J. a linear accelerator
   K. cobalt 60

L. an afterloading brachytherapy device
M. technetium 99m

9. Which one of the following statements about the radioisotope selected for inclusion in radiopharmaceuticals is not correct?
J. It should have a short half-life.
K. It should emit alpha or beta rays.
L. It should emit gamma rays in the range 100–250 keV.
M. All the atoms should be radioactive.

10. Which one of the following statements best describes what 'ionising radiation' is?
J. High-frequency electromagnetic radiation.
K. Charged particles that are emitted from radioisotopes.
L. Radiation that is emitted from a radioactive nucleus.
M. Radiation that can remove electrons from matter.

11. Radioactivity is the emission from the nucleus of an atom of
J. electrons or beta particles or gamma rays
K. alpha or beta particles or X-rays
L. electrons or beta particles or X-rays
M. alpha or beta particles or gamma rays

12. A radioisotope with a short half-life (say 5 hours) is
J. highly radioactive
K. weakly radioactive
L. of high penetrating ability
M. of low penetrating ability

13. In the nuclear reaction: ${}^{60}_{27}Co \longrightarrow {}^{0}_{0}\gamma + X$, the symbol 'X' represents
J. ${}^{60}_{28}Co$
K. ${}^{69}_{27}Co$
L. ${}^{60}_{27}Co$
M. ${}^{60}_{26}Co$

14. Which of the following is not a form of ionising radiation?
J. beta particles
K. gamma rays
L. infrared rays
M. X-rays

15. Brachytherapy as a form of radiation therapy has an advantage over external beam therapy (also called teletherapy) because
J. in brachytherapy, the radiation does not have to pass through healthy tissue to reach the tumour
K. in brachytherapy, there is the choice of using electrons as well as gamma rays
L. in teletherapy the energy of the radiation is limited to the energies available from the radioisotope
M. in teletherapy the total radiation dose must be given all at the one session

16. It is possible to trace metabolic pathways in the body using radioactive isotopes of the naturally occurring elements in the body because, radioactive isotopes
J. are used in such small quantities that they produce no toxic effects
L. have a very short half-life so soon decay to safe levels
L. are chemically identical to non-radioactive isotopes of the same element
M. are physically identical to non-radioactive isotopes of the same element

17. For *in vivo* diagnosis using a nuclear medicine technique, radioisotopes that emit low-energy gamma radiation are preferred to other radioisotopes because
J. other forms of radiation are emitted with too much energy
K. high-energy gamma radiation is not penetrating enough
L. most of the radiation will emerge from the patient's body
M. sources of X-rays require more extensive technical support than gamma sources

18. The 'relative biological effectiveness' (RBE) of radiation depends on the
J. recommended maximum permissible dose of radiation
K. amount of radiation absorbed by the whole body
L. dose of radiation that is actually absorbed in the tissue
M. energy deposited in the tissue per millimetre of distance travelled through the tissue

19. The intensity of gamma radiation decreases as the inverse square of the distance. This statement means that if the distance doubles, then the intensity
J. doubles
K. is halved
L. is four times as great
M. is one quarter as great

20. The use of staff of child-bearing age to nurse patients with implanted radioactive sources should be avoided because
J. such sources are highly radioactive
K. there is a risk of damage to the gametes of the staff
L. younger people are more at risk of developing radiation-induced cancers
M. implanted sources cannot be adequately shielded

CHAPTER 15

Commercial Chemicals and Human Health

The use of chemicals for the treatment of disease is one of the oldest human technologies. It began, thousands of years ago, as the preparation of complex mixtures from animal, vegetable and mineral sources. These mixtures varied greatly in their composition and most of them were useless.

For the last few decades the technology of chemical therapy has been dominated by the use of carefully formulated mixtures containing strictly controlled quantities of a single active ingredient. Many of these active ingredients are synthetic chemicals not found in nature. This modern approach to chemical therapy has enjoyed some spectacular successes and some of these are outlined in the first section of this chapter. On the other hand, the use of chemical therapy has, occasionally, gone badly wrong and some examples of this are also given.

The harm which is occasionally done by the use of therapeutic chemicals simply highlights the fact that all these substances are toxic. Many of them are best regarded as poisons having beneficial effects which outweigh their toxic effects. This feature of therapeutic chemicals is the reason for the inclusion of the chapter's second section which serves as an introduction to toxicology, the science of poisons.

In terms of volume, therapeutic chemicals make up a relatively small proportion of commercial chemicals. In agriculture and manufacturing industry they are used on a much greater scale and in ways which have seen them become contaminants of the general environment. Initially, concern about the capacity of this category of commercial chemicals to cause human injuries was restricted to the occupational setting and to people directly involved in their manufacture and use. In recent years though, it has been realised that some commercial chemicals present a risk to public health because of their presence in soil, air, water and food. The final section of this chapter gives an account of the uses and possible effects of some of these chemicals.

Learning Objectives

At the completion of this chapter you should be able to:

1. Discuss a number of compounds which, through their use as medicines, have significantly improved the human condition over the last 150 years.
2. Discuss some examples of serious harm caused by the use of medicines and the effect which such episodes have had on government regulation of medicines in countries like Australia.
3. Define the terms poison, acute poisoning, chronic poisoning, effective dose, threshold dose and Threshold Limit Value.
4. Outline the body's physical and biochemical defence mechanisms against toxic chemicals.

5. Discuss the basis for current concerns about the health effects of environmental lead in Australia, with particular reference to the situation which currently exists at Port Pirie, South Australia.
6. Discuss the basis for current concern over depletion of the earth's ozone layer and outline the health effects which this might be having now or those which might arise in future.
7. Discuss the diseases caused by exposure to asbestos, state the property of asbestos responsible for its toxicity and describe some situations in which asbestos exposure may occur.

15.1 Commercial Chemicals as Medicines

In the introduction the term **therapeutic chemical** has been used. This has the same meaning as the common term medicine and therapeutic chemicals or medicines may be defined as *substances which are taken for the purpose of preventing or altering the course of a disease*. In turn, a **disease** may be defined as *a morbid process or state which is accompanied by a characteristic set of symptoms*. The terms medicine and drug are often taken to have the same meaning but drug is a broader term than medicine. A **drug** may be defined as *any substance other than food which, when taken into the body, affects the living organism in some way*. From these definitions we see that *all medicines are drugs but not all drugs are medicines*. This distinction between drugs and medicines will be maintained throughout the following discussion.

15.1.1 *History of the Use of Medicines*

The earliest civilisations left written descriptions of the medicines which they used. Most of these must have been useless. For example, an ancient Egyptian medicine highly recommended for the treatment of blindness was a mixture of pig eyes, antimony, red ochre and honey. It was poured into the sufferer's ear. Any benefits which a person received from the use of this, and many other, ancient medicines can only have been due to either **spontaneous recovery** or **the placebo effect**. Spontaneous recovery occurs because of the inbuilt recuperative powers which we all possess. These are sufficient to get us over most of the diseases which we contract and sometimes they allow a person to recover from an illness which is usually fatal. The placebo effect occurs when people show an improvement in their condition after taking a substance which normally has no therapeutic benefit, but which they believe might be an effective remedy for their problem. This common, but mysterious, effect is a response to the mere act of taking a medicine.

Not all the ancient remedies can be dismissed as ineffective. For example, a medicine used for the treatment of night blindness was made from the livers of oxen. We now know that liver contains vitamin A and that a deficiency of this substance is the cause of night blindness. An ancient medicine used for the relief of pain and other discomforts was an extract of the opium poppy. These extracts contain the compound now known as morphine. Even now, thousands of years after it first came into use as a plant extract, morphine remains the most effective means available for the relief of deep-seated pain such as that which accompanies many forms of cancer. The number of effective medicines described in ancient historical records makes it likely that modern science has something to learn from a study of the medicines used today by the world's primitive people and this possibility occupies the attention of some scientists and physicians.

Although there were some effective medicines discovered in the period 4000 BC–1800 AD it is true to say that advances were slow and they did not have much impact on the outcome of most diseases and injuries. During this long period any person's chances of recovering from a serious disease or injury depended mainly on the quality of nursing care available to them. If a person had someone available to keep them clean, warm and fed, and if they were in good health prior to the occurrence of the disease or injury, their chances of recovery were as good as they could be. This situation did not start to change until the nineteenth century. Some of the most important developments which took place then were:

1. The development of the science of synthetic chemistry which gave access to a wide range of new compounds, some of which had useful therapeutic properties.

2. The development of anaesthetics. These improved the effectiveness of surgical procedures and greatly enlarged the range of procedures which could be attempted with some prospect of success.

3. The use of pure substances in place of complex and variable extracts. This allowed the physician to

control the dose of active ingredient a person was receiving as medicines were administered. Even more importantly, it helped establish the idea that particular, pure substances caused particular effects in the living organism.

4. The development of the germ theory of disease. This stimulated the use of antiseptics in surgery and improvements in the standards of personal and public hygiene.

15.1.2 *Anaesthetics*

The surgery carried out before about 1850 is best described as a series of savage, screaming encounters between the surgeons and their patients. A typical scene from those days is portrayed in Figure 15.1. The surgeon is shown halfway through the job of removing his patient's lower leg. The 'anaesthetist' is the person with his hand wrapped in cloth and standing nearby. He was often a retired boxer and at the start of the procedure he would step forward, at a signal from the surgeon, and strike the patient a hard blow to the head, rendering him unconscious! In those days the essence of the surgeon's skill was speed. He had to accomplish as much as he could during the brief period in which his patient was, at least to some degree, insensible to the fearsome pain which the surgery caused. If the patient regained consciousness before the surgery was completed the anaesthetist would step forward again and administer another dose of his crude anaesthetic.

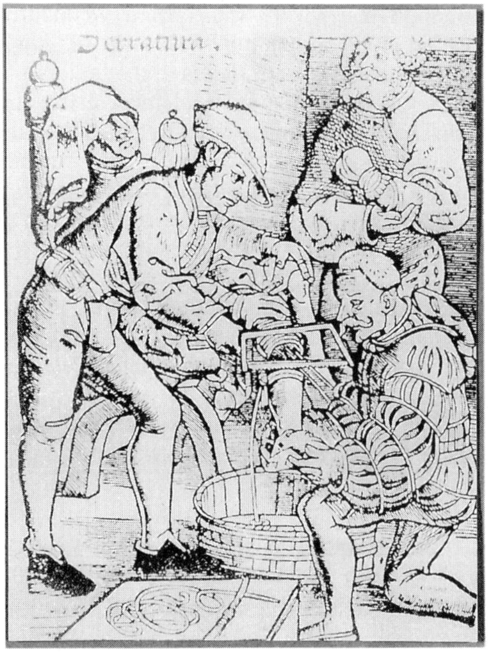

Figure 15.1 *Surgery in the sixteenth century*

All this began to change dramatically in 1846 when the American physician, William Morton, used **ether** as an anaesthetic during the extraction of a patient's tooth. This compound had been available since 1540. Its ability to alter consciousness had been noted many times but never exploited. However, soon after Morton's demonstration, ether became established in surgical practice in the United States.

In England, in 1847, **chloroform** was introduced as an anaesthetic by James Simpson. This compound was of more recent origin than ether, having been made for the first time in 1832. Simpson had witnessed the use of ether in the United States but was concerned by the large amount of it that was sometimes required to produce anaesthesia. This concern led him to investigate the anaesthetic properties of other volatile organic compounds. His experiments involved him inhaling the vapours of these compounds. He found chloroform to be superior to ether and his advocacy of the compound led to it becoming the anaesthetic most commonly used in Great Britain until about 1870. Structural formulae for ether and chloroform are given in Figure 15.2.

Simpson used chloroform to relieve women of the pain of childbirth. This was welcomed by his patients, but he was subjected to criticism by some clergymen who claimed that he was contravening the will of God. They argued that God had intended that women should suffer pain during childbirth. This criticism and argument continued until 1853. In that year Queen Victoria requested, and was given, chloroform in the hour before the birth of Prince Leopold. This brought to an abrupt end all criticism of the use of anaesthesia during childbirth. If it was appropriate for use by Victoria, Queen of England, Empress of India and Head of the Church of England, it was appropriate for any woman to use!

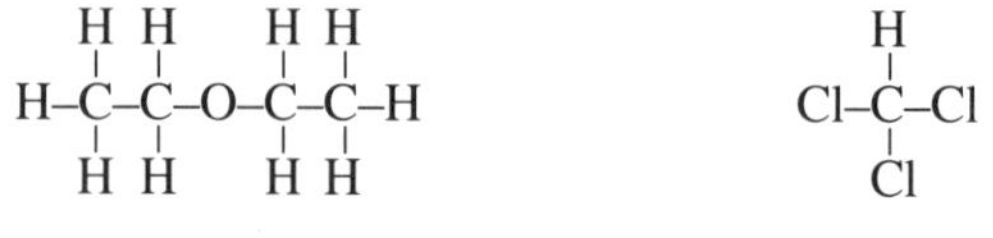

ether chloroform

Figure 15.2 *Structural formulae for ether and chloroform*

Even when chloroform use was at its height in Great Britain it was apparent to many physicians that ether was a far safer anaesthetic than chloroform. And yet chloroform continued in common use in some parts of the world until the early years of the twentieth century. This is rather surprising because it is a very hazardous substance which is capable of causing sudden death from heart failure. Within just a few months of its introduction it had caused the death of a fifteen-year-old girl who was anaesthetised for removal of a toe-nail. Three months earlier the same girl had had her other toe-nail removed under ether anaesthesia and had suffered no ill-effects. By 1863 the number of deaths caused in Great Britain by chloroform had reached the impressive total of 123 and many of these occurred during quite minor operations. The total number of deaths caused by chloroform must have been much greater than this because chloroform was also very popular in other parts of the world and was widely used for many years after 1863.

Perhaps the willingness of physicians to use such a hazardous substance as chloroform, for so long, simply reflects the great advance which chemical anaesthesia represented when it was introduced. Although chloroform claimed many lives it saved others and it spared thousands of people from excrutiating pain.

15.1.3 *Magic Bullets*

When the germ theory of disease is combined with the idea that a particular, pure substance might produce a particular effect in a living organism, the possibility arises of finding a pure substance which might kill the germ responsible for a disease without harming the person infected. The term **magic bullet** was coined to express this possibility and magic bullets have been responsible for most of the advances made this century in our ability to cure, or at least slow the progress of, diseases from which many people suffer. The names and structural formulae for several different magic bullets are shown in Figure 15.3. The development and action of each of these is discussed below.

Salvarsan, the First of the Magic Bullets. At the turn of this century the sexually transmitted disease **syphilis** was very common and when contracted it caused a long illness which led invariably to a premature and undignified death. In 1912, the German scientist, Paul Ehrlich, and his Japanese co-worker, Sachahiro Hata, announced their discovery of a substance which was effective against syphilis and which they called **arsphenamine**. It was sold as a medicine under the name **Salvarsan** as a cure for syphilis and proved effective in many cases. Although most medicines are organic compounds the names by which they are known are often unrelated to their correct chemical name. This is the case for many of the names which you will encounter in this chapter.

Ehrlich was led to his discovery by his observations, made years earlier, on the ability of certain compounds to selectively stain some cell components. These compounds were very useful in distinguishing the components of cells and have been used for that purpose ever since. Ehrlich reasoned that if compounds could be found which stained cells in different ways then it should be possible to find others which were selectively toxic. He was already aware of an arsenic compound which had been shown to have a favourable, although slight, effect on a human infection caused by a protozoan (single-celled organism). There were some similarities between this organism and the bacterium responsible for syphilis and so Ehrlich and his co-workers made many different arsenic compounds and tested each for anti-syphilitic activity. This led them to the discovery of arsphenamine (Salvarsan).

Treatment of syphilis with Salvarsan was not without its hazards. Arsenic compounds are toxic to humans and in the early years of its use Salvarsan killed many people while it cured others. However, the severity of the disease was such that people accepted the risk of death associated with the treatment in preference to the certainty of death without it.

Prontosil and Sulphanilamide. After the discovery of a cure for syphilis in 1912, no discoveries of similar consequence were made until 1935. In that year another German, Gerhard Domagk, observed that a compound which had been synthesised for use as a textile dye was able to cure severe bacterial infections in mice. The compound was known as **Prontosil** (see Figure 15.3). Domagk was greatly excited by his discovery and sought permission from his employers to embark on a study of Prontosil's capacity to cure similar infections in humans. Permission was denied, but almost immediately a strange twist of fate occurred. Domagk's young daughter pricked herself with a needle and, as a result, contracted a life-threatening infection as was common among children in those days. She was hospitalised, and near death, when Domagk urged her doctors to administer Prontosil. They agreed and the child made a remarkable recovery.

In spite of this dramatic demonstration of the efficacy of Prontosil the matter was not pursued in Germany.

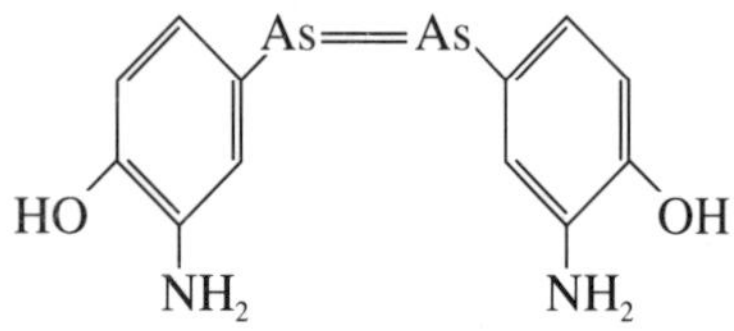

arsphenamine (Salvarsan)

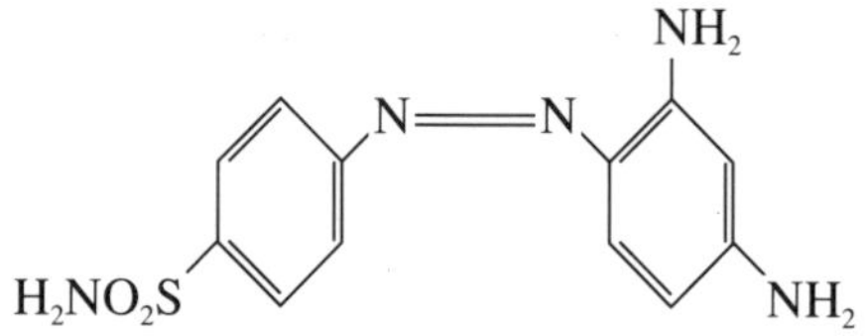

Prontosil

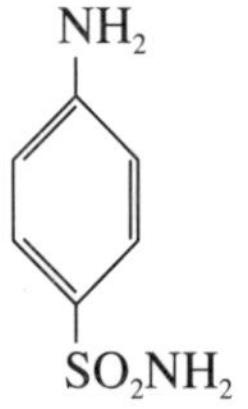

sulphanilamide

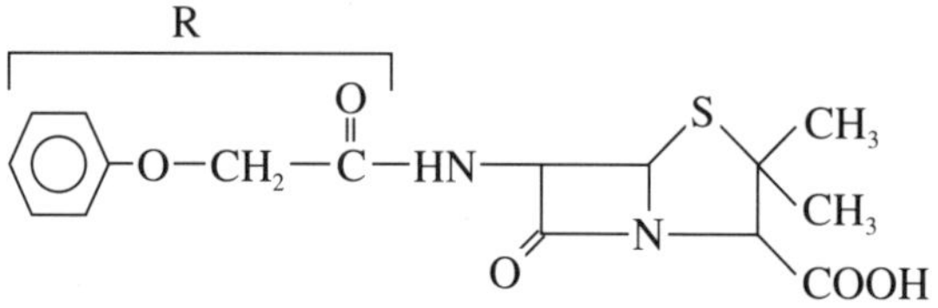

penicillin

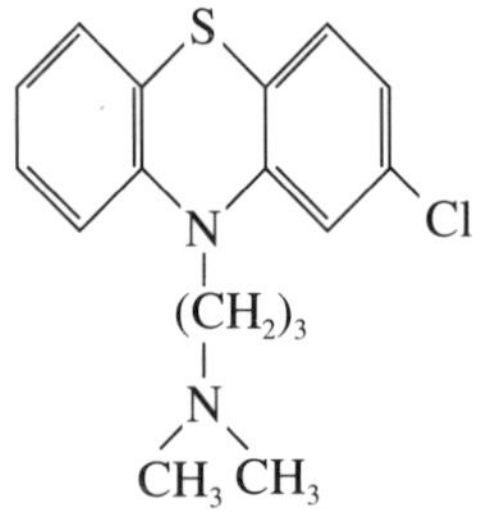

chlorpromazine

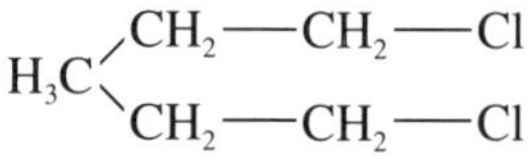

chlormethinum

Figure 15.3 *Magic bullets*

But in 1936, Prontosil was used in a clinical trial in London where it saved the lives of many women who had contracted blood infections (puerperal fever or childbed fever) while giving birth. In the meantime, it had been observed that Prontosil was not active against bacteria outside the body unless it was first subjected to reduction. This suggested that Prontosil itself was not active against bacteria but was converted inside the human body to another substance which was. This other substance was soon shown to be **sulphanilamide** (see Figure 15.3).

Sulphanilamide owes its anti-bacterial activity to its close resemblance to the amino acid, **p-aminobenzoic acid** (see Figure 15.4). This amino acid is essential for many bacteria. They use it to make **folic acid** (see Figure 15.4) which they then employ in the synthesis of amino acids and nucleotides. When sulphanilamide is present the bacterium mistakes it for p-aminobenzoic acid and uses it in place of that compound. This produces a substance similar to, but different from, folic acid. The substance is able to interact with the active sites of enzymes which the bacteria use for amino acid and nucleotide synthesis but it does not allow the normal reaction to proceed. In terms of the lock and key theory of enzyme action outlined in Section 13.8.5 the sulphanilamide causes the bacteria to produce a key which only fits the lock well enough to jam it. This 'jammed lock' causes the death of the bacterium by denying it a supply of essential compounds.

Sulphanilamide is a relatively toxic compound for humans. Furthermore, it had been synthesised and patented many years prior to the discovery of its anti-bacterial properties. The patent had lapsed and this meant that no company could obtain a fresh patent on the compound in 1936. These things together prompted a search for less toxic compounds of similar structure to sulphanilamide and having its anti-bacterial action. A number of these were discovered and brought into regular use. This family of medicines became known as the **sulphonamides** or the **sulphur drugs**. Two examples are **sulphapyridine** and **sulphathiazole**

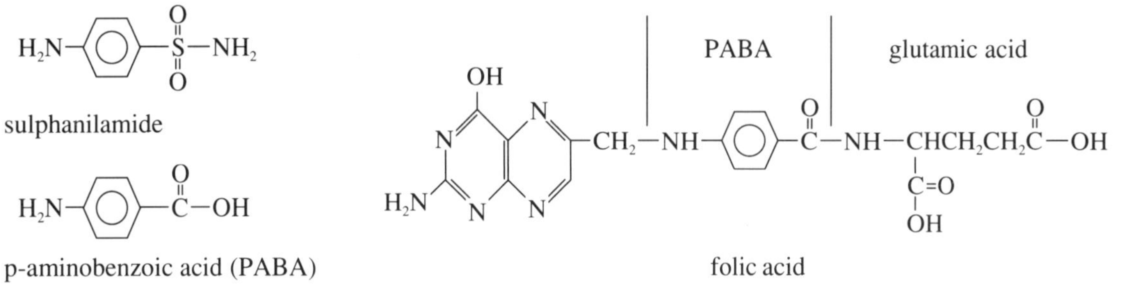

Figure 15.4 *Structural formulae for p-aminobenzoic acid and folic acid*

which have the structural formulae shown in Figure 15.5.

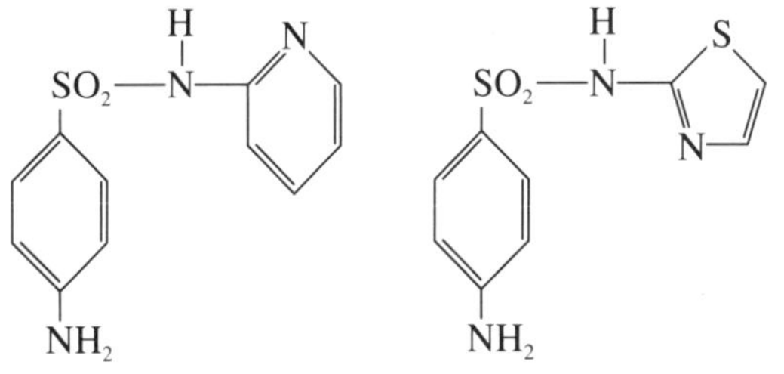

Figure 15.5 *Structural formulae for sulphapyridine and sulphathiazole*

Penicillin, the First Antibiotic. Although the sulphonamides represented a great step forward in the treatment of infectious disease they were not effective against all bacterial infections. In 1940, the first of a new type of anti-bacterial substance was made available through the efforts of Howard Florey and Ernst Chain (see Section 1.1.7). This was **penicillin**, a substance produced by a mould. Its toxicity was very low and it was remarkably effective against many organisms which were not vulnerable to the sulphonamides. It was the first example of the use of a substance produced by one microorganism to treat infections caused by other microorganisms. Penicillin turned out to be the first of many such substances and they became known collectively as the **antibiotics**. The structural formula of the original penicillin is shown in Figure 15.3. The section of the molecule designated 'R' may be varied by altering the composition of the medium on which the mould grows. In this way a whole family of penicillins has been made available and they are still the most effective agents available for the treatment of bacterial infections.

A distinguishing feature of bacteria is their possession of a comparatively rigid cell wall. Its function is to withstand quite large osmotic pressures which build up inside the organism due to concentration of solutes in its internal solution. Penicillins exert their effects against bacteria by interfering with the construction of this wall. They do so by interfering with the action of a specific enzyme responsible for the formation of covalent bonds between the large molecules out of which the cell wall is made. Formation of these bonds is essential in order for the cell wall to achieve the required rigidity. The cells in mammalian tissues are enclosed by membranes which are quite different to the walls of a bacterial cell and this explains why even massive doses of penicillin are well tolerated by most people.

Chlorpromazine and Mental Illness. In the 100 years prior to 1950 the number of people hospitalised for the treatment of mental illness increased steadily, year by year. Most of these people were suffering from a **psychosis**. This is the name given to any condition in which people lose touch with reality to such an extent that they cannot cope with the demands of ordinary life. These people may experience hallucinations, delusions, paranoia and dramatic swings in mood. An untreated psychosis is disabling and sufferers usually require hospitalisation. The conditions found in many psychiatric hospitals prior to 1950 were terrible, as the following description indicates.

> The major problem was violence. It was the violence of beat-up patients, beat-up staff, rooms torn apart, windows broken, toilets stuffed, clothes torn off, excrement thrown around and the all-day dehumanization of everyone. It was a time when knives and forks could not be provided at meals — curtains, wall pictures and anything but nailed-down furniture were not possible to use. There

were the "pack" rooms with their row on row of slabs and tubs for what was euphemistically called "hydrotherapy". There were the seclusion rooms furnished with nothing but a mattress and an out-of-reach light bulb where a creature, nude or in rags, paced like a caged animal, shouting back at his hallucinations. There were the insulin suite, the lobotomy ward — and always the interminable locking and unlocking of every door in the place. In such a chaotic situation the "good" patients were the mute, posturing catatonics. ('The Major Tranquilizers', *Drug Abuse and Alcoholism Newsletter, Vista Hill Foundation*, 4, No. (10): 1 (Nov. 1975). Quoted in Liska, 1981, p. 210.)

In 1954 all this began to change with the discovery of **chlorpromazine**. When this substance was administered to patients who had been severely agitated or violent, they became calm. Others who had been deeply withdrawn into their own private dream world where communication was impossible emerged so that psychiatric treatment of their condition could be attempted. Within a few years the population of pyschiatric hospitals began to decline for the first time in more than a century. This was not because chlorpromazine cured psychosis but it did, in many cases, control the symptoms to such an extent that the person affected was able to lead a fairly normal life.

The structural formula for chlorpromazine is given in Figure 15.3. Once its therapeutic usefulness had been confirmed there was a massive effort directed towards the synthesis of compounds having related structures, in the hope that some of these would also be therapeutically useful. This hope was realised and there are now about 20 compounds closely related to chlorpromazine which can be used for the treatment of psychoses. This family of medicines is often referred to as the **phenothiazines**. The structural feature which they all have in common is the three ring system of chlorpromazine with atoms of nitrogen and sulphur in the middle ring. They differ in the nature of the side chain attached to the nitrogen atom of the ring and in the atom, or set of atoms, located at the position occupied by chlorine in chlorpromazine.

The phenothiazines are believed to exert their antipsychotic effects by influencing the transmission of nerve impulses across the **synapse** (the narrow gap which exists between the extremities of connecting neurones). This transmission involves compounds called **neurotransmitters**. As the nerve impulse reaches the synapse it stimulates release of the neurotransmitter from storage sites on that side of the synapse. The neurotransmitter then diffuses across the synapse and makes contact with specialised sections of the cell membrane (**receptors**) of the neurone on the other side of the synapse. The neurotransmitter acts on these receptors to trigger passage of the nerve impulse along that neurone. This is illustrated in Figure 15.6.

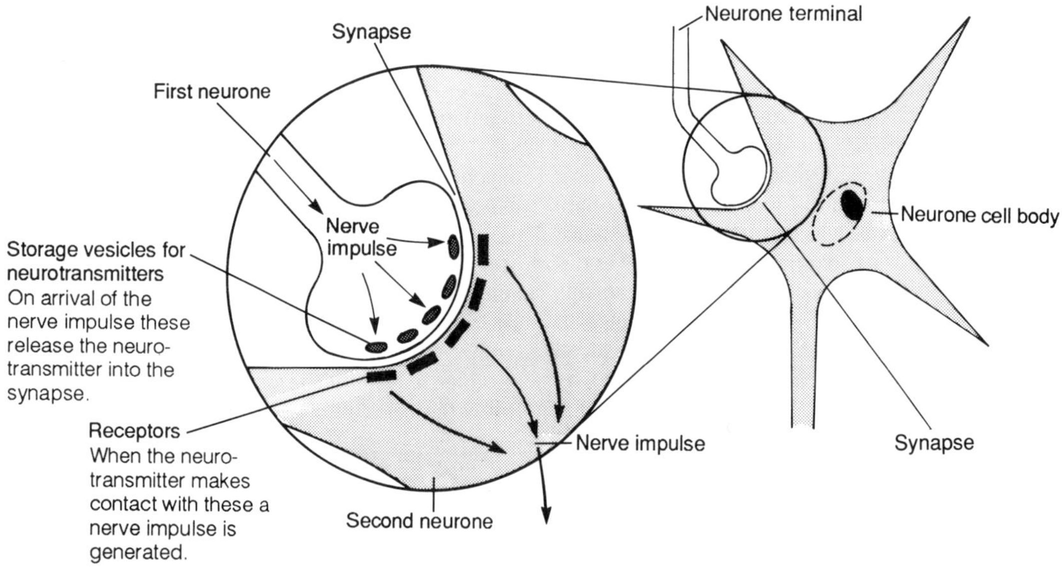

Figure 15.6 *Passage of a nerve impulse across the synapse*

There are several different neurotransmitters which have been identified and one of these is **dopamine** (see Figure 15.7). It is responsible for the transmission of nerve impulses between neurones in the higher centres of the brain. This is the neurotransmitter affected by chlorpromazine and the other phenothiazines. They attach to dopamine receptors but do not trigger passage of the nerve impulse. Furthermore, a receptor to which a phenothiazine molecule is attached cannot be stimulated by dopamine. In this way, the phenothiazines reduce the activity of neurones controlled by dopamine and this leads to a reduction in psychotic symptoms. This account of the action of the phenothiazines is based on the **Dopamine Theory of Schizophrenia** (schizophrenia is one of the most common categories of psychosis) which maintains that schizophrenia and other psychoses are due to a greater-than-normal activity of the neurones controlled by dopamine.

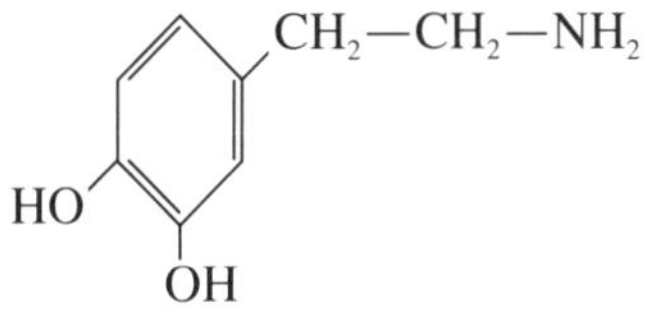

Figure 15.7 *Structural formula for the neurotransmitter dopamine*

The anti-psychotic medicines must be taken for very long periods of time, sometimes for decades. It is now apparent that this long-term use may often be accompanied by serious side effects. These include tremors, involuntary movement of the limbs and grotesque, uncontrolled movements of the jaws and tongue.

Medicines Against Cancer — the Nitrogen Mustards. The disease most feared by people today is **cancer**. The first non-surgical method for its treatment became available soon after radium had been discovered in 1903 by Marie and Pierre Curie. This was not a chemical treatment because it depended on the toxicity of the radiation emitted by radium rather than on the chemical behaviour of the substance.

The first significant step in the chemical treatment of cancer occurred with the development of a group of medicines known as the **nitrogen mustards**. These compounds are vessicants (they produce blisters on contact with the skin) and were developed during World War II for use as chemical weapons. During testing of their biological action they were observed to produce atrophy (wasting away) of lymphoid tissue and bone marrow. This led to their use in the treatment of leukemia and cancers of the lymphatic system.

The nitrogen mustards have an ability to form covalent bonds with sections of biological molecules, particularly nucleic acids. The effect of this bond formation is the attachment of alkyl radicals to the nucleic acids and for this reason the nitrogen mustards are often called **alkylating agents**. Cancer is a disease characterised by a rapid increase in cell numbers and this requires rapid replication of DNA since each new cell must contain its own set of DNA molecules identical to those present in the original cell from which the cancer has developed. The effectiveness of the nitrogen mustards against cancer is due to the presence in their molecules of two groups of atoms capable of forming bonds with nucleic acids. This makes it possible for the nitrogen mustard to form a 'bridge' between different strands of DNA molecules thus impeding DNA and cell replication.

All cells contain DNA and so all cells are vulnerable to damage by the nitrogen mustards. They are not very selective medicines and the extent to which they can be used is limited by their toxicity. Their enhanced toxicity for cancer cells compared to normal cells is due mainly to the high rate of DNA replication in cancer cells. Some normal tissues, including bone marrow, gastrointestinal epithelium and hair follicles also rely on rapid replication of DNA. These normal tissues are often adversely affected by treatments involving the nitrogen mustards (and other anti-cancer medicines). For example, hair loss and gastrointestinal upsets are common side effects of such treatment.

15.1.4 *Some Disasters of Chemical Therapy*

There is no such thing as a completely safe medicine. Even penicillin has been responsible for the deaths of some people due to a severe allergic reaction which it causes in a small proportion of the population. To this type of largely unavoidable danger in the use of medicines must be added other dangers arising from the fallibility of the people responsible for producing, testing and distributing them, and from the limitations of the scientific techniques available for detecting their adverse effects. Set out below are brief descriptions of three episodes from the history of medicine which illustrate these dangers.

Elixir Sulphanilamide. Two disadvantages of sulphanilamide are its low solubility in water or water/alcohol mixtures (elixirs) and an unpleasant taste. This made the medicine difficult to administer to children. In the United States, in 1937, a drug company 'solved' this problem by dissolving sulphanilamide in ethylene glycol (HO–CH_2–CH_2–OH). The company sold the solution obtained under the name **Elixir Sulphanilamide**. Ethylene glycol, which we use today as an anti-freeze agent in the radiators of motor vehicles, is a cruel and deadly poison. In a short period after it was released for sale in the United States, Elixir Sulphanilamide killed more than one hundred Americans, many of them young children. The company responsible for this tragedy could only be prosecuted for false advertising: it had called its product an elixir when food and drug regulations required that all elixirs must have a water/alcohol mixture as the solvent. The company was fined $26 000, no criminal charges were laid and no compensation was made to the families of victims. The head of the company described the incident as a regrettable and unfortunate accident. He pointed out, quite correctly, that his company had violated no law.

As news of the Elixir Sulphanilamide tragedy and its aftermath spread across America, people were outraged at the weakness of regulations governing the production, testing and sale of substances intended for human consumption. It became widely known that this was due to the effectiveness of a powerful political lobby representing the interests of manufacturers. This lobby had, for over 30 years, stalled the introduction of stricter regulations by pushing the argument that their industry could be relied upon to regulate itself. The Elixir Sulphanilamide episode provided mighty ammunition for the opponents of this lobby and it was swept away, almost overnight. This was the beginning of the era of strict government control over the commercial use of all chemicals which people consume in their food or as medicines.

Thalidomide and Phocomelia. Thalidomide, the structural formula of which is shown in Figure 15.8, was first prepared in Germany in 1954. It quickly became popular as an hypnotic (sleep inducer) because it seemed to have no effects other than the production of sleep. It was much less toxic than other substances then in use as hypnotics and therefore presented a much smaller risk when being used by people with a suicidal inclination. Prior to 1960 the only adverse effect of thalidomide that had been identified was inflammation of nerves. This had been sufficient to cause health authorities in the United States to ban the medicine even while it was on sale in Europe, Japan, Australia and elsewhere. However, by this time it was common for physicians in these countries to prescribe thalidomide for pregnant women with sleeping difficulties.

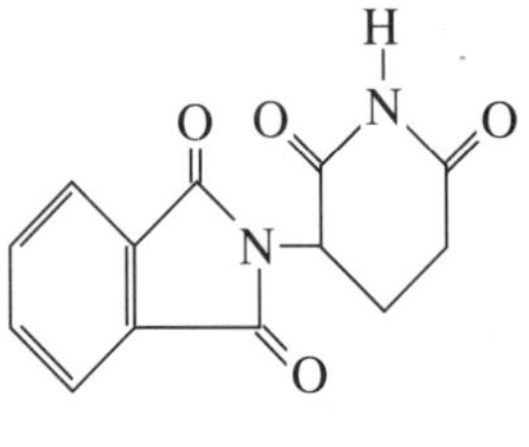

Figure 15.8 *Structural formula of thalidomide*

In 1960 there began a terrible epidemic of **phocomelia**, a condition in which children are born with small flipper-like limbs. This is normally a very rare condition, but in 1962 in Germany hundreds of cases were suddenly seen. This experience was repeated in many other countries. Thalidomide was soon identified as the causative agent and this medicine, which had seemed so safe, was revealed as a powerful **teratogen**, a substance able to affect the development of the growing foetus. It caused phocomelia whenever it was taken by a woman between days 35 and 50 of her pregnancy. The total number of children born with thalidomide-induced phocomelia was about 10 000.

This was a disaster of quite a different sort to the Elixir Sulphanilamide episode. That had been an example of gross negligence, but the thalidomide tragedy called into question the reliability of scientific medicine. The manufacturers of thalidomide claimed that the tragedy could not have been foreseen. The uncomfortable truth was that science had become complacent about the possibility of teratogenic injury caused by medicines. So few examples had been documented that this type of toxicity was not taken seriously. The experiments performed to detect it were poorly designed and carried out more as a ritual required to satisfy health authorities than as a serious attempt to detect subtle effects which were known to be theoretically possible.

Needless to say, the experience with thalidomide jolted medical science and health authorities out of their complacency. Today, the possibility of teratogenic injury caused by medicines is taken very seriously.

Diethylstilbestrol (DES). This substance is a **synthetic estrogen**. The estrogens are the compounds responsible for the development of secondary sexual characteristics in females. They also act to produce a suitable environment for fertilisation, implantation and nutrition of the early embryo. The structural formula for DES is shown in Figure 15.9 along with that of a natural estrogen. The comparison shows that while DES has a different structure to the natural estrogen there is a similarity. It is now believed that in the human body DES is transformed into a compound which more closely resembles a natural estrogen. This involves the creation of additional rings within the DES molecule by the formation of new bonds between some of its different parts.

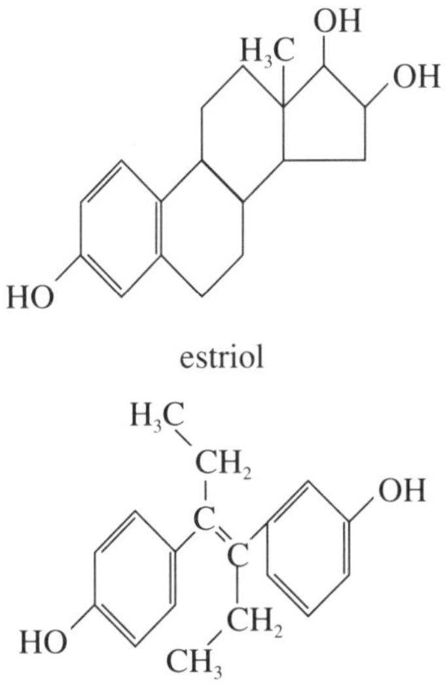

Figure 15.9 *DES and a natural estrogen*

Use of DES commenced in the 1940s and continued into the 1970s. The different purposes for which it has been used include:

1. As an additive in cattle feed. Here it promotes growth and shortens the time needed to prepare animals for sale.
2. As a 'morning after' contraceptive. A large dose of DES is taken the morning after sexual intercourse and this prevents any fertilised egg from implanting.
3. In cases of rape or incest where it serves the same purpose as outlined in 2.
4. As a means of reducing the risk of miscarriage in the early stage of a pregnancy.

By the late 1960s there was considerable evidence available to indicate that the last use of DES listed above was responsible for a rare form of vaginal cancer occurring in young women whose mothers had received the medicine during their pregnancies.

This is an example of an undesirable effect of a medicine which would have been very hard to detect prior to its use by physicians. Furthermore, the long delay between consumption of the medicine and the appearance of the disease which it causes ensured that it was administered to many women before the danger was apparent. Careful screening of medicines and a conservative approach to their introduction can reduce this type of risk but never eliminate it altogether.

15.1.5 *Control of Therapeutic Chemicals*

Each developed country has one or more agencies in which it invests the authority to control the use of medicines within its borders. In the United States this authority is the Food and Drug Administration (FDA) and in Australia it is the Australian Drug Evaluation Committee (ADEC) which has been established by the Commonwealth Government's Department of Health. Because of the much greater size of the medicines industry in the United States, United Kingdom and Europe, compared to the Australian industry, the role of ADEC is mainly one of evaluating advice obtained from the large overseas agencies.

For the FDA to give its approval for the clinical trialling of a new medicine, the sponsor of the medicine must ensure that all the following information is available for evaluation:

1. description of the chemical formula of the drug and the methods used in synthesis, purification, quality control and potency measurement;
2. form of administration, route of administration and proposed dosage;
3. details of the drug's absorption, distribution, metabolism, excretion and dose–effect relationships;
4. details of toxicologic investigations carried out in a variety of species, both by acute and chronic administration. The type and number of animals used in these investigations must be specified;
5. details of experiments performed to rule out the possibility of teratogenic action of the medicine if it is to be prescribed for women of child-bearing age.

Even if all this information indicates that the medicine is safe it will not be allowed into general use unless the sponsor can also demonstrate that it is superior to the medicines already available for the same purpose. This is a far cry from the situation which prevailed in the United States in 1937 when Elixir Sulphanilamide went on sale, or in Germany in 1935 when Gerhard Domagk, without reference to any outside authorities, was able to persuade doctors to administer Prontosil to his daughter.

Most people, having in mind the unnecessary suffering which has been caused in the past by the use of some medicines, are prepared to support the maintenance of these strict controls over their development and use. However, it is a sobering thought to know that these same controls which protect us from the toxic effects of medicines must also delay, and occasionally prevent, the introduction of new, useful medicines. This is an inescapable dilemma but the modern trend towards erring in the direction which reduces the chance of injuries caused by therapy is consistent with the ancient teachings of Hippocrates, the father of medicine. Twenty five centuries ago, he told his followers that they must 'above all, do no harm'.

This conservative approach to the introduction of new medicines is currently under considerable pressure from groups who wish to accelerate the development of medicines against AIDS (acquired immune deficiency syndrome). Already, these groups have been able to persuade the FDA to modify its approval procedures in ways which will allow such medicines to be introduced more rapidly.

15.2 Toxicology, the Science of Poisons

Toxicology is the study of the action of poisons on living organisms. It is not an exact science in the same sense that anatomy, physiology, physics and chemistry are exact sciences. This is definitely the case when the living organism involved is a human being. The subject matter of toxicology is the adverse effects which poisons produce. An exact science may only develop when a wide range of experiments can be performed to test predictions and discover new phenomena. It is simply not permitted to perform experiments on human beings in which serious, adverse effects are produced by poisons deliberately administered by the investigator. For these reasons many of the conclusions drawn about the effects of poisons on human beings are based on opinion and inference rather than on direct observation.

15.2.1 *Definition of a Poison*

It is very hard to define a poison in precise terms. One may say that a substance is a poison if small doses of it cause harm to living tissue. However, in this simple definition, the reference to dosage is critical. Nearly every substance is capable of causing harm to living tissue if the dose is high enough. For example, a child given two tablespoonfuls (about 40 g) of sodium chloride (salt) would quite likely die unless the material is quickly removed from the body by vomiting.

Experience shows that one simply cannot distinguish precisely between poisonous and non-poisonous substances. This point is well illustrated by the element copper. Small quantities of copper are required to maintain a human being in good health. In larger quantities it becomes highly toxic. For example, water-dispensing devices (water coolers, hot water services) with copper plumbing have, in some circumstances, been known to impart sufficient copper to the water to make it toxic when used for drinking. There is a disease known as Wilson's disease in which copper accumulates to toxic levels in the body. This disease must be treated with drugs which promote elimination of copper in the urine.

It is even difficult to distinguish between poisonous and non-poisonous doses of the same substance. The reason for this is that people differ in their susceptibility to the toxic effects of chemicals.

Acute Versus Chronic Poisoning. Acute poisoning involves exposure to a single large dose of a poison. Its effects are usually dramatic and unmistakable. Acute poisonings occur most frequently as acts of suicide or as accidents. Chronic poisoning involves repeated exposures to small doses over a long period of time. Its effects may not become noticeable until after serious damage has occurred. Chronic poisoning is the main concern in occupational and public health settings.

15.2.2 *Effective Dose, Threshold Dose and Threshold Limit Values*

The critical importance of dosage in determining the toxicity of a substance brings us to consider the terms effective dose, threshold dose and threshold limit value.

Effective Dose. A poison may only exert its toxic effects if it gains entry to some part of the body and is then absorbed into the bloodstream, or, in some other way, becomes closely associated with tissue. By

effective dose is meant the amount of material which is involved in this absorption–association process.

Threshold Dose. Toxicologists have traditionally accepted the notion that, for most substances, there exists an effective dose below which the substances elicit no biological reaction from living tissue no matter how long exposure continues. This is called the **threshold dose**. The concept of a biological threshold for substances is illustrated in Figure 15.10.

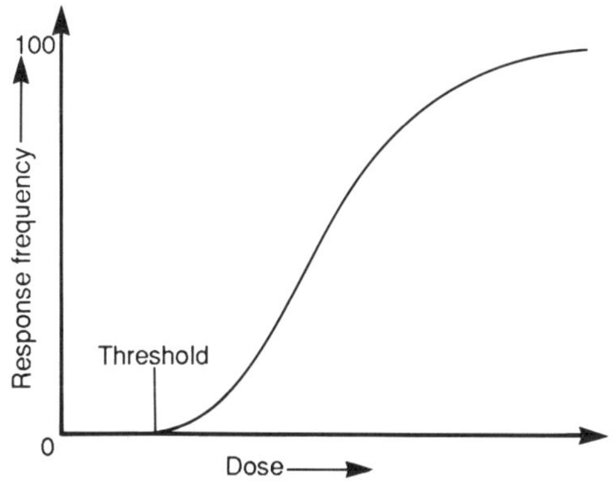

Figure 15.10 *The threshold dose*

The magnitude of the threshold dose varies from substance to substance and for a single substance it may vary from one person to another. It is the task of toxicologists to ensure that people handling chemicals in industry do not receive effective doses of those chemicals which exceed the threshold. The approach adopted has been to set limits on the concentrations to which people may be exposed and these limits are called **Threshold Limit Values** (TLVs). They have the following important features:

1. They are concentrations in air. This is because about 90% of all occupational poisonings result from the inhalation of contaminated air.
2. They represent conditions under which it is believed that nearly all workers may be exposed day after day without adverse effect.
3. They are set on the assumption that workers will be exposed for no more than eight consecutive hours and then be free from exposure for sixteen hours.
4. They do *not* provide a reliable indicator of the hazard existing when workers are exposed to mixtures of toxic chemicals.

15.2.3 *Physical Defence Mechanisms Against Toxic Chemicals*

The human body is under constant challenge from toxic substances entering through the respiratory tract, the gastrointestinal tract and the skin. Most of the time this challenge is successfully met by the body's defensive mechanisms and it is only when these are impaired or overwhelmed that damage occurs. The defence mechanisms of the body may be categorised as either physical or biochemical. Physical defence mechanisms usually depend on the normal structure and function of the body system or organ which the toxic substance first encounters.

The Respiratory Tract. This may be considered as consisting of three sections: **nasopharynx, tracheo-bronchial area** and **alveoli** (see Figure 15.11). Toxic material in air entering the respiratory tract is dealt with by processes of **filtration, inactivation/destruction** and **removal**. Large particles in air are filtered out of the incoming air stream by hair at the entrance to the nose. Further along, particles become embedded in the secretions of mucous glands and are washed out of the upper respiratory tract by the action of cilia which line the bronchial and nasal passages. The cough and sneeze reflexes also assist. In this way, particles larger than 10 μm in diameter are largely prevented from penetrating to the alveolar area of the respiratory tract. However, such penetration may occur if the action of cilia is impaired or if particle diameter is smaller than 10 μm (pollen grains and the carbon particles in smoke may be this small).

Another mechanism which operates to prevent penetration of foreign material via the respiratory tract is **bronchospasm**: contracting of muscles which surround the bronchial tree. This reduces the size of the bronchial passages and impedes the movement of the invading material. Of course, it also impedes breathing and so produces respiratory distress.

The final barrier between the bloodstream and toxic materials contained in inspired air is provided by alveolar tissue. This tissue is very delicate, having a thickness of about 2.5 μm. It has associated with it macrophage cells which are capable of inactivating much of the material which reaches the alveolar area. The alveolar cells are also lined with a surfactant. This is mainly responsible for allowing the alveoli to expand during inspiration but it also assists in reducing contact between alveolar tissue and toxic material present in inspired air.

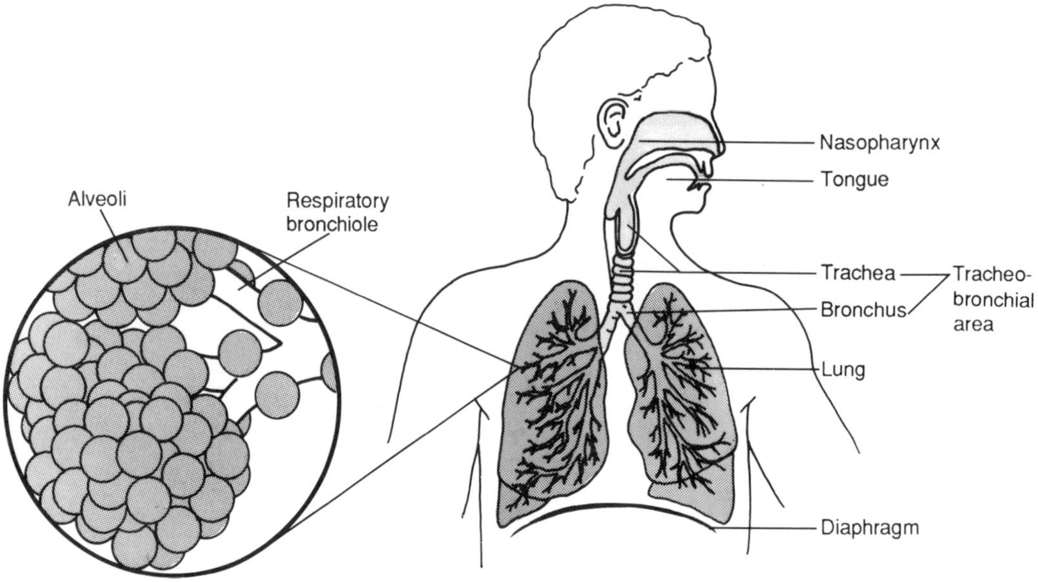

Figure 15.11 *The respiratory tract*

The processes described above are effective against particles present in air but not against gaseous substances which it may contain. Whereas the penetration of particles into the respiratory tract is controlled largely by their size, the penetration of gases is determined by the solubility of the gas in water. If a gas is highly soluble in water (for example, ammonia and sulphur oxides) it will dissolve in the water which lines the upper structures of the respiratory tract and in this way be prevented from penetrating deeply. Of course, these gases may cause damage to tissue in the regions where they dissolve. Gases which do not dissolve readily in water (for example, nitrogen dioxide, hydrocarbons) will penetrate into the alveolar region and may then enter the bloodstream.

The Gastrointestinal Tract. This system provides a means of entry for toxic substances present in food and water. The absorption of most toxic substances entering the gastrointestinal tract occurs in the small intestine. In this region is found an enormous number of small finger-like structures called **villi**. They project into the intestinal space and provide a large surface area for the absorption of all material present in that part of the intestine.

When toxic agents enter the gastrointestinal tract they may trigger the response of vomiting and in this way the body rids itself of them. Alternatively, the response may be for more rapid movements of the intestine to occur so that the material is rapidly expelled in faeces.

The Skin. This provides a physical barrier to the entry of many of the toxic substances present in air and water. However, it is permeable to some compounds and there have been many instances of people being severely, or even fatally, injured when chemicals spill onto clothing or skin and then are not immediately removed.

15.2.4 *Biochemical Defence Mechanisms of the Body*

The body's biochemical defence mechanisms consist of a variety of chemical processes which transform the toxic substance into other compounds. This process is known as **biotransformation** and the compounds formed are known as **metabolites**.

The most important site for biotransformation is the liver, but it occurs to some extent in all tissues. The prominent role which the liver plays in biotransformation is due to its ability to produce a wide range of enzymes in response to the presence of foreign substances. These enzymes bring about the biotransformation. There are two types of biotransformation: conjugation and non-synthetic biotransformation.

Conjugation. This involves chemical combination of the foreign compound with an **endogenous** compound (a compound found normally in the body). Endogenous compounds which participate in conjugation are usually carbohydrates or amino acids or compounds closely related to one of these classes. Some examples are shown in Figure 15.12.

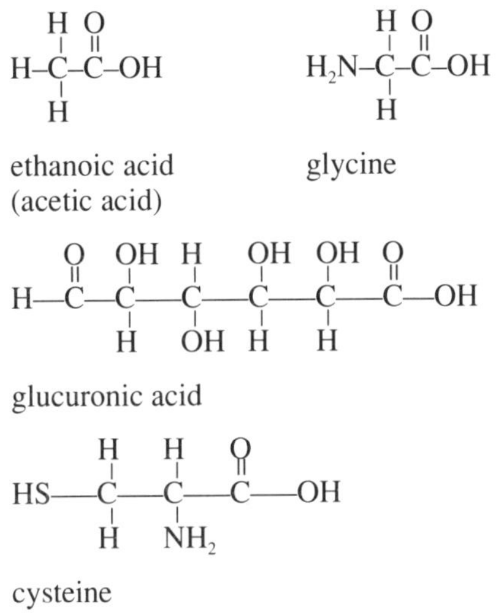

Figure 15.12 *Endogenous compounds involved in conjugation*

The most important features of conjugation are:

1. It converts the foreign compound to a metabolite which is more soluble in water and less soluble in lipid. This is due to the fact that the foreign compound is joined to a molecule containing –OH and –NH groups of atoms.
2. It converts the foreign compound to a metabolite which is less toxic.
3. The foreign compound is easily regenerated from its conjugated form.

Overall, the effects of conjugation on a foreign compound are a reduction in its toxicity and an increase in its rate of excretion in urine. The protective effect of this is obvious. An alternative term often used in place of conjugation is **synthetic biotransformation**.

Non-synthetic Biotransformation. This type of process leads to a permanent alteration in the chemical nature of the foreign compound. In contrast to conjugation, non-synthetic biotransformation often leads to the formation of a metabolite which is more toxic and less soluble in water than the original compound. Non-synthetic biotransformation is usually followed by conjugation and excretion.

In cases where biotransformation leads to the formation of a more toxic metabolite the amount of damage caused depends on how quickly the metabolite undergoes conjugation and then excretion. If this occurs rapidly, very little of the toxic metabolite will survive long enough to cause damage. If the process is slow, or the levels of exposure are very high, then the toxic metabolite may be present for long enough, and at levels high enough, to be damaging.

A scheme which summarises the interaction of foreign compounds with the chemical defence mechanisms of the body is set out in Figure 15.13.

15.3 Commercial Chemicals as Contaminants of the Environment

The commercial chemicals which contaminate the environment may either be naturally occurring (for example, asbestos and lead) or synthetic (for example, chlorinated hydrocarbon insecticides and chlorofluorocarbons). In both cases it is usually the scale on which the substance is used which gives rise to the problem. For example, in the period 1950–1967 in the United States over one million tonnes of the chlorinated hydrocarbon insecticide DDT (this is an acronym for the compound's chemical name, dichlorodiphenyltrichloroethane) was produced and used for the control of insect pests. Closer to home, the lead smelter at Port Pirie in South Australia has processed millions of tonnes of ore since it began operation in 1889. During this time over 160 000 tonnes of lead-containing material has been emitted by the smelter and much of this has settled over the surrounding town and countryside.

Industrial/agricultural activities on this scale alter the chemical composition of the environment. These changes, together with a whole range of corresponding real and imaginary health effects, are now regularly reported in the popular media. From these reports it is easy to form the impression that the industries which produce and use chemicals do not take enough care and that it is this lack of care which is responsible for the environmental contamination which they cause.

In some instances this is a fair criticism, but it is very important to realise that many industries do take

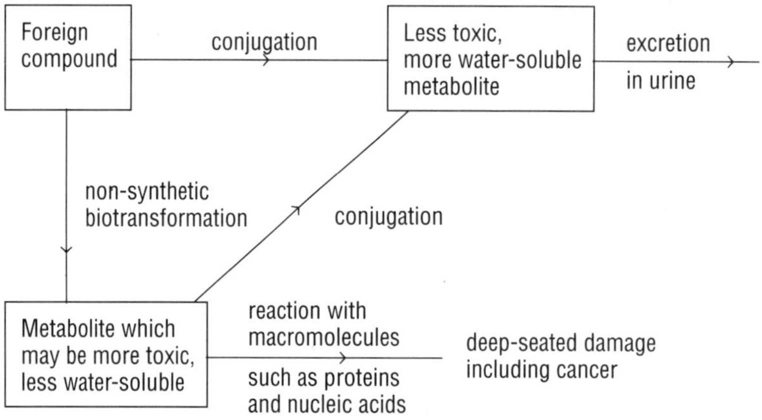

Figure 15.13 *Metabolism of foreign compounds*

a great deal of care over their use of chemicals. Even so, chemical contamination of the environment still occurs and it always will occur no matter how much trouble is taken with attempts at prevention. Some change in the chemical composition of our environment is the inevitable price we must pay if we wish to have the comforts and advantages of a modern, industrialised society. The only realistic aim which we can have is to ensure that the problems caused by chemical contamination of the environment are kept at a level where they are well and truly offset by the benefits the corresponding activity provides for the people affected.

Any substance which is present in air, soil and water will find its way into our bodies where it may cause illness if the amount is high enough. This is the most common way in which environmental contaminants influence human health but it is not the only way. Health effects may arise indirectly from some other change in the environment caused by the contaminant. We shall now consider cases which illustrate both of these possibilities.

15.3.1 *Lead in the Australian Environment*

Lead occurs most commonly in nature as the sulphide ore, **galena (PbS)**, although it is occasionally found as the uncombined metal (native metal). It is relatively easy to extract lead from its ores and processes for achieving this were developed over 2000 years ago.

In ancient Rome metallic lead was used by well-to-do Romans in cooking vessels, in pipes for the transport of drinking water and for many other purposes. It has been suggested that the Roman aristocracy poisoned itself with lead and that this contributed to the fall of the Roman Empire (see Gilfillan, S. C., 'Lead poisoning and the fall of Rome', *Journal of Occupational Medicine*, vol. 7, 53–60, 1965). This suggestion is supported by the high lead levels found in the bony remains of Romans who lived around the time of the empire's demise. It is also supported by historical records which show that there was a declining birth rate among aristocratic Romans during this same period: chronic lead poisoning is known to reduce fertility. Lead also causes mental illness and this might account for some of the bizarre behaviour displayed by the last Roman emperors.

Lead is a very useful material and the metal, together with many of its compounds, continues in use today. Metallic lead is used in the manufacture of chemical engineering equipment, screens for protection against radiation, car batteries and on roofs. The compound red lead (Pb_3O_4) is used as a rust inhibitor in paint. Another compound, lead tetraethyl [$Pb(C_2H_5)_4$], is used as a petrol additive. The extensive use made of lead and its compounds has produced increases in the levels of lead to which many people are exposed day after day throughout their lives.

The toxicity of lead is well known and its impact on public health is constantly monitored. Thus, in 1981 the Australian Academy of Science published a report entitled 'Health and Environmental Lead in Australia'. In 1983–84 the South Australian Health Commission published several reports on lead pollution at Port Pirie. Much of what is written below has been based on these reports.

Lead in the Atmosphere of Cities. The level of lead in the pristine (uncontaminated) atmosphere has been estimated as less than 0.01 $\mu g/m^3$. The maximum level recommended by the National Health and Medical Research Council (NHRMC) is 1.5 $\mu g/m^3$ (averaged over a three-month period). Thus, we accept a level of lead in the air which is more than 150 times the pristine level. Measurements performed in 1977/78 near busy roads in a number of Australian cities showed that in some places the lead concentration in air was more than twice the maximum level recommended by the NHMRC.

Over 90% of the lead in the atmosphere of cities comes from the lead tetraethyl used in petrol. As the petrol burns in the engine the lead tetraethyl first forms lead oxide. The petrol also contains dibromoethane and dichloroethane which react with the lead oxide to form lead chlorobromide. This is more volatile than lead oxide and is swept from the engine in the exhaust gases. In this way the build up of lead in the engine is prevented, but at the cost of substantial lead emissions to the atmosphere. The fate of the lead additive in petrol is as follows:

1. 60–65% is emitted as lead chlorobromide particles in the exhaust gases;
2. 5–10% is emitted as unchanged lead tetraethyl;
3. approximately 20% is retained in sump oil (which is eventually burned or dumped).

Most of the lead emitted by vehicle exhausts is in the form of particles ranging in diameter from 1–5 μm. These particles eventually settle out of the air. The larger ones settle out more quickly and are deposited close to the road, but the smaller ones may spread high and wide from the point of emission. It is generally observed that lead concentration in air declines rapidly with increasing distance from the roadside and with decreasing traffic density.

Lead tetraethyl went on sale as a petrol additive in the United States in 1923 following its development by Thomas Midgely, an engineer for General Motors. In 1925 it was voluntarily removed from sale by the manufacturer after it had caused the severe poisoning of 70 workers. Ten of these died. On 20 May 1925 a committee was appointed by the US government to investigate the health hazards involved in the use of lead tetraethyl in petrol. In January 1926 the committee reported that there were no good grounds for prohibiting the use of lead tetraethyl in petrol and it immediately went back on sale and has been used ever since.

All the while, there has been concern over the possibility that lead additives in petrol might be having an undesirable effect on public health and pressure has steadily mounted for this use to be discontinued. As a result, all vehicles now being manufactured in Australia, or imported into the country, are designed to run on unleaded petrol and all service stations must supply unleaded petrol as well as that which contains lead. There can be no doubt that the shift to unleaded petrol will reduce the concentration of lead in the atmosphere of Australian cities. Similar action taken in West Germany in 1976 saw lead levels in air fall by a factor of about three within three years.

Lead in Soil and Dust. The pristine levels of lead in soil have been estimated at 10–16 mg/kg. The values found in rural areas of Australia are usually in this range or are close to it. However, levels of lead found in samples of dust obtained in city areas are often dramatically greater than the pristine level. This accumulation of lead is undoubtedly caused by the lead additives in petrol. Many children attending schools in the inner areas of Australian cities are in close contact with dust which contains lead at concentrations which are hundreds of times as great as the pristine level. It is quite possible that children in such an environment could be taking significant quantities of lead into their bodies.

Lead in Food. Most of the food which Australians eat is grown in rural areas where the levels of lead in the soil and atmosphere are low. It is therefore not surprising, as well as reassuring, to know that measurement of the lead levels in Australian foodstuffs usually gives values well below the level of concern.

Where food is found to have a high lead level it is usually due to use of lead-based agricultural chemicals, or to the food being grown close to a highway, or being sold in open markets where it has picked up leaded dust from the atmosphere. Lead may also enter food during processing, particularly when the food is being canned. It has been estimated that canned foods add 15% extra lead to an average daily lead intake.

Lead in Water and Drink. The estimated pristine level of lead in fresh water is 0.5 $\mu g/l$. In Australia today fresh water supplies usually contain 10–20 $\mu g/l$ of lead and the recommended maximum level for drinking water is 50 $\mu g/l$. Carbonated soft drinks sold in Australia have an average lead content of 160 $\mu g/l$ and that for beer is 130 $\mu g/l$. Thus it can be seen that the level of lead present in drinking water and common beverages is well above the estimated pristine level in fresh water.

In some parts of the world lead enters drinking water through contact with plumbing materials which contain lead. This source of lead is not important in

Australia because lead has rarely been used in this way.

Absorption of Lead by Australians. Lead absorption follows ingestion or inhalation. The amounts ingested and inhaled by an adult male each day have been estimated at about 500 μg and 30 μg respectively. Of the lead ingested about 11% (50 μg) enters the bloodstream. The rest is eliminated in faeces. For inhaled lead, about 40% (12 μg) enters the bloodstream. The source of inhaled lead is almost entirely the lead additives in petrol.

The total lead absorption for an adult living in an urban area is about 40–70 μg/day and for a two-year-old child is about 45–70 μg/day. Children take in less lead than adults but absorb it more efficiently.

Distribution of Lead Within the Body. Once lead is absorbed from the lungs, or from the gastrointestinal tract, it enters the bloodstream and is, from there, distributed as follows:

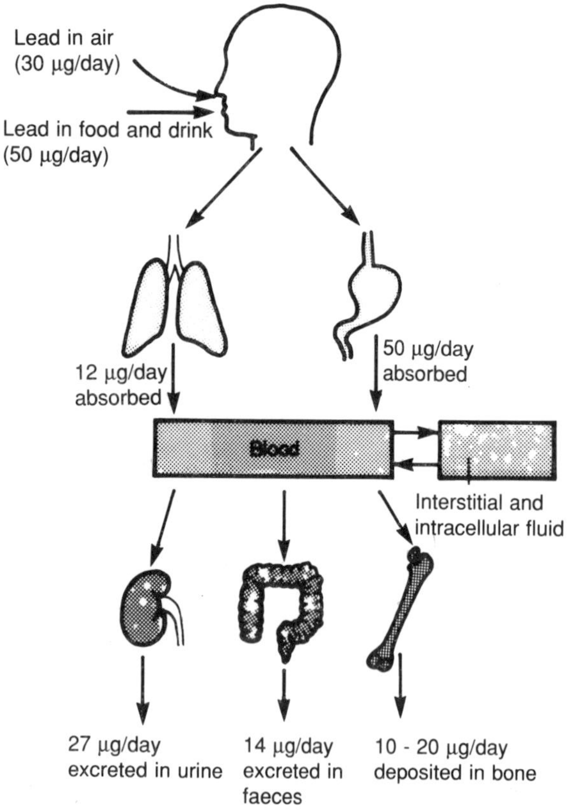

Figure 15.14 *Distribution of lead within the body* (see Errata)

1. it is taken to the other extracellular fluid compartments;
2. it becomes attached to red blood cells;
3. it is taken up by soft tissues;
4. it is taken up and stored in bone;
5. it is excreted in urine and faeces.

This is summarised in Figure 15.14.

You can see from Figure 15.14 that the amount of lead absorbed each day is greater than the amount excreted. Over a lifetime, most of the absorbed lead which stays in the body accumulates in bone. At birth, a human has about 0.2 mg of lead in the bones. At age 50 this has increased to about 200 mg. Thus, the lead content of bone increases 1000 times while body weight increases about 20–25 times. This protects the body because lead in bone is inert and does not exert any toxic effects.

15.3.2 *Lead in the Environment at Port Pirie*

The South Australian city of Port Pirie has a population of 17 000 people. Its main industry is a lead smelting and refining plant established in 1889 to process the output of the Broken Hill mines.

There is a long history of concern about the health effects of lead in Port Pirie. In the period 1910–1925 the effects of lead on workers was the subject of parliamentary enquiries and of a Royal Commission. In the 1970s a team from the Commonwealth Scientific and Industrial Research Organisation (CSIRO) investigated the distribution of lead and other heavy metals in Port Pirie and the surrounding region. They found significantly increased levels of lead in many locations. In 1981 some Port Pirie children were found to have excessive lead absorption and this led community leaders to request blood tests for all children in the city. Of the children eligible, 1239 (50%) were tested and 87 (7%) of these had blood lead levels greater than 30 μg/100 ml which is regarded as the level of concern. For children in the age group 3–5 years 16% displayed this level. At the present time the NHMRC is funding a long-term study of the Port Pirie environment and its effect on child development including effects during pregnancy.

Elevated levels of lead have been found at Port Pirie in soil, house dust, rain water tanks and on home-grown vegetables. The areas most affected are those closest to the smelter. The concentration of lead in home-grown vegetables at Port Pirie is about 10 times greater than that found in vegetables grown in Adelaide.

The concentrations of lead in the soil and dust found in the homes of children who had blood lead levels above the level of concern (30 μg/100 ml) were greater than the concentrations found at the homes of children with blood lead levels below this.

The main source of the lead which contaminates the environment at Port Pirie is the lead smelter. It has been estimated that in the period 1889–1974 the smelter stack has emitted 160 000 tonnes of lead waste. The rate of emission was greatest in the early years of operation and has declined rapidly since 1974. At present the rate of emission is about 50 tonnes/year. Other sources of lead in the Port Pirie environment are:

1. vehicle exhausts (5 tonnes/year);
2. lead-based paint peeling from old structures;
3. lead dust carried away from the smelter on the bodies and clothes of workers.

Health Significance of Lead at Port Pirie. There have been no recent cases of people suffering acute lead poisoning in Port Pirie. Symptoms of such poisoning include abdominal pain, metallic taste in the mouth, vomiting, diarrhoea and coma. Chronic lead poisoning has fewer dramatic symptoms which include loss of appetite, weight loss, constipation, loss of recently developed skills, behavioural disturbances and lead-line on the gums. Even this less severe level of lead poisoning has not been observed in recent times at Port Pirie. However, there is still great concern about the health significance of the elevated lead levels found there. This concern is based on some evidence that lead absorption below the level needed to produce the symptoms of poisoning does still produce subtle effects including some impairment of intellectual development.

A study described in the *New England Journal of Medicine* in 1979 compared the intellectual performance of people having elevated blood lead levels (high lead population) with that of people having normal levels (low lead population). The main findings of this study were that:

1. the median IQ score (this is the score which is exceeded by half of the population) for the high lead population is about 10 points less than that for the low lead population;
2. among the high lead population about 14% of people have scores less than or equal to 80, which is the score corresponding to intellectual impairment. In the low lead population this percentage is about 3–4;
3. among the low lead population about 5–10% of people have IQ scores greater than, or equal to, 125, which is the score corresponding to superior intelligence. In the high lead population this percentage is zero.

(Needleman, H. L. and others, *New England Journal of Medicine*, vol. 300, 584–695, 1979.)

Of course, a study like this does not allow one to identify particular individuals who have suffered intellectual impairment as a result of lead absorption. It simply indicates that *some* members of the high lead group have suffered in this way. In 1983, the South Australian Government engaged an American expert, Dr P. J. Landrigan, to give an opinion on the Port Pirie situation. He expressed his concern in the following question:

> Can Port Pirie afford the permanent, albeit invisible loss, from the group of children with blood levels of greater than 40 μg/100 ml of the one child in twenty with truly superior intelligence; and can Port Pirie afford, for the group of children with blood lead levels of greater than 40 μg/100 ml, a concomitant quadrupling in the number of children with intellectual impairment?

As part of its investigation of the lead pollution problem at Port Pirie the South Australian Health Commission compared the environment and behaviour of children having elevated blood lead levels with those of children having levels below the level of concern. This comparison revealed that elevated blood lead levels were correlated significantly with the following environmental and behavioural factors:

1. location of residence;
2. number of family members working at the smelter;
3. frequency of placing objects in the mouth;
4. nail-biting;
5. dirty clothing;
6. dirty hands;
7. eating lunch at home.

The relative importance of each of these factors was assessed and the most important one, by far, was the location of residence.

Controlling the Lead Problem at Port Pirie. In his report to the South Australian Government Landrigan made recommendations under three headings:

1. changing the environment;
2. changing the behaviour of children and their families;
3. relocation of people from the worst affected areas.

Landrigan's suggestions for changing the environment included the following:

1. sealing of all pathways and roads to reduce dust circulation;

2. planting of lawns, shrubs and trees in open areas, again to reduce dust circulation;
3. removal of accumulated ceiling dust from houses to reduce lead absorption occurring in the home;
4. removal of dust accumulated in carpets and reduction of general household dust by frequent vacuuming and washing;
5. removal of all lead-based paint from the interior of houses;
6. replacement of contaminated garden soil.

Suggestions for changing behaviour included:

1. advising people not to eat home-grown vegetables;
2. encouragement of a diet high in calcium, iron, zinc and low in fat. Such a diet leads to reduced retention of lead in the body;
3. changes to work practices at the smelter to ensure that workers shower and change clothes before leaving for home;
4. education of children to reduce nail-biting, increase frequency of hand-washing before meals and reduce the consumption of non-food items.

Landrigan made it clear that the most effective action would be to relocate families from the affected areas. The main problem with this is the cost and thus far there has been no large-scale relocation program announced. However, the South Australian Government has funded a program in which houses in the affected area were thoroughly decontaminated.

15.3.3 *Childhood Lead Poisoning*

In countries like Australia and the United States lead poisoning of adults is very rare, but childhood lead poisoning remains as a significant disease. Children living in areas close to lead processing industries, such as the Port Pirie smelters, are at risk because of the general environmental pollution which such industries cause. Other children may be at risk from lead present in their immediate surroundings. For example, lead may be found in newspapers and comic books, crayons and pencils (this does not refer to the 'lead' in lead pencils which is not lead at all, but graphite, a form of carbon), toothpaste containers and some types of ceramic kitchenware.

By far the most important cause of lead poisoning among children is the ingestion of lead-based paints which occurs when children live in old houses where the paint is peeling from the walls. This creates lead dust which a child may unintentionally ingest. It may also produce large flakes of paint which the child eats intentionally. Children who display this behaviour of frequently eating non-food items are said to be suffering from the condition of **pica** and they are very much at risk when they live in an environment contaminated with lead.

Household items and paints which contain lead have been the subject of considerable government legislation in Australia. Items such as those mentioned earlier (newspapers, crayons, pencils) which are manufactured in Australia or imported into the country must not contain significant amounts of lead. Paints which are sold for general use now contain little or no lead. Some specialised paints are still manufactured which contain lead in appreciable quantities but they are subject to strict rules which govern their labelling and use. For example, such paints are never used on the interior of buildings. All this legislative activity ensures that there is no addition to the risk of lead poisoning from materials used in the past. However, old materials still present a risk where children live in close proximity to them.

15.3.4 *Treatment of Lead Poisoning*

Lead and the other heavy metals exert their toxic effects by attaching to protein molecules via –SH (thiol) groups in the side chains of the protein. This causes denaturation. Treatment of heavy-metal poisoning involves the use of medicines known as

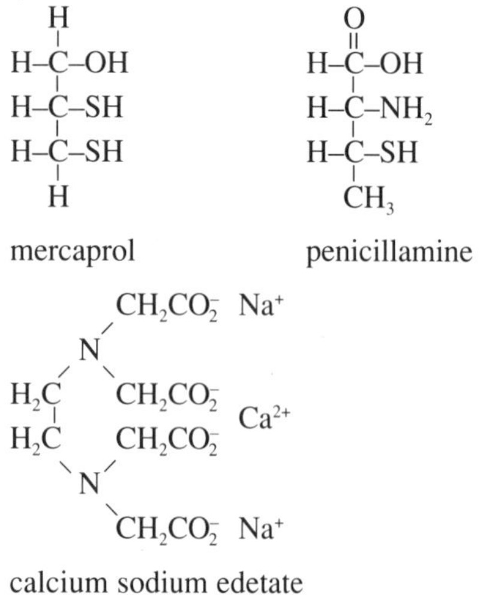

Figure 15.15 *Structural formulae for some chelating agents*

chelating agents. The molecules of these medicines all contain two or more of the groups of atoms –SH, $-NH_2$ or $-CO_2^-$ which are able to attach to the heavy-metal ion and displace it from its association with protein. This reverses the denaturation. Once it has attached to the chelating agent, the heavy-metal ion is liable to excretion in urine and faeces.

The chelating agents most often used as medicines are **mercaprol, sodium calcium edetate** and **penicillamine**. Structural formulae for these compounds are shown in Figure 15.15.

The action of a heavy metal on protein, and the way in which a chelating agent reverses this action, are illustrated in Figure 15.16. You will notice that the chelating agent and the heavy metal form a cyclic structure. This is why the medicines are called chelating agents. The word 'chelate' comes from a Greek word which means 'claw' and it is used to describe these medicines because they act after the fashion of a claw in their interaction with heavy-metal ions.

Chelating agents are quite hazardous medicines. The reason for this is that they are prone to attach to the body's essential metal ions as well as to heavy metals. This may significantly alter the distribution and rate of excretion of the essential metal ions. The consequences of this can be serious and so chelating agents are only administered under strict medical supervision (usually in hospital).

If a child's blood lead level is not too far above the level of concern then chelating agents are not likely to be used. Instead, the source of the exposure will be identified and steps taken to ensure that it is removed. If this is difficult the child is moved to an uncontaminated environment while the problem is solved.

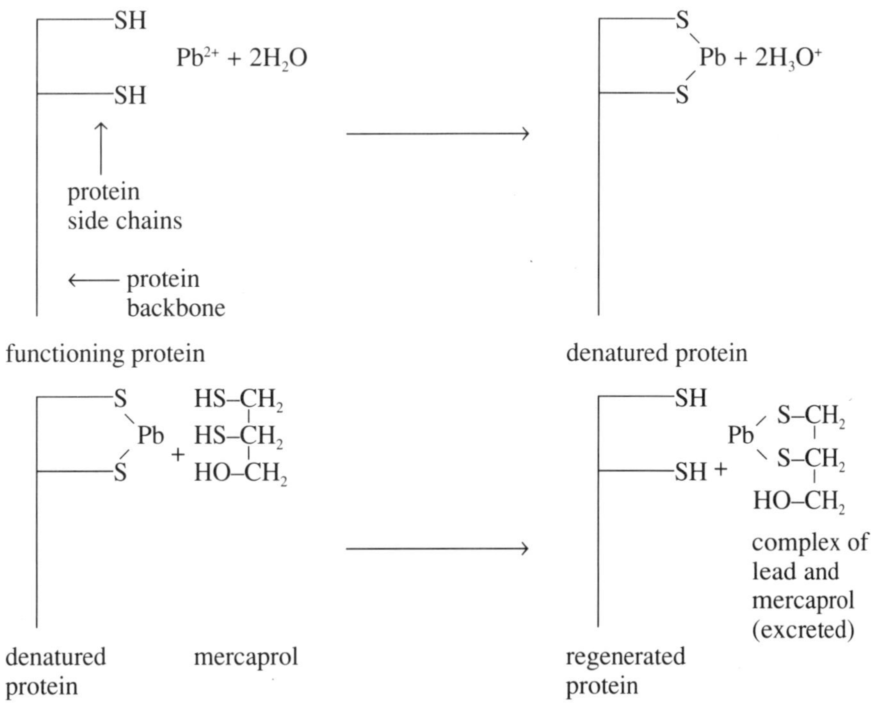

Figure 15.16 *Action of a chelating agent*

15.3.5 *Chlorofluorocarbons and the Earth's Ozone Layer*

Ozone. Most of the elemental oxygen present in the atmosphere is in the form of diatomic molecules, O_2. However, there is also a small amount of oxygen present in the form of triatomic molecules, O_3. These two forms of oxygen have quite different properties (see Table 15.1) and they are said to be **allotropes** of oxygen. This term is used to describe forms of an element in which the atoms are arranged differently. Many elements exist as allotropes. Graphite (the 'lead' in your pencil) and diamond are allotropes of carbon; phosphorus exists in two forms, red and white phosphorus; sulphur exists in three allotropic forms called rhombic, monoclinic and amorphous.

Table 15.1 *Properties of the oxygen allotropes*

Name	Oxygen	Ozone
formula	O_2	O_3
melting point (°C)	–218	–250
boiling point (°C)	–183	–112
odour	none	strong
toxicity	low	high

The allotrope of oxygen having three atoms in its molecules is called **ozone** and it is a substance of great contemporary interest. It forms from diatomic oxygen as a result of the absorption of energy. This energy may be supplied by electromagnetic radiation, by the passage of electricity through the oxygen sample or by reactive particles present in the sample.

The Earth's Ozone Layer. You have probably heard the saying 'a place for everything and everything in its place'. The meaning of this phrase is well illustrated by the different ways in which ozone can have an impact on human health.

The 'proper' place for ozone is in the **stratosphere** which is that portion of the atmosphere found between 10 and 50 km above the surface of the earth. We live in the **troposphere** which extends from the earth's surface to the stratosphere. All the effects which we call weather occur exclusively in the troposphere which is a constantly moving, mixing mass of air. In contrast to the troposphere, the stratosphere is much more stable. Most of the earth's ozone is found at altitudes of between 15 and 35 km and this section of the stratosphere is often called the **ozone layer**. The energy required for formation of ozone in the stratosphere is supplied by ultraviolet (UV) radiation from the sun. This is radiation having wavelengths in the range 100–400 nm. For the purpose of our discussion it is useful to divide this radiation into three categories according to wavelength. These are:

UV-A, 315–400 nm (lower energy)
UV-B, 280–315 nm (intermediate energy)
UV-C, 100–280 nm (higher energy)

The shorter wavelength (higher energy) UV-C radiation is absorbed by diatomic oxygen molecules and causes them to break apart forming single oxygen atoms. Thus,

$$O_2 + \underset{\text{radiation}}{\text{energy as UV-C}} \longrightarrow O + O \quad \text{(Reaction 15.1)}$$

Single oxygen atoms do not have a stable number of electrons and this makes them highly unstable and prone to reaction. They increase their stability by joining to oxygen molecules and as they do so some of their energy is released into the surroundings as heat. Thus,

$$2O + 2O_2 \longrightarrow 2O_3 + \text{energy as heat} \quad \text{(Reaction 15.2)}$$

If we add these two equations together we obtain

$$O_2 + \text{energy as UV-C radiation} + 2O + 2O_2 \rightarrow 2O + 2O_3 + \text{energy as heat}$$

and this becomes

$$3O_2 + \underset{\text{radiation}}{\text{energy as UV-C}} \longrightarrow 2O_3 + \text{energy as heat} \quad \text{(Reaction 15.3)}$$

The equation for Reaction 15.3 shows that when UV-C radiation is absorbed by oxygen of the stratosphere it brings about the formation of ozone and the release of heat. In this way virtually all UV-C radiation is prevented from reaching the surface of the earth. Absorption of this category of radiation depends on the presence of diatomic oxygen in the stratosphere and the amount of this is so great that there is no prospect of any significant increase in the amount of UV-C radiation reaching the earth's surface. However, diatomic oxygen does not absorb much UV-A or UV-B radiation and it is ozone which prevents a lot of this radiation from reaching the earth's surface.

Ozone absorbs UV-B radiation and the energy of the radiation causes it to split into oxygen molecules and single oxygen atoms. Thus,

$$O_3 + \underset{\text{radiation}}{\text{energy as UV-B}} \longrightarrow O_2 + O \quad \text{(Reaction 15.4)}$$

The oxygen molecules and oxygen atoms formed in this way can recombine to form ozone and when they do heat is released. Thus,

$$O_2 + O \longrightarrow O_3 + \text{energy as heat} \qquad \text{(Reaction 15.5)}$$

The net effect of these two processes is the conversion of UV-B radiation into heat and in this way about 50% of this category of radiation is prevented from reaching the surface of the earth. Neither oxygen nor ozone absorbs much UV-A radiation and more than 90% of the UV radiation which reaches the surface is in this category. This radiation (UV-A) is not regarded as being harmful.

We have now seen that the interaction of UV radiation with the oxygen and the ozone of the stratosphere prevents a large proportion of UV radiation from reaching the surface of the earth. In addition, the interaction has the effect of converting the radiation into heat and this makes the stratosphere warmer than the upper reaches of the troposphere.

Vulnerability of the Ozone Layer. Even where ozone concentrations are highest within the ozone layer the substance is still only a minor component of the atmosphere. Thus, while we are protected from UV-C radiation by the enormous amount of oxygen present in the atmosphere our protection against UV-B depends on a much smaller quantity of ozone. Some idea of the fragility of our planet's ozone screen is given by the fact that if all the ozone in the atmosphere was used to form a layer of gas having the same pressure as the pressure of the atmosphere at ground level then the layer would be about 4 mm thick!

The reason why the concentration of ozone in the atmosphere is so low is that the substance is unstable and is readily converted back into diatomic oxygen by reaction with other components of the atmosphere. This may simply involve its direct reaction with some of the single atoms of oxygen present in the atmosphere. Thus,

$$O_3 + O \longrightarrow 2O_2 \qquad \text{(Reaction 15.6)}$$

However, the atmosphere contains other reactive particles including OH, H, NO, Cl and Br. These may also contribute to the destruction of ozone. Thus,

$$X + O_3 \longrightarrow XO + O_2 \qquad \text{(Reaction 15.7)}$$

where X = OH, H, NO, Cl or Br.

Unfortunately, this is not the end of the matter. All the particles OH, H, NO, Cl and Br are not permanently consumed by Reaction 15.7, but may be regenerated by reaction with single oxygen atoms. Thus,

$$XO + O \longrightarrow X + O_2 \qquad \text{(Reaction 15.8)}$$

Reactions 15.7 and 15.8 accomplish the same thing as Reaction 15.6 (the conversion of ozone into diatomic oxygen via reaction with single oxygen atoms), but more efficiently. They are said to make up a **catalytic cycle** and this term is used because the reactive particle X which destroys an ozone molecule in Reaction 15.7 is regenerated in Reaction 15.8 and so remains available to destroy another ozone molecule, then another and so on.

The amount of ozone present in the stratosphere at any time is determined by the balance reached between the rate of production of ozone (Reactions 15.1 and 15.2) and its rate of destruction (Reactions 15.6–15.8). The rate of destruction is very much dependent on the concentrations of the particles OH, H, NO, Cl and Br which are present in the stratosphere. These particles are capable of acting as catalysts in the destruction of ozone and so relatively small changes in their concentrations might be expected to bring about quite large changes in the ozone concentration and, consequently, large changes in the amount of UV-B radiation reaching the earth's surface.

This possibility was well publicised during the 1970s when several nations were considering the production of large fleets of supersonic passenger aircraft. These aircraft must, in order to make efficient use of fuel, fly through the stratosphere where wind resistance is low, otherwise their operation is uneconomic. Opponents of this development were quick to point out that exhaust gases of these aircraft would contain significant concentrations of the gas, nitrogen monoxide, NO (often called nitric oxide). It was estimated that a single supersonic passenger aircraft would add about 3 tonnes of nitrogen monoxide to the stratosphere during each hour of flight and at one stage it was proposed to have hundreds of them in regular operation. This raised the possibility of rapid ozone depletion on a massive scale and became a factor (though not the only one) in the decision by the United States government to withdraw its support for the construction and use of the aircraft. As it turned out only the Russians and an Anglo-French consortium went ahead with the project and then only at a token level.

Ozone at the Earth's Surface. While ozone is highly desirable as a component of the stratosphere and has its place there, at ground level it is out of place and its presence is most unwelcome. Ozone is highly toxic to plants and animals. In human beings it is a severe irritant of the respiratory tract and is partly responsible for the effects of **photochemical smog** which often builds up in cities as a result of the action of sunlight on the compounds present in car exhaust emissions.

As well as its adverse health effects ozone causes economic loss mainly through its effects on plants, on rubber and on some textiles. These effects occur at ozone concentrations less than those required to produce adverse health effects in people. They were first noticed in 1950, at the start of the Korean War, when the United States army attempted to use vehicle tyres which had been stored unused since the end of the Second World War. The tyres had developed badly cracked surfaces and had lost much of their flexibility. They failed after only a few hundred kilometres of use. It was soon shown that the deterioration of the tyres was due to a chemical reaction between low levels of ozone in the atmosphere and the rubber of which the tyres were made. Rubber kept in a stretched condition was particularly susceptible to this type of damage. The problem was solved by the development of substances which, when added to the rubber, prevented its reaction with ozone.

The effect of ozone on untreated rubber is the basis of a simple method used by air pollution inspectors for the estimation of the concentration of ozone in air. The inspector carries a stretched rubber band and examines it periodically to count the number of cracks which have appeared in its surface. The rate at which these cracks appear provides a rough estimate of the ozone concentration.

Chlorofluorocarbons (CFCs) and the Ozone Layer. Strictly speaking, a chlorofluorocarbon is an organic compound in which the only elements present are carbon, chlorine and fluorine. In practice, some compounds which contain hydrogen and/or bromine as well as these three elements are also referred to as CFCs.

CFCs were brought into commercial use in the United States in 1931 in response to a need which had developed in the refrigeration industry. Prior to 1931 most refrigerators used ammonia (NH_3) or sulphur dioxide (SO_2) as the substance responsible for producing the cooling effect. Both of these compounds are highly toxic and corrosive. As refrigeration units became common in small retail businesses and in homes it became important to replace the ammonia or sulphur dioxide with some less hazardous substance. Thomas Midgley, the General Motors engineer who had discovered the anti-knock properties of lead tetraethyl in 1921, again came to the fore. He pioneered the use of dichlorodifluoromethane and trichlorofluoromethane as replacements for ammonia and sulphur dioxide in refrigeration equipment. They were effective cooling agents and, as well, were non-toxic, non-corrosive, non-flammable, odourless and could be produced quite cheaply. In short, they were ideal. Their structural formulae are shown in Figure 15.17.

dichlorodifluoromethane trichlorofluoromethane

Figure 15.17 *Structural formulae for two CFCs*

As the years went by more and more uses were found for CFCs and other similar compounds. By 1974 the annual world production of the compounds had reached about 8×10^5 tonnes and more than half of this was being used as aerosol propellant. Other uses were as refrigerants, as blowing agents in the manufacture of rigid polymer foams, as solvents, as fire extinguishing agents and even as an inhalation anaesthetic. The compound used for this last application is halothane which has the structural formula shown in Figure 15.18. You can see that its molecules contain a bromine atom and a hydrogen atom, which means that it is not a true CFC.

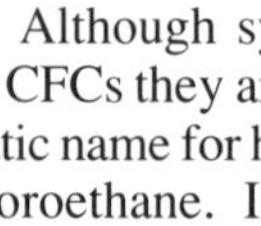

Figure 15.18 *Structural formula for halothane, the inhalation anaesthetic*

Names for CFCs. Although systematic names are easily devised for all CFCs they are rather lengthy. For example, the systematic name for halothane is 1-bromo-1-chloro-2,2,2-trifluoroethane. In industry they are usually referred to using a numerical code. For example, dichlorodifluoromethane has the code 12 (one-two, not twelve) and trichlorofluoromethane has the code 11. The rules of this code are as follows:

1. The first digit equals the number of carbon atoms in the molecule *minus one* and is omitted when the value is zero.

2. The next digit equals the number of hydrogen atoms in the molecule *plus one*.
3. The next digit equals the number of fluorine atoms in the molecule.
4. If bromine atoms are present the capital letter B is written next, followed by the digit which equals the number of bromine atoms in the molecule.
5. The number of chlorine atoms in the molecule equals the number of valencies which are left unused on carbon atoms after rules 1–4 have been applied.

In spite of its obvious perversity this system is the one commonly used. To make things even more peculiar the code may be preceded by a trade name or by a letter designating the intended use for that particular batch. For example, dichlorodifluoromethane manufactured by the Dupont company is known as Freon-12 because Freon is the Dupont trade name for chlorofluorocarbons. A sample of the same compound intended for use as a propellant might be called P 12. Structural formulae, numerical codes and common uses for several CFCs and related compounds are given in Table 15.2.

As CFC use reached its peak in the 1970s it was shown that the compounds were present in the atmosphere all over the earth. In 1973, two American scientists, Sherwood Rowland and Mario Molina, began an investigation of their likely fate. Before the end of that year they were convinced that CFCs posed a significant threat to all forms of life on earth.

Table 15.2 *CFCs and related compounds: structural formulae, code numbers and uses*

Structural formula	Code	Uses
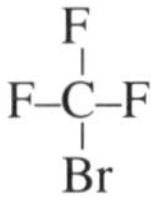	13B1	fire extinguishers, refrigerant
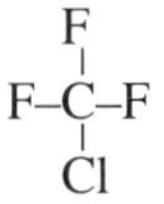	13	refrigerant
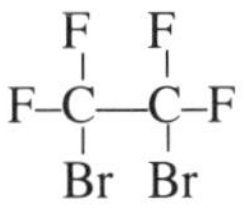	114B2	fire extinguishers
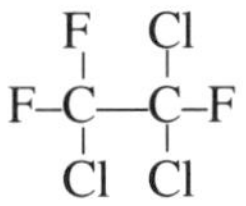	113	solvent, refrigerant
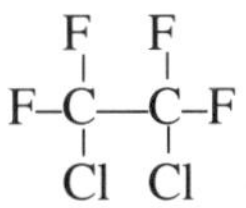	114	propellant, refrigerant

Rowland and Molina began by considering the three things that may happen to a molecule in the atmosphere. It may absorb sunlight and be broken down. It may dissolve in water and be removed from the atmosphere by rain. Or it may be destroyed by chemical reaction with other components of the atmosphere. The CFCs did not absorb much of the sunlight reaching the troposphere, they were not soluble in water and they were chemically inert. This introduced the possibility that they might persist in the atmosphere long enough for them to move out of the troposphere and into the stratosphere where they would be exposed to the effect of high-energy UV-C radiation.

When Rowland and Molina exposed a sample of a CFC to UV-C radiation in a laboratory experiment they found that its molecules were broken apart and that one of the fragments formed was a single chlorine atom (see Reaction 15.9). This was one of the particles known to be a catalyst for the destruction of ozone via Reactions 15.7 and 15.8.

$$CF_2Cl_2 + \text{UV-C} \longrightarrow CF_2Cl + Cl$$

(Reaction 15.9)

Rowland and Molina suggested that CFC use might produce sufficient additional chlorine atoms in the stratosphere to bring about a significant reduction in its ozone content and, consequently, a significant increase in the amount of UV-B radiation reaching the earth's surface. Measurements of the actual ozone concentrations in the stratosphere, carried out in the 1970s, confirmed that ozone concentrations were in decline and this produced a call for CFCs to be banned from all uses which allowed them to escape into the atmosphere. The latest development in this story occurred in 1985 when measurements of the ozone levels in the stratosphere above Antartica showed a dramatic decline during spring. This quickly became known as the **ozone hole**. Data collected before and after 1985 have been used to confirm the validity of the ozone hole as a new and real effect. There seems to be no doubt now that something has happened in the stratosphere to increase the rate of destruction of ozone. The most likely explanation is an increase in the statospheric concentration of single chlorine atoms arising from CFC molecules.

This is particularly significant for Australians. Each year in November/December the ozone hole over

Antarctica 'fills-in' as a result of the movement of ozone-rich air from the Equator towards the South pole. This movement displaces the ozone-poor air away from Antarctica towards the earth's middle latitudes where the southern part of Australia is located. In December 1987, measurements showed that ozone concentrations over Antarctica increased while those over Southern Australia and New Zealand decreased. So, at the time of the year when people in southern Australia are most exposed to radiation from the sun, the ozone layer over that region is significantly depleted.

As a response to this threat to the ozone layer governments in many countries have moved to restrict the manufacture and use of CFCs. The effectiveness of these moves remains to be seen but in the short term there is nothing which can be done about the CFCs already in the atmosphere. They will last for many years and, if they are altering the ozone layer, their effects will also last many years.

Adverse Health Effects of Ozone Layer Depletion. The immediate effect of ozone layer depletion is an increase in the amount of UV-B radiation reaching the earth's surface. It has been estimated that each 1% decline in stratospheric ozone concentration leads to a 2% increase in UV-B. It is well known that this radiation causes damage to the skin.

UV-B and Skin Cancer. Skin cancers are usually divided into two groups. The first group consists of **basal** and **squamous cell carcinomas** which have the following characteristics:

1. They constitute about 30% of all cancers and 95% of all skin cancers.
2. Their mortality rate is 1–2%.
3. They occur almost exclusively on parts of the body exposed most to the sun: face, exposed parts of the head, hands
4. Their incidence is greatest near the equator, among people working out of doors and among light-skinned people.
5. Their incidence increases with increasing age.

Given some of these characteristics there is no doubting the existence of a relationship between exposure to UV radiation and the occurrence of the cancers. By comparing the incidence of cancers in populations from parts of the world where UV-B levels are different, it is possible to estimate the effect which a given change in the level of exposure has on the incidence of the disease. On this basis it has been estimated that a 2% increase in exposure to UV-B will increase the incidence of basal and squamous cell carcinomas by 3–6%. Although the mortality rate for these cancers is low because they do not usually spread to other organs of the body, they can affect large areas of skin and be highly disfiguring.

The other category of skin cancer is known as **cutaneous** or **malignant melanoma**. This constitutes only about 5% of skin cancers but its mortality rate is 30–40%, which makes it a very serious disease indeed. Although exposure to UV-B is also a factor in the development of malignant melanoma the relationship here is not so clear cut. This is shown by the facts that the disease often affects skin which is not exposed much to the sun and it occurs more frequently among people working indoors. An explanation which has been suggested for this is that melanoma is caused by a few severe exposures rather than constant low-level exposure. It is argued that parts of the body not often exposed to the sun are just those parts likely to suffer occasional severe exposures. Likewise, people who work most of the time indoors are more likely to be burned badly when they venture out of doors. They are also more likely to be affluent and able to afford holidays in sunny climates.

Although it is more difficult to estimate the effect of increasing UV-B exposure on the incidence of melanoma it appears that a 10% increase in exposure would produce a 5–10% increase in the incidence.

The incidence of skin cancer of all types has been increasing throughout this century and has accelerated over the last few years. It is important to realise that this cannot be due to depletion of the ozone layer. Skin cancers take many years to develop and ozone layer depletion is a very recent phenomenon. The increase in skin cancer which we are seeing now is due mainly to lifestyle. This does not make ozone depletion any less important. On the contrary, it probably means that the worst is yet to come. We can be sure that depletion of the ozone layer has already created a store of additional skin cancers which will eventually show up.

Another effect which UV-B causes is cataract (opacity of the lens of the eye). There is also some evidence that it suppresses the activity of the immune system. It is possible that this is an important component of the action of UV-B in causing cancer: if the immune system is suppressed then this would reduce the body's capacity to destroy cancers at an early stage of their development.

The ozone layer is likely to remain depleted for many years into the future. The main prospects for slowing the increase in incidence of skin cancers and other UV-induced disease is through identification of high-risk individuals and education/counselling designed to produce changes in lifestyles which reduce exposure.

15.3.6 *Diseases Caused by Asbestos*

The 4 March 1985 issue of the American Chemical Society's weekly journal, *Chemical and Engineering News*, had as the headline for its cover story 'Asbestos, the Fibre that's Panicking America'. The American Chemical Society is the largest scientific society in the world, with a membership of about 130 000 chemists and engineers. It is a conservative organisation not normally given to sensationalism in its communication with members and the public. That such a headline should be used in its most widely circulated journal is an indication of the seriousness of the health problems caused by asbestos.

In Australia, as well as America, asbestos causes panic among people who believe that they might be exposed to it. They have good reason to be worried because there is no doubt that asbestos has caused more serious human injuries than any other commercial substance (except, of course, tobacco and alcohol, but at least in the case of these substances the injuries which people suffer are self-inflicted). It has probably caused more human injuries than all other commercial chemicals put together. It has been estimated that in the United States alone 250 000 people will have died from asbestos-related diseases by the end of this century. Most of these deaths will be the consequence of exposure which occurred during the period 1940–1980.

Asbestos is a silicate mineral which exists as fibres. Its physical nature is most vividly described by a term used in the French-speaking regions of Canada where it is called *pierre coton* which means 'cotton stone'.

Asbestos is chemically inert, non-flammable and resistant to corrosion. The fibrous nature of asbestos allows it to be woven into cloth and rope and to then be used in the manufacture of soft products such as blankets, hand mittens, curtains and clothing. These products are rarely used today, but once they were very common. Most fire blankets and fire curtains were made from asbestos, boilermakers were often supplied with asbestos mittens for the handling of hot rivets, and asbestos cloth was used in the manufacture of fireproof clothing. Asbestos is also incorporated into many hard products such as wall sheeting, pipes, floor tiles and brake linings for motor vehicles.

An enormous amount of asbestos has been used as insulation in buildings, in ships and in the manufacture of machinery. In the technical sense asbestos is an ideal insulating material. It is a very poor conductor of heat and can resist the effects of prolonged exposure to high temperatures, moisture and corrosive chemicals. Furthermore, it will not burn and so is a good fire retardant. Asbestos is available in the form of rope, cloth and as a loose product. The rope and cloth forms of asbestos are well suited for the insulation of pipes since they can be wound tightly around them. The loose form of asbestos is convenient for the insulation of floor and roof spaces in buildings because it can be sprayed into place.

People at Risk from Asbestos. Most asbestos injuries are occupational in origin. The first official concerns about this type of injury among workers were expressed in 1898 in a British Government Annual Factory Inspectors' Report. In those days, and up until about 20 years ago, it was very common for asbestos miners and asbestos process workers to be exposed to high concentrations of asbestos fibres in the air which they breathed. These workers often brought home enough asbestos dust on their clothing to put other family members at risk when the clothing was shaken to remove the dust prior to washing.

Some workers, not directly involved in the handling of asbestos themselves, have suffered injury due to the presence of asbestos in their work environment. Sailors are in this category due to the fact that asbestos has been very widely used as pipe insulation in ships. It is often not enclosed and is subject to disturbance during maintenance work. This, together with the fact that ships are very hard to ventilate, makes it possible for the air inside a ship to become heavily contaminated with asbestos fibres. The risk of asbestos-related disease among sailors was highlighted recently in Australia when it became known that the Governor of New South Wales, Sir David Martin, was suffering from the disease, **mesothelioma**, which is known to be caused by asbestos. Sir David served for many years in ships of the Royal Australian Navy and there is no doubt that his disease was caused by exposure to the asbestos present in those ships. Sir David died shortly after the public announcement of his illness.

Diseases Associated with Asbestos. The first disease identified as being caused by exposure to asbestos was **asbestosis**. This was recognised in 1930 in the United Kingdom. It is caused by chronic exposure to asbestos fibres in air and it involves extensive formation of scar tissue on the lungs. This scar tissue reduces the effectiveness of gas exchange in the lungs, and the work which the heart is forced to do in pumping blood through them is greatly increased. Since most people only rarely make full use of their lung capacity asbestosis may go unnoticed for years. However, the lung capacity of an asbestosis sufferer will eventually be reduced to such an extent that dyspnea (difficulty in breathing) and shortness of breath become unmistakable.

Other symptoms of asbestosis include a persistent dry cough, loss of appetite, increased vulnerability to infections and a 'ground glass' appearance of the lower region of the lung when an X-ray photograph is taken.

Asbestosis has a latency period of about 10 years which means that the disease is not usually diagnosed until 10 years after exposure commences. A person may live for many years after asbestosis has been diagnosed but the eventual outcome is usually death from heart or respiratory failure.

Mesothelioma. This disease was first recognised as being caused by asbestos in 1960 in South Africa. It is a rare form of cancer affecting the mesothelium, which is the membrane enclosing the lungs (pleural mesothelium), the heart (pericardial mesothelium) and lining the peritoneal cavity (peritoneal mesothelium). Cancers of the mesothelium are so rare among people who have no history of exposure to asbestos that the disease is taken a 'marker disease' for asbestos exposure. The pleural and peritoneal sections of the mesothelium are most frequently affected.

The symptoms of pleural mesothelioma include: chest pain, difficulty in breathing, persistent cough, loss of weight, loss of appetite and vomiting. The pleural mesothelium, which is usually about as thick as a thin sheet of paper, may become several centimetres thick as the tumour grows. In peritoneal mesothelioma the common symptoms are: abdominal pain, constipation and weight loss. The latency period for mesothelioma is about 30 years. Death usually occurs within about 12 months of diagnosis.

Asbestos, Smoking and Typical Cancers. Asbestosis and mesothelioma are conditions which are only seen in people with a history of asbestos exposure. However, these diseases are not the only ones known to be associated with asbestos exposure. Cancer of the lung, larynx and bowel all occur more frequently among people with a history of exposure to asbestos than among the unexposed population.

In lung cancer there is a very strong interaction between smoking and exposure to asbestos. A smoker who is also exposed to asbestos runs a much greater risk of developing lung cancer than a person who smokes, but is not exposed to asbestos, or than a person who is exposed to asbestos but does not smoke. In fact, most smokers who are exposed to asbestos will develop lung cancer and so smoking is usually forbidden in any work place where asbestos is used. In cancer of the larynx there is also an interaction between smoking and asbestos exposure.

Asbestos Toxicity. Considering that asbestos is such an inert substance, its ability to cause serious illness is somewhat surprising. The cause of asbestos toxicity is not clear, but the size of its fibres is thought to be an important factor. Fibres of intermediate size are the most toxic. It appears that very small asbestos fibres are engulfed by macrophage cells present on the surface of the alveoli and then removed from the lungs. Large fibres seem to settle out, or are filtered out, of inhaled air before it reaches the lungs. The fibres of intermediate size which reach the alveoli and remain there, probably produce their toxic effects by physical irritation of tissue over a long period. If this is so then the substances proposed for use in place of asbestos need to be chosen very carefully. The problem is that any substance which can be used as a substitute for asbestos is likely to have similar physical characterisitics and if it does it may turn out to be just as toxic. .

There are a number of different types of asbestos and, in decreasing order of the amounts used, these are: **chrysotile** (white asbestos), **crocidolite** (blue asbestos), **amosite** (brown asbestos) and **anthophyllite**. Health authorities in Australia consider crocidolite, or blue asbestos, to be the most dangerous form. In South Australia the use of crocidolite is completely forbidden by industrial legislation. Crocidolite was the form of asbestos mined at the infamous Wittenoom mine in Western Australia. This mine operated from 1938 until 1966. More than 100 mine workers at Wittenoom subsequently developed pleural mesothelioma. The steady accumulation of these cases during the 1970s attracted a great deal of public attention in Australia. This marked the beginning of the development of a high level of awareness among the Australian public and the trade union movement of the hazards of asbestos. In 1978, the Western Australian government decided to close the nearby town of Wittenoom and move its residents elsewhere.

Although crocidolite may be more toxic than other forms of asbestos they are all very dangerous if inhaled. In America, health authorities have decided to treat all forms of asbestos as if they are equally hazardous.

Dose–Response Relationship for Asbestos. Asbestos is one of very few substances which does not exhibit a threshold. All exposures to asbestos are considered capable of causing harm. In pristine air the concentration of asbestos is about 0.01 nanograms per cubic metre (a nanogram (ng) is 10^{-9} g). In a typical urban environment the concentration is likely to be about 3 ng/m^3. So, asbestos is another substance which is often present in the human environment at concentrations far higher than those found in a pristine environment.

The Public Health Risk of Asbestos. The general public is at some risk from asbestos because of its widespread use in buildings. If it is present in the building in a form which allows asbestos fibres to enter the air then there is a real risk to any person who enters the building, and the risk will increase as the time a person spends in the building increases. If the asbestos in a building is in a form in which it cannot escape into the air then it poses no immediate danger.

Public awareness of the dangers posed by asbestos is now so great that whenever it becomes known that asbestos is present in a building there is likely to be a demand made for its immediate removal. It is quite common to hear that people have refused to continue working in a building where asbestos is present or that parents are keeping their children home from school because the school buildings contain asbestos.

A great deal of effort (and money) is currently being devoted to the removal of asbestos from public and commercial buildings. This is called **asbestos abatement** and it is a growth industry. Some asbestos abatement work has been criticised as doing more harm than good. This is quite possibly true in cases where the asbestos being removed is in a form where it would not normally be capable of entering the air. For example, sheets of asbestos used as wall lining. Provided these sheets are hard and kept painted they present no danger. However, such sheets can easily be damaged and partly converted to dust when they are removed from a building. If the dust formed in this way is allowed to enter the air then it might well constitute a bigger hazard than the original asbestos. This, however, is not an argument against asbestos abatement. It simply highlights the need to ensure that all asbestos abatement work is carried out in ways that prevent asbestos dust from entering the atmosphere.

In this chapter we have seen that commercial chemicals have produced many important impacts on human health. For an overwhelming majority of the people affected, the impact has been positive. Nevertheless, there are now more than enough well-documented examples of injuries caused by commercial chemicals to justify the concern which many people have expressed about their use. There is no doubt that people will become more and more conscious of the possible health effects of commercial chemicals: those to which they are exposed at work, those which they take as medicines and those which are contaminants of the general environment.

Bibliography

Albert, A. *Selective Toxicity: The Physico-chemical Basis of Therapy* (sixth edition). Chapman and Hall, London, 1981.

Australian Academy of Science. *Health and Environmental Lead in Australia.* Australian Academy of Science, Canberra, 1981.

Banks, R. E. *Organofluorine Chemicals and their Industrial Applications.* Ellis Horwood, Chichester, 1979.

Bickel, L. *Rise Up to Life.* Angus and Robertson, London, 1972.

Duncum, Barbara M. *The Development of Inhalation Anaesthesia With Special Reference to the Years 1846–1900.* Oxford University Press, London, 1947.

Landrigan, P. *Lead Exposure, Lead Absorption, and Lead Toxicity, in the Children of Port Pirie: A Second Opinion.* South Australian Health Commission, Adelaide, 1983.

Lewis, M. J. *Task Force on Lead Contamination of the Environment of Port Pirie.* South Australian Health Commission, Adelaide, 1983.

Lead Implementation Group. *Report of the Lead Implementation Group.* South Australian Health Commission, Adelaide, 1983.

Liska, K. *Drugs and the Human Body with Implications for Society.* Macmillan, New York, 1981.

McCullock, J. *Asbestos: Its Human Cost.* Queensland University Press, St Lucia, 1986.

Refshauge, W. (ed.). 'The ozone layer and health', *Transactions of the Menzies Foundation*, **15**, 1989.

Zurer, Pamela. 'Asbestos: The fiber that's panicking America', *Chemical and Engineering News*, **63**(9), 4 March, pp. 28–41, 1985.

Questions

1. Explain, using examples, what is meant by the term 'magic bullet'.
2. A new medicine, which has been established as being as effective as an older one, may not obtain the

approval of the health authorities. If these authorities do agree that the new medicine is as effective as the old one how would they justify their refusal to approve its use?

3. Outline the body's defence mechanisms (physical and biochemical) against toxic chemicals.

4. Outline the fate of lead which is ingested or inhaled.

5. Explain the action of chelating agents (medicines used for the treatment of poisoning by lead and other heavy metals). What hazard is associated with use of these medicines?

6. At Port Pirie in South Australia there is a concern that some people are being affected by exposure to lead. Who are the people most at risk, what is the nature of the risk and what is being done to eliminate or reduce the risk?

7. The earth's atmosphere prevents a lot of the sun's ultraviolet radiation from reaching the earth's surface. Outline the processes involved in this screening action of the atmosphere.

8. It now appears that chlorofluorocarbons (CFCs) in the atmosphere are seriously affecting its ability to screen out ultraviolet radiation. How are the CFCs doing this?

9. What are the main undesirable health effects likely to be caused by increased levels of ultraviolet radiation at the earth's surface? What steps can be taken to reduce these effects?

10. Asbestos is considered to be the cause of more human injuries than any other commercial chemical. What properties and uses of asbestos are responsible for this?

Answers to Exercises and Questions

Chapter 1

Exercises

1.1 **(a)** The resistance equals the voltage divided by the current **(b)** Cardiac output = stroke volume × heart rate

1.2 Equation 1.1 $F = \frac{W}{D}$; $D = \frac{W}{F}$

Equation 1.4 $V = I \times R$; $I = \frac{V}{R}$

Equation 1.5 $s = \frac{Q}{m \times \Delta T}$; $m = \frac{Q}{s \times \Delta T}$; $\Delta T = \frac{Q}{m \times s}$

1.3

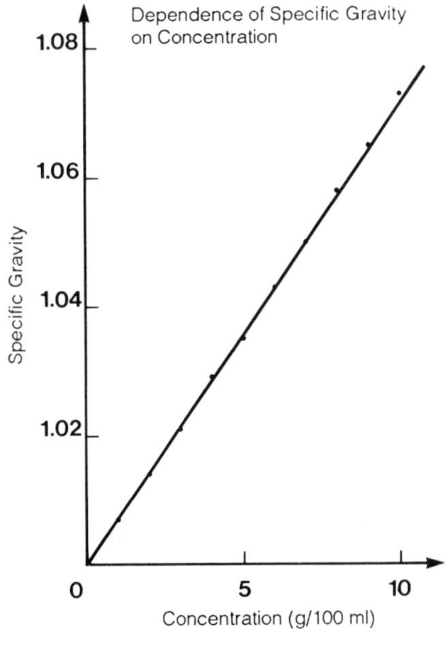

Questions

1. M; **2.** L; **3.** J; **4.** L; **5.** J; **6.** M; **7.** K

8. **(a)** Physical change **(b)** Chemical change **(c)** Physical change

11. **(a)** Absolute errors are 0.5 cm and 0.05 kg **(b)** Percentage errors are

$$\text{height, } \frac{0.5}{163} \times 100 = 0.3$$

$$\text{mass, } \frac{0.05}{60.5} \times 100 = 0.08$$

(c) $\text{BMI} = \frac{60.5}{1.63 \times 1.63} = 22.7709$

Number of significant figures in height is three and in the mass is three. Therefore the BMI should have only three significant figures and is written as 22.8.

12. **(a)** The instructor's measurement is the best estimate for the true value. She is a highly skilled person who has performed this type of measurement many times.

(b) If every student had obtained values within a range of two we would say that the measurements were as precise as could be expected given the limitations of the measuring instrument. There is one value which is very different to all the others and so precision is not as good as we might expect. If every student had reported values within one of the instructor's value we would say that the measurements were as accurate as we could expect given the limitations of the measuring instrument. Of the six measurements, three meet this criterion and so accuracy is not as good as we could expect. The instructor would certainly ask the student who obtained the value of 15 to repeat the measurement.

(c) All the values reported by the students are less than the instructor's value and this suggests the possibility that the students are making a systematic error as they perform the measurement. The instructor would take a close look at the technique being used to see if this error could be identified.

14. **(a)** Unsafe **(b)** Safe **(c)** Unsafe **(d)** Safe

15. The symbol μg is too easily mistaken for mg particularly if the prescription has been written by hand. A milligram is a thousand times larger than a microgram.

Chapter 2

Exercises

2.1 **(a)** Na_2O **(b)** MgO **(c)** $CaCl_2$ **(d)** K_2S

2.2 **(a)** 1 **(b)** 4 **(c)** 3 **(d)** 3 **(e)** 2 **(f)** 1

2.3 **(a)** CH_4 **(b)** H_2S **(c)** CO_2 **(d)** CCl_4 **(e)** NH_3 **(f)** O_2F

2.4 **(a)**

```
  H
  |
H–C–H
  |
  H
```

(b) H–S–H **(c)** O=C=O

(d)

```
   Cl
   |
Cl–C–Cl
   |
   Cl
```

(e)

```
H–N–H
  |
  H
```

Questions

1. M; **2.** M; **3.** M; **4.** L; **5.** J; **6.** J; **7.** M; **8.** L; **9.** M; **10.** L; **11.** J

12. $^{4}_{2}He$ represents an atom of helium containing 2 protons, 2 electrons and 2 neutrons; $^{18}_{8}O$ represents an atom of oxygen containing 8 protons, 8 electrons and 10 neutrons; $^{23}_{11}Na$ represents an atom of sodium containing 11 protons, 11 electrons and 12 neutrons; $^{40}_{19}K$ represents an atom of potassium containing 19 protons, 19 electrons and 21 neutrons; $^{56}_{26}Fe$ represents an atom of iron containing 26 protons, 26 electrons and 30 neutrons.

13. Molecules must be escaping from this sample of solid otherwise it could not have an odour. The forces acting between its particles must be relatively weak and this shows that it must be a covalent, molecular compound.

14. It is pure water that has a low electrical conductivity. Water on the hands and on the floor will not be pure. It will dissolve ionic compounds through its contact with the skin and floor. These will make it a good conductor of electricity because they will provide it with appreciable numbers of charged particles which are free to move about.

15. The statement is false. The melting of water has no effect on the forces holding hydrogen and oxygen atoms together *within* molecules. These forces are covalent bonds. They are very strong and melting has no effect on them. Melting only disrupts the forces which act *between* molecules and it is these forces which are weak.

16. The substance must be covalent, molecular. It is soluble but does not conduct electricity in solution. It cannot be ionic because if it was its solution would conduct electricity. Although some molecular, covalent compounds have an odour, not all do and so lack of odour does not tell us much about the nature of a substance.

17. (a) S=C=S (b) Cl–S–Cl

(c)

```
  F
  |
F–C–F
  |
  F
```

(d)

```
Cl–N–Cl
   |
   Cl
```

Chapter 3

Exercises

3.1

Table 3.3 *Chemical formulae for some compounds*

Compound	Formula	Elements present	Ratio of atoms
water	H_2O	H, O	2:1
sodium chloride (common salt)	NaCl	Na, Cl	1:1
carbon dioxide	CO_2	C, O	1:2
hydrogen peroxide	H_2O_2	H, O	2:2 (1:1)
alcohol	C_2H_6O	C, H, O	2:6:1
calcium carbonate (limestone)	$CaCO_3$	Ca, C, O	1:1:3
calcium phosphate	$Ca_3(PO_4)_2$	Ca, P, O	3:2:8

3.2

Table 3.4 *Formulae for some common ions*

Ion	Formula	Elements present	Ratio of atoms
hydroxide ion	OH^-	H, O	1:1
bicarbonate ion	HCO_3^-	H, C, O	1:1:3
phosphate ion	PO_4^{3-}	P, O	1:4
sodium ion	Na^+	Na	—
calcium ion	Ca^{2+}	Ca	—
ammonium ion	NH_4^+	N, H	1:4

3.3

Reactants	Products	Balanced equations
1. carbon dioxide, CO_2 water, H_2O	glucose, $C_6H_{12}O_6$ oxygen, O_2	$6CO_2 + 6H_2O \rightarrow C_6H_{12}O_6 + 6O_2$
2. urea, CON_2H_4 water, H_2O	ammonia, NH_3 carbon dioxide, CO_2	$CON_2H_4 + H_2O \rightarrow 2NH_3 + CO_2$
3. Calcium hydroxide, $Ca(OH)_2$ hydrogen chloride, HCl	calcium chloride, $CaCl_2$ water H_2O	$Ca(OH)_2 + 2HCl \rightarrow CaCl_2 + 2H_2O$

Questions

1. C_2H_6 is a molecular formula. It cannot be an empirical formula because it does not state the simplest whole number ratio of atoms present in the compound. The empirical formula would be CH_3. A structural formula for ethane would be

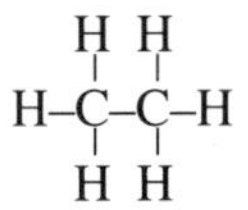

2. **(a)** carbon, hydrogen chlorine (1:1:3)
(b) Sodium, hydrogen, carbon, oxygen (1:1:1:3)
(c) Carbon, oxygen, nitrogen, oxygen (1:1:2:4)
(d) Copper, nitrogen, oxygen (1:2:6)
(e) Hydrogen, phosphorus, oxygen (3:1:4)
(f) Carbon, hydrogen, oxygen (2:4:2 or 1:2:1)
3. **(a)** Nitrogen dioxide **(b)** Chromium(II) oxide **(c)** Chromium(III) oxide **(d)** Sodium carbonate **(e)** Potassium monohydrogenphosphate
(f) Sodium permanganate
4. **(a)** K_3PO_4 **(b)** $Na_2C_2O_4$ **(c)** PCl_5 **(d)** P_2O_3 **(e)** CO **(f)** $MnCl_2$
5. **(a)** $2N_2 + 3H_2 \rightarrow 2NH_3$
(b) $CH_4 + 2O_2 \rightarrow CO_2 + 2H_2O$
6. All relative atomic mass values have been rounded off to the nearest whole number except chlorine which has been taken as 35.5.
(a) Formula is $C_8H_9NO_2$, relative formula mass is $8 \times 12 + 9 \times 1 + 1 \times 14 + 2 \times 16 = 151$; mass of 1 mole is 151 g.
(b) Formula is $Ca(OH)_2$, relative formula mass is $1 \times 40 + 2 \times 16 + 2 \times 1 = 74$; mass of 1 mole is 74 g.
(c) Formula is NH_4Cl, relative formula mass is $1 \times 14 + 4 \times 1 + 1 \times 35.5 = 53.5$; mass of 1 mole is 53.5 g.
(d) Formula is $C_7H_6O_2$, relative formula mass is $7 \times 12 + 6 \times 1 + 2 \times 16 = 122$; mass of 1 mole is 122 g.

Chapter 4

Questions

1. L; **2.** L; **3.** K; **4.** M; **5.** K; **6.** M; **7.** M; **8.** L; **9.** J; **10.** K; **11.** K

Chapter 5

Questions

1. L; **2.** K; **3.** J; **4.** M; **5.** M; **6.** J; **7.** K; **8.** L; **9.** J; **10.** M; **11.** L; **12.** L; **13.** L; **14.** K; **15.** J

Chapter 6

Questions

1. J; **2.** L; **3.** M; **4.** L; **5.** M

10. Two litres of water have a mass of 2 kg or 2000 g. The heat accompanying evaporation of water is calculated from

$$\begin{aligned} \text{heat} &= \text{mass} \times \text{latent heat of vaporisation} \\ &= 2000 \times 2280 \text{ J} \\ &= 4560 \text{ kJ} \end{aligned}$$

11. The heat accompanying a change in temperature of sample of matter (in this case human tissue) is calculated from

$$\text{heat} = \text{mass} \times \text{specific heat} \times \text{temp. change}$$

This can be rearranged to give

$$\begin{aligned} \text{temp. change} &= \frac{\text{heat}}{\text{mass} \times \text{specific heat}} \\ &= \frac{4560 \times 1000}{70 \times 1000 \times 4} \\ &= 16\ °\text{C} \end{aligned}$$

A temperature change even half this value is likely to be fatal!

Chapter 7

Questions

1. L; **2.** L; **3.** K; **4.** M; **5.** J; **6.** M; **7.** L; **8.** L; **9.** K; **10.** K

11. (a) Solution **(b)** Mechanical suspension **(c)** Colloidal suspension

12. (a) (i) Concentration $= \frac{4}{150} \times 100 = 2.7\%$ (w/v)

(ii) Concentration $= \frac{110}{2000} \times 100 = 5.5\%$ (w/v)

(b) (i) Mass of solute $= \frac{\text{concentration} \times \text{volume}}{100}$

Mass of solute $= \frac{6 \times 250}{100} = 15$ g

(ii) Mass of solute $= \frac{15 \times 75}{100}$

$= 11.3$ g (11 g to two sig. figs)

(c) Use the expression

$$\begin{matrix}\text{vol.} \\ \text{before dil.}\end{matrix} \times \begin{matrix}\text{conc.} \\ \text{before dil.}\end{matrix} = \begin{matrix}\text{vol.} \\ \text{after dil.}\end{matrix} \times \begin{matrix}\text{conc.} \\ \text{after dil.}\end{matrix}$$

(i) $250 \times 8 =$ vol. after dil. $\times 5$

vol. after dil. $= \frac{250 \times 8}{5} = 400$ ml

Add $400 - 250 = 150$ ml of water

(ii) $75 \times 15 =$ vol. after dil. $\times 5$

vol. after dil. $= \frac{75 \times 15}{5} = 225$ ml

Add $225 - 75 = 150$ ml of water

(d) 0.9% (w/v) means 0.9 g dissolved in each 100 ml of solution. In 1 litre there will be $10 \times 0.9 = 9$ g dissolved. The molar mass of sodium chloride is $23 + 35.5 = 58.5$ g and so in each litre of solution there will be $9/58.5 = 0.15$ moles of sodium chloride dissolved.

Concentration is 0.15 mol/l (0.2 mol/l to one sig. fig.).

13. (b) Density is 1.2 g/ml or 1.2 kg/l

15. Nitric acid; ammonium chloride; sodium acetate; ammonia. You have to assume that equal numbers of moles of each substance have been dissolved.

17. A and B are both acids. A is a stronger acid than B.

18. (a) The pH will increase to 9.5. **(b) (i)** The pH will fall slightly. The actual amount by which it falls depends on the quantity of acid added

(ii) The value of the ratio will fall.

Chapter 8

Questions

1. M; **2.** L; **3.** L; **4.** K; **5.** L; **6.** L; **7.** K; **8.** J; **9.** M; **10.** K; **11.** J; **12.** L; **13.** L; **14.** K; **15.** J; **16.** L; **17.** M; **18.** J; **19.** M

Chapter 9

Questions

1. J; **2.** L; **3.** M; **4.** M; **5.** K; **6.** J; **7.** L; **8.** K

11. **(a)** Hypertonic **(b)** Hypotonic
(c) Hypertonic **(d)** Hypotonic

13. **(a)** Molar mass of calcium chloride is 40 + (2 × 35.5) = 111 g; therefore we have dissolved

$$\frac{55.5}{111} = 0.5 \text{ moles}$$

$$\text{Concentration in mol/l} = \frac{0.5}{0.4} = 1.25$$

(b) When calcium chloride dissolves it forms separate Ca^{2+} and Cl^- ions (a total of three ions from each $CaCl_2$ unit).

conc. in osmol/l = conc. in mol/l × no. of ions in the formula
= 1.25 × 3
= 3.75

(c) Concentration of an ion expressed in equivalents is related to its concentration expressed in moles by

conc. in equivalents/l = conc. in mol/l × magnitude of the charge on the ion

For Ca^{2+} this becomes

conc. in equivalents/l = 1.25 × 2
= 2.5

For Cl^- this becomes

conc. in equivalents/l = 2.5 × 1
= 2.5

Total concentration of solution in equivalents per litre is 5.0

Chapter 10

Questions

1. K; **2.** M; **3.** L; **4.** M; **5.** L; **6.** L; **7.** M; **8.** K; **9.** M; **10.** J; **11.** K; **12.** K; **13.** J; **14.** M; **15.** J; **16.** J; **17.** K

Chapter 11

Questions

1. L; **2.** K; **3.** J; **4.** J; **5.** M; **6.** J; **7.** L; **8.** L; **9.** K

Chapter 12

Questions

1. J; **2.** L; **3.** L; **4.** K; **5.** M; **6.** M; **7.** K; **8.** J

Chapter 13

Exercises

13.1 Butyl radical and pentyl radical
13.2 Propanoic acid and ethanol
13.3 Ethyl propanoate
13.4 Position 1, one carbon atom, one hydrogen atom; position 2, one carbon atom, one hydrogen atom; position 3, one carbon atom; position 4, one carbon atom, two hydrogen atoms

Questions

1. J; **2.** L; **3.** L; **4.** J; **5.** J; **6.** M; **7.** M; **8.** M; **9.** J; **10.** M

12. **(a)** Carboxylic acid and ester **(b)** Amide and ether **(c)** Amide and phenol
(d) Ester and phenol

13. **(a)** Estrone is a ketone and estradiol is not. In estradiol the ketone group of estrone has been changed to an alcohol. These differences are reflected in the names of the two compounds by their endings. Estrone ends in 'one' as the names of all ketones do. Estradiol ends in 'ol' as the names of all alcohols do. The compound is called estra<u>di</u>ol because its molecules contain two alcohol groups.
(b) Estriol has an additional alcohol group compared to estradiol and this is reflected in the 'tri' section of its name.
(c) The synthetic estrogen is diethylstilbestrol. This is apparent from the fact that it has quite a different structure to the other three estrogens.

(d) All four compounds are members of the phenol family.

14. **(a)** Alkane **(b)** Alkene **(c)** Aromatic hydrocarbon **(d)** Alcohol **(e)** Ester **(f)** Aldehyde

15. **(a)** 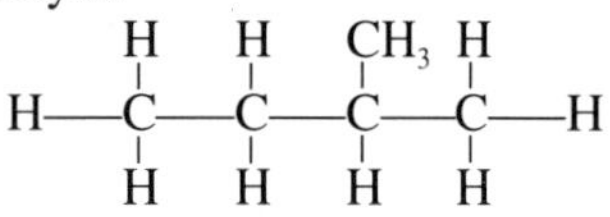

(b) 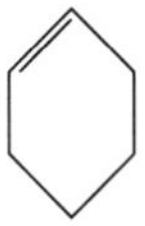

(c) 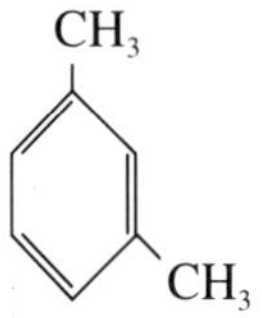

(d) 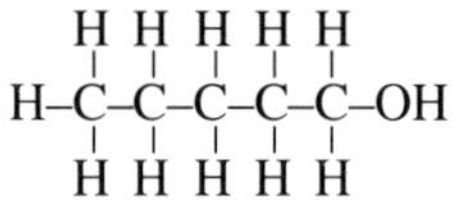

(e) 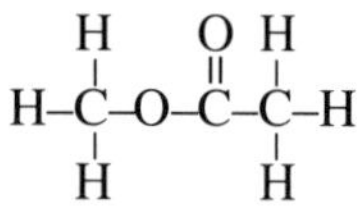

(f) 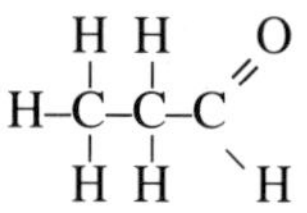

Chapter 14

Questions

1. J; **2.** L; **3.** M; **4.** J; **5.** M; **6.** L; **7.** K; **8.** J; **9.** K; **10.** M **11.** M; **12.** J; **13.** L; **14.** L; **15.** J; **16.** M; **17.** L; **18.** M; **19.** M; **20.** K

Errata

Please note the following errata to figures:

p. 79, Figure 4.1. The figure should be laterally inverted so that east faces west.
p. 85, Figure 4.7. For 40° read 20°.
p. 142, Figure 7.4. For potassium chloride ($KClO_4$) read potassium chlorate ($KClO_3$).
p. 233, Figure 10.16. For net osmotic pressure at the arteriole and (left), read 0.4kPa. For net osmotic pressure at the venule end (right), read –0.9kPa.
p. 344, Figure 14.7. Insert a Greek gamma label between thin foil and lead.
p. 345, Figure 14.8. Transpose the labels above Tc_{43} (left and right).
p. 374, Figure 15.14. For Lead in food and drink (50 μg/day), read Lead in food and drink (500 μg/day).

Index

PERIODIC TABLE

Key

Atomic number Name Symbol Relative atomic mass Electron structure

Transition metals

I A	II A							
1 Hydrogen **H** **1·01** 1								
3 Lithium **Li** **6·94** 2,1	4 Beryllium **Be** **9·01** 2,2							
11 Sodium **Na** **22·99** 2,8,1	12 Magnesium **Mg** **24·31** 2,8,2							
19 Potassium **K** **39·10** 2,8,8,1	20 Calcium **Ca** **40·08** 2,8,8,2	21 Scandium **Sc** **44·96** 2,8,9,2	22 Titanium **Ti** **47·90** 2,8,10,2	23 Vanadium **V** **50·94** 2,8,11,2	24 Chromium **Cr** **52·00** 2,8,13,1	25 Manganese **Mn** **54·94** 2,8,13,2	26 Iron **Fe** **55·85** 2,8,14,2	27 Cobal **Co** **58·93** 2,8,15,
37 Rubidium **Rb** **85·47** 2,8,18,8,1	38 Strontium **Sr** **87·62** 2,8,18,8,2	39 Yttrium **Y** **88·91** 2,8,18,9,2	40 Zirconium **Zr** **91·22** 2,8,18,10,2	41 Niobium **Nb** **92·91** 2,8,18,12,1	42 Molybdenum **Mo** **95·94** 2,8,18,13,1	43 Technetium **Tc** **98·91** 2,8,18,13,2	44 Ruthenium **Ru** **101·07** 2,8,18,15,1	45 Rhodiu **Rh** **102·9** 2,8,18,1
55 Caesium **Cs** **132·91** 2,8,18,18,8,1	56 Barium **Ba** **137·34** 2,8,18,18,8,2	**57-71** **Lanthanides**	72 Hafnium **Hf** **178·49** 2,8,18,32,10,2	73 Tantalum **Ta** **180·95** 2,8,18,32,11,2	74 Tungsten **W** **183·85** 2,8,18,32,12,2	75 Rhenium **Re** **186·2** 2,8,18,32,13,2	76 Osmium **Os** **190·2** 2,8,18,32,14,2	77 Iridiu **Ir** **192·2** 2,8,18,32
87 Francium **Fr** **[223]** 2,8,18,32,18, 8,1	88 Radium **Ra** **[226]** 2,8,18,32,18, 8,2	**89-103** **Actinides**						

Lanthanides

57 Lanthanum **La** **138·91** 2,8,18,18,9,2	58 Cerium **Ce** **140·12** 2,8,18,20,8,2	59 Praseody- mium **Pr** **140·91** 2,8,18,21,8,2	60 Neodymium **Nd** **144·24** 2,8,18,22,8,2	61 Promethium **Pm** **[145]** 2,8,18,23,8,2	62 Samari **Sm** **150·4** 2,8,18,24

Actinides

89 Actinium **Ac** **[227]** 2,8,18,32,18, 9,2	90 Thorium **Th** **232·04** 2,8,18,32,18, 10,2	91 Protactinium **Pa** **231·04** 2,8,18,32,20, 9,2	92 Uranium **U** **238·03** 2,8,18,32,21, 9,2	93 Neptunium **Np** **237·05** 2,8,18,32,22, 9,2	94 Plutoni **Pu** **[244]** 2,8,18,32 9,2